Competency Based Questions and Answers in

Physiology

for First MBBS Professional Examination

Compiled and Designed as per CBME Guidelines | Competency Based
Undergraduate Curriculum for the Indian Medical Graduate

Competency Based
Questions and Answers in
Physiology

for First MBBS Professional Examination

Compiled and Designed as per CBME Guidelines | Competency Based
Undergraduate Curriculum for the Indian Medical Graduate

Sushrutha Academy
Bengaluru

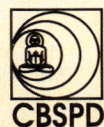

CBSPD

CBS Publishers & Distributors Pvt Ltd

New Delhi • Bengaluru • Chennai • Kochi • Kolkata • Lucknow • Mumbai
Hyderabad • Jharkhand • Nagpur • Patna • Pune • Uttarakhand

Competency Based
Questions and Answers in

Physiology

for First MBBS Professional Examination

Compiled and Designed as per CBME Guidelines |
Competency Based Undergraduate Curriculum for the
Indian Medical Graduate

ISBN: 978-81-947082-5-4

First Edition: 2021
Reprint: 2022, 2023, 2024

Published by Satish Kumar Jain and produced by Varun Jain for

CBS Publishers & Distributors Pvt Ltd
4819/XI Prahlad Street, 24 Ansari Road, Daryaganj, New Delhi 110 002, India
Ph: 011-23289259, 23266838

Website: www.cbspd.com
e-mail: delhi@cbspd.com

Corporate Office: 204 FIE, Industrial Area, Patparganj, Delhi 110 092, India
Ph: 0114934 4934   Fax: 011-4934 4935   e-mail: publishing@cbspd.com; publicity@cbspd.com

Branches

- **Bengaluru:** Seema House 2975, 17th Cross, K.R. Road, Banasankari 2nd Stage, Bengaluru 560 070, Karnataka, India
  Ph: +91-80-26771678/79   Fax: +91-80-26771680   e-mail: bangalore@cbspd.com
- **Chennai:** 7, Subbaraya Street, Shenoy Nagar, Chennai 600 030, Tamil Nadu, India
  Ph: +91-44-26680620, 26681266   Fax: +91-44-42032115   e-mail: chennai@cbspd.com
- **Kochi:** 42/1325, 1326, Power House Road, Opp KSEB, Power House, Ernakulam, Kochi, 682 018, Kerala, India
  Ph: +91-484-4059061-65,67   Fax: +91-484-4059065   e-mail: kochi@cbspd.com
- **Kolkata:** 147, Hind Ceramics Compound, 1st Floor, Nilgunj Road, Belghoria, Kolkata 700 056, West Bengal, India
  Ph: +91-33-25633055/56   e-mail: kolkata@cbspd.com
- **Lucknow:** Basement, Khushnuma Complex, 7-Meerabai Marg (behind Jawahar Bhawan), Lucknow 226 001, UP, India
  Ph: +91-522-4000032   e-mail: tiwari.lucknow@cbspd.com
- **Mumbai:** PWD Shed, Gala no. 25/26, Ramchandra Bhatt Marg, Next to JJ Hospital Gate no. 2,
  Opp. Union Bank of India, Noorbaug, Mumbai 400 009, Maharashtra, India
  Ph: +91-22-66661880/89   e-mail: mumbai@cbspd.com

Representatives

• **Hyderabad**	0-9885175004	• **Jharkhand**	0-9811541605	• **Nagpur**	0-8692091830
• **Patna**	0-9334159340	• **Pune**	0-9664372571	• **Uttarakhand**	0-9716462459

Printed at: Goyal Offset Works Pvt. Ltd, Kundli, Sonipat, Haryana

to

Ancient Gurus of Bharat

Contributors

M Shilpa MD
Associate Professor
Department of Physiology
Sri Siddhartha Institute of Medical Sciences
and Research Centre
T Begur, Nelamangala, Bengaluru Rural

Madhurima K Nayak MS, DNB
Consultant Ophthalmologist
Yenepoya Specialty Hospital
Kodailbail, Mangaluru

HK Parimala MD
Assistant Professor
Department of Physiology
KIMS, Bengaluru

U Kirthana Kunikullaya MD, DNB, MAMS
Assistant Professor
Department of Physiology
MS Ramaiah Medical College, Bengaluru

CN Veena MD
Associate Professor
Department of Physiology
Dr Chandramma Dayananda Sagar Institute of Medical
Education and Research
Deverakaggalahalli, Kanakapura Road
Ramanagara Dt., Karnataka

K Praveen Kumar MSc, PhD
Associate Professor
Department of Physiology, TRIHMS, Naharlagun
Arunachal Pradesh

Preface

"Assessment drives learning"

The purpose of assessment is not just to assess learning but also assist learning. The new CBME curriculum proposed by the Medical Council of India (MCI) calls for an outcome-based teaching-learning approach and transition from just acquisition of knowledge to application and practice of knowledge. Assessments need to be designed to suit the newer teaching-learning methods and to assess if the required competency has been achieved or not.

The purpose of bringing out this book is to introduce the I MBBS students to the new format of questions that is most likely to be asked during the internal assessment and the university examination and also equip them to face these exams without fear. Students can use this book for self-assessment of learning, preparing for internal assessment and university examination.

The book has been compiled by group of teachers who have undergone MCI recognized training in revised basic medical education technologies and advanced course in medical education. The questions in this book have been arranged according to competencies as listed in the MCI curriculum document. Various types of questions including structured long essays, modified essays, short answers, and multiple choice questions are added. These questions have been framed according to the guidelines set by the MCI with appropriate use of verbs at each level of Bloom's taxonomy of cognitive domain. The questions not only assess recall but also higher levels of learning.

We would like to acknowledge all the people who are involved in the preparation of this book especially Shri SK Jain (Chairman), Shri Varun Jain (Managing Director), Shri YN Arjuna (Vice President—Publishing, Editorial and Publicity), Ms Ritu Chawla (GM Production), and Ms Jassi, and of CBS for their all-time support and bringing out this book in record short time.

We hereby wish all the readers of the book all the best in their endeavors.

Happy reading!

Sushrutha Academy
sushruthaacademy@protonmail.com

Contents

Details of the Number of Questions and MCQs Included as per the Competency

S. No.	Competency No.	Competency details	Long essays	Short essays	Short answers	MCQs
1. General Physiology						
1.	PY 1.1	Describe the structure and functions of a mammalian cell	—	—	03	5
2.	PY 1.2	Describe and discuss the principles of homeostasis	—	02	02	3
3.	PY 1.3	Describe intercellular communication	—	01	01	3
4.	PY 1.4	Describe apoptosis-programmed cell death	—	01	05	1
5.	PY 1.5	Describe and discuss transport mechanisms across cell membranes	—	01	—	6
6.	PY 1.6	Describe the fluid compartments of the body, its ionic composition and measurements	—	01	—	4
7.	PY 1.7	Describe the concept of pH and buffer systems in the body	—	02	—	1
8.	PY 1.8	Describe and discuss the molecular basis of resting membrane potential and action potential in excitable tissue	—	02	01	2
9.	PY 1.9	Demonstrate the ability to describe and discuss the methods used to demonstrate the functions of the cells and its products, its communications and their applications in clinical care and research.	—	01	—	1
2. Haematology						
10.	PY 2.1	Describe the composition and functions of blood components	—	01	—	1
11.	PY 2.2	Discuss the origin, forms, variations and functions of plasma proteins	—	02	02	2
12	PY 2.3	Describe and discuss the synthesis and functions of haemoglobin and explain its breakdown. Describe variants of haemoglobin	—	—	02	3
13	PY 2.4	Describe RBC formation (erythropoiesis and its regulation) and its functions	02	—	—	1
14	PY 2.5	Describe different types of anaemias and jaundice	01	02	—	2
15	PY 2.6	Describe WBC formation (granulopoiesis) and its regulation	—	01	02	5
16	PY 2.7	Describe the formation of platelets, functions and variations.	—	02	—	3
17	PY 2.8	Describe the physiological basis of hemostasis and anticoagulants. Describe bleeding and clotting disorders (hemophilia, purpura)	02	05	02	4
18	PY 2.9	Describe different blood groups and discuss the clinical importance of blood grouping, blood banking and transfusion	—	04	—	1

S. No.	Competency No.	Competency details	Long essays	Short essays	Short answers	MCQs
19	PY 2.10	Define and classify different types of immunity. Describe the development of immunity and its regulation	—	05	02	1
20	PY 2.11	Estimate Hb, RBC, TLC, RBC indices, DLC, blood groups, BT/CT	—	07	—	2
21	PY 2.12	Describe test for ESR, osmotic fragility, hematocrit. Note the findings and interpret the test results, etc.	—	03	—	2
22	PY 2.13	Describe steps for reticulocyte and platelet count.	—	—	03	2
		3. Nerve and Muscle Physiology				
23	PY 3.1	Describe the structure and functions of a neuron and neuroglia; discuss nerve growth factor and other growth factors/cytokines	—	03	—	5
24	PY 3.2	Describe the types, functions and properties of nerve fibers	02	08	06	7
25	PY 3.3	Describe the degeneration and regeneration in peripheral nerves	01	02	04	5
26	PY 3.4	Describe the structure of neuromuscular junction and transmission of impulses	01	03	01	5
27	PY 3.5	Discuss the action of neuromuscular blocking agents	—	01	02	5
28	PY 3.6	Describe the pathophysiology of myasthenia gravis	—	02	01	5
29	PY 3.7	Describe the different types of muscle fibres and their structure	—	03	02	5
30	PY 3.8	Describe action potential and its properties in different muscle types (skeletal and smooth)	01	10	13	5
31	PY 3.9	Describe the molecular basis of muscle contraction in skeletal and in smooth muscles	02	08	03	5
32	PY 3.10	Describe the mode of muscle contraction (isometric and isotonic)	—	02	02	5
33	PY 3.11	Explain energy source and muscle metabolism	—	03	03	5
34	PY 3.12	Explain the gradation of muscular activity	—	—	02	4
35	PY 3.13	Describe muscular dystrophy: Myopathies	—	02	01	5
36	PY 3.14	Perform ergography	—	02	—	5
37	PY 3.15	Demonstrate effect of mild, moderate and severe exercise and record changes in cardiorespiratory parameters	—	01	—	5
38	PY 3.16	Demonstrate Harvard step test and describe the impact on induced physiologic parameters in a simulated environment	—	01	—	4
39	PY 3.17	Describe strength–duration curve	—	—	01	5
40	PY 3.18	Observe with computer assisted learning (i) Amphibian nerve–muscle experiments (ii) Amphibian cardiac experiments	—	—	—	6

S. No.	Competency No.	Competency details	Long essays	Short essays	Short answers	MCQs
60	PY 5.10	Describe and discuss regional circulation including microcirculation, lymphatic circulation, coronary, cerebral, capillary, skin, foetal, pulmonary and splanchnic circulation	—	05	—	5
61	PY 5.11	Describe the pathophysiology of shock, syncope and heart failure	01	—	01	5
62	PY 5.12	Record blood pressure and pulse at rest and in different grades of exercise and postures in a volunteer or simulated environment	02	01	—	—
63	PY 5.13	Record and interpret normal ECG in a volunteer or simulated environment	—	—	01	—
64	PY 5.14	Observe cardiovascular autonomic function tests in a volunteer or simulated environment	—	01	—	—
65	PY 5.15	Demonstrate the correct clinical examination of the cardiovascular system in a normal volunteer or simulated environment	—	01	—	—
66	PY 5.16	Record arterial pulse tracing using finger plethysmography in a volunteer or simulated environment.	—	02	—	—
6. Respiratory Physiology						
67	PY 6.1	Describe the functional anatomy of respiratory tract	—	01	02	5
68	PY 6.2	Describe the mechanics of normal respiration, pressure changes during ventilation, lung volume and capacities, alveolar surface tension, compliance, airway resistance, ventilation, V/P ratio, diffusion capacity of lungs	06	07	03	7
69	PY 6.3	Describe and discuss the transport of respiratory gases: Oxygen and carbon dioxide	—	03	02	6
70	PY 6.4	Describe and discuss the physiology of high altitude and deep-sea diving	—	01	—	5
71	PY 6.5	Describe and discuss the principles of artificial respiration, oxygen therapy, acclimatization, and decompression sickness.	—	—	01	4
72	PY 6.6	Describe and discuss the pathophysiology of dyspnea, hypoxia, cyanosis, asphyxia; drowning, periodic breathing	—	02	03	5
73	PY 6.7	Describe and discuss lung function tests and their clinical significance	—	—	01	3
74	PY 6.8	Demonstrate the correct technique to perform and interpret spirometry	—	—	02	—
75	PY 6.9	Demonstrate the correct clinical examination of the respiratory system in a normal volunteer or simulated environment	—	01	—	—
76	PY 6.10	Demonstrate the correct technique to perform measurement of peak expiratory flow rate in a normal volunteer or simulated environment	—	01	—	—

S. No.	Competency No.	Competency details	Long essays	Short essays	Short answers	MCQs
93	PY 9.2	Describe and discuss puberty: Onset, progression, stages; early and delayed puberty and outline adolescent clinical and psychological association.	—	01	03	5
94	PY 9.3	Describe male reproductive system: Functions of testis and control of spermatogenesis and factors modifying it and outline its association with psychiatric illness	—	01	04	6
95	PY 9.4	Describe female reproductive system: (a) Functions of ovary and its control; (b) Menstrual cycle—hormonal, uterine and ovarian changes	01	01	02	7
96	PY 9.5	Describe and discuss the physiological effects of sex hormones		01	01	5
97	PY 9.6	Enumerate the contraceptive methods for male and female. Discuss their advantages and disadvantages	—	02	03	5
98	PY 9.7	Describe and discuss the effects of removal of gonads on physiological functions	—	—	02	4
99	PY 9.8	Describe and discuss the physiology of pregnancy, parturition and lactation and outline the psychology and psychiatry—disorders associated with it.	—	04	02	6
100	PY 9.9	Interpret a normal semen analysis report including (a) sperm count, (b) sperm morphology and (c) sperm motility, as per WHO guidelines and discuss the results	—	—	03	5
101	PY 9.10	Discuss the physiological basis of various pregnancy tests	—	—	01	5
102	PY 9.11	Discuss the hormonal changes and their effects during perimenopause and menopause	—	01	01	5
103	PY 9.12	Discuss the common causes of infertility in a couple and role of IVF in managing a case of infertility.	—	02	01	5

10. Neurophysiology

S. No.	Competency No.	Competency details	Long essays	Short essays	Short answers	MCQs
104	PY 10.1	Describe and discuss the organization of nervous system	—	01	04	6
105	PY 10.2	Describe and discuss the functions and properties of synapse, reflex, receptors	—	05	03	10
106	PY 10.3	Describe and discuss somatic sensations and sensory tracts.	01	06	02	7
107	PY 10.4	Describe and discuss motor tracts, mechanism of maintenance of tone, control of body movements, posture, and equilibrium and vestibular apparatus	02	08	04	11
108	PY 10.5	Describe and discuss structure and functions of reticular activating system, autonomic nervous system (ANS)	—	01	02	5

S. No.	Competency No.	Competency details	Long essays	Short essays	Short answers	MCQs
109	PY 10.6	Describe and discuss spinal cord, its functions, lesion and sensory disturbances	01	—	01	6
110	PY 10.7	Describe and discuss functions of cerebral cortex, basal ganglia, thalamus, hypothalamus, cerebellum and limbic system and their abnormalities	05	03	06	9
111	PY 10.8	Describe and discuss behavioral and EEG characteristics during sleep and mechanism responsible for its production	—	02	01	6
112	PY 10.9	Describe and discuss the physiological basis of memory, learning and speech	—	04	04	6
113	PY 10.10	Describe and discuss chemical transmission in the nervous system. (Outline the psychiatry element.)	—	01	—	5
114	PY 10.11	Demonstrate the correct clinical examination of the nervous system: Higher functions, sensory system, motor system, reflexes, cranial nerves in a normal volunteer or simulated environment	—	—	01	—
115	PY 10.12	Identify normal EEG forms	—	01	—	—
116	PY 10.13	Describe and discuss perception of smell and taste sensation	01	03	—	5
117	PY 10.14	Describe and discuss pathophysiology of altered smell and taste sensation	—	—	02	2
118	PY 10.15	Describe and discuss functional anatomy of ear and auditory pathways and physiology of hearing	01	04	03	5
119	PY 10.16	Describe and discuss pathophysiology of deafness. Describe hearing tests	—	02	02	5
120	PY 10.17	Describe and discuss functional anatomy of eye, physiology of image formation, physiology of vision including colour vision, refractive errors, colour blindness, physiology of pupil and light reflex	—	07	08	9
121	PY 10.18	Describe and discuss the physiological basis of lesion in visual pathway	01	—	—	3
122	PY 10.19	Describe and discuss auditory and visual evoke potentials	—	—	01	5
123	PY 10.20	Demonstrate (i) testing of visual acuity, colour and field of vision, (ii) hearing, (iii) testing for smell, and (iv) taste sensation in volunteer/simulated environment	—	—	01	—

11. Integrated Physiology

S. No.	Competency No.	Competency details	Long essays	Short essays	Short answers	MCQs
124	PY 11.1	Describe and discuss mechanism of temperature regulation	—	01	02	5
125	PY 11.2	Describe and discuss adaptation to altered temperature (heat and cold)	—	01	—	5
126	PY 11.3	Describe and discuss mechanism of fever, cold injuries, and heat stroke	—	—	03	6

S. No.	Competency No.	Competency details	Long essays	Short essays	Short answers	MCQs
127	PY 11.4	Describe and discuss cardiorespiratory and metabolic adjustments during exercise; physical training effects	—	—	03	5
128	PY 11.5	Describe and discuss physiological consequences of sedentary lifestyle	—	02	03	6
129	PY 11.6	Describe physiology of infancy	—	—	01	5
130	PY 11.7	Describe and discuss physiology of aging; free radicals and antioxidants			03	6
131	PY 11.8	Discuss and compare cardiorespiratory changes (isometric and isotonic) with that in the resting state and under different environmental conditions (heat and cold)	01	01	01	5
132	PY 11.9	Interpret growth charts	—	—	02	5
133	PY 11.10	Interpret anthropometric assessment of infants	—	—	01	5
134	PY 11.11	Discuss the concept, criteria for diagnosis of Brain death and its implications	—	—	01	5
135	PY 11.12	Discuss the physiological effects of meditation	—	—	01	5
136	PY 11.13	Obtain history and perform general examination in the volunteer/simulated environment.	—	—	01	5
137	PY 11.14	Demonstrate basic life support in a simulated environment	—	—	01	6
		Total Content	**50**	**244**	**255**	**621**

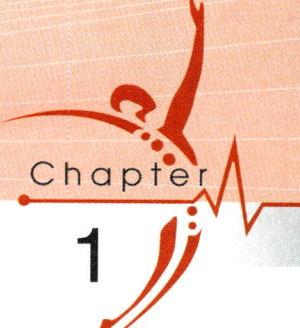

General Physiology

SHORT ANSWERS

1. Write the functions of plasma membrane.

- It is a protective membrane that encloses cell body
- It is also called cell membrane or plasmalemma.

Functions

1. **Protective function:** The cell membrane protects the cell organelles and cytoplasm from external substances by forming a mechanical barrier.
2. **Permeability:** Since the plasma membrane is selectively permeable to some substances and impermeable to others.
3. **Exchange of gases:** Oxygen and carbon dioxide can diffuse into and out of the cell through cell membrane as they are soluble in the cell membrane.
4. **Absorption:** Some substances are absorbed through cell membrane, especially nutrients.
5. **Excretion:** Some unwanted excretory wastes are thrown out of the cell through plasma membrane.
6. **Maintenance of shape and size of cell:** It prevents water accumulation and maintains cell size through NAK ATPase channels.

2. Which organelle is called suicide bag of the cell? What type of enzymes does it contain? And what is its function?

Organelle

- Lysosome is called the suicide bag of the cell.

- These are membrane bound vesicles within the cytoplasm of a cell.

Enzymes

1. **Amylases:** They digest carbohydrates
2. **Proteases:** They digest proteins
3. **Lipases:** They digest lipids
4. **Nucleases:** They digest nucleic acids

Functions

1. Degradation of macromolecules that have been engulfed by phagocytosis, pinocytosis or endocytosis.
2. Degradation of damages organelles is carried out by lysosome by formation of autophagolysosome.
3. Removal of excreted products is done by lysosomes.
4. Some lysosomes have been found to have secretory function. Examples are perforin and granzymes which can destroy microbes, serotonin by mast cells carry out allergic response and melanin secretion from melanocytes.

3. What are the peculiarities of mitochondrial DNA?

Mitochondria

- Are called powerhouse of the cell
- It has an outer membrane which encloses the cytosol

- The inner membrane is thrown into numerous folds which have 5 enzymes required for Krebs cycle.

Mitochondrial DNA

- The matrix of the mitochondria houses the DNA.
- Most of the DNA is packed within the nucleus. But a small portion is enclosed within the mitochondria.
- It is around 16,500 Da in mass.
- It is inherited from the mother as only nucleus of the sperm takes part in zygote formation and other cell organelles are derived from the egg.
- This DNA is responsible for production of enzymes that takes part in respiratory cycle and specific for cells having mitochondria.
- Due to its small size and ease to isolate, it has been a target for genome sequencing projects.
- It lacks introns as against DNA in the nucleus.
- Also, it has the ability of translation using a single t-RNA sequence.

1.2 DESCRIBE AND DISCUSS THE PRINCIPLES OF HOMEOSTASIS

SHORT ESSAYS

1. Explain the different feedback mechanisms operating to maintain homeostasis with examples.

- Homeostasis is a phenomenon of maintenance of constant internal environment.

Feedback Mechanisms

- Any change in pattern of any system activates sensors
- These signals reach a control centre.
- The effectors bring about the necessary change by causing the required action.

1. Negative Feedback Mechanism

- A change in homeostasis causes to inhibit the natural activity to bring the change under control
- Example: Thyroid hormone regulation

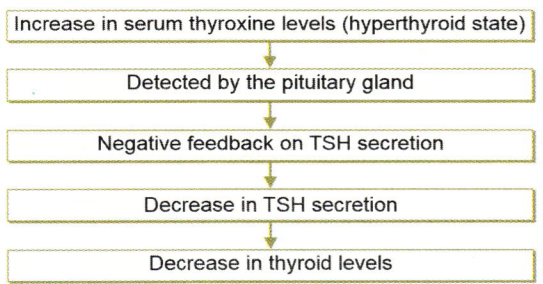

Fig. 1.1

- The same holds good for FSH regulation also.
- Another example of negative feedback is water regulation.

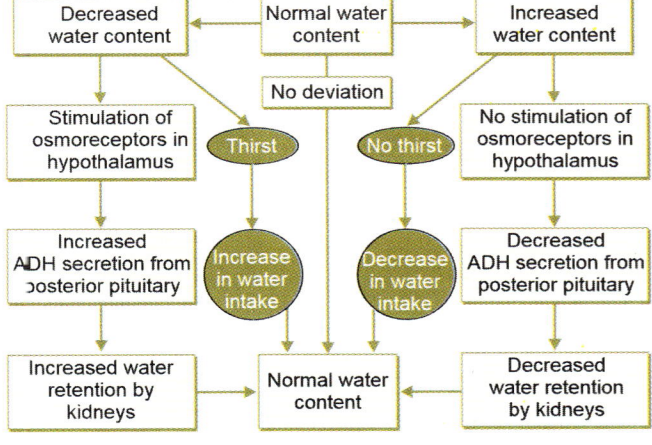

Fig. 1.2

2. Positive Feedback Mechanism

- In this type of feedback, there is increase in the activity in the same direction.
- Examples are blood clotting, labor, milk ejection reflex.

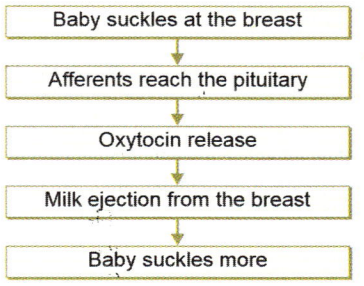

Fig. 1.3

2. What is milieu intérieur? What are the mechanisms which help in maintaining fluid osmolality?

Milieu Intérieur

- Milieu intérieur literally means internal environment.
- Claude Bernard, a scientist in the 19th century explained that multicellular organisms live in a perfectly organized and coordinated environment—which he called milieu intérieur.
- It is the extracellular fluid which house various types of cells and contains many nutrients, ions and various other structures required for sustenance of cells.
- It is further divided as blood and interstitial fluid.

Homeostasis in Maintaining Fluid Osmolarity

1. ADH Mechanism

- Hypothalamus plays an important role in detecting osmolarity of blood through osmoreceptors.
- Osmoreceptors sense a variation-decrease or an increase in osmolarity in the blood.

Increase in blood osmolarity

- May be due to water loss or due to inadequate solutes in blood
- When the osmolarity is increased, thirst increases and the osmoreceptors are stimulated.
- Thirst causes the person to drink more water
- This causes stimulation of posterior pituitary to secrete antidiuretic hormone.

- ADH acts on the distal convoluted tubule to absorb more water through increased formation of aquaporin channels and increases water reabsorption.
- This causes dilution of ECF and decreases in osmolarity.

Decrease in blood osmolarity

- May be due to water loss or due to inadequate solutes in blood
- When the osmolarity is increased, thirst increases and the osmoreceptors are stimulated.
- Thirst causes the person to drink more water
- This causes stimulation of posterior pituitary to secrete antidiuretic hormone.
- ADH acts on the distal convoluted tubule to absorb more water through increased formation of aquaporin channels and increases water reabsorption.
- This causes dilution of ECF and decreases in osmolarity.
- The reverse happens in decreased osmolarity.

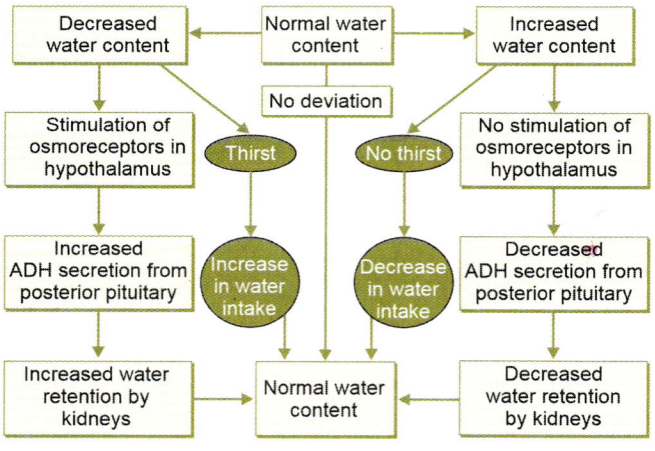

Fig. 1.4

2. RAAS Mechanism

- Renin is a hormone secreted by juxtaglomerular cells.
- It is secreted when there is a decrease in Na$^+$ concentration in the thick ascending limb. Sympathetic stimulation also causes renin release.
- Most of the actions are produced due to formation of angiotensin II.

Action on adrenal cortex

- Renin stimulates the adrenal cortex to produce aldosterone.

- Aldosterone is a mineralocorticoid and increases sodium retention and thus increases osmolarity.

Action on glomerular apparatus

- It constricts the afferent arteriole and decreases the blood flowing into the glomerulus and thus decreases glomerular filtration. This increases the ECF volume.
- It leads to contraction of the glomerular mesangial cells, thereby decreasing the surface area of glomerulus.
- It increases sodium reabsorption from the proximal tubules.

Action on brain

- Angiotensin II increases water intake by stimulating the thirst center.
- It increases the release of ADH from posterior pituitary.

SHORT ANSWERS

1. Explain negative feedback mechanisms with 2 examples.

Feedback Mechanisms

- Any change in pattern of any system activates sensors.
- These signals reach a control centre.
- The effectors bring about the necessary change by causing the required action.

Negative Feedback Mechanisms

- A change in homeostasis causes to inhibit the natural activity to bring the change under control
- *Example:* Thyroid hormone regulation

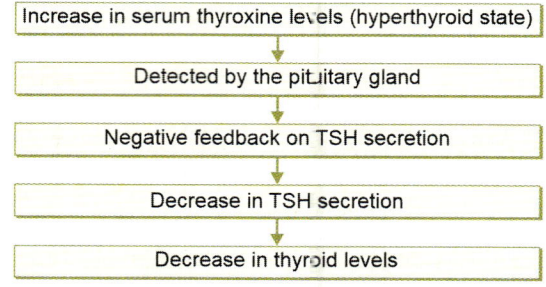

Fig. 1.5

- The same holds good for FSH regulation also.
- Another example of negative feedback is water regulation.

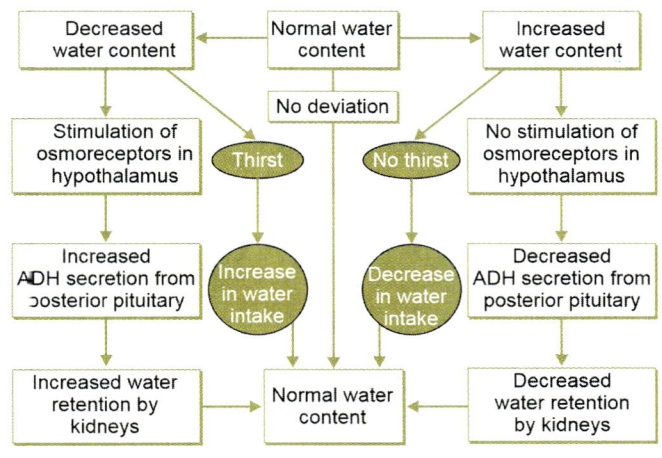

Fig. 1.6

2. Define homeostasis. Give the examples for positive feedback mechanisms.

- Homeostasis is a phenomenon of maintenance of constant internal environment.

Positive Feedback Mechanisms

- In this type of feedback, there is increase in the activity in the same direction.
- *Examples are:*

  1. **Blood clotting**

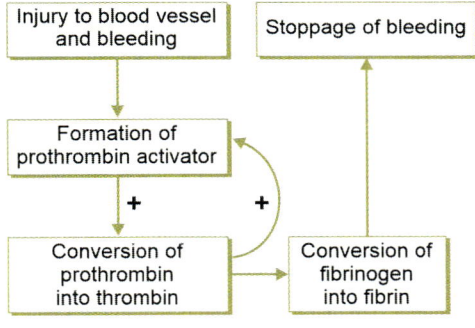

Fig. 1.7

2. **Labor**

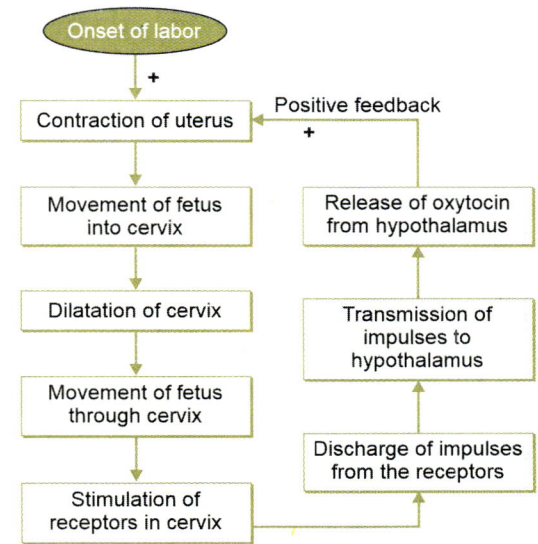

Fig. 1.8

3. **Milk ejection reflex**

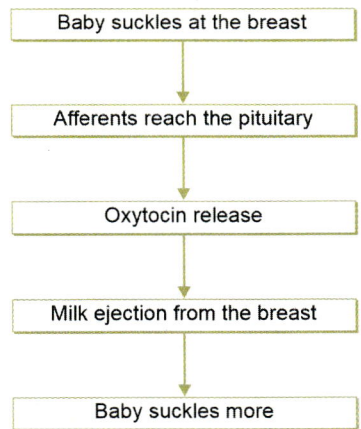

Fig. 1.9

1.3 DESCRIBE INTERCELLULAR COMMUNICATION

SHORT ESSAYS

1. Explain the types of intercellular communication. Mention one physiological significance of each.

Types of Intercellular Communication

Also called cell junctions.

1. Tight Junctions (Fig. 1.10)

- Also called zona occludens, it is an intercellular occluding junction between two cells which does not allow passage of macromolecules.
- Each tight junction consists of one-half ridge from each cell and the junction occupies the space between the two cells.
- They only allow specific molecules to pass through it.

Physiological importance

i. **Blood–brain barrier:** Tight junctions between capillaries form blood–brain barrier which does not allow penetration of chemicals across it thus protects the brain from harmful chemicals present in the blood.

ii. **Gastrointestinal tract:** Tight junctions in the epithelium of the mucosa of the stomach do not permit entry of substances to be absorbed excepting a few lipid-soluble substances like alcohol.

iii. **Renal tubular cells**
- Tight junctions are present on the luminal side of the tubular cells which allow Na^+ ions and water to diffuse in.
- They are sensitive to ADH and control the amount of water absorption.

2. Gap Junctions (Fig. 1.11)

- These are intercellular junctions that allow passage of ions and smaller molecules between two cells.
- These are present in the cardiac muscle and basal epithelium of the gut mucosa.

Physiological significance

- They help in fast conduction of action potential. As a result, multiple cells with gap junctions function as a single unit—syncytium. These are found very commonly in smooth muscles of viscera like gut, bile ducts, uterus and many blood vessels.

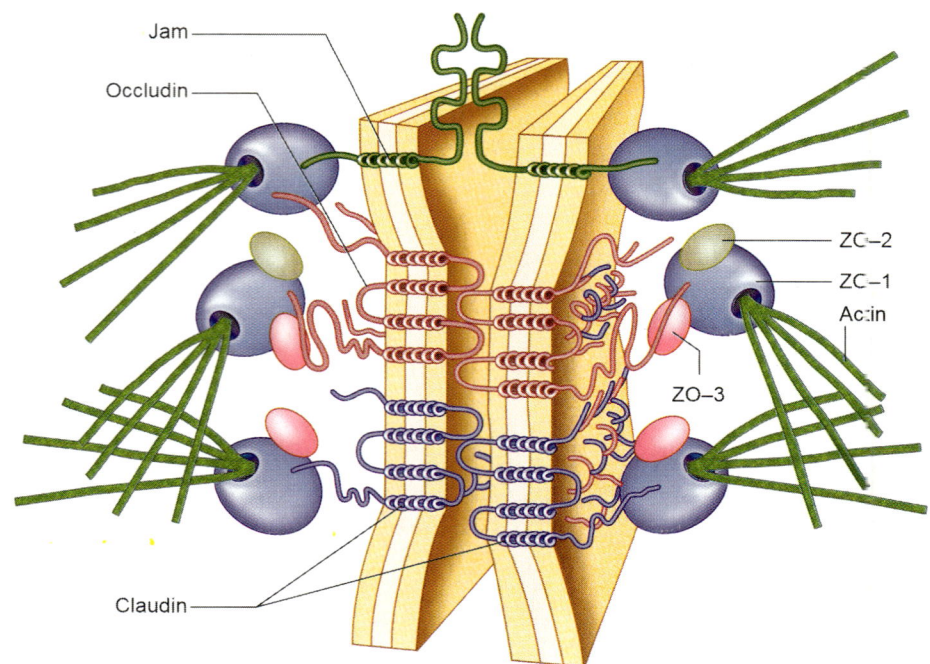

Fig. 1.10

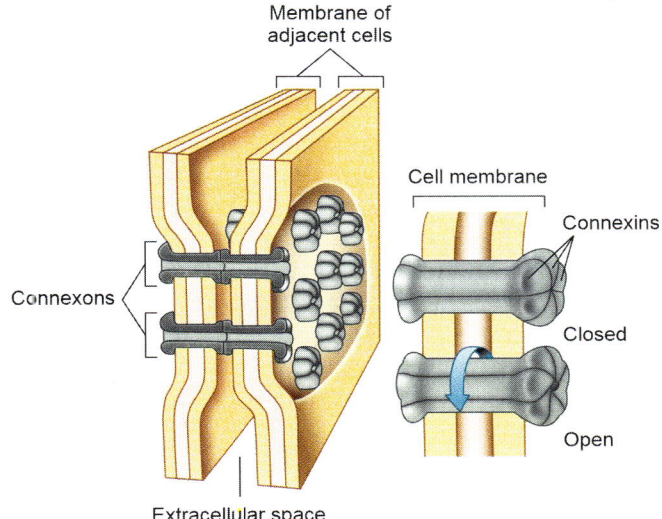

Fig. 1.11

- The cardiac muscles also are connected by gap junctions. They act like a syncytium such that cardiac cells are connect with each other. The heart is divided into atrial and ventricular syncytium by a fibrous band. As a result, action potential is conducted at the same time through all fibers of atria. Similarly, all muscle fibers of the ventricle contract together.

- In smooth muscle of the gut, these smooth muscles are connected with other by gap junctions, lengthwise such that peristalsis waves are conducted lengthwise.

- Estrogen acts on the uterine muscle to increase in gap junctions and forms a syncytium. During parturition, the whole uterus contracts as single unit.

3. Anchoring Junctions (Fig. 1.12)

- These form connections between actin filaments of one cell to another, just below tight junctions.
- The proteins responsible for this are called cadherins.
- Desmosomes are cell-to-cell junction, where intermediate filaments are held together. There is thickening of membrane intervening between two cells.

Physiological significance

- Adherent junctions are present in the intercalated discs between cardiac muscles. During contractions the cells are held together tightly.
- They are also present in epidermis.

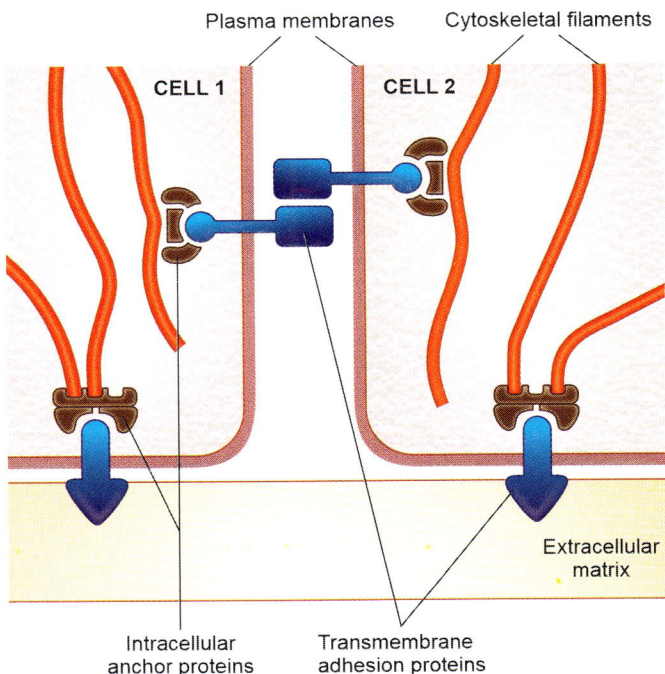

Fig. 1.12

SHORT ANSWERS

1. What are gap junctions? What is its physiological significance?

Gap Junctions

- These are intercellular junctions that allow passage of ions and smaller molecules between two cells.
- These are present in the cardiac muscle and basal epithelium of the gut mucosa.

Physiological Significance

- They help in fast conduction of action potential. As a result, multiple cells with gap junctions function as a single unit—syncytium. These are found very commonly in smooth muscles of viscera like gut, bile ducts, uterus and many blood vessels.
- The cardiac muscles also are connected by gap junctions. They act like a syncytium such that cardiac cells are connect with each other. The heart is divided into atrial and ventricular syncytium by a fibrous band. As a result, action potential is conducted at the same time through all fibers of atria. Similarly, all muscle fibers of the ventricle contract together.
- In smooth muscle of the gut, these smooth muscles are connected with other by gap junctions, lengthwise such that peristalsis waves are conducted lengthwise.
- Estrogen acts on the uterine muscle to increase in gap junctions and forms a syncytium. During parturition, the whole uterus contracts as single unit.

1.4 DESCRIBE APOPTOSIS—PROGRAMMED CELL DEATH

SHORT ESSAY

1. What is apoptosis? Give its physiological importance with examples.

Apoptosis

- Apoptosis is defined as programmed cell death.
- It is under genetic control, and thus referred to as 'cell suicide'.
- It is not associated with inflammation.
- It is related to the word 'ptosis'—which means 'fall'

Physiological Significance

1. Intrauterine life
   - It helps in normal development of organs.
   - It helps to sculpt organs, create the interdigital web spaced.
2. In adulthood
   - About 10 billion cells die every day to maintain stem cell homeostasis
   - In the bone marrow, millions of copies of stem cells are produced. They are destroyed by apoptosis to maintain normal miles.
3. If a cell is damaged by radiation or virus, the cell is destroyed mediated by P53 gene. Its importance has shown by the loss of P53 gene leading to an increased propensity to cancers where there is altered genetic make-up introduced by a mutagenic stimulus.
4. It is necessary for regression of certain ducts during sex differentiation in fetus (e.g. wolffian duct). Also, failure to absorb one of such ducts can lead to fistulae.
   Example: Patent urachus, patent ductus arteriosus.
5. Apoptosis of auto-aggressive T cells is needed to prevent autoimmune conditions.
6. Apoptosis is an important cause for shedding of endometrium during menstruation.
7. Increased apoptosis leads to pathological neurodegeneration as in Alzheimer's disease, Parkinson's disease and AIDS.
8. Decreased apoptosis leads to malignancies and autoimmune conditions.

1.5 DESCRIBE AND DISCUSS TRANSPORT MECHANISMS ACROSS CELL MEMBRANES

SHORT ANSWERS

1. Define

A. Osmotic pressure
B. Osmosis
C. Osmolality

A. Osmotic Pressure

- It is the pressure created by solutes in the fluid which drive fluid towards the region containing them by osmosis.
- Each solute has its own osmotic pressure.

B. Osmosis

Passive movement of water or other solvent molecules across a semipermeable membrane from a region of higher concentration to a region of lower concentration along the concentration gradient is called osmosis.

C. Osmolality

- It is a measure of a fluid's ability to create osmotic pressure.
- It is also called osmolar concentration of a solution.

2. Explain Facilitated Diffusion

Facilitate Diffusion

- It is a type of diffusion across a semipermeable membrane where water-soluble larger molecules are transported with the help of a carrier protein, irrespective of the concentration gradient.

- Based on the carrier protein, there are two types:
  1. **Channel proteins:** A passageway is formed by proteins which lead to fast passage of small ions and water molecules.
     Example: Potassium ions in nerve fiber, water molecules.
  2. **Uniporters:** They carry a single molecule at a time along a concentration gradient. Binding of the molecule causes conformational change in the protein.
     Example: Sugars, aminoacids.

3. What do mean by secondary active transport? Give examples.

Secondary Active Transport

- Transport of a molecule or an ion across a semipermeable membrane with the help of another ion (usually sodium) and a carrier protein.
- It can be in the same direction as sodium or in opposite direction.
- When both the ions are being transported, it is called co-transport and when the ions are transferred in opposite directions, it is called counter-transport.

Examples
1. **Sodium co-transport (Fig. 1.13)**
   - The carrier protein called symport takes both the ions in the same direction.

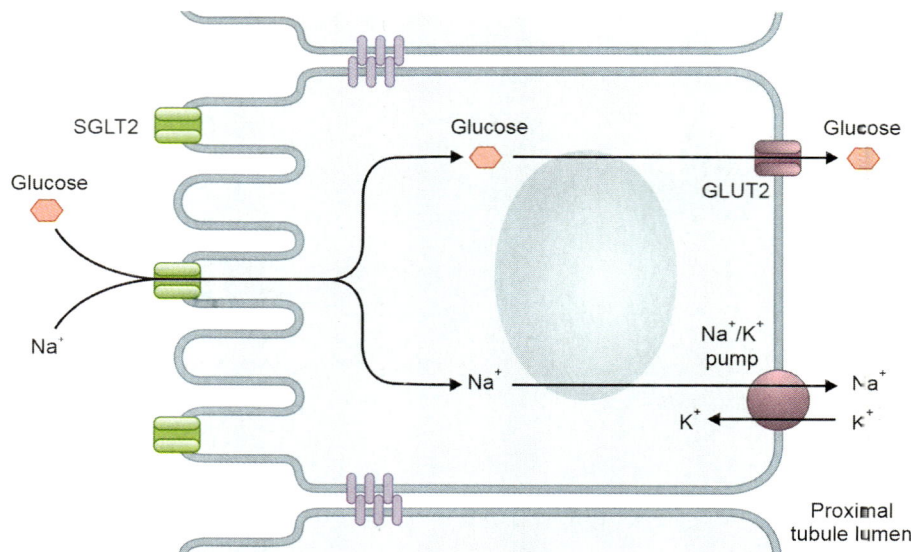

Fig. 1.13

- In proximal convoluted tubules of the kidney, the sodium and glucose molecules are carried towards the inside of the cell at the same time.
- Iron, urea, iodine and amino acids are also co-transported with sodium in the proximal convoluted tubules.
- The carrier protein has two sites for attachment of these substances.
- When both the substances attach, the carrier protein undergoes conformational change and leads to inward turning of the protein.
- Then the molecules detach from the carrier protein and transported into the intracellular space.

2. **Sodium counter-transport mechanism (Fig. 1.14)**
   - The carrier protein is called antiport.
   - Sodium is exchanged for various molecules along with sodium.

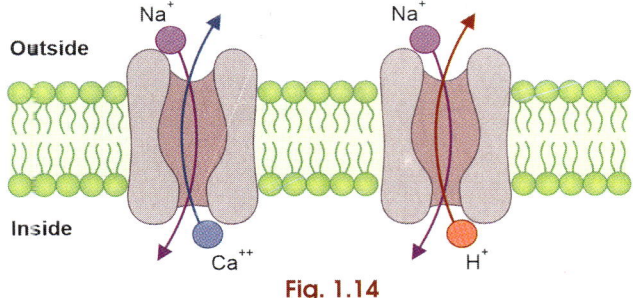

Fig. 1.14

- Sodium calcium channels are present in all cells. In this, sodium influxes along with efflux of calcium at the same time.
- Others are $Na^+ - H^+$ counter-transport in renal tubular cells, sodium–magnesium, $Na^+ - K^+$, $Ca^{++} - Mg^{++}$, $Ca^{++} - K^+$ counter-transport mechanisms.

4. Explain Na⁺ –K⁺ transport mechanism and give its physiological importance (Fig. 1.15).

Na–K Transport Mechanism

- They are transported by active transport across the cell membrane with the help of a carrier protein and use of ATP.
- It is called the Na–K-ATPase pump.
- It transports sodium from inside the cell to outside and brings in potassium from outside to inside.

Physiological Importance

- This pump is very important to maintain the integrity and volume of the cell. Na⁺ ions have more affinity to water molecules. Increase in Na⁺ ions cause the cell to swell and die.
- As three sodium ions are removed for every 2 potassium ions, a negativity is created within the cell. This helps in creating a negative potential which is the basis for many activities like action potential in neurons and muscle fibers. Hence, this pump is said to be electrogenic.

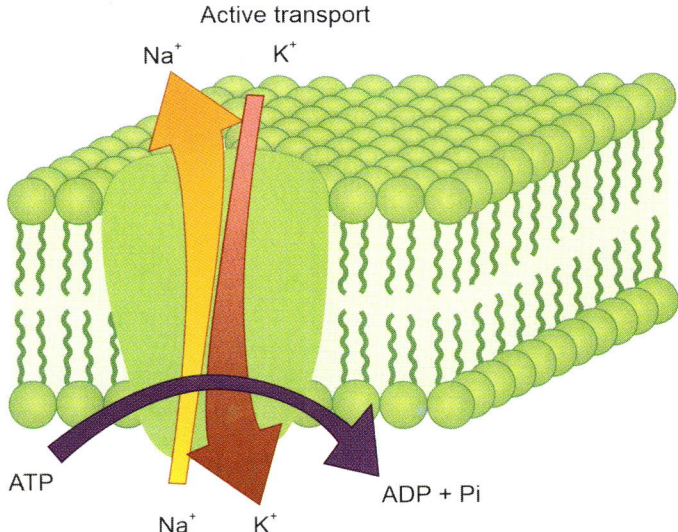

Active transport against concentration gradient with input of energy

Fig. 1.15

5. What is the physiological importance of tight junctions? Explain with 2 examples.

Tight Junctions: Physiological Importance

- Also called zona occludens, it is an intercellular occluding junction between two cells which does not allow passage of macromolecules.
- Each tight junction consists of one-half ridge from each cell and the junction occupies the space between the two cells.
- They only allow specific molecules to pass through it.

Examples

1. **Blood–brain barrier:** Tight junctions between capillaries form blood–brain barrier which does not allow penetration of chemicals across it thus protects the brain from harmful chemicals present in the blood.

2. **Gastrointestinal tract:** Tight junctions in the epithelium of the mucosa of the stomach do not permit entry of substances to be absorbed excepting a few lipid-soluble substances like alcohol.

3. **Renal tubular cells**
   - Tight junctions are present on the luminal side of the tubular cells which allow Na^+ ions and water to diffuse in.
   - They are sensitive to ADH and control the amount of water absorption

1.6 DESCRIBE THE FLUID COMPARTMENTS OF THE BODY, ITS IONIC COMPOSITION AND MEASUREMENTS

SHORT ESSAYS

1. Define osmosis. When RBCs are suspended in hypotonic solution what happens to the cells? Mention 2 examples for isotonic solutions.

Osmosis

- Osmosis is defined as passive movement of water molecules across a semipermeable membrane from a region of higher concentration to a region of lower concentration along the concentration gradient.
- It should flow towards the region of higher concentration of solutes.
- 0.9% solution is considered isotonic. Solutions with concentration of NaCl lesser than that are considered hypotonic and concentration more than 0.9% are considered hypertonic.

RBC Suspended in Hypotonic Solution

- When RBCs are suspended in hypotonic solution, water enters the RBC and causes lysis of the cell. This is called osmotic fragility.
- Normal osmotic fragility of nRBC is 0.45% for older RBCs and 0.35% for younger RBCs.

Hypotonic

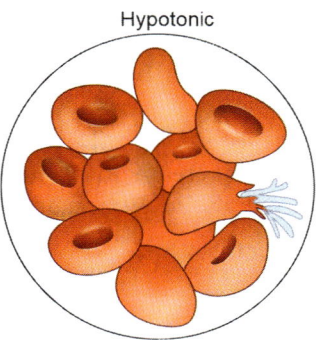

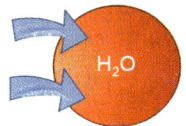

Fig. 1.16

Examples for Isotonic Solutions

- 0.45% saline is considered half-normal saline. It is used in conditions called diabetic ketoacidosis to rehydrate the cells.

1.7 DESCRIBE THE CONCEPT OF pH AND BUFFER SYSTEMS IN THE BODY

SHORT ESSAYS

1. What is metabolic acidosis? Why does it occur in diabetes mellitus?

Metabolic Acidosis

- It is an acid–base imbalance in the body characterized by increase in organic acids in the blood due to metabolic derangements.

Diabetic Ketoacidosis

- It is a complication of type 1 diabetes or insulin dependent diabetes.
- It is potentially fatal
- In this type, there is absolute deficiency of insulin.
- It is characterized by increased ketones in the body.

Pathophysiology (Figs 1.17 and 1.18)

It is precipitated by a stress or an infection which causes excess counter-regulatory hormones in blood.

2. What are the different mechanisms with which pH is regulated in the body?

Mechanisms of pH Regulation

- Acid–base balance is key regulator for maintenance of homeostasis. A lot of enzymes are dependent on normal pH of the body

- Normal pH of ECF is 7.38–7.42

$$pH = \log \frac{1}{H^+}$$

where H^+ is the concentration of hydrogen ions or protons
- An increase in pH causes alkalosis and a decrease in pH causes acidosis.
- Whenever there is a disturbance in the pH, there are three compensatory mechanisms that kick in:
  1. Acid–base buffer mechanism
  2. Respiratory mechanism
  3. Renal mechanism

1. Acid–Base Buffer Mechanism

- An acid–base buffer is a combination of a weak acid with a strong base salt
- It acts immediately. It is of three types:
  i. **Bicarbonate buffer system**
     - It consists of a weak acid, carbonic acid and a base salt-sodium bicarbonate.
     - Its pK is 6.1. It is not a very strong buffer but is very efficient due to both acid and base buffers work separately and simultaneously.

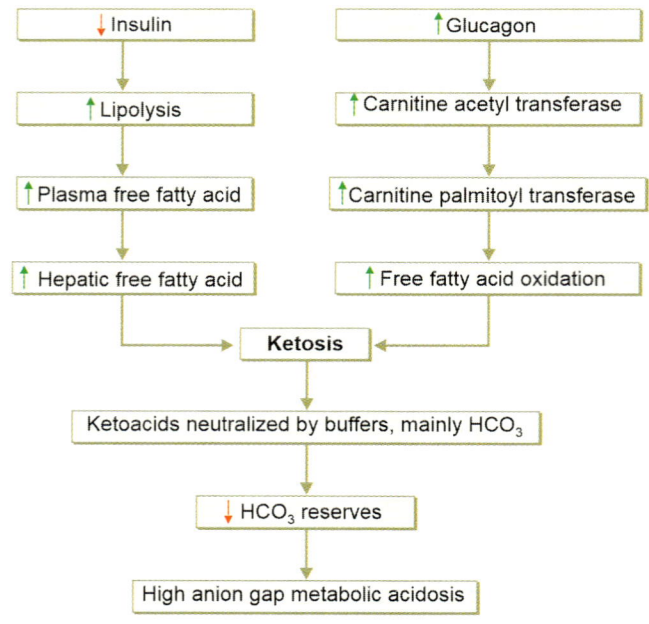

Fig. 1.17

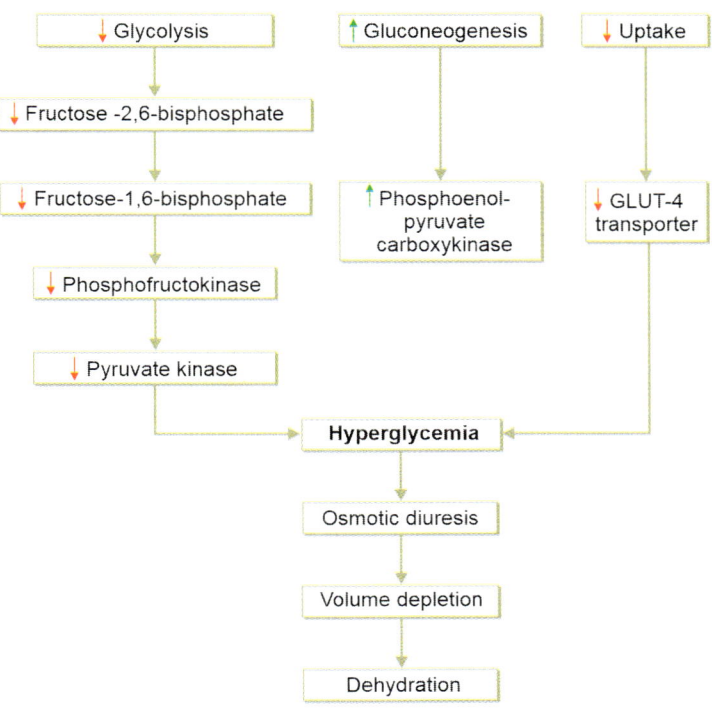

Fig. 1.18

- In acidic environment
  - o When the pH decreases in situations where there is excess H+, it combines with $NaHCO_3$ to form carbonic acid and Na^+.
  - o Carbonic acid (H_2CO_3) is a weak acid and readily dissociates into CO_2 and H_2O.
- In alkaline environment
  - o When there is excess HCO_3, the milieu becomes alkaline.
  - o The H_2CO_3 acts as the buffer. The OH^- ion of the base combines with H^+ of the carbonic acid and forms water.
  - o Na^+ combines bicarbonate to form $NaHCO_3$

ii. *Phosphate buffer system*
  - This buffer system consists of a weak acid: Dihydrogen phosphate as acidic substance and sodium dihydrogen phosphate as the salt—NaH_2PO_4
  - It has a pK of 6.8. hence more powerful than bicarbonate system.
  - It consists of disodium hydrogen phosphate as the base—Na_2HPO_4
  - It mainly operates in the intracellular fluid and renal tubules.

- In RBCs it is present as potassium dihydrogen phosphate and dipotassium hydrogen phosphate.
- In acidic environment
  - o When a strong acid like HCl is added to fluid consisting of phosphate buffer, hydrogen ions combine with Na_2HPO_4 to form NaH_2PO_4 (sodium dihydrogen phosphate)
- In alkaline environment
  - o When a strong base-like NaOH is added to a fluid consisting of phosphate buffer, OH^- combines with NaH_2PO_4 to form disodium hydrogen phosphate.

iii. *Protein buffer*
  - It is present in plasma and erythrocytes.
  - The proteins which take part in buffer system are hemoglobin (most powerful), C-terminal carboxy group and N-terminal amino end of glutamic acid, side chain amino group of lysine, imidazole ring of histidine.
  - They have a pK of 7.4. hence, they are powerful.
  - When a deoxygenated hemoglobin molecule is exposed to low pH, it readily combines with hydrogen ions.

2. Respiratory Mechanism

- When pH of the blood falls, there is an increase in hydrogen ions.
- It combines with bicarbonate in blood to form, H_2O and CO_2.
- CO_2 is easily blown out by hyperventilation by the lungs. Hyperventilation is caused by chemoreceptors which are triggered by hydrogen excess.

3. Renal Mechanisms (Fig. 1.19)

- In presence of acidosis, kidneys excrete hydrogen ions and retain bicarbonate ions.
- In cases of metabolic acidosis, kidneys play an important role in preventing metabolic acidosis, by excreting excess H^+ ions
- It is done by 3 methods:

  i. **Bicarbonate mechanism**
     - Excess bicarbonate and H^+ in urine combine to form H_2CO_3 (unstable). It dissociates to form H_2O and CO_2 which enter the tubular cell.
     - In presence of carbonic anhydrase, they form H_2CO_3 which is catalyzed into H^+ and HCO_3^-
     - Bicarbonate ions enter the interstitium
     - The H^+ ions are exchanged for Na^+ at the luminal end.

  ii. **Phosphate mechanism**
     - In the tubular lumen, Na_2HPO_4 splits into Na^+ and $NaHPO_4^-$

  - In the tubular cell, $H_2O + CO_2 = H_2CO_3$. It splits immediately into H^+ and HCO_3^-
  - The H^+ is exchanged for Na^+
  - The H^+ combines with $NaHPO_4^-$ to sodium dihydrogen phosphate

  iii. **Ammonia mechanism**
     - Ammonia is generated with the tubular cell from glutamine.
     - It is transported to the tubular lumen in exchange for Na^+
     - The hydrogen that is normally excreted combines with ammonia to form ammonium
     - Thus, for each molecule of ammonia formed one H^+ is excreted and NCO_3^- is retained.

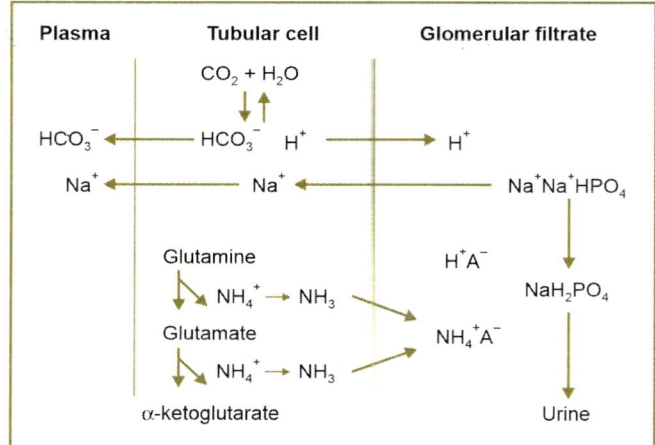

Fig. 1.19

1.8 DESCRIBE AND DISCUSS THE MOLECULAR BASIS OF RESTING MEMBRANE POTENTIAL AND ACTION POTENTIAL IN EXCITABLE TISSUE

SHORT ESSAYS

1. The resting membrane potential of a nerve is –70 mV. Substantiate.

Resting Membrane Potential

- It is the potential difference across the membrane of a neuron prior to beginning of an action potential and its value is –70 mV. That means the potential inside the nerve fibre is –70 mV lower than its exterior.
- The factors involved in maintaining this potential is the ionic gradient created across the membrane.
- It is mainly maintained through Na-K pump and Na-K leaky channels (Fig. 1.20).

Role of Sodium Potassium Active Pumps

- It is a powerful pump that continuously pumps K^+ ions inside the cell and Na^+ ions outside the cell with the help of ATP.
- It is an electrogenic pump, in the sense that, it pumps 3 Na^+ ions out and allows two K^+ ions inside the cell.
- As a result, a negative charge is created. Also, a gradient is created.

Na$^+$ (extracellular)	142 mEq/L	Ratio: 0.1
Na$^+$ (intracellular)	14 mEq/L	(inside:outside)
K$^+$ (extracellular)	4 mEq/L	Ratio: 35
K$^+$ (intracellular)	140 mEq/L	(inside:outside)

Role of Leak Channels

- These provide leakage of ions across the membrane and are 100 times more permeable to potassium influx.

- As a result, passive influx of sodium ions is much less compared to passive outflux of potassium ions.
- Further efflux of potassium ions is prevented by relative positivity outside the cell which prevents its efflux and negativity within the cell which keeps the potassium within.

2. Explain the ionic basis of the action potential in skeletal muscle

Ionic Basis of Action Potential

- Action potential is a series of electrical changes that occur in membrane potential when the muscle or nerve is stimulated (Fig. 1.21).
- Voltage-gated sodium and potassium channels play an important role in causing an action potential.
- It has three phases: Latent phase, depolarization and repolarization.

Latent Period

- It is the time taken when no change takes place in the membrane potential after applying a stimulus.
- There is no change in resting membrane potential (–90 mV)
- It is 0.5–1 ms in length.
- *Stimulus artifact:* It occurs at the time of application of stimulating electrode due to leakage of current from the stimulating electrode to the recording electrode. It occurs prior to latent period.

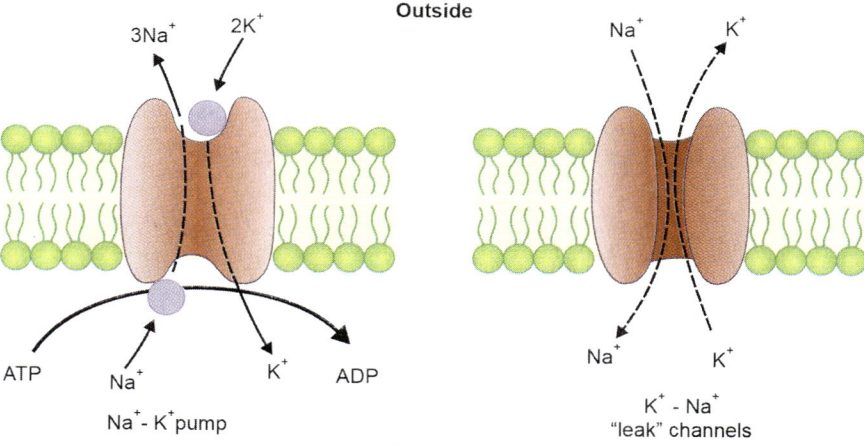

Fig. 1.20

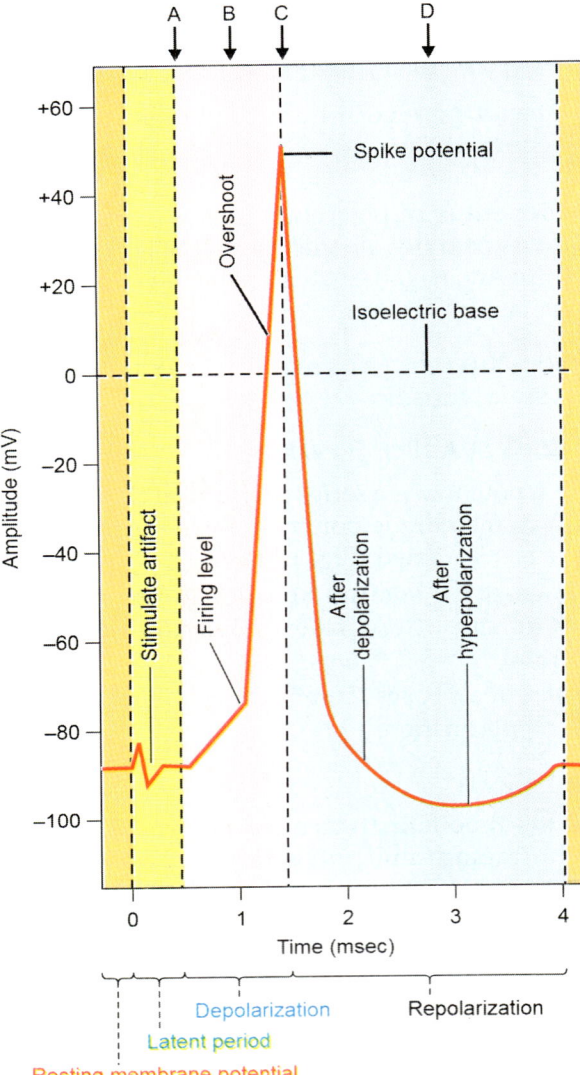

Fig. 1.21

A. Opening of sodium channels leading to influx of sodium ions, B. opening of more and more sodium channels causing influx of Na+, C. closure of sodium channels and opening of potassium channels leading to efflux of potassium, D. continued efflux of potassium ions leading to increase in negativity inside the cell

Depolarization

- It is a positive wave. For the first 15 mV it is very slow.
- Ionic basis for initial depolarisation: Represented by A in the diagram: It is due to opening of new sodium channels.
- After about 15 mV of depolarization, there is an increase in slope of the depolarization wave. Depolarization crosses the isoelectric point (0 mV) and overshoots by +55 mV.
- Ionic basis for firing level: Opening of more and more sodium channels. It is represented by B in the diagram.

Repolarization

- It is marked by reversal of potential from positive to negative. Ionic basis: Closure of sodium ions and opening of potassium ions. It is marked C in the diagram.
- It is followed by slow repolarization. Ionic basis: Open potassium ions leading to continuous influx of potassium ions.
- It is then followed by a slow hyperpolarization. Ionic basis: Potassium channels remain open for longer than sodium channels leading to further efflux of sodium ions leading to hyperpolarization. It is represented as D in the diagram.

SHORT ANSWER

1. Give the normal resting membrane potential of nerve, skeletal muscle and smooth muscle.

- Resting membrane potential is the difference between the electrical potential that exists within and outside a cell prior to excitation.
- Also called transmembrane potential.

Nerve	– 70 mV
Skeletal muscle	– 90 mV
Smooth muscle	– 50 to –60 mV

1.9 DEMONSTRATE THE ABILITY TO DESCRIBE AND DISCUSS THE METHODS USED TO DEMONSTRATE THE FUNCTIONS OF THE CELLS AND ITS PRODUCTS, ITS COMMUNICATIONS AND THEIR APPLICATIONS IN CLINICAL CARE AND RESEARCH

SHORT ESSAY/SHORT ANSWER

1. Explain patch clamp technique.

- It is a method to measure ion current across biological membranes.
- It was discovered in 1992 and is useful for studying ion potential across cell membranes.

Procedure (Fig. 1.22)

- The cells isolated for the body and is isolated in a dish.
- It is placed in culture media and placed in the incubator.
- A micropipette with an opening of around 0.5 micron is placed on the surface of the cell under a microscope.
- It is filled with saline solution.
- A recorder is fitted to the pipette and is connected to an amplifier.
- The pipette is applied firmly to the surface of the cell and gentle suction is created.
- The part of the cell membrane within the pipette is called the patch.

Methods of Studying Ion Potentials (Fig. 1.23)

1. **Cell attached patch:** The cell is intact and allows flow of current through the channels under the micropipette.

2. **Inside-out patch**
   - When the pipette is gently pulled out, a part of the cell is broughtout.
   - Now the inside of the cell is exteriorized.
   - Then, this part of the cell along with the pipette is placed in another solution.
   - This procedure helps to understand effects of different ionic concentration on the cell membrane.

3. **Whole cell patch**
   - If the pipette is advanced further, the solution in the pipette mixes with the ICF.
   - When the mixing is complete, an equilibrium is reached.
   - It is useful in studying current flow through all channels.

4. **Outside-out patch**
   - From the whole cell patch, a portion of the membrane is torn away from the cell.
   - Immediately, the free ends of the torn membrane seal to form a vesicle.
   - The vesicle is placed in a bath solution and the fluid within the cell behaves like ICF.

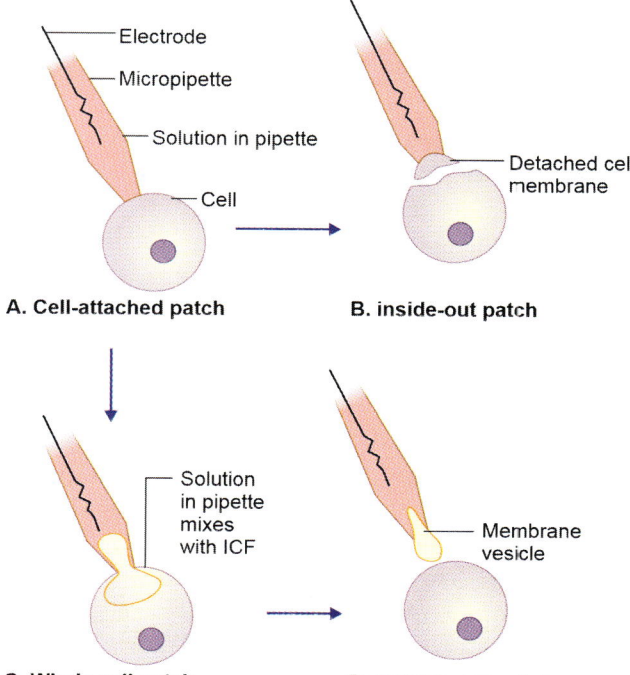

A. Cell-attached patch   B. inside-out patch

C. Whole cell patch   D. Outside-out patch

Fig. 1.23

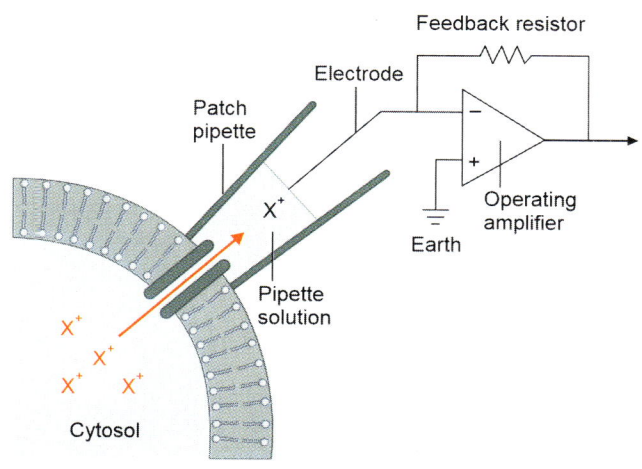

Fig. 1.22

Haematology

2.1 DESCRIBE THE COMPOSITION AND FUNCTIONS OF BLOOD COMPONENTS

SHORT ESSAY

1. How do you classify body fluid compartments? How do you measure ECF volume experimentally?

Classification of Body Fluid Compartments

- It is mainly divided into an intracellular compartment (forms 55% of 40 L, that is 22 L) and an extracellular compartment (forms 45% of 40 L, that is 18 L).
- The extracellular space is subdivided into the following:
  – Interstitial space (20%)
  – Plasma (7.5%)
  – Fluid in bones (7.5%)
  – Fluid in cartilage (7.5%)
  – Transcellular fluids (2.5%)
    o CSF, intraocular, synovial space, digestive juices, urinary tract fluid, peritoneal fluid, pericardial fluid and pleural fluid.

Measurement of ECF Volume

- Solutes that pass through the capillary membrane but remain extracellular are used to measure ECF volume.
- Examples are radioactive sodium, chloride, bromide, saccharides like inulin, mannitol, raffinose and sucrose. These saccharides remain unmetabolized in blood.

- A known quantity of any of these substances is injected into blood.
- It mixes with the fluid of all sub-compartments of ECF within 30–60 minutes.
- A sample of blood is taken as blood represents a part of ECF.
- Indicator dilution method is used to calculate volume of extracellular fluid.

Volume of ECF =

$$\frac{\text{Mass of substance injected} - \text{amount lost in urine}}{\text{Concentration of the substance in plasma}}$$

- Some marker substances like sodium, chloride, insulin, and sucrose diffuse uniformly in all the sub-compartments of ECF.
- Hence, the volume of ECF calculated by using these substances is referred as sodium space, chloride space, inulin space and sucrose space.

Example

- 500 ml of mannitol is injected into blood
- After 30 minutes, urine is collected. It contains 10 g of mannitol
- The plasma concentration of mannitol is 3.2 mg/100 ml. Thus, ECF is:

$$= \frac{500\,\text{mg} - (10\%\ \text{of}\ 500\,\text{mg})}{3.2\,\text{mg}/100\,\text{ml}}$$

$$= \frac{450\,\text{mg}}{3.2\,\text{mg}/100\,\text{ml}} = \frac{450\,\text{mg}}{32\,\text{mg/L}} = 14.1\,\text{L}$$

2.2 DISCUSS THE ORIGIN, FORMS, VARIATIONS AND FUNCTIONS OF PLASMA PROTEINS

SHORT ESSAYS

1. Describe the formation, composition, circulation and functions of lymph in the body.

- Lymph is a fluid ubiquitous to life.
- It is produced during the transit of interstitial fluid from various organs and it collects various products of metabolism as well as circulating immune cells and ferries them to the regional lymph nodes.

Formation of Lymph

- It is formed by filtration of the interstitial fluid, due to the high permeability of lymph capillaries.
- When blood passes through the capillaries in the tissues, 90% of it passes into venous end of capillaries.
- The remaining 10% of the fluid passes into lymph capillaries, which have a permeability higher than that of blood capillaries.
- So, the composition of lymph is more or less similar to that of interstitial fluid including protein content.
- The blood capillaries are impervious to the proteins due to their large size. So, these larger proteins enter lymph vessels.
- Proteins and fats are added from the liver and GIT. Thus, lymph in larger vessels additionally has more proteins and lipids.
- In the lymph nodes, water is absorbed. Thus, lymph gets concentrated.

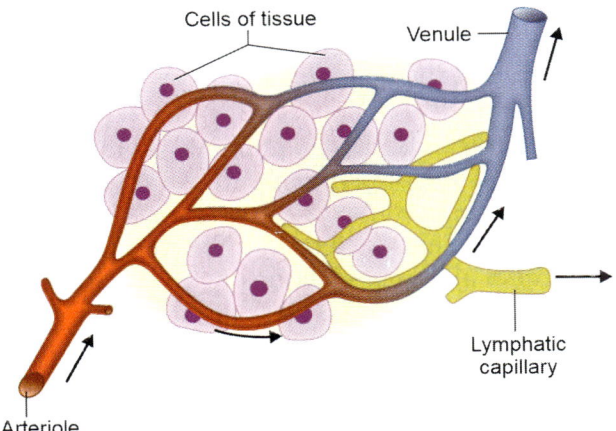

Fig. 2.1

Rate of Lymph Flow

- Approximately 120 ml of lymph flows into blood per hour throughout the body.
- Of this, about 100 ml/hour flows through thoracic duct and 20 ml/hour flows through the right lymphatic duct.

Composition of Lymph

It is mostly composed of water (95%) and solids make up for the remaining 5%.

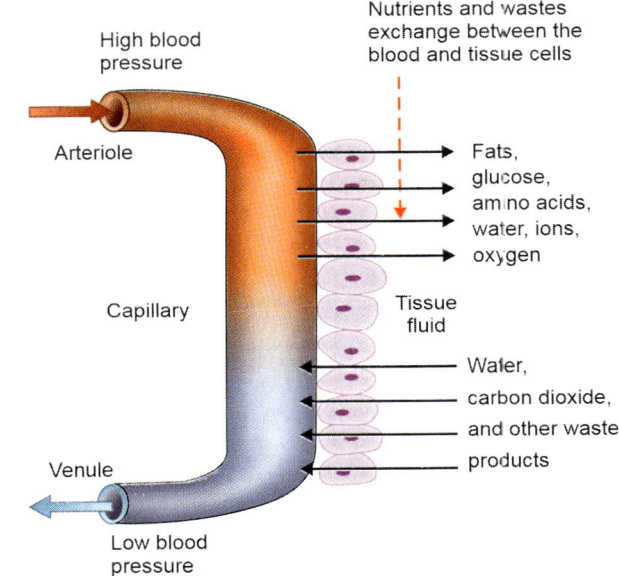

Fig. 2.2

Proteins	Albumin, globulin, fibrinogen, all clotting factors, enzymes, antibodies
Lipids	Chylomicrons and lipoproteins
Carbohydrates	Glucose
Nitrogenous wastes	Urea, creatinine
Electrolytes	Na, K, Ca, bicarbonate, chloride
Cellular content	Lymphocytes

Lymph Circulation

- All parenchymal organs in the human body except the brain have a network of lymphatics.
- The lymphatic capillaries are formed by a single layer of endothelial cells resting on a thin basement membrane.

- The endothelial cells are connected by specialized intercellular junctions, containing platelet endothelial cell adhesion molecule 1 (PECAM1) and vascular endothelial cadherin (VE cadherin).
- The lymph capillaries have one-way valves to facilitate entry of proteins, fluids, macromolecules, small molecules and immune cells.
- The directional flow of lymph is also maintained through unidirectional bicuspid valves, positioned along the collectors, which open and close synchronously with the contraction of the lymph vessel.
- The part of the lymphatic collectors present between the two sets of valves is called a lymphangion.
- Contraction of a distal lymphangion towards the proximal to the lymph node, in synchrony with directional valve closure, leads to unidirectional lymph transport (towards the heart).

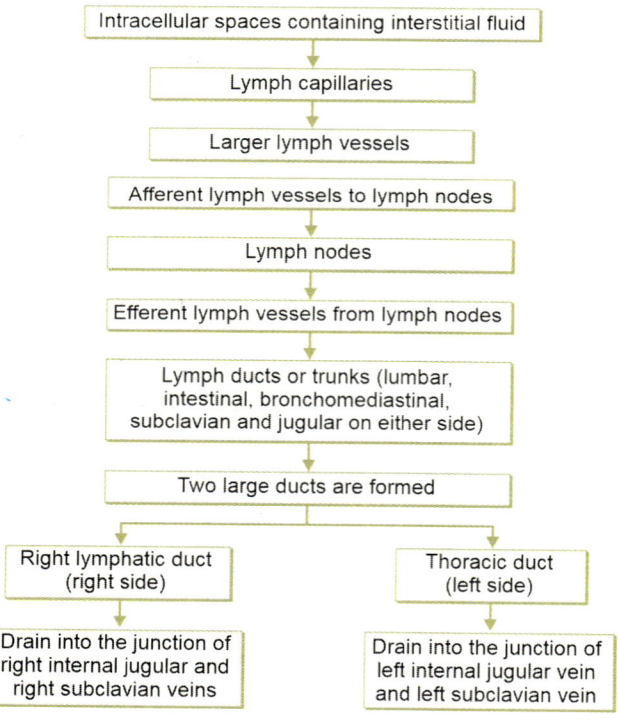

Fig. 2.3

Functions of Lymph

1. To redistribute proteins from interstitial spaces into blood.
2. Redistribution of fluid in the body.

3. Immune function: Removal of bacteria, toxins, and other foreign bodies from tissues through lymph by drainage. It also helps in transport of lymphocytes.
4. Lymph flow is responsible for maintaining structural and functional integrity of a tissue.
5. Intestinal fat absorption is dependent solely on lymph.

2. Enumerate the plasma proteins. Explain its functions.

Plasma Proteins

Serum albumin	3.5–5.0 gm/100 ml (4.8 g%)
Serum globulin	1.5–2.5 gm/100 ml
Fibrinogen	150–300 mg/100 ml

Functions of Plasma Proteins

1. **Albumin:** Highest concentration
   - It helps in transport of various compounds in the blood from one site to another.
   - It also helps to bind drugs and improve their lifespan in the blood.
   - Albumin cannot be filtered by kidneys. They stay in the blood. As a result, they exert an osmotic pressure due to their polar nature and retain water in the ECF. Its value is about 25 mm Hg.
   - Albumin has buffering action due to which it plays an important role in acid–base balance.
   - Increases blood viscosity.
   - They serve as reserve proteins in case of prolonged fasting.
   - They help in formation of trephones which are required for nourishment of leukocytes.
   - Albumin serves as a reliable laboratory indicator for acute liver dysfunction.

2. **Globulin**
   - They are important in immunity as they help in formation of gamma globulins (immunoglobulins). Antibodies are important in fighting against many bacteria and viruses.
   - Alpha and beta globulins help in transport of metals.
   - Help in maintaining osmotic pressure in the blood as they cannot be filtered by kidneys.
   - Globulins increase the tendency for rouleaux formation. It is important factor for ESR measurement.

- Globulins help in maintaining red blood cells suspended in the plasma. It is called suspension stability.
- They serve as reserve proteins in case of prolonged fasting.
- They help in formation of trephones which are required for nourishment of leukocytes.

3 **Fibrinogen**
- Helps in coagulation
- They increase the tendency for rouleaux formation. It is important factor for ESR measurement.
- They help in maintaining red blood cells suspended in the plasma. It is called suspension stability.
- They serve as reserve proteins in case of prolonged fasting.
- They help in formation of trephones which are required for nourishment of leukocytes

SHORT ANSWERS

1. What is the importance of albumin–globulin ratio? What is its normal value? Mention two conditions where this ratio gets reversed.

Albumin–Globulin Ratio

It is the ratio of plasma levels of albumin to globulin.

Normal Value

It is normally 2:1

Importance

- Albumin is primarily produced by liver and has a half-life of 21 days.
- It is not excreted in urine and if found in urine signifies renal dysfunction.
- So, a decrease in albumins seen in liver dysfunction like hepatitis and cirrhosis and in kidney diseases like diabetic nephropathy, nephrotic syndrome and others.
- Also, albumin has more oncotic pressure compared to globulin. As a result, in states of decreased albumin in blood, there is more water retention leading to pedal edema, ascites and pulmonary edema.

A:G ratio is reversed in:
1. Cirrhosis of liver (decreased albumin production)
2. Multiple myeloma increased (globulin production).

2. What is oncotic pressure? What determines the oncotic pressure?

Oncotic Pressure

- It is osmotic pressure exerted by the plasma proteins in blood
- It is the pressure exerted by solutes in a fluid and tends to draw fluid from another solution separated by a semipermeable membrane.
- Increased oncotic pressure indicates increased pressure to draw fluid into the solution.
- Normal values
  - Normal colloidal osmotic pressure of plasma is 28 mm Hg
  - 19 mm is exerted by plasma proteins
  - 9 mm by Donnan effect (sodium, potassium, and other cations)

Determinants of Oncotic Pressure

- **Number of molecules of the solute:** More the molecules, more is the oncotic pressure.
- **Its permeability through the membrane:** Lesser the permeability, more is the pressure exerted.
- **Pore size in the basement membrane of capillaries:** In certain conditions, these may be increased due to damage to the endothelium.

Albumin

- It is a highly negative charged plasma protein with high concentration in plasma.
- It is the smallest of all plasma proteins and thus maximum in concentration per unit volume.
- It is the main determinant of colloidal osmotic pressure or oncotic pressure and contributes to 80% of the total oncotic pressure.

2.3 DESCRIBE AND DISCUSS THE SYNTHESIS AND FUNCTIONS OF HAEMOGLOBIN AND EXPLAIN ITS BREAKDOWN. DESCRIBE VARIANTS OF HAEMOGLOBIN

SHORT ANSWERS

1. Describe the pathophysiology of thalassemia and its types.

Pathophysiology of Thalassemia

- Each hemoglobin molecule has a heme compound with 4 protein chains—2 alpha and 2 beta chains.
- This variation is due to the amino acid sequence
- Thalassemia is a group of disorders due to faulty production or absence of these globin or amino acid chains resulting from a gene mutation responsible for production of globin chains.
- In alpha thalassemia, there is fault in the alpha chain and in beta thalassemia, beta chain is faulty.
- As a result of absence or ineffective production of one chain, there is over production of its counter-part which precipitates in the RBC precursor and leads to its lysis.
- This causes ineffective erythropoiesis.
- As a result, there is anemia.

Types

1. **Alpha thalassemia**
   i. Alpha thalassemia major
   ii. Alpha thalassemia minor
2. **Beta thalassemia**
   i. Beta thalassemia minor
   ii. Beta thalassemia major

2. What is haemoglobinopathies? Explain beta thalassemia.

Hemoglobinopathy

It is a genetic disorder characterized by one or more abnormal polypeptide chains of hemoglobin.

Types

1. **Hemoglobin S**
   - It is found in sickle cell anemia.
   - In this type of hemoglobin, the β-chains are normal
   - However, in the β-chains, there is a point mutation causing substitution of amino acid valine instead of glutamic acid.

2. **Hemoglobin C**
   - The β-chains are abnormal. In the sixth position, the glutamic acid is substituted by lysine.
   - As a result, the hemoglobin is less soluble and forms crystals. There is an increase in viscosity of blood and increased cellular rigidity.
   - It causes hemoglobin C disease, which is characterized by mild hemolytic anemia and splenomegaly.

3. **Hemoglobin M**
   - It is the abnormal hemoglobin present in the form of methemoglobin.
   - It occurs due to a variety of mutation of genes of α-, β- and γ-chains, resulting in abnormal replacement of amino acids. The resultant hemoglobin is resistant to reduction.
   - It presents in babies as blue baby syndrome.

4. **Hemoglobin E**
   - Here also the β-chains are abnormal. In the 26th position, glutamic acid is replaced by lysine.
   - It can coexist with sickle cell or thalassemia.
   - It causes hemoglobin E disease which is also characterized by mild hemolytic anemia and splenomegaly.

Beta Thalassemia

- Thalassemia is a group of disorders due to faulty production or absence of these globin or amino acid chains. It occurs due to mutation of genes responsible for production of globin chains.
- Each hemoglobin molecule has a heme compound with 4 protein chains—2 alpha and 2 beta chains. This variation is due to the amino acid sequence.
- In alpha thalassemia, there is fault in the alpha chain and in beta thalassemia, beta chain is faulty. As a result of absence or ineffective production of one chain, there is over production of its counter-part which precipitates in the RBC precursor and leads to its lysis.
- This causes ineffective erythropoiesis. As a result, there is anemia.
- Also, there is increased lysis of RBCs causing hemolytic anemia, jaundice and hepatospleno-megaly.

- Due to ineffective erythropoiesis, there is expansion of bone marrow in an effort to produce more RBCs. Therefore, these children have hyperostosis.

Types

1. **Beta thalassemia minor:** This disease is asymptomatic, as only one gene is affected. They may have mild anemia but have the propensity to pass on the disease to their offspring.
2. **Beta thalassemia major:** In this disease, both alleles are mutated. As a result, there is severe anemia and require treatment.

Treatment

These children usually require frequent blood transfusions.

2.4 DESCRIBE RBC FORMATION (ERYTHROPOIESIS AND ITS REGULATION) AND ITS FUNCTIONS

LONG ESSAYS

1. **Define erythropoiesis. Explain the site, duration, steps of erythropoiesis, and factors affecting it.   (1 + 5 + 2 + 2 marks)**

Erythropoiesis

Erythropoiesis is defined as origin, development and maturation of erythrocytes or red blood cells.

Duration

It takes 7 days for new RBCs to form.

Steps of Erythropoiesis (Fig. 2.4)

- RBCs are produced from hematopoietic stem cells in the bone marrow
- The steps are:
  - Uncommitted pluripotent hematopoietic stem cells (PHSC) (capable of producing all types of blood cells)
  - Committed PHSC (destined to produce RBCs)
  - Colony forming myelocytes—they give rise to all types of cells other than lymphocytes
  - Colony forming unit-erythrocytes (CFU-E)
- The changes that occur are:
  i. Decrease in the size of the cell
  ii. Disappearance of nucleus and nucleolus
  iii. Appearance of hemoglobin
  iv. Change in staining pattern of the cytoplasm.

1. **Proerythroblast:** Large cell, of diameter around 20 micron. Huge nucleus which occupies most of the space within the cell. Cytoplasm is basophilic, nucleus has two nucleoli, does not contain hemoglobin.

2. **Early normoblast:** Formed by multiple division of proerythroblast, slightly smaller, diameter of 15 micron, nucleoli disappear, chromatin network condenses.

3. **Intermediate normoblast:** Further reduction in size (10–12 micron), further condensation of chromatin network, hemoglobin starts appearing and hence stains with both acidophilic and basophilic stains (polychromatic erythroblast).

4. **Late normoblast:** Diameter of cell is around 8–10 microns, nucleus is very small and is called ink spot nucleus, chromatin is very much condensed, hemoglobin increases and cell stains mostly acidic (orthochromic erythroblast).

5. **Reticulocyte:** Immature RBC, cytoplasm contains remnant of organelles in the form of reticulum/network, stains with supravital stain. They enter peripheral blood. Its concentration is 1% in adults, 2–6% in children in peripheral blood. It takes 5 days to produce a reticulocyte.

6. **Mature RBC:** It takes 2 more days for the reticulocyte to mature. Its diameter is 7.2 microns. Nucleus is lost and shape is biconcave.

Site and Duration of Erythropoiesis

Sites

In fetal life	In newborn babies, children, and adults	
It occurs in three stages 1. Mesoblastic stage: First two months of intrauterine life, the yolk sac is the primary site of production of RBCs 2. Hepatic stage: From 3–6 months of intrauterine life, liver, spleen and lymphoid organs are the sites of erythropoiesis. 3. Myeloid stage: In the last three months, RBC production takes place in bone marrow and liver.	In post-natal life, erythropoiesis takes place only in the bone marrow. Up to 20 years: Bone marrow of all long bones and flat bones	After 20 years: Bone marrow of long bones: Become yellow marrow and contain fat. Main site of erythropoiesis is flat bone marrow like sternum, ileum, skull bones, vertebrae, ribs, and ends of long bones.

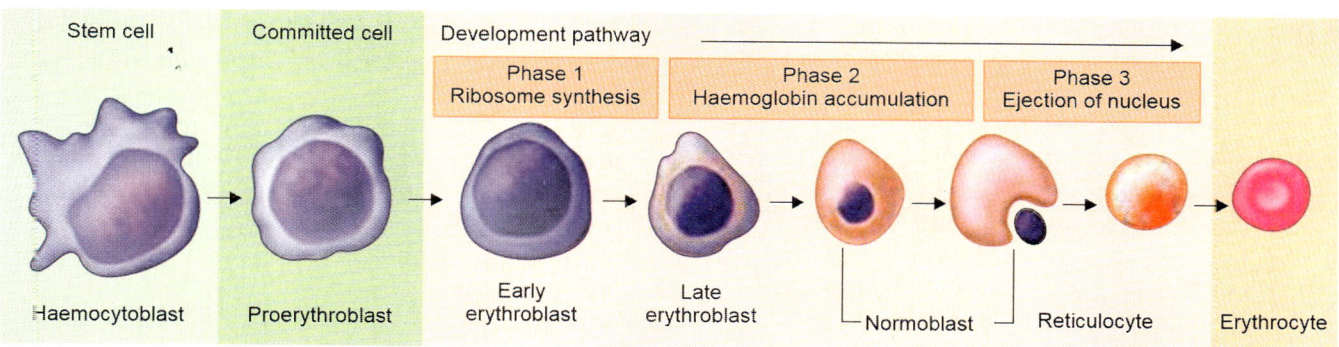

Fig. 2.4

Factors Affecting Erythropoiesis

1. **General factors**
   - Erythropoietin: Most important, it is hormone secreted by peritubular capillaries of kidneys, its secretion is stimulated by hypoxia.
   - Thyroxine
   - Hematopoietic growth factors like interleukins and stem cell factors
   - Vitamins like B, C, D, E
2. **Maturation factors**
   - Vitamin B_{12}
   - Folic acid
   - Intrinsic factor of Castle
3. **Factors necessary for hemoglobin formation**
   - Proteins and amino acids
   - Iron
   - Copper
   - Cobalt and nickel

2. What is erythropoietin? Where is it synthesized? Describe its functions. What are the other factors which influence erythropoiesis?

Erythropoietin

- Erythropoietin is a hormone responsible for generation of red blood cells.
- It is a cytokine by chemical nature

Site of Production

- Erythropoietin is secreted by the endothelial cells of the peritubular capillaries of kidneys.
- Partly secreted by liver and brain.
- The ratio of production by kidney to liver is 9:1.

Stimulants for Production

1. Hypoxia—most important factor.
   - Hypoxia 'release of hypoxia inducible factor 'binds to EPO 5' hypoxia response element' increase in EPO transcription
2. Alkalosis due to high altitude
3. Androgens

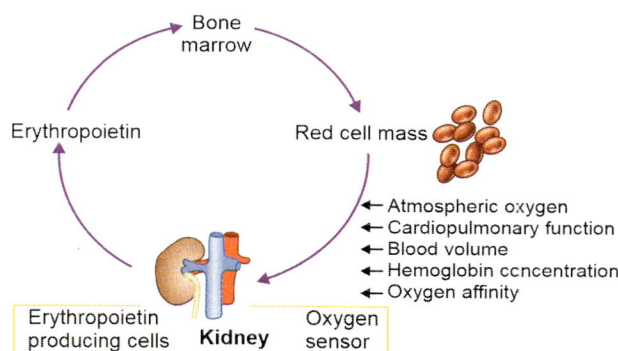

Fig. 2.5

Functions

1. Erythropoietin stimulates the bone marrow to produce red blood cells (RBCs).
2. It induces proliferation and differentiation of erythroid progenitor cells mainly targeting the colony stimulating factor-E.
3. Its gene expression is mainly stimulated by ischemia which causes hypoxia inducible factor which in turn stimulates production of erythropoietin.
4. The steps in erythropoiesis which are extremely dependent on erythropoietin are conversion of CFU-E to proerythroblast and subsequently to early erythroblast.

5. Non-erythropoietic role of erythropoietin
   - It has cardioprotective action during cardiac ischemia by stimulating angiogenesis. Also it has anti-apoptotic properties which prevent post-ischemia death of cardiac myocytes.
   - It has a neuroprotective role in CNS and PNS, retina. It facilitates nerve regeneration.
   - It has a protective role in reperfusion injury in brain, kidney, liver, retina and intestine.
6. Clinical uses of erythropoietin
   - Anemia due to chronic kidney disease
   - Anemia of cancer
   - Illegally used for doping by athletes to increase performance
   - Has been tried in ischemic optic neuropathy—not yet approved.

Other Factors which Influence Erythropoiesis

1. Erythropoietin is the most important influence
2. General factors
   - Thyroxine
   - Interleukins
   - Stem cells factors (STEEL)
   - Vitamins B, C, D, E
3. Maturation factors
   - Vitamin B_{12}
   - Folic acid
   - Intrinsic factor of Castle
4. Factors necessary for the Hb formation
   - Proteins and amino acids
   - Iron
   - Copper
   - Cobalt, nickel

2.5 DESCRIBE DIFFERENT TYPES OF ANAEMIAS AND JAUNDICE

LONG ESSAY

1. A 35-year-old female is diagnosed to have anemia. Her peripheral smear showed macrocytic hypochromic red cells.

A. What is your diagnosis in this case? Define anemia.

B. Give the morphological classification of anemia.

C. Explain blood indices and give its normal values.

D. If treatment with iron and Vit B$_{12}$ does not improve the clinical condition, how would you treat the patient and why?

A. Diagnosis

- Megaloblastic anemia
- Anemia is defined as decreased hemoglobin, decreased RBC count or packed cell volume.

B. Morphological Classification of Anemia

Based on RBC size and color in anemia (Fig. 2.6).

Type	Size of RBC	Color of RBC	Causes
Microcytic hypochromic	<72 microns	Less than 1/3rd of the RBC is red	Iron deficiency anemia
Macrocytic normochromic	>110 microns	>2/3rds of RBC are red	Vitamin B$_{12}$ deficiency
Macrocytic hypochromic	>110 microns	Less than 1/3rd of the RBC is red	Folic acid deficiency

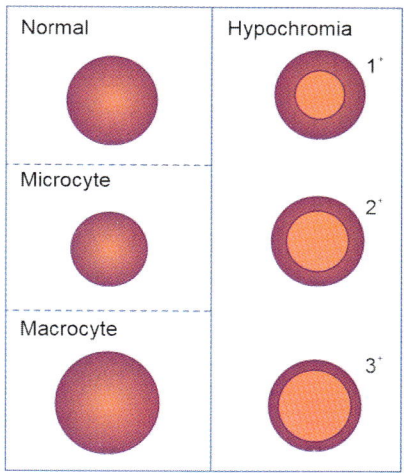

Fig. 2.6

C. Blood Indices and its Normal Values

Blood indices	Description	Normal value
MCV or mean corpuscular volume	It is the average volume of a single RBC and is expressed in cubic microns	
	Variants: Microcyte (small), macrocyte (large) and normocyte.	78–90 cu mic.
MCH or mean corpuscular hemoglobin	It is the average mass of hemoglobin per RBC.	27–32 pg
MCHC or mean corpuscular hemoglobin concentration	It is the mass of hemoglobin per unit volume of RBC.	30–38%
	When it is normal: Normochromic	
	Variants: Hypochromic (decreased percentage), hyperchromic (increased percentage)	
Color index	Ratio between the percentage of hemoglobin and percentage of RBCs in the blood.	0.8–1.2
RDW or red cell distribution width	Measure of range of variation of volume of red cell.	11.5–14.5%

D. Folate is also a factor which can cause megalo-blastic anemia when in deficiency. So, this patient has to be supplemented with folic acid also.

SHORT ESSAYS

1. Explain the fate of hemoglobin. What is jaundice? Classify with examples. (3+2 marks)

Fate of Hemoglobin

- RBC has a lifespan of 120 days after which it undergoes lysis in the spleen.
- Hemoglobin is released into plasma and broken down into heme and globin by the reticuloendothelial cells.
- Globin is recycled for *de novo* synthesis of hemoglobin.
- Heme is broken down into iron and porphyrin.
- Iron is taken up for formation ferritin and hemosiderin and stored. It is reused for hemoglobin synthesis.
- The porphyrin is degraded into unconjugated bilirubin and then converted into biliverdin.
- The bilirubin thus formed is transported in blood in association with albumin.
- After circulation in blood for a few hours, the unconjugated bilirubin is taken up by hepatocytes and it undergoes a process called conjugation in the liver.
- Now conjugated bilirubin is water-soluble and is excreted in the bile and later into feces as stercobilinogen.

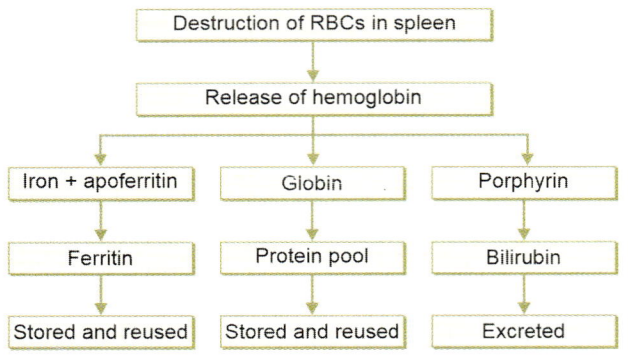

Fig. 2.7

Jaundice

- It is a clinical condition characterized by increased bilirubin in blood (hyperbilirubinemia)—unconjugated or conjugated or both.

- It usually manifests when total bilirubin exceeds 2 mg/dl as icterus (yellowish discoloration of sclera) and yellowish discoloration of skin. Other manifestations are yellowish discoloration of urine, generalised pruritus and pale colour of feces (in conjugated bilirubinemia).

Classification of Jaundice

Based on the Component of Bilirubin Elevated

1. Unconjugated hyperbilirubinemia
2. Conjugated hyperbilirubinemia

Based on the Pathology

1. Prehepatic jaundice
   - The cause is increased breakdown of heme and the liver function is normal.
   - Examples are hemolytic anemia, malaria, thalassemia, autoimmune conditions.
2. Hepatic jaundice
   - Due to damage to the hepatocytes, the liver cells are not able to conjugate bilirubin
   - Examples are infectious hepatitis, alcoholic hepatitis, exposure to toxic substance, cirrhosis of liver.
3. Posthepatic jaundice
   - Due to obstruction of outflow of bile due to stones or fibrosis of the bile duct.
   - As a result, there is no disturbance in conjugation and the conjugated bilirubin leaks into the circulation as it is diluted.
   - Examples are gall stones, primary biliary cirrhosis, carcinoma of biliary system or pancreas.

2. A child aged 5 years comes with a history of severe anemia. He was later diagnosed to be suffering from sickle cell anemia.
   - **A. What is the pathophysiology of sickle cell anemia?** (2 marks)
   - **B. What are the different types of Hb? (2 marks)**
   - **C. Why is HbF raised in such patients? (1 mark)**

A. Pathophysiology of Sickle Cell Anemia

- In sickle cell anemia, the amino acid valine is substituted for glutamic acid at one point in each of the two beta chains.
- This forms the hemoglobin S.

- When this type of hemoglobin is exposed to low oxygen, it forms elongated crystals inside the red blood cells that are sometimes 15 micrometers in length.
- This causes decreased flexibility of the RBCs to course through arterioles.
- As a result, they result in breakage of RBCs and thus cause hemolysis and anemia.
- This condition is called sickle cell anemia.

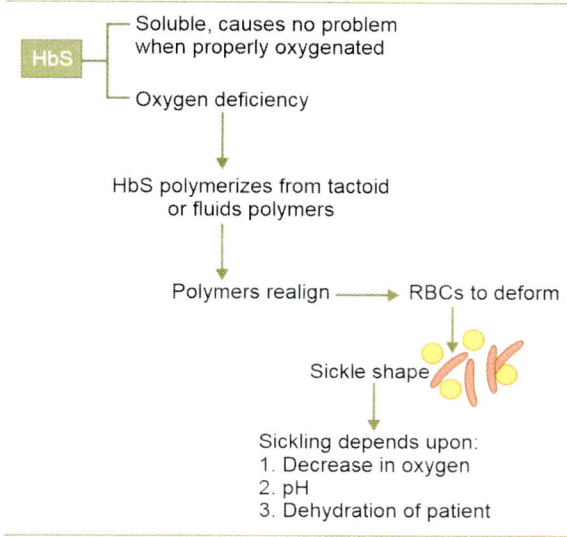

Fig. 2.8

B. Different Types of Hemoglobin

- Each heme molecule binds with a globin molecule to form a hemoglobin chain.
- 4 such chains are bound loosely to form a hemoglobin molecule.

- There are four types of globin chains—alpha, beta, gamma and delta.
- Depending on that variations in hemoglobin have been described.

Hemoglobin A	2 alpha chains and 2 beta chains
Hemoglobin A2	2 alpha chains and 2 delta chains
Hemoglobin F	2 alpha chains and 2 gamma chains
Hemoglobin S	2 normal alpha chains and 2 beta chains with valine replacing glutamic acid

- Others are hemoglobin C (lysine substitutes glutamic acid in beta chain 6th amino acid), hemoglobin M and hemoglobin E (lysine substitutes glutamic acid in beta chain 26th amino acid).
- Based on hemoglobin derivatives:
  - *Oxyhemoglobin:* Bound to oxygen
  - *Carboxyhemoglobin:* Bound to carbon monoxide
  - *Methemoglobin:* Ferric state of iron atom in hemoglobin
  - *Sulfhemoglobin:* Combination of hemoglobin to hydrogen sulfide

C. Hemoglobin F in Sickle Cell

- Hemoglobin F is fetal hemoglobin and has high affinity to oxygen
- At birth, 80% of Hb is HbF. During the first 6 months of life, it decreases to about 5% of total.
- HbF level may remain elevated in children with anemia and beta thalassemia, as a compensatory measure.

2.6 DESCRIBE WBC FORMATION (GRANULOPOIESIS) AND ITS REGULATION

SHORT ESSAYS

1. What are the functions of neutrophils? Explain the steps of phagocytosis.

Functions of Neutrophils

1. Neutrophils play an important role in the defense mechanism.
2. They are the first line of defense against the invading microorganisms.

Steps of Phagocytosis (Fig. 2.9)

- It is the process by which substances larger than macromolecules are engulfed into the cells.
- *Phago* = eat, *cyte* = cell.
- Cells capable of phagocytosis: Macrophages, neutrophils and monocytes.
- The cell sends cytoplasmic extensions around the bacteria or foreign body—pseudopodia.
- The edges of the pseudopodia surround the bacteria.
- The edges evaginate around the bacteria and engulf it.
- The bacteria are now converted into an endosome.
- The lysosome fuses with the endosome to form the endolysosome.
- It releases hydrolytic enzymes to digest the particles.

2. Classify WBC. Explain leucocytosis and leucopenia with 4 examples each

WBC Classification

Based on presence of granules in the cytoplasm, WBCs are classified as granulocytes and agranulocytes (Fig. 2.10).

1. **Granulocytes**
   - These cells have a granular cytoplasm.
   - They are further divided based on staining properties
     - Neutrophils (take up both acidic and basic stains)
     - Eosinophils (the granules take up acidic stain)
     - Basophils (the granules take up basic stain)

2. **Agranulocytes**
   - These cells do not have granules in the cytoplasm
   - They are of two types:
     i. *Monocytes:* The nucleus is one side and cytoplasm occupies majority of the cell
     ii. *Lymphocytes:* The nucleus is huge and occupies most of the cytoplasm.

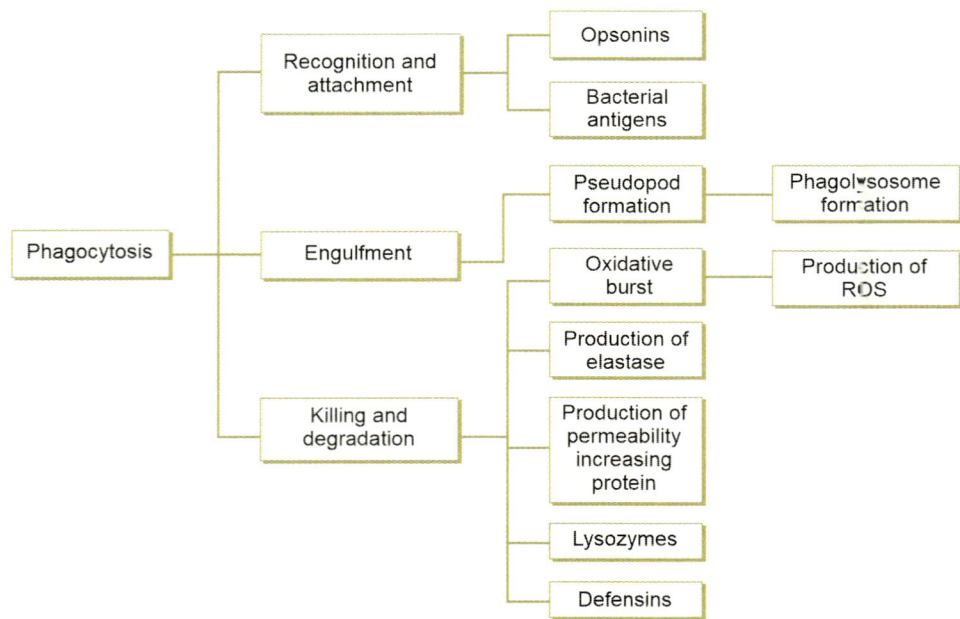

Fig. 2.9

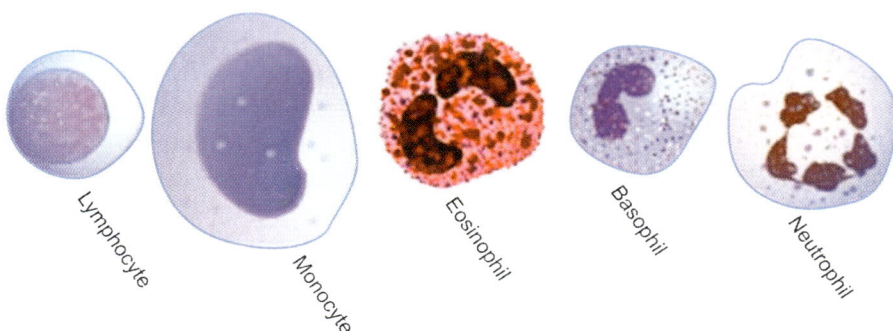

Fig. 2.10

Leukocytosis	Leukopenia
• Increased in quantity of all types of leukocytes (total leukocyte count) in blood more than 11,000/mm³	• Decreased quantity of all types of leukocytes (total leukocyte count) in blood less than 4000/mm³
• Causes for leukocytosis	• Causes for leukopenia
1. Bacterial infections	1. Pernicious anemia
2. Tuberculosis	2. Bone marrow aplasia
3. Leukemia	3. Dengue
4. Allergy	4. Malignant infiltration of bone marrow
	5. Viral infections

SHORT ANSWERS

1. Describe the contents and functions of eosinophil granules.

Eosinophilic Granules

- Eosinophils are a type of white blood cells which defend against parasites, foreign bodies and allergens.
- Eosinophils are differentiated on microscopy by the presence of crystalline granules in the cytoplasm.
- These granules are sources of diverse cationic proteins.

Contents and Functions

Eosinophil peroxidase	Against helminths, bacteria, and tumor cells
Major basic protein	It is highly effective against helminths. It destroys them by causing ballooning and detachment of tegmental sheath
Eosinophil cationic protein	It is a strong neurotoxin and 10 times more potent than MBP It kills by complete lysis of helminths
Eosinophil derived neurotoxin	It is directed against myelin sheath
Interleukins 4 and 5	They are inflammatory cytokines

2. Explain reticuloendothelial system.

Reticuloendothelial System

- They form a system of cells and tissue concerned with providing defence to the body. They mainly consist of primitive phagocyte cells.
- The reticular cells found in:
  - Endothelium of blood vessels and lymphatics
  - Connective tissue of spleen, liver, lungs, lymph nodes and bone marrow

Classification

1. **Fixed reticuloendothelial cells or tissue macrophages**
   - Also called fixed histiocytes as they are seen in particular tissues.
   - Examples of such locations are:
     - Connective tissue like pleura, omentum, mesentery
     - Reticulum of spleen, bone marrow and lymph node
     - Lungs
     - Blood sinusoids in liver—Kupffer cells
     - CNS: Meningiocytes in meninges and microglia

2. **Wandering reticuloendothelial cells**
   - *Free histiocytes of blood:* Neutrophils, monocytes
   - *Free histiocytes of tissue:* Fixed histiocytes become wandering during an emergency

Functions

1. Phagocytic function
2. Secretion of bactericidal agent
3. Secretion of interleukins
4. Secretion of growth factor

2.7 DESCRIBE THE FORMATION OF PLATELETS, FUNCTIONS AND VARIATIONS

SHORT ESSAYS

1. Explain the properties and functions of Platelets.

Properties

1. **Adhesiveness**
   - It is the property by which platelets stick to a rough surface.
   - When endothelium is damaged, the collagen is exposed, the platelets get adhered to the collagen and get activated.
   - These activated platelets secrete serotonin and thromboxane A_2, which activate more and more platelets.

2. **Aggregation**
   - When platelets are activated, they form long filamentous pseudopodia called filopodia which help them to form clumps of aggregations.
   - They thus form a plug which arrests bleeding temporarily.

3. **Agglutination**
   - Agglutination is formation of clumps ⸱⸱
   - It is caused by platelet agglutinins and platelet activating factor.

Functions

1. Formation of intrinsic prothrombin activator helps in initiating the coagulation cascade.
2. The cytoskeletal proteins help in contraction of the platelets and thus help in clot retraction.
3. The activated platelets secrete serotonin which causes vasoconstriction and decreases blood flow following an injury.
4. Also, due to their adhesiveness, the platelets seal the damage in the blood vessels.
5. They form a temporary platelet plug prior to formation of a coagulum and arrest bleeding.
6. Platelet derived growth factor helps in repair of damaged blood vessels.
7. Platelets have a property of agglutination and thus engulf foreign bodies and destroy them.

2. Explain the types of granules present in platelets and mention its functions.

- Platelets are anucleate discoid cells mainly involved in hemostasis.
- The cytoplasm of platelets contains various organelles, microtubules, filaments and granules.
- The granules present in platelets are of two types:
  1. Alpha granules
  2. Dense granules.

Alpha Granules

- These are unique for platelets
- Most abundant type of granules, 50–80 per cell
- The main content of these granules is proteins associated with various functions.

Hemostasis	von Willebrand factor, factor V
Membrane associated proteins	αIIβ3, p-selectin
Inflammatory	CXCL1, interleukin-8
Wound healing	Vascular endothelial growth factor, fibroblast growth factor

Dense Granules

- Second most abundant to alpha granules, 3–8 per cell.
- They are so-called as they are dense in appearance on electron microscopy.

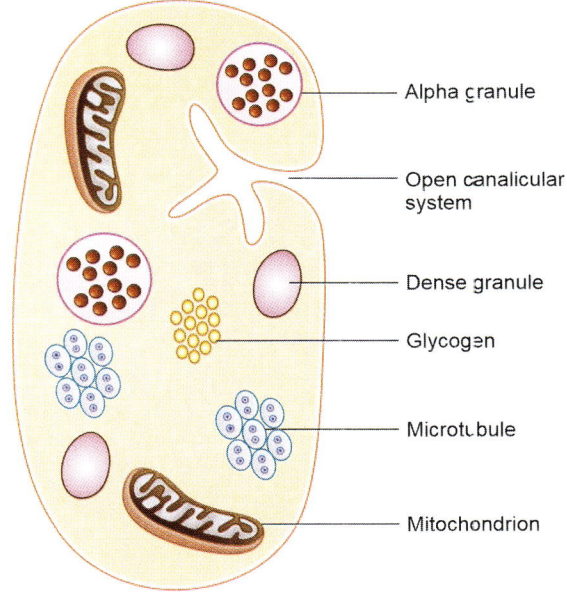

Fig. 2.11

- They are also unique to platelets and called lysosome related organelles (LRO).
- They mainly contain bioactive amines like histamine, serotonin.
- They also contain adenine nucleotides, pyrophosphates and polyphosphates.
- They are rich in calcium.

Other Granules

- Besides alpha and dense granules, there are other granules.
- They contain 1–3 lysosomes per cell and also peroxisomes.
- There are T granules which express toll-like receptors on surface.

2.8 DESCRIBE THE PHYSIOLOGICAL BASIS OF HEMOSTASIS AND ANTICOAGULANTS. DESCRIBE BLEEDING AND CLOTTING DISORDERS (HEMOPHILIA, PURPURA)

LONG ESSAYS

1. A 50 years old chronic alcoholic comes to medicine OPD with history of excessive bleeding following a fall. What are the clotting factors synthesised in the liver? Explain the steps of hemostasis. Explain any 4 tests to diagnose bleeding and clotting disorders.

(3 + 4 + 3 marks)

Clotting Factors Synthesized in Liver

- Liver is a major source of clotting factors.
- The hepatocytes synthesize factors fibrinogen, prothrombin, V, VII, IX, X, XI, XII, protein C, protein S.
- The endothelium of the sinusoids synthesizes von Willebrand factor, factor VIII.
- Vitamin K is stored in liver.

Steps of Hemostasis

- Factors involved in blood clotting
  - Substances necessary for clotting are called clotting factors.
    Factor I: Fibrinogen
    Factor II: Prothrombin
    Factor III: Thromboplastin (tissue factor)
    Factor IV: Calcium
    Factor V: Labile factor (proaccelerin or accelerator globulin)
    Factor VI: Presence has not been proved
    Factor VII: Stable factor
    Factor VIII: Antihemophilic factor (antihemophilic globulin)
    Factor IX: Christmas factor
    Factor X: Stuart-Prower factor
    Factor XI: Plasma thromboplastin antecedent
    Factor XII: Hageman factor (contact factor)
    Factor XIII: Fibrin-stabilizing factor (fibrinase).
- Stages of blood coagulation

Stage 1: Formation of Prothrombin Activator

- Formation of prothrombin activator is the first step of hemostasis. It converts prothrombin into thrombin.
- Formation of prothrombin activator occurs through two pathways:

I. *Intrinsic pathway*

- In this pathway, platelets initiate the formation of prothrombin activator.
- Sequence of events:

> When a blood vessel ruptures during an injury endothelium is damaged and underlying collagen gets exposed
> ↓
> Factor XII (Hageman factor) meets exposed collagen, it is converted into activated factor XII in the presence of kallikrein and high molecular weight (HMW) kinogen
> ↓
> The activated factor XII activates factor XI to activated factor XI in the presence of HMW kinogen.
> ↓
> Activated factor XI activates factor IX in the presence of factor IV (calcium).
> ↓
> Activated factor IX activates factor X in the presence of factor VIII and calcium.
> ↓
> When platelet meets collagen of damaged blood vessel, it gets activated and releases phospholipids.
> ↓
> Activated factor X reacts with platelet phospholipid and factor V to form prothrombin activator. This needs the presence of calcium ions.
> ↓
> Factor V is also activated by positive feedback effect of thrombin
> ↓
> Prothrombin activator converts prothrombin to thrombin. Thrombin converts fibrinogen to fibrin which bind together along with calcium ions to forma fibrin clot.

II. *Extrinsic pathway*

- Formation of prothrombin activator is initiated by tissue thromboplastin.
- Sequence of events

> When tissues that are damaged during injury release tissue thromboplastin (factor III).
> ↓
> Actiavtion of factor X in presence of factor VII by the glycoprotein and phospholipid components of thromboplastin
> ↓
> Reaction between activated factor X + factor V + phospholipid component of tissue thromboplastin (in presence of calcium) to form prothrombin activator.

Stage 2: Conversion of Prothrombin into Thrombin

- Prothrombin activator that is formed in intrinsic and extrinsic pathways converts prothrombin into thrombin in the presence of calcium (factor IV).
- Formation of thrombin is a positive feedback mechanism. It initiates more and more conversion of prothrombin to thrombin.
- The initially formed thrombin activates Factor V.
- Factor V in turn accelerates formation of prothrombin activator by both intrinsic and extrinsic pathways.

Stage 3: Conversion of Fibrinogen into Fibrin

- The final stage of blood clotting involves the conversion of fibrinogen into fibrin by thrombin.

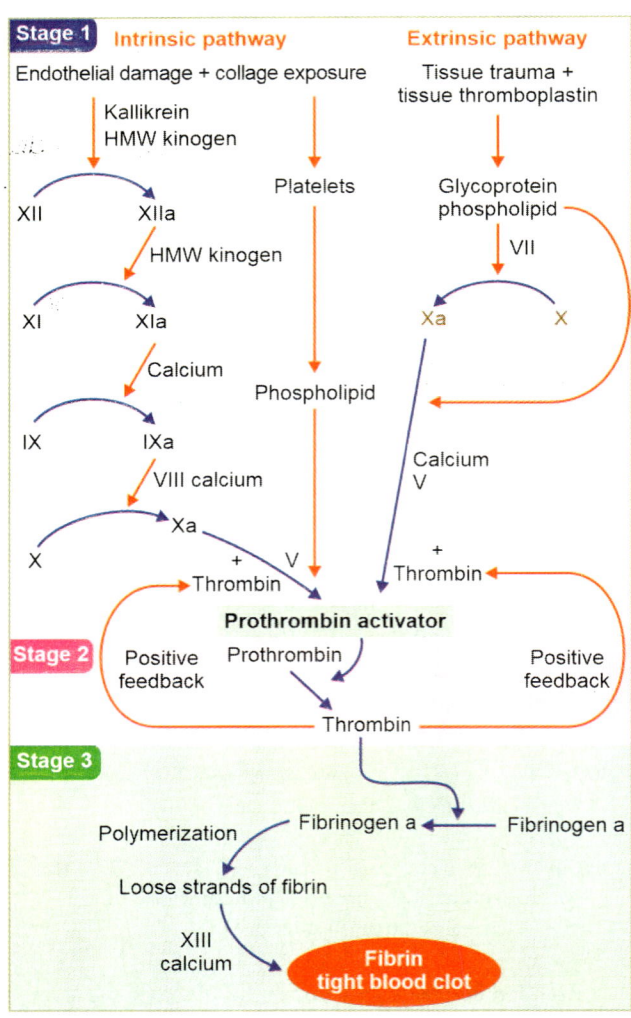

Fig. 2.12

- Sequence of events
  - Thrombin activates fibrinogen by removing 2 pairs of polypeptides from each fibrinogen molecule. The activated fibrinogen is also called fibrin monomer.
  - These monomers polymerize with each other to form loosely arranged strands of fibrin.
  - Later these loose strands are modified into dense and tight fibrin threads by fibrin-stabilizing factor (factor XIII) in the presence of calcium ions. All the tight fibrin threads are aggregated to form a meshwork of stable clot.

Tests to Diagnose Bleeding and Clotting Disorders

- Mainly used to diagnose bleeding and clotting disorders and for understanding the response to therapy.

1. **Bleeding time**
   - It is the time from the time of cut or injury to the skin and cessation of bleeding.
   - It is performed clinically by making a nick with the tip of a needle and measuring the time till when the bleeding continues.
   - Normal value: 3–6 minutes
   - It is a measure of platelet function and bleeding time is increased in von Willebrand's disease, thrombocytopenia, thrombasthenia.

2. **Clotting time**
   - It is the time measured from oozing of blood following a cut or injury till clot formation.
   - It is performed clinically by making a nick with the tip of a needle and collecting blood in a capillary tube. The capillary tube is broken from one end every 10 seconds till clot formation is seen.
   - It is prolonged in hemophilia, vitamin K deficiency (liver cirrhosis).

3. **Prothrombin time, international normalized ratio (INR)**
   - It is time taken for blood to clot after addition of tissue thromboplastin to it.
   - It is to measure the total prothrombin in blood.
   - The blood is collected from the patient and oxalate is added. It chelates the calcium and thus prevents clotting.

- Immediately, large quantities of thromboplastin and calcium are added. The calcium nullifies the effect of oxalate and clotting mechanism take place by extrinsic pathway.
- Normal value is 9 seconds.
- It is increased in deficiency of I, V, VII and X. It is normal in hemophilia.
- INR (international normalized ratio): It is the rating of the patient's PT with an average.

Normal people	INR is 1
On anticoagulant therapy and atrial fibrillation	INR should be between 2 and 3
Patients with valvular heart disease	INR should be between 3 and 4

4. aPTT or activated partial thromboplastin time
- Phospholipid long with calcium, kaolin is added to blood. Kaolin is a surface activator and acts as a platelet substitute.
- Normal duration is 30–45 seconds.
- It is mainly used for monitoring patients on anticoagulants.

2. A young boy aged 10 years came with history of swelling of his knee joint. He also complains of excessive bleeding during an injury. His doctor suspects it to be hemophilia.

A. What is the pathophysiology of haemophilia? What are its types?

B. Explain intrinsic mechanism of coagulation.

A. Pathophysiology of Haemophilia (Fig. 2.13)
- It is a genetically inherited disorder of the clotting system due to absence or deficiency of clotting factor VIII (in 85% of patients), or factor IX or factor XI.
- As a result, they are not able to form prothrombin activator through the intrinsic pathway.
- These patients have propensity to spontaneously bleed and thus present with hemarthrosis (bleeding into joints), hematuria and increased period of bleeding following trivial trauma.

Types of Haemophilia
1. Classical hemophilia or hemophilia A—due to deficiency of factor VIII
2. Hemophilia B or Christmas disease—due to deficiency of factor IX
3. Hemophilia C—due to deficiency of factor XI

B. Intrinsic Pathway of Coagulation (Fig. 2.14)
- Blood clotting involves three main steps: Formation of prothrombin activator, conversion of prothrombin to thrombin and conversion of fibrinogen to fibrin.
- Prothrombin activator is needed for conversion of prothrombin to thrombin.
- It occurs through two ways——intrinsic pathway and extrinsic pathway.
- Intrinsic pathway is initiated by platelets.

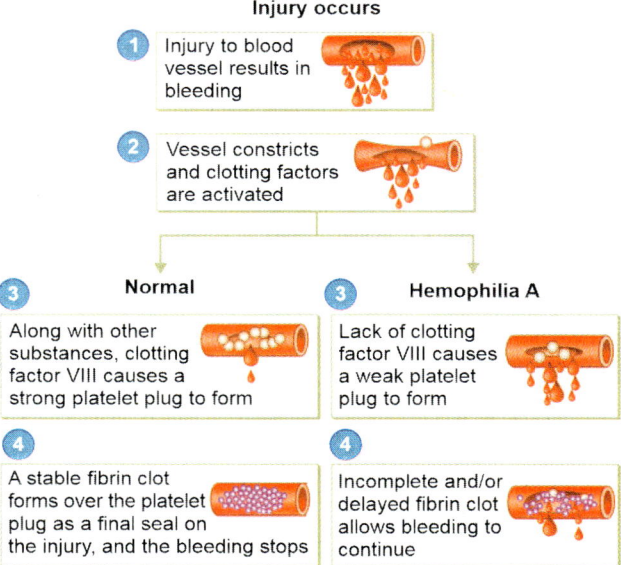

Injury occurs

1. Injury to blood vessel results in bleeding

2. Vessel constricts and clotting factors are activated

Normal

3. Along with other substances, clotting factor VIII causes a strong platelet plug to form

4. A stable fibrin clot forms over the platelet plug as a final seal on the injury, and the bleeding stops

Hemophilia A

3. Lack of clotting factor VIII causes a weak platelet plug to form

4. Incomplete and/or delayed fibrin clot allows bleeding to continue

Fig. 2.13

When a blood vessel ruptures following trauma, its endothelium is disrupted and underlying collagen gets exposed
↓
Factor XII (Hageman factor) meets exposed collagen, it is converted into activated factor XII in the presence of kallikrein and high molecular weight (HMW) kinogen
↓
The activated factor XII activates factor XI to activated factor XI in the presence of HMW kinogen.
↓
Activated factor XI activates factor IX in the presence of factor IV (calcium).
↓
Activated factor IX activates factor X in the presence of factor VIII and calcium.
↓
When platelet meets collagen of damaged blood vessel, it gets activated and releases phospholipids.
↓
Activated factor X reacts with platelet phospholipid and factor V to form prothrombin activator. This needs the presence of calcium ions.
↓
Factor V is also activated by positive feedback effect of thrombin
↓
Prothrombin activator converts prothrombin to thrombin.
↓
Thrombin converts fibrinogen to fibrin which bind together along with calcium ions to form a fibrin clot.

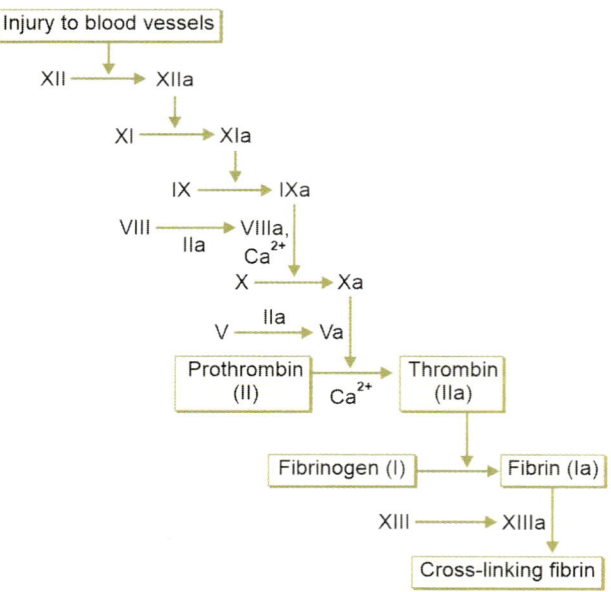

Fig. 2.14

SHORT ESSAYS

1. Explain anticlotting mechanisms. Why is aspirin given as a prophylactic drug to prevent cardiovascular incidents?

A. Prevention of Blood Clotting in Normal Vascular System

1. **Endothelial surface factor**
   - Endothelial cell surface is smooth. It presents contact activation of the intrinsic clotting pathway.
   - Glycocalyx, a mucopolysaccharide is present as a coating on the endothelial cell surface. It repels platelets and others clotting factors.
   - Thrombomodulin, a protein bound to the endothelium, binds to the thrombin, and forms a complex. Thus, it reduces the amount of thrombin available for clotting. Also, the complex activates protein C which further inactivates factor V and factor VIII.
   - All the above three methods fail when there is damage to the endothelium.

2. **Physical factors**
   - It includes a continuous blood flow through the vascular channels which prevents clotting.

3. **Antithrombin action of fibrin and antithrombin**
   - When a clot forms from fibrin, 80–90% of thrombin gets adhered to the clot thereby decreasing the availability of thrombin. Thus, excessive clot formation elsewhere in the body is prevented.
   - The left-out thrombin combines with antithrombin III which blocks action of thrombin

4. **Heparin**
   - Produced in very low concentration by the liver in physiological conditions
   - When heparin combines with antithrombin III, the effect of the latter to block the action of thrombin is increased by 100 folds.
   - It is also produced by pericapillary basophilic mast cells. They are present in lungs and liver.
   - This feature of heparin makes its usefulness as a therapeutic agent in clotting disorders.

B. Aspirin in Clotting Disorder

- Aggregation of platelets to form a platelet plug forms.
- Aspirin is a salicylate which is a non-steroidal anti-inflammatory drug.

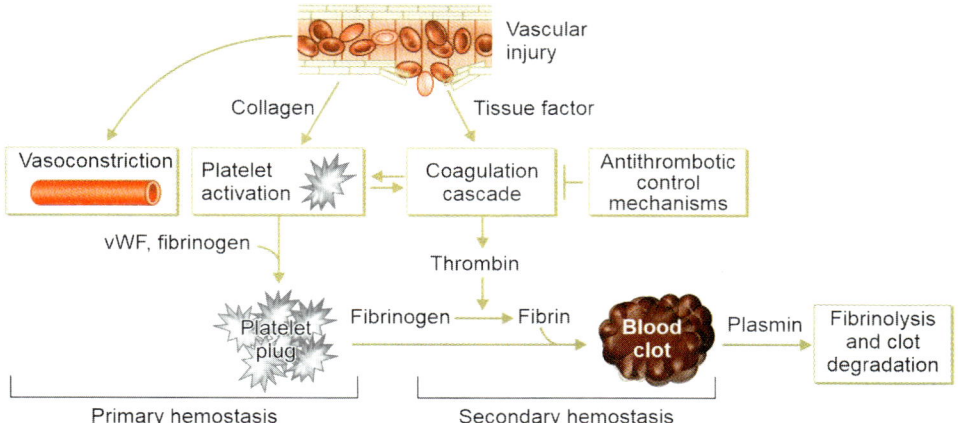

Fig. 2.15

- Thromboxane is an imported chemical responsible for platelet aggregation and clot formation.
- Aspirin inhibits thromboxane and thus clot formation. Thus, it is used in ischemic heart disease to reduce clot formation.

2. Explain the steps in hemostasis. What is the role of Vit K in hemostasis?   (3 + 2 marks)

Steps in Hemostasis (Fig. 2.15)

1. **Vasoconstriction**
   - It is a local phenomenon and occurs immediately after injury to blood vessel.
   - When there is breach in the basement membrane, the collagen is exposed.
   - Platelets attach to the exposed collagen and get activated. These activated platelets secrete various chemokines like serotonin and thromboxane A_2 which cause vasoconstriction.
   - This limits blood loss and hence is a protective response.

2. **Platelet plug formation**
   - The activated platelets secrete thromboxane A2 and ADP.
   - These recruit more platelets and activate them.
   - These sticky platelets form a temporary plug and arrest bleeding.

3. **Coagulation of blood**
   - Blood clotting involves three main steps: Formation of prothrombin activator, conversion of prothrombin to thrombin and conversion of fibrinogen to fibrin.

- Prothrombin activator is needed for conversion of prothrombin to thrombin.
- It occurs through two ways—intrinsic pathway and extrinsic pathway.
- Intrinsic pathway is initiated by platelets.

Role of Vitamin K in Blood Clotting

- It is essential for formation of several clotting factors like II, VII, IX and X.
- Also helps in production of fibrinogen and prothrombin.
- It is also essential for maturation of these factors. Coagulation factors are produced in their naive forms. Post-translational modification of these factors requires gamma carboxylation of the glutamic acid residues.
- Thus, deficiency of vitamin K as in liver failure causes spontaneous bleeding.

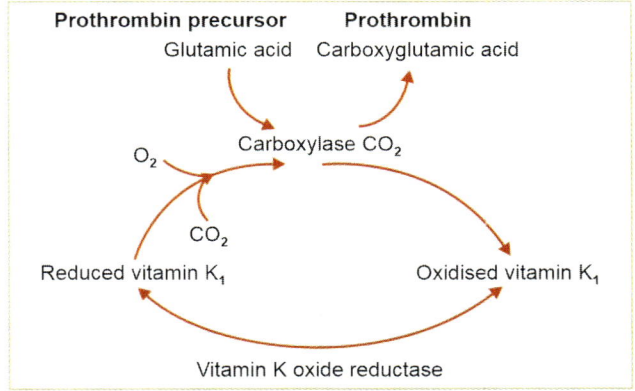

Fig. 2.16a

3. Give an account of the process of blood coagulation. Name any two anticoagulants and describe their mode of action.

Process of Blood Coagulation

- Coagulation is defined as the process in which blood loses its fluidity and becomes a gel-like mass within a few minutes of being shed out or collected in a container.
- Factors involved in blood clotting
  - Substances necessary for clotting are called clotting factors.
  - Thirteen clotting factors are identified:
    1. Factor I: Fibrinogen
    2. Factor II: Prothrombin
    3. Factor III: Thromboplastin (tissue factor)
    4. Factor IV: Calcium
    5. Factor V: Labile factor (proaccelerin or accelerator globulin)
    6. Factor VI: Presence has not been proved
    7. Factor VII: Stable factor
    8. Factor VIII: Antihemophilic factor (anti-hemophilic globulin)
    9. Factor IX: Christmas factor
    10. Factor X: Stuart-Prower factor
    11. Factor XI: Plasma thromboplastin antecedent
    12. Factor XII: Hageman factor (contact factor)
    13. Factor XIII: Fibrin-stabilizing factor (fibrinase).
- Stages of blood coagulation (Fig. 2.16b)
  Stage 1: Formation of prothrombin activator
  Stage 2: Conversion of prothrombin into thrombin
  Stage 3: Conversion of fibrinogen into fibrin

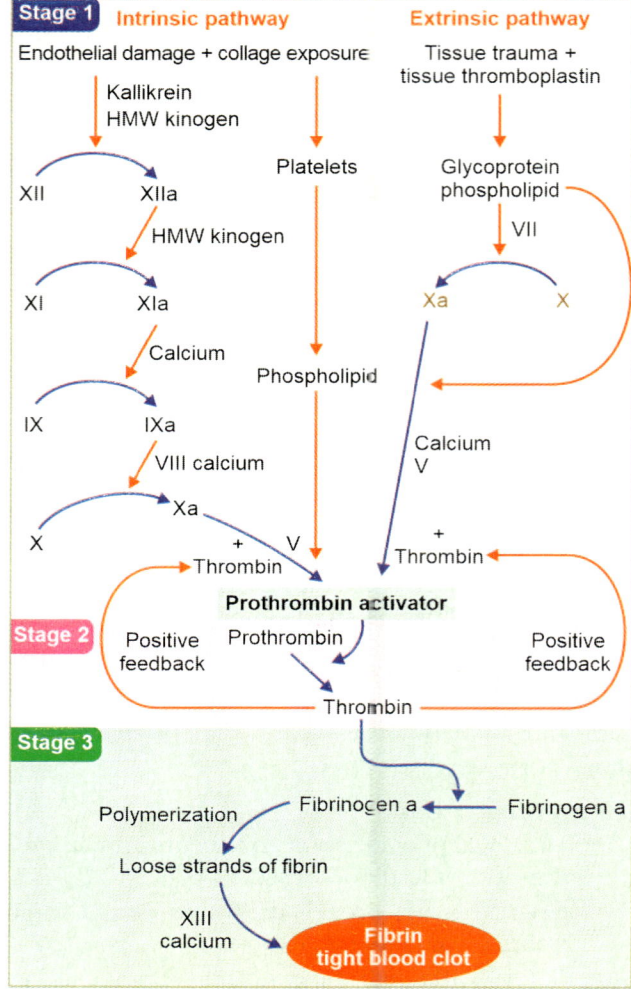

Fig. 2.16b

Anticoagulants

- Substances which prevent coagulation of blood are called anticoagulants.
- Anticoagulants can be used to prevent blood clotting both *in vivo* and *in vitro*. *In vitro:* use is for diagnostic purposes and *in vivo:* for therapeutic purposes.

1. **Heparin**
   - Heparin is a naturally occurring anticoagulant in the body.
   - It is produced by wandering mast cells present immediately outside the capillaries in many tissues or organs that contain more connective tissue; mostly in lungs and liver.
   - Basophils also secrete heparin.

Mechanism of action of heparin (Fig. 2.17)
- Prevents blood clotting by blocking the activity of antithrombin. It directly suppresses the activity of thrombin
- Combines with antithrombin III (a protease inhibitor presents in circulation) and thrombin to form a complex. Hence, thrombin becomes inactive
- Inactivates the active form of other clotting factors like IX, X, XI and XII

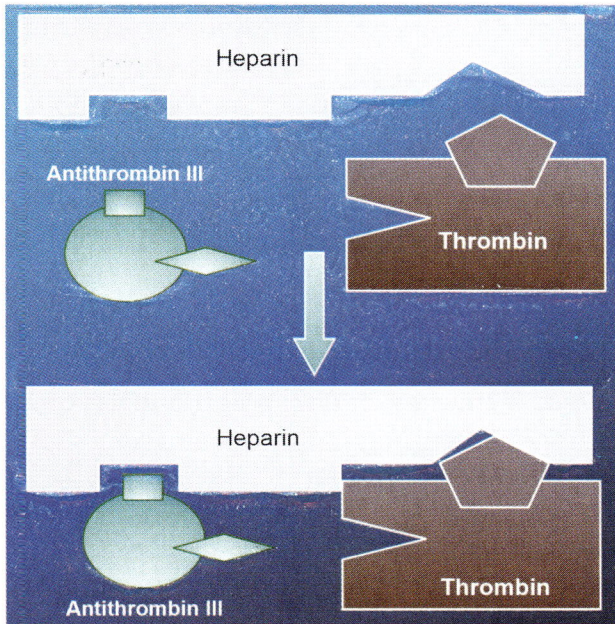

Fig. 2.17

2. **Coumarin derivatives:** Warfarin and dicoumarol are the derivatives of coumarin.

Mechanism of action
- Prevent blood clotting by inhibiting the action of vitamin K.
- Vitamin K is essential for the formation and activation of various clotting factors, namely II, VII, IX and X.

4. Explain the following:
A. Purpura
B. Haemophilia
C. Thrombasthenia

A. Purpura
- These are minute bleeding spots under the dermis due to decreased ability of the platelets to control bleeding.
- These lesions appear as purple spots under the skin in various parts of the body
- These patients have a prolonged bleeding time.
- They usually manifest when platelet count is decreased than $50,000/mm^3$
- When there are larger bleeding spots, it is called ecchymosis.

Causes
- **Thrombocytopenia:** Decreased platelets. It can be due to increased destruction or decreased production.
- **Idiopathic thrombocytopenic purpura:** It is a specific disease characterised by autoimmune mediated destruction of platelets leading to increased bleeding tendency.
- **Thrombasthenic purpura:** There is structural and functional abnormality of platelets.

Treatment
Replenish with platelets by blood transfusion.

B. Hemophilia
Causes
- It is a genetically inherited disorder of the clotting system due to absence or deficiency of clotting factor VIII (in 85% of patients), or factor IX or factor XI.
- As a result, they are not able to form prothrombin activator through the intrinsic pathway.

Classification
1. Classical haemophilia or haemophilia A—due to deficiency of factor VIII
2. Hemophilia B or Christmas disease—due to deficiency of factor IX
3. Hemophilia C—due to deficiency of factor XI

Symptoms
- These patients have propensity to spontaneously bleed and thus present with hemarthrosis (bleeding into joints), haematuria and increased period of bleeding following trivial trauma.
- Minor surgical procedures like tooth extraction also can lead to severe hemorrhage.

Laboratory Findings
- Increased clotting time
- Decreased or absent respective clotting factor

Treatment
Fresh frozen plasma to replace the clotting factors.

C. Thrombasthenia
It literally means weak platelets.

Causes

- The platelets are structurally and functionally abnormal, but the count is normal.
- Glanzmann's thrombabasthenia is a rare inherited disorder characterised by decreased quality and quantity of the glycoprotein IIb/IIIA.
- It is required to attach von Willebrand factor to the damaged endothelium and to the platelets. Also, it is required for integration of fibronectin, fibrinogen to form a complex.
- As a result, formation of platelet plug is almost impossible.

Symptoms

- There are episodes of bleeding following minor injuries and procedures.
- Severe menorrhagia
- Severe hemorrhage following parturition

Laboratory Investigations

- Prolonged bleeding time, clotting time
- Failure of the platelets to aggregate in presence of L-epinephrine, ADP, collagen and arachidonic acid

Treatment

Factor VIIa is helpful. It is given through fresh frozen plamsa infusion.

5. What is the role of streptokinase given in the treatment of acute myocardial infraction.

(5 marks)

- Acute myocardial infarction results due to ischemia of a portion of the cardiac muscle due to sudden decrease in blood supply as a result of a thrombotic occlusion of the coronary arteries.
- Streptokinase is an enzyme procured from bacteria (beta hemolytic streptococcus) which helps in clot lysis.
- It can be administered by intravenous route or by intracoronary administration to lyse the clot.
- Streptokinase combines with plasminogen to activate it to plasmin (Fig. 2.18).
- Plasmin breaks the fibrin into degradation products and thus the coronary circulation is re-established.
- The action is very rapid as the half-life is 30–60 minutes.
- Other drugs with similar action are urokinase, tissue plasminogen activator, staphylokinase and desmoteplase.

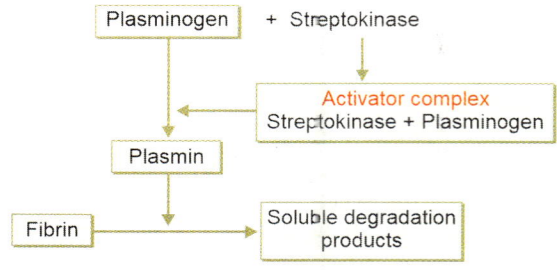

Fig. 2.18a

SHORT ANSWERS

1. What is the role of von Willebrand's factor in blood clotting?

von Willebrand's Factor

- It is a factor involved in clotting secreted by damaged endothelium of blood vessels.
- It enhances adhesion of platelets to collagen which is exposed due to injury.
- Following this, platelets get activated and form platelet plugs.
- Also, vasoconstriction is induced by secretion of serotonin and blood clotting is initiated by activation of prothrombin.
- von Willebrand factor also stabilizes factor VIII in plasma by preventing its degradation by activated protein C.

von Willebrand's Disease

- It is a bleeding disorder characterized by episodes of bleeding following to minute trauma.
- It is due to decreased platelet adhesion and decreased activation of factor VIII.

2. Describe the mechanism of the anticoagulants, heparin and warfarin.

Anticoagulants

- Chemicals which prevent coagulation of blood are called anticoagulants
- Anticoagulants used to prevent blood clotting both *in vivo* and *in vitro*.

1. **Heparin**
   - Heparin is a naturally produced anticoagulant in the body.
   - It is produced by mast cells which are the wandering cells present immediately outside the capillaries in many tissues or organs that contain more connective tissue, mostly in liver and lungs.
   - Basophils also secrete heparin.

Mechanism of action of heparin
- Prevents blood clotting by blocking the activity of antithrombin. It directly suppresses the activity of thrombin

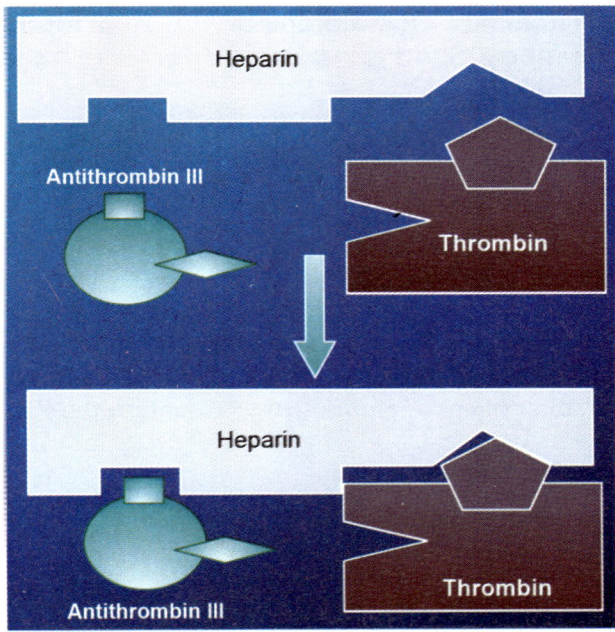

Fig. 2.18b

- Combines with antithrombin III and thrombin to form a complex. Hence, thrombin becomes inactive
- Inactivates the active form of other clotting factors like IX, X, XI and XII

2. **Coumarin derivatives:** Warfarin and dicoumarol are the derivatives of coumarin.

Mechanism of action
- Prevent blood clotting by inhibiting the action of vitamin K.
- Vitamin K is essential for the formation and activation of clotting factors like II, VII, IX and X.

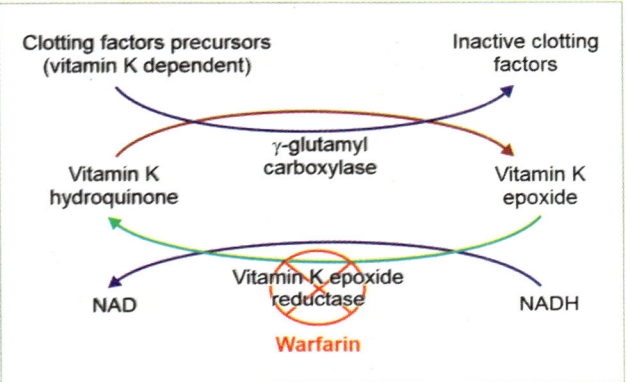

Fig. 2.19

2.9 DESCRIBE DIFFERENT BLOOD GROUPS AND DISCUSS THE CLINICAL IMPORTANCE OF BLOOD GROUPING, BLOOD BANKING AND TRANSFUSION

SHORT ESSAYS

1. A Rh–ve female marries a Rh +ve male. Her 1st pregnancy was uneventful. During her 2nd pregnancy she had stillbirth. The fetus was swollen, abdomen bloated and tender.
   A. What is this clinical entity called? (1 mark)
   B. Why does it occur? (2 marks)
   C. What are the different blood group antigens and antibodies in ABO and Rh system?

A.

- This clinical condition is called erythroblastosis fetalis or hemolytic disease of the newborn—a condition in which maternal specific antibodies are targetted against Rh antigen of the fetus leading to destruction of fetal RBCs and death.

B. Cause for Erythroblastosis Fetalis

- It occurs when a Rh negative mother carries a Rh positive fetus (Rh factor is a dominant trait and is expressed when inherited from father).
- During the first pregnancy, the red blood cells of the Rh positive fetus do not enter the maternal blood and therefore do not elicit an immune response. During parturition and during separation of placenta, the fetal RBCs enter maternal blood and the mother produces antibodies within one month of delivery.
- When the mother conceives again with a Rh positive baby (baby has Rh antigen on RBCs), the antibodies can now freely enter fetal circulation through placental vessels.
- These antibodies lead to destruction of red blood cells. As a result, the child develops severe anemia and jaundice (due to increased bilirubin from hemolysis) and usually culminates in death.

C. Types of Blood Group

Blood group	Antigen on RBC	Antibody in serum
A positive	A, Rh	Anti-B
A negative	A	Anti-Rh, anti-B
B positive	B, Rh	Anti-A
B negative	B	Anti-A, anti-Rh
O positive	Rh	Anti-A, anti-B
O negative	–	Anti-A, anti-B, anti-Rh
AB positive	A, B, Rh	–
AB negative	A, B	Anti-Rh

2. Explain the following:
   A. Landsteiner's law (2 marks)
   B. Principle of crossmatching (2 marks)
   C. Bombay blood group (1 mark)

A. Landsteiner's Law

- Karl Landsteiner is the father of blood grouping
- The antigens were called agglutinogen and the antibody was called agglutinin
- These experiments were discovered based on the results from agglutination tests
- If an antigen/agglutinogen is present on the surface of RBC, then the respective antibody/agglutinin is absent in the plasma.
- If an antigen/agglutinogen is absent on the RBC, then the corresponding antibody/agglutinin is present in the plasma.
- The second rule is an exception for Rh factor.
- Based on this law, blood groups are divided

Blood Types	Agglutinogens	Agglutinins
A	A	Anti-B(β)
B	B	Anti-A(α)
AB	A and B	–
0	–	Anti-A and anti-B

B. Principle of Crossmatching (Fig. 2.20)

- Agglutination tests are used to determine the type of blood group using anti-A and anti-B serum.
- The principle is based on Landsteiner's law: If the blood contains agglutinogen A, then if agglutinin A is added, there is agglutination. The same is for agglutinogen.
- Based on this there are 4 groups: A, B, AB and O.
- Crossmatching is done when the patient has to be transfused with donor's blood.
- It has to be always done prior to blood transfusion, even if the blood groups of both the individuals are known.
- It is done by mixing recipient's sera and donor RBCs.
- The mixture is incubated for 1 hour and the centrifuged.
- If there is agglutination, the recipient's blood is found incompatible.

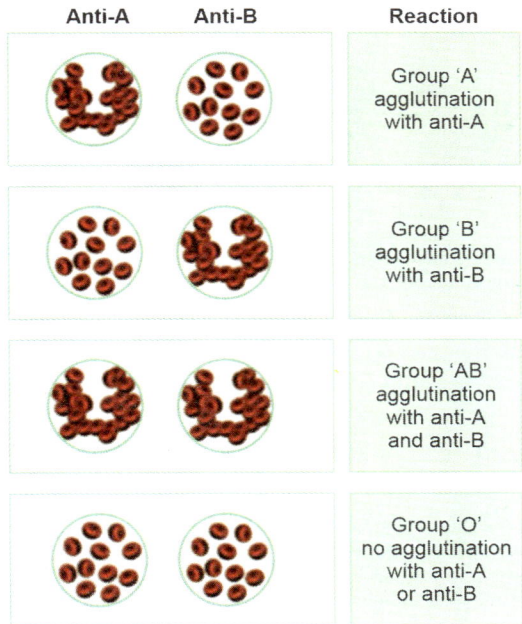

	Anti-A	Anti-B	Reaction
			Group 'A' agglutination with anti-A
			Group 'B' agglutination with anti-B
			Group 'AB' agglutination with anti-A and anti-B
			Group 'O' no agglutination with anti-A or anti-B

Fig. 2.20

Blood group	Antigen on RBC	Antibody in serum
A positive	A, Rh	Anti-B
A negative	A	Anti-Rh, anti-B
B positive	B, Rh	Anti-A
B negative	B	Anti-A, anti-Rh
O positive	Rh	Anti-A, anti-B
O negative	–	Anti-A, anti-B, anti-Rh
AB positive	A, B, Rh	–
AB negative	A, B	Anti-Rh

C. Bombay Blood Group

- It is the rarest phenotype of blood group.
- These individuals have a clinical blood group O ad do not have H antigen on the RBC surface. They have the gene for A and B antigens but are not able to express due to the lack of H antigen.
- They have antibodies to H, A and B antigens.
- Thus, they can donate blood to any of the groups of ABO system but cannot receive blood from one member other than Bombay blood group.

3. Classify blood groups. Describe physiology of ABO and Rh blood group systems. Explain Landsteiner's law. (2 + 2 + 1 marks)

Blood Groups: Classification

- The most common classification of blood group is the ABO system.
- They are based on the antigen that is present on the surface of RBCs.
- There are four blood groups: A, B, AB and O. If the RBC has antigen A, it is designated as blood group A. if the RBCs has antigen B, then the blood group is B. If both the antigens are present on RBC, then the blood group is AB. If neither is present, then it is O.
- Based on presence or absence of Rh antigen on the RBC surface, the groups are designated as 'positive' or 'negative'

Physiology of ABO and Rh Blood Group Systems

- It is based on the fact that antigens present on the surface of the RBCs would react with the antibodies in the serum and get agglutinated and destroyed.
- The surface antigens are inherited. The H antigen is expressed on the chromosome 19. Depending on whether N-acetylglucosamine or galactose is attached to it, the surface antigen becomes A or B.
- The expression of the surface antigen is handled by a single gene—ABO which has three alleles: i, I^A, I^B
- For the blood group to be expressed, either allele is sufficient. They exist as codominant genes.

	Phenotype	Genotype
Blood group A	AA, AO	$I^A I^A$, I^A, i
Blood group B	BB, BO	$I^B I^B$, I^Bi
Blood group AB	AB	IA, IB
Blood group O	OO	ii

Similarly, Rh antigen is present on the surface of the RBC in 85% of population. It is also called D antigen.

Presence of it makes the blood group positive and absence of it makes the blood group negative.

It is also inherited as a codominant gene.

- I^A inheritance cause expression of surface antigen A, IB causes expression of antigen B and i allele does not lead to expression of either surface antigens.

A, B, O Inheritance			
Allele from Parent 1	Allele from Parent 2	Child's genotype	Child's phenotype
A	A	AA	A
A	O	AO	A
A	B	AB	AB
B	A	AB	AB
B	B	BB	B
B	O	BO	B
O	O	OO	O

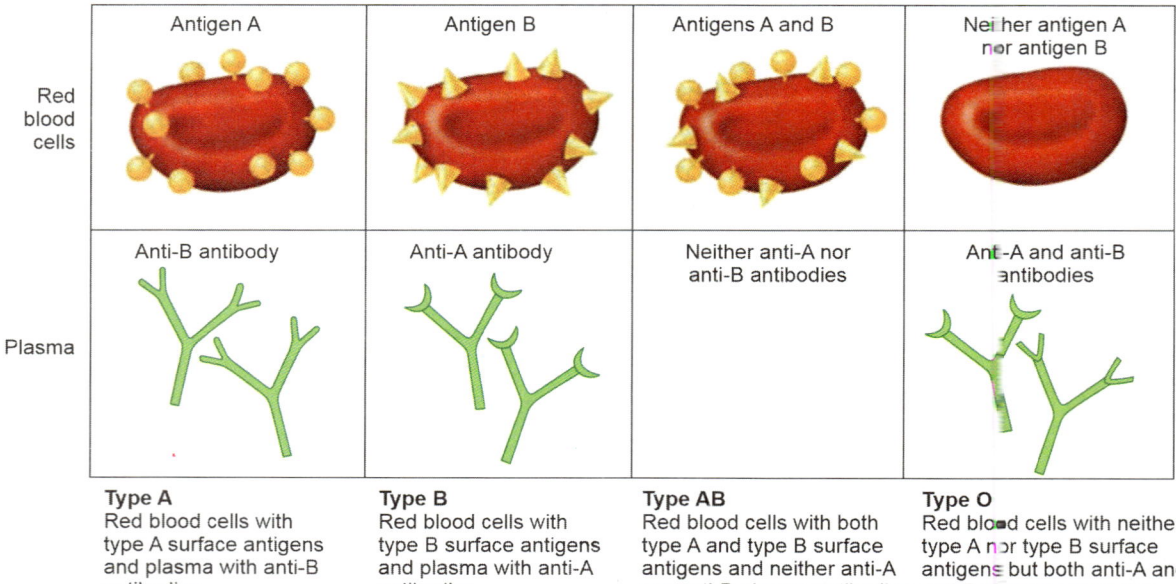

Fig. 2.21

- Blood group has an antigen A on the surface of the RBC and anti-B antibody in the serum. Presence of antigen A excludes the possibility of antibody to it in the body. The physiological basis for this is, the anti-B antibody destroys B antigen carrying cells in developmental period. Thus, they are not expressed (Fig. 2.21).
- Same hold good for Rh antigen. Presence of Rh antigen on the RBC surface excludes the antibody being present in the serum.
- Whenever the serum containing respective antibody is added to the RBCs, there is an antigen–antibody reaction occurring leading to destruction of the RBC.
- It is a type II hypersensitivity reaction.

Landsteiner's Law

- Karl Landsteiner is the father of blood grouping
- The antigens were called agglutinogen and the antibody was called agglutinin
- These experiments were discovered based on the results from agglutination tests
- If an antigen is present on the surface of RBC, then the respective agglutinin is absent in the plasma.
- If an agglutinogen is absent on the RBC, then the corresponding agglutinin is present in the plasma.
- The second rule is an exception for Rh factor.
- Based on this law, blood groups are divided

Blood Types	Agglutinogens	Agglutinins
A	A	Anti-B(β)
B	B	Anti-A(α)
AB	A and B	–
0	–	Anti-A and anti-B

4. What are the hazards of mismatched blood transfusion?

Blood transfusion is the process of transferring blood or blood components from one person (the donor) into the intravascular compartment of another person (the recipient).

Mismatched Blood Transfusion

- These reactions occur due to an error while assessing the blood group or wrong crossmatching.
- It can be due to ABO incompatibility or Rh incompatibility.
- The reactions may be mild causing only fever and hives (skin disorder characterized by itching) or may be severe leading to renal failure, shock and death.
- Reactions occur between donor's RBC having a particular agglutinogen and recipient's plasma containing antibodies or agglutinins. Vice versa does not happen due to dilution of donor RBCs.
- Donor RBCs are agglutinated resulting in transfusion reactions.

Signs and Symptoms of Transfusion Reactions

1. Non-hemolytic transfusion reaction

- Non-hemolytic transfusion reaction develops within a few minutes to hours after the commencement of blood transfusion.
- It is due to allergic response to blood and the products used for storage
- Common symptoms are fever, dyspnoea and severe pruritus.

2. Hemolytic transfusion reaction: Hemolytic transfusion reaction may be acute or delayed.

Immediate Reaction

- The acute hemolytic reaction occurs within few minutes of transfusion due to massive hemolysis.
- Symptoms include fever, chills, palpitations, hypotension, dyspnoea, wheezing, nausea, vomiting, red urine, chest pain, back pain and rigor.
- Complement release causes the systemic effects.
- Some patients may develop pulmonary edema and congestive cardiac failure.

Delayed Reaction

- Delayed hemolytic reaction occurs from 1 to 5 days after transfusion.
- The hemolysis of RBCs results in release of large amount of hemoglobin into the plasma.

- This leads to the following complications:

i. *Jaundice*
   - When the RBCs undergoes lysis, hemoglobin released. It is then converted to porphyrins and bilirubin.
   - When the serum bilirubin level increases above 2 mg/dL, jaundice occurs.
   - The unconjugated bilirubin is elevated

ii. *Cardiac shock*
   - Haemoglobin released into the plasma increases its viscosity which increases the workload on the heart leading to heart failure.
   - Moreover, toxic substances released from haemolysed cells lead to hypotension and circulatory failure.

iii. *Renal shutdown*
   - The toxic substances released during hemolysis cause constriction of blood vessels in kidney.
   - In addition, the toxic substances along with free hemoglobin are filtered through glomerular membrane and enter renal tubules which cause obstruction.
   - This causes cessation of urine formation and leads to azotemia.
   - This may culminate in death if not treated with dialysis.

2.10 DEFINE AND CLASSIFY DIFFERENT TYPES OF IMMUNITY. DESCRIBE THE DEVELOPMENT OF IMMUNITY AND ITS REGULATION

SHORT ESSAYS

1. What is antigen presenting cell? Explain humoral mediated immunity.   (1 + 4 marks)

Antigen Presenting Cells

- They are special types of cells which induce release of antigens from various organisms and then present them to helper T cells.
- They are 3 types: Macrophages, dendritic cells and B lymphocytes.
- They are helpful in cell-mediated immunity.
- The invading organisms are engulfed or trapped by these cells. They digest the antigens and form short segments of peptides which move to the surface of the cells where they bind with MHC molecules. These are presented to helper T cells which later lead to cell mediated and humoral immunity.

Humoral Mediated Immunity

- Humoral immunity is defined as immunity mediated through antibodies.
- Antibodies are secreted into the blood and lymph by B lymphocytes.
- They are nothing but gamma globulins directed against specific antigens.

Mechanism of Humoral Immunity

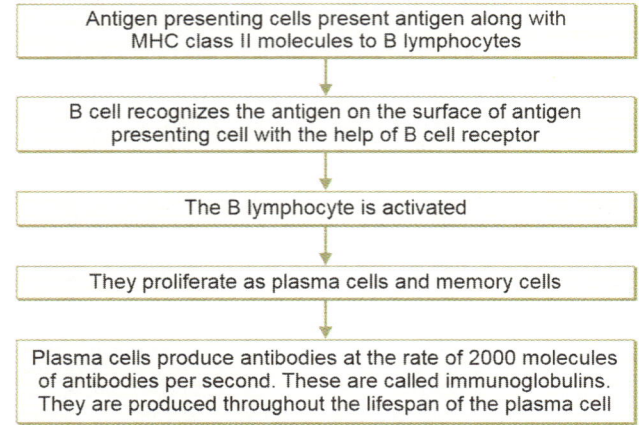

Antigen presenting cells present antigen along with MHC class II molecules to B lymphocytes
B cell recognizes the antigen on the surface of antigen presenting cell with the help of B cell receptor
The B lymphocyte is activated
They proliferate as plasma cells and memory cells
Plasma cells produce antibodies at the rate of 2000 molecules of antibodies per second. These are called immunoglobulins. They are produced throughout the lifespan of the plasma cell

Fig. 2.22

- Memory cells produced become inactive and are stored in the lymphoid tissue. They get activated during a second attack by the same organism. This

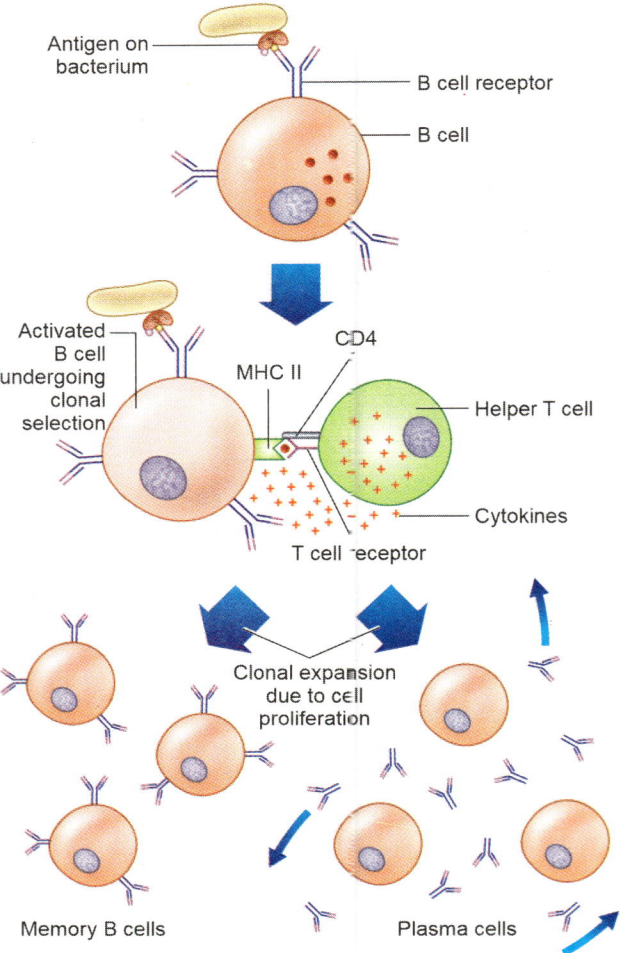

Fig. 2.23

time the antibodies are faster and more in number. This forms the basis for vaccination.

2. Define autoimmunity. What are the theories that explain autoimmunity?

Definition

- Autoimmunity is defined as a condition in which body mounts an immune response against own cells and tissues recognized as antigens.
- Normally, body's own cells and tissues are not recognized as antigens due to a process called tolerance.
- Autoimmunity develops because of failure of tolerance mechanisms.

Theories

1. Epitope spreading

- During the mechanism of tolerance, only a few antigens are selected and presented to the immune system.
- The host antigens which are not presented to the immune system are called cryptic epitopes.
- During a severe inflammatory response, the antigen presenting cells present these cryptic epitopes to the immune system leading to an immune response.

2. Molecular mimicry

- An infection with a virus or a bacterium causes activation of a set of antibodies.
- These antibodies recognize other antigens which are like the antigens against which they were originally targeting.
- This is explained in Hashimoto's thyroiditis, Graves' disease, and rheumatic fever.

3. Sequestered antigen

- These are host antigens which have been protected from immunity by a protective capsule and never been exposed to the immune system.
- Examples are sperm, uvea and lens protein.
- This is explained by post-traumatic orchitis, post-traumatic iritis and phacoanaphylactic glaucoma.

4. Nonspecific activation:
Certain highly inflammatory molecules nonspecifically activate lymphocytes which are inactive towards self-antigens.

5. Genetic factors:
MHC gene produce certain MHC alleles that specific affinity towards self-antigens and incite an inflammatory response.

3. Describe the following:
A. Sequestered antigens
B. Forbidden clones
C. Autoimmune disease

A. Sequestered Antigens

- These are host antigens which have been protected from immunity by a protective capsule and never been exposed to the immune system.
- During development, they do not interact with the circulation.
- Examples are sperm, uvea and lens protein.
- These are considered foreign by the body when introduced into the circulation and elicit a humoral and cell-mediated immunity.

- This is explained by post-traumatic orchitis, post-traumatic iritis and phacoanaphylactic glaucoma.
- An entity called sympathetic ophthalmia is explained by this theory.
- When there is injury to ciliary portion of the eye causing exposure of uveal tissues, these antigens enter the circulation.
- Antibodies are formed against these cells which attack uveal tissue of both eyes leading to blinding panuveitis in both eyes.

B. Forbidden Clones

- Some B lymphocytes which are produced in response to self-antigens are destroyed by apoptosis
- This is called forbidden clone.
- In some autoimmune conditions, persistence of these B cells is retained and gives rise to antibody reaction.
- These self-activated forbidden clones of lymphocytes produce antibodies which are organ specific or nonspecific.
- This is explained in causation of many diseases like rheumatoid arthritis, polymyositis, systemic lupus erythematosus, multiple sclerosis, idiopathic thrombocytopenic purpura.

C. Autoimmune Disease

- Autoimmunity is defined as a condition in which body mounts an immune response against own cells and tissues recognized as antigens.
- Normally, body's own cells and tissues are not recognized as antigens due to a process called tolerance.
- Autoimmunity develops because of failure of tolerance mechanisms.
- It can be organ specific or organ nonspecific

Role of HLA

- These are a group of proteins encoded by a cluster of genes present on the long arm of chromosome 6.
- Some specific HLA and MHC molecules are associated with some autoimmune conditions.
- They increase the antigen presentation and recognise self-antigens as a stranger. These help in transporting the antigen from within the cell to the cell surface and thus helps in recognising them as antigens.

Examples of Autoimmune Conditions

1. Insulin dependent diabetes mellitus
2. Myasthenia gravis
3. Graves' disease
4. Hashimoto's thyroiditis
5. Rheumatoid arthritis
6. Multiple sclerosis
7. Systemic lupus erythematosus

4. Explain clonal selection and clonal deletion theory in autoimmunity.

- Autoimmunity is generally defined as a phenomenon in which antibodies or T cells react with autoantigens.
- Clone: A group of identical cells derived from a single cell.

Clonal Selection (Fig. 2.24)

- A hypothesis which states that an individual lymphocyte (specifically, a B cell) expresses receptors specific to the distinct antigen, determined before the antibody ever encounters the antigen. Binding of Ag to a cell activates the cell, causing a proliferation of clone daughter cells.
- The clonal selection hypothesis has become a widely accepted model for how the immune system responds to infection and how certain types of B and T lymphocytes are selected for destruction of specific antigens invading the body.
- Clonal selection of lymphocytes:
  - A hematopoietic stem cell undergoes differentiation and genetic rearrangement to produce
  - Immature lymphocytes with many different antigen receptors.
  - Antigens from the body's own tissues are destroyed, while the rest mature into:
    o Inactive lymphocytes. Most of these will never encounter a matching
    o Foreign antigen, but those that do are activated and produce
    o Many clones of themselves

Clonal Deletion Theory (Fig. 2.25)

- It is a mechanism involved in immune tolerance
- According to this theory, during embryonic development, T cells maturing in the thymus acquire the ability to distinguish self from non-self. These T cells are then eliminated by apoptosis for the tolerant individual.

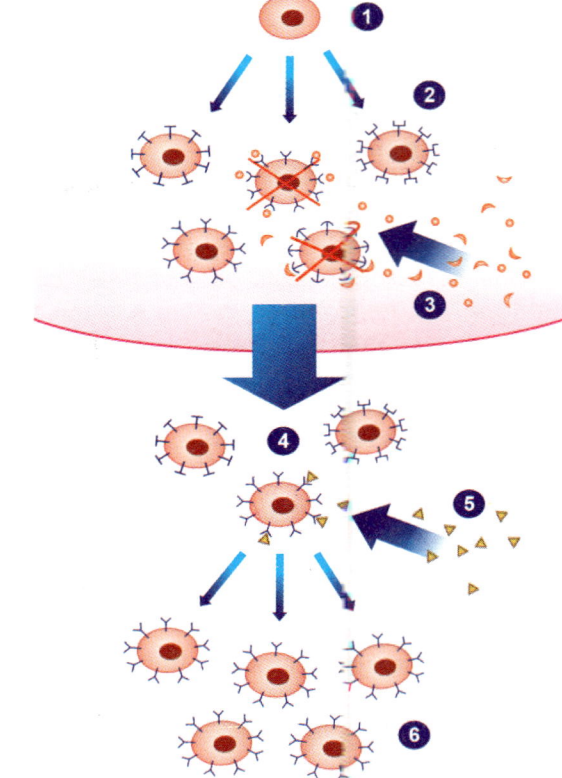

Fig. 2.24

- Clonal deletion can help protect individuals against autoimmunity.
- Clonal deletion is thought to be the most common type of negative selection.

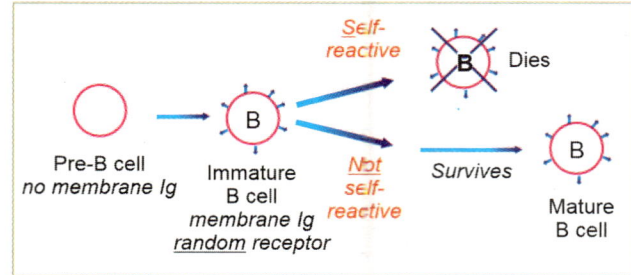

Fig. 2.25

5. Explain cell-mediated immunity. What are the different types of cells involved in it? What is T-T and T-B cooperation? (5 marks)

Cell-mediated Immunity

- It is the immune response mounted by T cells.
- It is the major defense mechanism against viruses, fungi and mycobacteria.
- It involves the following steps

1. Antigen presenting cells (Fig. 2.26)

- When a pathogen enters the blood stream or a tissue, it is engulfed by the macrophage—the first line of defense.
- They phagocytose the pathogen and express their antigen on their surface.
- Antigen presenting can also be done by dendritic cells which trap the antigen without engulfing them.
- These antigens are broken into small fragments and presented along with a protein called major histocompatibility complex (MHC).

2. Activation of helper cells

- Helper cells recognize the antigen presented by the antigen presenting cells.
- Th1 cells are associated with cell-mediated immunity
- They secrete interleukin 2 which activates other T cells and gamma interferon which stimulates phagocytic activity of NK cells, macrophages and cytotoxic cells.

3. Cytotoxic T cells

- The cytotoxic cells attach to the pathogen and enlarge
- They release lysosomal enzymes and destroy the invading organisms.

T-T Cooperation and T-B Cooperation

T-T cooperation (Fig. 2.27)

- It is a part of cell-mediated immunity and is protective against fungi, viruses and certain bacteria
- An antigen that enters the body is processed and presented by the antigen presenting cell along with MHC class II molecule.
- This is recognized by lymphocytes with a TCR- T cell receptor
- They differentiate into CD4+ and CD8+ cells.
- CD8 cells differentiate into cytotoxic T cells and suppressor T cells (T_c and T_s)
- CD4 cells differentiate into helper T cells and delayed hypersensitivity cells (T_h and T_d)
- This differentiation is interdependent, and this is called T-T cooperation.

T-B Cooperation (Fig. 2.28)

- It is the interaction between cell mediated and humoral immunity
- When the antigen is presented by the antigen presenting cell to the helper T cells, Th2 cells secrete two interleukins—IL-2 and B cell growth factor
- This causes proliferation of B cells and their conversion into plasma cells.
- Two types of B cells are formed.

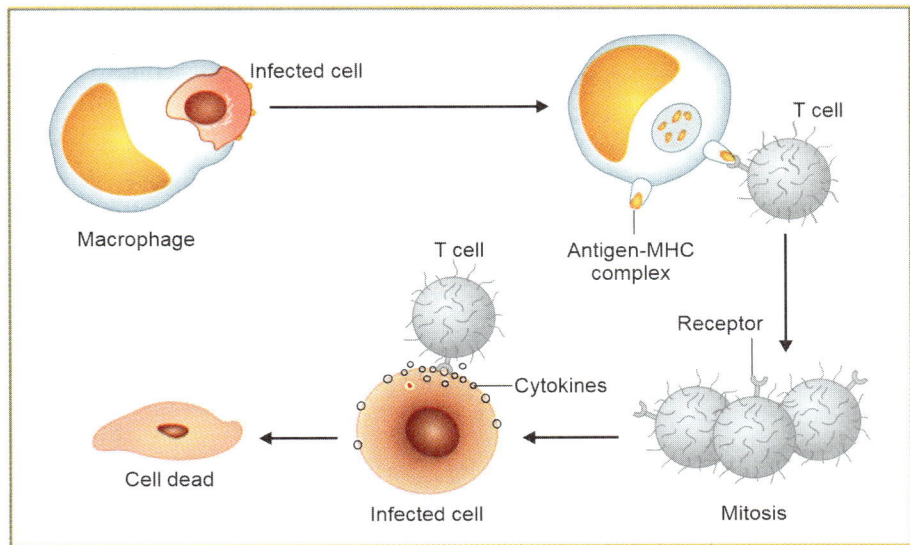

Fig. 2.26

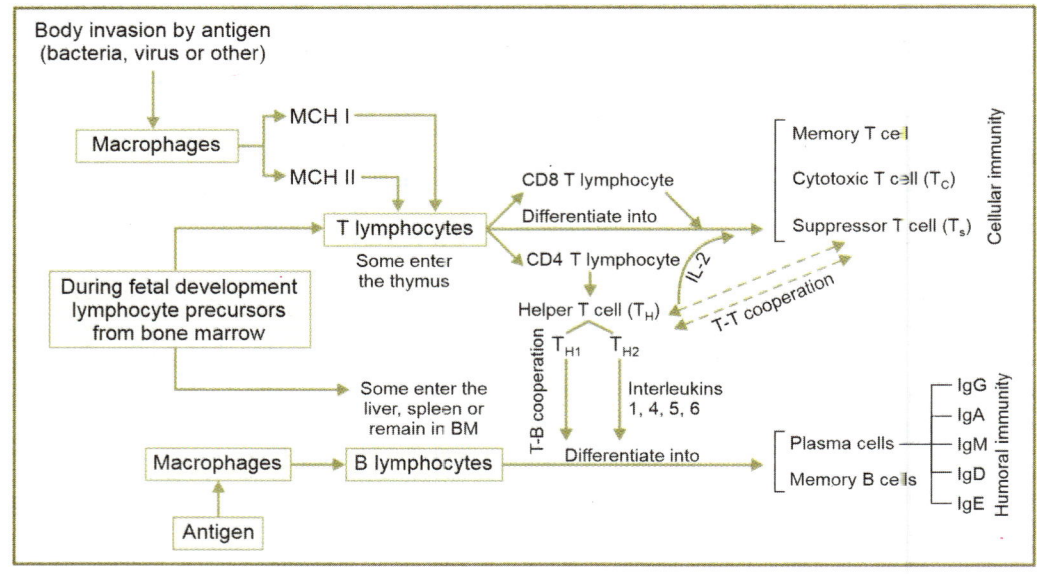

Fig. 2.27

Fig. 2.28

1. **Plasma cells**
   – When B lymphocyte is converted into plasma cells, the cytoplasm increases
   – It becomes granular and secretes antibodies.
   – They are of 5 types: IgA, IgG, IgM, IgE, IgD.

2. **Memory B cells**
   – A small portion of B lymphocytes does not enlarge but remains small and get distributed in the lymphoid tissue
   – They are more specific to the antigen and offer immunity when there is a second attack
   – Till then, they remain inactive.

SHORT ANSWERS

1. What are antibodies? Name the different types of antibodies.

Antibodies

They are proteins produced by plasma cells or activated B lymphocytes in response to an antigen.

Different Types of Antibodies

IgA (alpha)	Provides local immunity
IgE (epsilon)	Provides allergic response
IgM (mu)	Recent immunity, helps in complement fixation
IgG (gamma)	Helps in complement fixation
IgD (delta)	Helps in recognition of antigen by B lymphocytes

2. Explain the types of hypersensitivity reactions.

- It is an abnormally exaggerated immune response to a chemical or physical or biological agent.
- It is mediated by proliferation and recruitment of specific types of cells.
- Based on the underlying mechanism, it is grouped into four types.

Type I Hypersensitivity or Anaphylactic Reaction

- Anaphylaxis means, hyperexaggerated immune response to an agent to which the body is already sensitized
- During the first exposure, when the allergen meets the body's immune system, antigen presenting cells present antigen to helper T cells.
- IgE antibodies are produced by the B cell in response to this
- During the next exposure, the IgE binds to receptors on the surface of basophils and mast cells
- This leads to rupture of granules to release of substances like histamine, leukotriene which cause a set of symptoms specific to anaphylaxis
- These chemical mediators cause severe vasodilatation leading to sudden lowering of blood pressure, laryngeal edema, acute diarrhea and urticaria on skin
- Examples are drug reaction, bee sting, Stevens-Johnson syndrome
- Hay fever and allergic rhinitis are mild forms

Type II Hypersensitivity or Cytotoxic Reaction

- It involves production of IgG antibodies
- Allergens are presented to helper cells in association with helper T cells
- IgG antibodies cause lysis of cells
- Examples are autoimmune hemolytic anemia and Rh incompatibility (erythroblastosis fetalis)

Type III Hypersensitivity Reaction

- In this type, a complex is formed between antigen and antibody.
- The antigen–antibody complex formed gets deposited in the tissue and causes inflammatory reaction.
- Examples are rheumatic fever, post-infectious glomerulonephritis, systemic lupus erythematosus.

Type IV Hypersensitivity Reaction

- In this type of hypersensitivity, there is immune response against an antigen is mounted in the form of mononuclear aggregation
- The helper cells involved are Th1 cells and activate CD8 cells
- In some conditions like tuberculosis and sarcoidosis, granuloma forms. In tuberculosis the central portion of the granuloma undergoes a process called caseation.

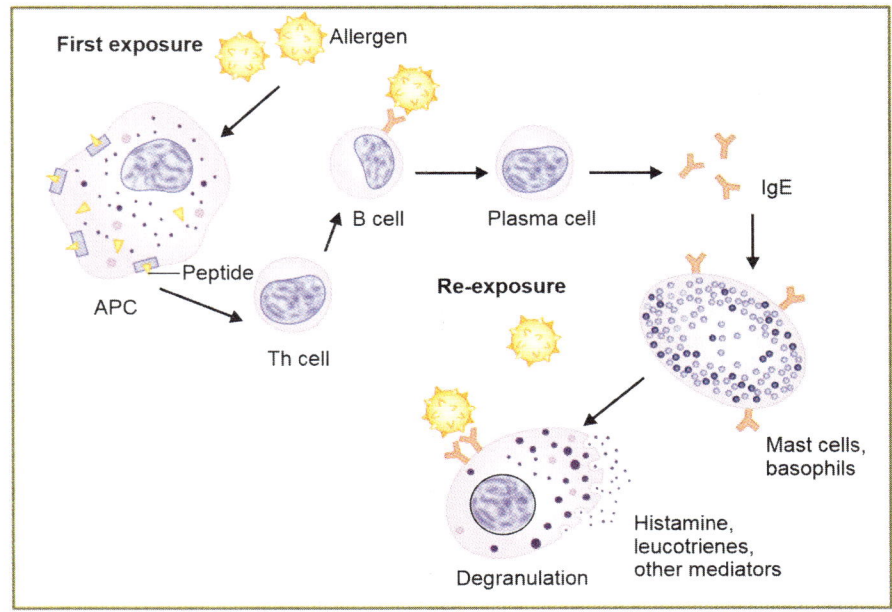

Fig. 2.29

2.11 ESTIMATE HB, RBC, TLC, RBC INDICES, DLC, BLOOD GROUPS, BT/CT

SHORT ESSAYS/SHORT ANSWERS

1. A 50-year-old female comes with the history of weakness, tiredness, on examination she has pallor. Which test will you perform to assess if she is anemic? Estimate the total leucocyte count (TLC) of your blood and report.

- In this patient who has signs of anemia, the first important test to be performed in blood hemoglobin levels.
- Others include blood indices like MCV, MCH, MCHC, RDW, serum iron, serum transferrin to classify the type of anemia.
- Other investigations should be performed to know the cause of anemia that is to know the site of blood loss.

Estimation of Total Leukocyte Count

Principle

- A sample of blood is diluted with a diluting fluid
- The purpose is to destroy the red cells and stain the nuclei of the leukocytes.
- The cells are then mounted in a counting chamber and counted.
- Their number in undiluted blood is reported as leukocytes/mm^3.

Apparatus

1. Microscope with 5–6 clean slides, coverslip
2. Counting chamber (Fig. 2.30)
3. Sterile lancet, cotton swab, 70% alcohol
4. WBC pipettes: White bead in bulb, and markings 0.5, 1.0, and 11. Two clean and dry pipettes, with free-rolling beads are taken (Fig. 2.31).
5. Turk's fluid—it is diluent fluid. It contains glacial acetic acid 1.5 ml (hemolyzes RBCs without affecting WBCs), gentian violet (1% solution) 1.5 ml (it stains the nuclei of leukocytes)
6. Distilled water to 100 ml.

Procedure

- After swabbing the fingertip with 70% alcohol, a knick in made with a sterile lancet by a quick movement.
- Discard the first two drops and collect a large drop with the help of pipette, suck blood till 0.5 mark and Turk's fluid till 11 mark.

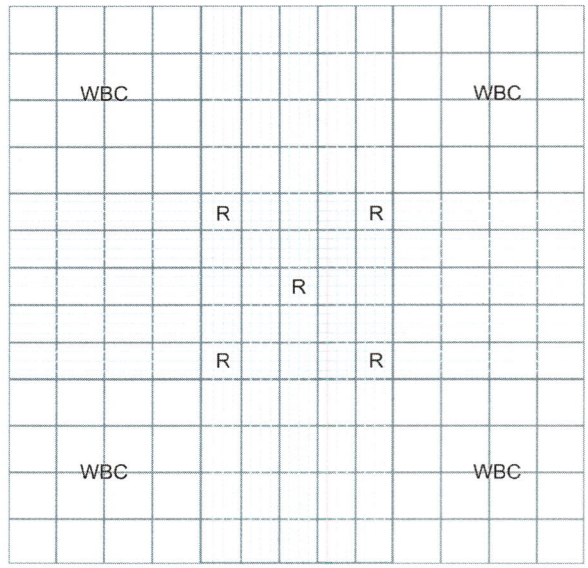

Fig. 2.30

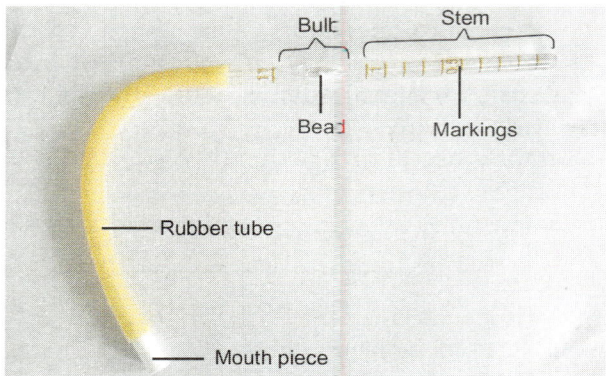

Fig. 2.31: Pipette

- The contents are mixed by rolling the pipette between both palms.
- Charging the chamber: After placing the coverslip, discard first two drops of the mixture and then charge the chamber at a 45° angle such that it completely covers the coverslip evenly.
- Allow the cells to settle for 3–4 minutes and then load the slide onto the microscope.
- Under low magnification, the leukocytes are seen as blue dots with a halo around them (nucleus stained with gentian violet with surrounding stained cytoplasm).
- Switch to high magnification to see the cells and their nuclei clearly. Some have lobed nuclei whereas others are non-lobed.

- The peripheral 4 large squares containing 16 boxes are counted for the number of cells in each chamber.

Calculation

- No. of cells counted = 79
- Area counted = 1 mm × 4 = 4 mm², depth = 1/10 mm
- Total volume in which WBCs are counted = 4/10 mm³
- Dilution = 1:20
- So, the number of WBCs in undiluted blood

$$= 79 \times 10/4 \times 20$$
$$= 79 \times 50 = 3950/mm^3$$

2. Determine the differential leucocyte count (DLC) of your blood and analyse the report.

Procedure of Estimation of Differential Count

Principle

- A blood film is stained with Leishman stain and WBCs are seen under a microscope
- Each WBC is identified and counted until 200 cells have been counted.
- Each type of cell is counted and then the percentage is calculated.
- It is multiplied by the total leukocyte count to get the absolute number.

Apparatus Required

1. Microscope with 5–6 clean slides
2. 70% alcohol
3. Cotton swabs
4. Sterile lancet
5. Glass dropper
6. Leishman's stain
7. Blotting paper
8. Distilled water

Procedure

Preparation of blood film

- After swabbing the fingertip with 70% alcohol, a nick in made with a sterile lancet by a quick movement.

- Hold a coverslip by its edges between your thumb and index finger, touch its center to the blood drop.
- Carefully drop the coverslip in the center of a glass slide.
- The blood drop will spread into a thick film by the weight of the coverslip.
- Apply Vaseline around the edges using a toothpick, to seal the capillary space under it. This will prevent evaporation of water and drying up of the preparation.
- Examine the preparation under low and high magnifications and record your observations.

Procedure

- The blood film is fixed and stained with supravital stain.
- The leukocytes are identified under oil immersion.
- Red cells—these are the most numerous and appear pink. They are non-nucleated and biconcave. Normally, the centre is pale.
- Leukocytes—5 main types of leukocytes are seen. They are identified based on their shape of nucleus and presence or absence of cytoplasmic granules.
- Platelets—these are minute, membrane bound round or oval bodies and may be in clumps.

Identification of Leukocytes

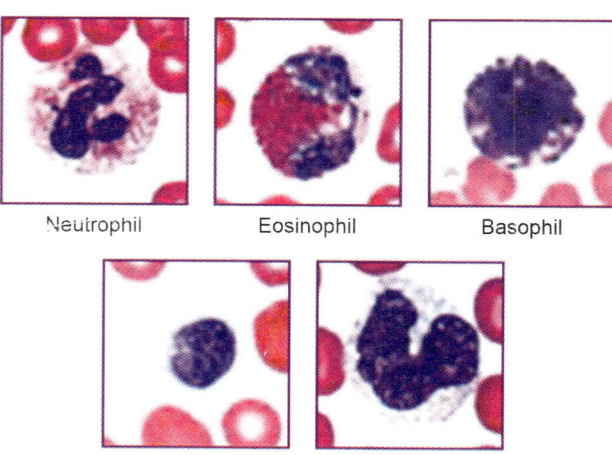

Neutrophil   Eosinophil   Basophil

Lymphocyte   Monocyte

Fig. 2.32

Cell type	Diameter (µm)	Nucleus	Cytoplasm	Cytoplasmic granules
Granulocytes				
Neutrophils (40–75%)	10–44 (1.5–2 × a RBC)	• Blue violet • 2–6 lobes, connected by chromatin threads seen clearly through cytoplasm	• Slate-blue in color	• Fine closely-packed violet pink • Not seen separately • Give groundglass appearance • Do not cover nucleus
Eosinophills (1–6%)	10–15	• Blue-violet • 2–3 lobes, often bilobed, lobes connected by thick or thin chromatin band Seen clearly through cytoplasm	• Eosinophilic • Light pink-red • Granular	• Large, coarse • Uniform-sized • Brick-red to orange • Seen separately • Do not cover nucleus
Basophils (0–1%)	10–15	• Blue-violet • Irregular shape, may be S-shaped, rarely bilobed • Not clearly seen, because overlaid with granules	• Basophilic • Bluish • Granular	• Large, very coarse • Variable-sized • Deep purple • Seen separately Completely fill the cell and cover the nucleus
Agranulocytes				
Monocytes (5–10%)	12–20 (1.5–3 × a RBC)	• Pale blue-violet • Large single • May be indented horse, or kidney shaped (can appear oval or round, if seen from the side)	• Abundant • Frosty • Slate-blue • Amount may be larger than that of nucleus	• No visible granules
Small Lymphocytes				
(20–40%)	7–9	• Deep blue-violet • Single, large, round, almost fills cell • Condensed, lumpy chromatin, gives 'ink-spot' appearance	• Hardly visible • Thin crescent of clear, ligh blue cytoplasm	• No visible granules
Large lymphocytes	10–15	• Deep blue-violet • Single, large, round or oval, almost fills cell • May be central or eccentric	• Large, crescent of clear, light blue cytoplasm • Amount larger than in small lymphocyte	• No visible granules

Findings

Neutrophils	156	78%
Lymphocytes	36	18%
Monocytes	4	2%
Eosinophils	4	2%
Basophils	0	0

Impression

The sample shows neutrophilia, indicating a bacterial infection.

3. Determine the differential leucocyte count (DLC) of your blood and report. Focus the eosinophil.

Principle

- A blood film is stained with Leishman stain and WBCs are scanned under a microscope
- Each WBC is identified and counted until 200 cells have been counted.
- Each type of cell is counted and then the percentage is calculated.
- It is multiplied by the total leukocyte count to get the absolute number.

Apparatus Required

1. Microscope with 5–6 clean slides
2. 70% alcohol
3. Cotton swabs
4. Sterile lancet
5. Glass dropper
6. Leishman's stain
7. Blotting paper
8. Distilled water

Procedure

Preparation of Blood Film

- After swabbing the fingertip with 70% alcohol, a nick in made with a sterile lancet by a quick movement.
- Hold a coverslip by its edges between your thumb and index finger, touch its center to the blood drop.
- Carefully drop the coverslip in the center of a glass slide.
- The blood drop will spread evenly into a thick film.
- Apply Vaseline around the edges using a toothpick, to seal the capillary space under it. This will prevent evaporation of water and drying up of the preparation.
- Examine the preparation under low and high magnifications and observe the cells.

Procedure

- The blood film is fixed and stained with supravital stain.
- The leukocytes are identified under oil immersion.
- *Red cells:* These are the most numerous and appear pink. They are non-nucleated and biconcave. Normally, the centre is pale.
- *Leukocytes:* 5 main types of leukocytes are seen. They are identified based on their shape of nucleus and presence or absence of cytoplasmic granules.
- *Platelets:* These are minute, membrane bound round or oval bodies and may be in clumps.

Identification of Leukocytes

Findings

Neutrophils	132	56%
Lymphocytes	36	18%
Monocytes	4	2%
Eosinophils	24	12%
Basophils	4	2%

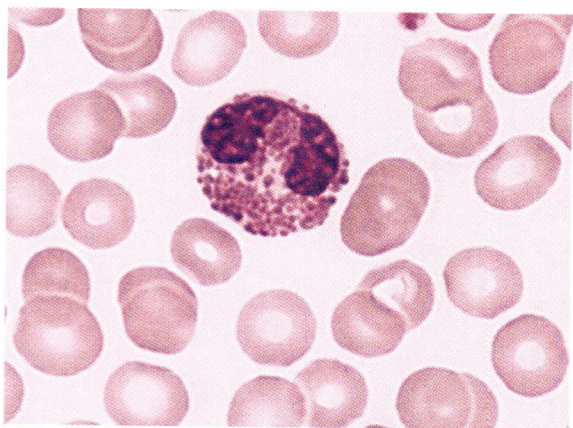

Fig. 2.33

- 10–15 micron size cell, with bilobed nucleus connected by a thin chromatin strand and eosinophilic granular cytoplasm.

Impression

The sample shows eosinophilia, indicating a worm infestation or allergy.

4. Estimate haemoglobin concentration and calculate the oxygen carrying capacity of your blood. Determine MCH for the given RBC count: 4.5 million cells/cu mm of blood. Also determine MCHC for the given PCV 45%.

Haemoglobin Estimation

Principle

- Haemoglobin in blood is converted into hematin by using hydrochloric acid
- It is brown in colour.
- The estimate of haemoglobin is made by matching the colour of hematin with the glass of the Sahli's apparatus.

Equipment

- Cotton swab, sterile lancet, 70% alcohol
- Sahli's hemoglobinometer (Fig. 2.34)
- It consists of a rectangular plastic box with a slot at the centre to place the calibrated hemoglobin tube.
- An opaque white sheet is placed behind to provide uniform illumination.
- The hemoglobin tube is a rectangular or cylindrical calibrated tube with yellow marking for measurement of Hb in g/dl on one side and percentage on the other side.

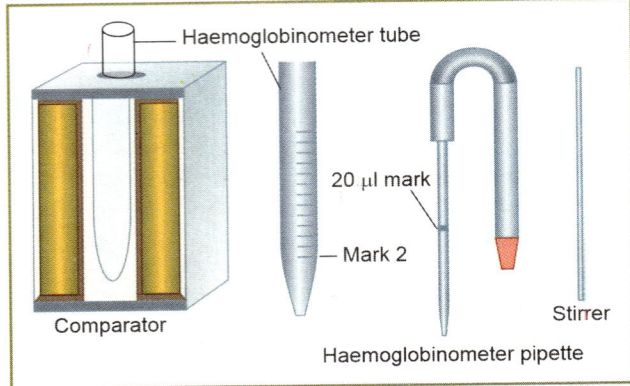

Fig. 2.34

- Hemoglobin pipette: It is capillary tube with a single mark for 20 cu mm.
- Glass stirrer
- Decinormal hydrochloric acid (N/10)
- Distilled water

Procedure

- Using a dropper, 8–10 drops of HCl are taken in the haemoglobin tube up to the 3 g mark.
- After swabbing the fingertip with 70% alcohol, a nick in made with a sterile lancet by a quick movement.
- Let go of the first two drops of blood and wait for a large bead of blood
- Pipette 0.2 ml of blood using the haemoglobin pipette
- Immediately push the drawn blood into the hemoglobinometer and rinse the blood with the same solution to remove all the blood
- Carefully, withdraw the tube and make sure no solution is wasted.
- Stir using the glass stirrer
- Let the tube stand for 6–8 minutes
- After this, start adding drop by drop of distilled water and gently stirring till the colour in the tube matches the standard color.
- The value of hemoglobin estimation of my blood is 13.8 g/dl.

Oxygen Carrying Capacity

- Oxygen carrying capacity of 1 g of hemoglobin is 1.34 ml of oxygen.
- Thus, oxygen carrying capacity of 13.8 g of hemoglobin is 18.49 ml of oxygen/dl.

MCH

$$MCH = \frac{Hb \text{ in } g\% \times 10}{RBC \text{ count in million/mm}^3}$$

$$MCH = 13.8 \text{ g/dl} \times 10 / 4.5 \text{ million cells/mm}^3$$
$$= 30.66 \text{ pg.}$$

MCHC

$$MCHC = \frac{Hb \text{ in } g \text{ per } 100 \text{ ml blood}}{PCV \text{ per } 100 \text{ ml blood}} \times 100$$

$$= \frac{Hb \text{ } g\%}{PCV\%} \times 100$$

$$MCHC = 13.8/45 \times 100 = 30.66\%$$

5. Determine the bleeding time of your blood and report.

Bleeding Time

Principle

- It is a platelet function test
- The time taken till bleeding stops after giving a cut is taken as bleeding time.

Equipment

- Cotton swab, 70% alcohol
- Sterile lancet

Procedure

- After cleansing the area (fingertip or earlobe) with an alcohol swab, firm pressure is applied on the pulp of the finger
- A deep prick of length 1–3 mm is made with a lancet.
- Remove the blood with a filter paper from the edges of the wound till blood disappears.
- The time duration till cessation of bleeding recorded.

Result

Bleeding time is 2 minutes 33 seconds: It is normal.

6. Determine the clotting time of your blood and report.

Clotting Time

Principle

- It is a test for clotting factors.
- Skin is made to bleed after a prick and the blood is collected in a capillary tube

- When blood comes in contact with an external surface like glass tube, it starts to clot.

Equipment

- Cotton swab, 70% alcohol
- Sterile lancet
- Capillary tube

Procedure

- After cleansing the area (fingertip or earlobe) with an alcohol swab, firm pressure is applied on the pulp of the finger
- A deep prick of length 1–3 mm is made with a lancet.
- Allow the first two drops of blood
- Collect the next large bead of blood into a capillary tube and note the time
- Hold the tube between your palms so that the body temperature is maintained to simulate physiological conditions
- Gently break the ends of the tube at 30 seconds intervals.
- When the blood starts to clot is seen as threads of at least 5 mm between the broken ends of the tube.
- The number of pieces of the capillary tube is counted.

Result

Clotting time is 3 minutes 40 seconds: It is normal.

7. Do the blood grouping and Rh typing of your blood and report?

Principle

- The RBCs have a surface antigen which is responsible for its blood group.
- The serum of the same individual lacks respective agglutinin or antibody

- When serum contain respective antibody is added the RBC, agglutination occurs.

Equipment

1. Sterile lancet, cotton swab, 70% alcohol
2. Clean glass slides-4–5 or a porcelain dish with 12 depressions
3. Microscope
4. Antisera A and antisera B, anti-Rh serum

Procedure

- Using a pencil, 3 different circles are marked on a glass slide.
- Mark them as A, B and Rh on top left of each circle.
- Another separate slide is kept aside for dilution. 8–10 drops of saline are placed on it.
- Under aseptic precautions, prick the tip of a finger and collect blood in the saline slide. Gently mix the blood.
- Put a drop of anti-A serum, anti-B serum and anti-Rh serum in the first slide, side by side in each circle.
- Added the diluted red blood cells to each.
- This can also be performed on separate slides.
- Mix them by gentle tilting movements.
- Wait for 8–10 minutes.
- Agglutination can be seen as clumping on naked eye. It can be confirmed under microscope.

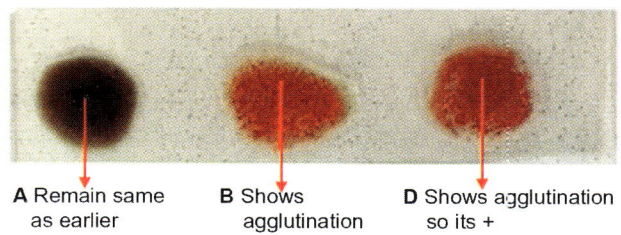

A Remain same as earlier   **B** Shows agglutination   **D** Shows agglutination so its +

Fig. 2.35

2.12 DESCRIBE TEST FOR ESR, OSMOTIC FRAGILITY, HEMATOCRIT. NOTE THE FINDINGS, INTERPRET THE TEST RESULTS, ETC.

SHORT ESSAYS

1. What is osmotic fragility? Mention 2 conditions where osmotic fragility is decreased. What is the pathophysiology in spherocytosis?

Osmotic Fragility

Susceptibility of an RBC to hemolysis or break easily when placed in a hypotonic solution is called osmotic fragility.

Conditions where Osmotic Fragility is Decreased

- Old RBCs
- Hereditary spherocytosis
- Autoimmune hemolytic anemia

Pathophysiology of Hereditary Spherocytosis

- It is a genetic condition in which the RBCs have a shorter lifespan due to their increased fragility
- They owe their increased fragility to multiple mutations that lead to abnormal membrane proteins.
- The RBCs acquire a small spherical shape and are referred to as microspherocytes
- They have a weak cytoskeleton and have poor osmotic fragility. They are unable to buffer certain intracellular and intravascular abnormalities
- This causes hemolysis and anemia. Since spleen is the graveyard for RBCs, there is splenomegaly

2. Explain the clinical importance of ESR. What are the methods used to determine ESR? Give its normal values.

ESR: Erythrocyte Sedimentation Rate

- It is a commonly performed laboratory investigation for inflammation.
- It is the rate at which erythrocytes settle down when allowed to stand in a vertical tube.
- Normally, RBCs are suspended in circulation due to their property of suspension stability. When mixed with an anticoagulant and made to stand in a vertical tube, the RBCs settle down due to gravity.

Importance

- It is an easy, non-expensive simple test
- It is a non-specific marker of inflammation

- A highly elevated value has an apparent cause like a malignancy, infection, or temporal arteritis.
- If mild increased ESR is an isolated or an accidental finding, without an apparent etiology, it should be repeated after a few months, rather than looking for an etiology.
- It can also be used in some diseases for monitoring disease progression and therapeutic result. (For example: Temporal arteritis, polymyalgia rheumatica, rheumatoid arthritis, Hodgkin's lymphoma.)

Physiological causes for raised ESR	Pathological causes for raised ESR
1. Females	1. Tuberculosis
2. Menstruation	2. Anemia (except sickle cell)
3. Pregnancy	3. Temporal arteritis
	4. Rheumatoid arthritis
	5. Rheumatic fever
	6. Malignancies
Physiological causes for decreased ESR	Pathological causes for decreased ESR
1. Infancy	1. Sickle cell anemia
2. Less in males	2. Polycythemia
	3. Leukocytosis
	4. Allergic conditions

- They are especially helpful in conditions like tuberculosis, rheumatoid arthritis, polymyalgia rheumatica and temporal arteritis. ESR is a supporting factor, not a key diagnostic test.

Methods to Determine ESR (Fig. 2.36)

Wintrobe's Method

- It is a short tube, 110 mm, with one end close
- It can be used to measure PCV also
- It is marked from above downwards from 0 to 100 for measuring ESR and the other way on the other side for measuring PCV.

Westergren's Method

- Westergren's tube is used to measure ESR
- It is 300 mm in length and open on both sides
- 1.6 ml of blood is mixed with 0.4 ml of 3.8% of sodium citrate and loaded into the tube and placed vertically

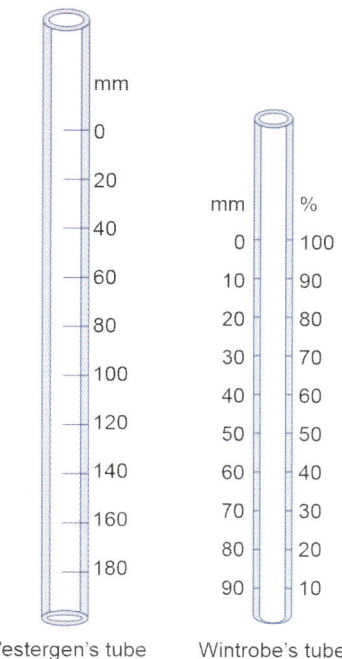

mm

Westergen's tube   Wintrobe's tube

Fig. 2.36

- It is left undisturbed for an hour
- It is marked from 0 to 200 from above downwards

Normal values

Westergren method	Wintrobe method
In males: 3 to 7 mm in 1 hour	In males: 0 to 9 mm in 1 hour
In females: 5 to 9 mm in 1 hour	In females: 0 to 15 mm in 1 hour
Infants: 0 to 2 mm in 1 hour	Infants: 0 to 5 mm in 1 hour

- In men: 0–10 mm/hour
- In women: 0–20 mm/hour

3. Define hematocrit. How to estimate hematocrit? Give its normal values. (5 marks)

Haematocrit

It is also known as packed cell volume. It is the percentage of blood occupied by red blood corpuscles.

Estimation of Haematocrit

Principle

- Blood is mixed with an anticoagulant and centrifuged
- RBCs being heavier settle down
- The plasma stays on top

Equipment

- **For venepuncture:** Cotton swab, alcohol rub, 5 mm syringe and 24 gauge 1 inch needle
- **Wintrobe tube:** It is a 11 cm long, heavy cylindrical tube which is closed at one end. It has a uniform diameter of 2 mm. It is calibrated from below upwards 0 to 10 for PCV measurement.
- **Pasteur pipette:** It is a thin nozzle with a glass rod and a rubber teat.
- **Centrifuge machine:** It should run at a speed of 3000 rpm.

Procedure

- Under aseptic precautions, 5 ml of blood is drawn from the antecubital vein into a sterile vacutainer with anticoagulant
- Fill the pasteur pipette with blood and place the tip of the nozzle at the bottom of the Wintrobe's tube

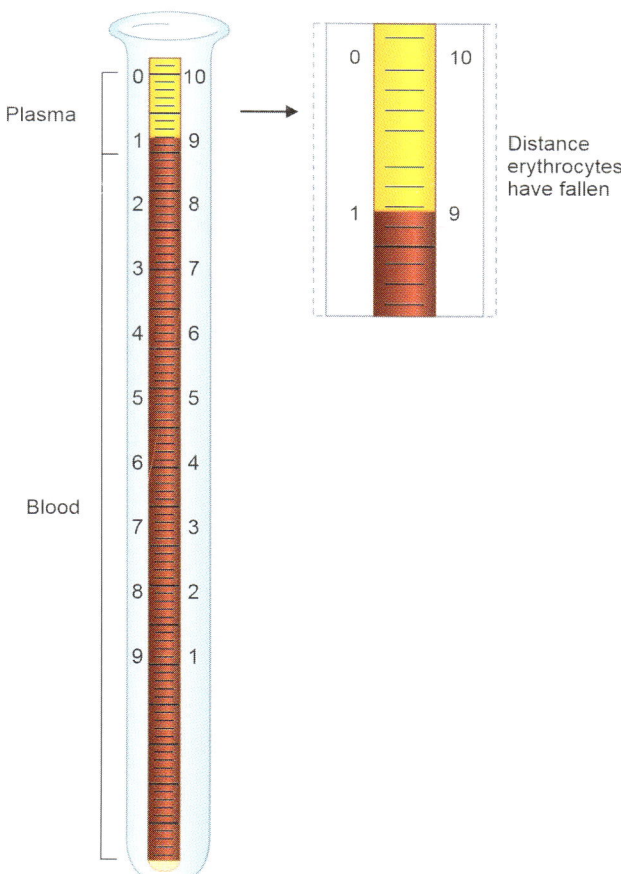

Fig. 2.37

- Slowly expel the blood into the tube
- Bring the blood till the exact 10 mark
- Close the mouth of the tube and place it in the rack and rotate the centrifuge at 3000 rpm for 30 minutes

Findings

- The RBCs settle at the bottom and the upper border corresponds to the PCV.

- The WBCs and platelets are the buffy coat—yellow in color
- Clear plasma stays at the top

Normal values

- Depends on the number of RBCs and shape of RBCs.
- Males: 38–50%
- Females: 36–45%

2.13 DESCRIBE STEPS FOR RETICULOCYTE AND PLATELET COUNT

SHORT ANSWERS

1. What are reticulocytes? What is the normal reticulocyte count? What is the strain used to identify them? Give 2 conditions where reticulocyte count is decreased?

(1 + 0.5 + 0.5 + 1 marks)

Reticulocytes (Fig. 2.38)

- Reticulocytes are immature RBCs which are slightly larger than mature RBCs.
- They are produced in the bone marrow and are let out into the circulation. They mature in peripheral blood.
- Their cytoplasm has reticular network formed by disintegrated organelles.

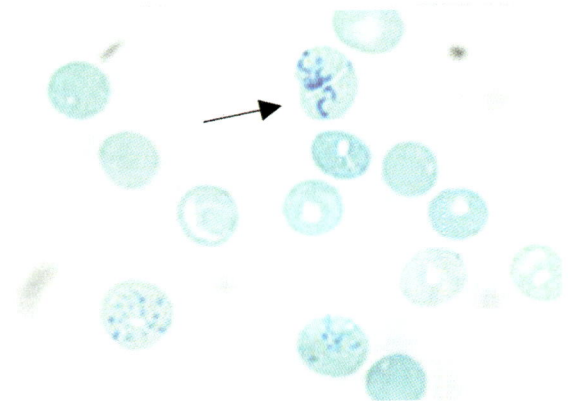

Fig. 2.39

2. Why is dengue called haemorrhagic fever? What is the normal platelet count? Mention 2 conditions where platelet count is reduced.

(1 + 1 + 1 marks)

Dengue Called Haemorrhagic Fever

- Dengue is a viral fever caused by dengue virus and transmitted by Aedes mosquito.
- One of its clinical subtypes—dengue hemorrhagic fever—is called so because it is associated with decreased platelet count and associated excessive bleeding or hemorrhage and death.

Normal Platelet Count

2,00,000–4,00,000 cells per mm^3

Causes for Decreased Platelet Count

1. Idiopathic thrombocytopenic purpura
2. Disseminated intravascular coagulation
3. Dengue
4. Aplastic anemia
5. Acute myeloid leukemia

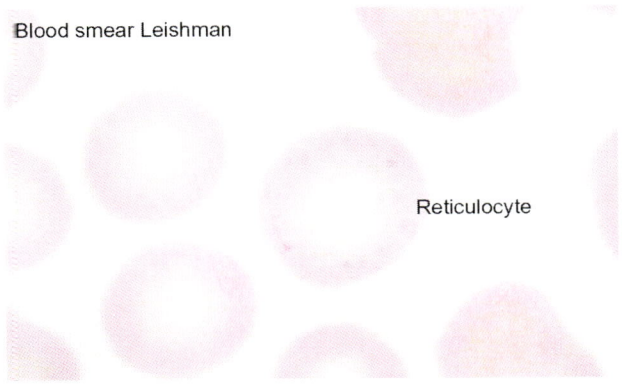

Blood smear Leishman

Reticulocyte

Fig. 2.38

Normal Count

Newborn	2–6% of total RBCs
Adults—peripheral blood	<1% of total RBCs

Identification (Fig. 2.39)

It is identified by supravital stain. It is stained with methylene blue which highlights the reticulin fibres.

Causes for Decreased Reticulocyte Count

1. Pernicious anemia
2. Aplastic anemia

3. A patient diagnosed with anemia, on treatment for 2 months. How do you assess if she is responding to treatment? Mention 2 conditions where reticulocyte count is increased.

Treatment of Anemia

- Immediate effect of treatment for anemia is seen as increased appetite. However, blood components take time to show changes.

- A desired effect of increase in 1 g/dl of hemoglobin is expected after 1 month of starting treatment for anemia.
- Increase in reticulocyte count and reticulocyte hemoglobin are seen to increase within one week of treatment with oral iron supplementation.
- Serum iron increases within 6 weeks of treatment.
- At the end of three months, complete blood count and blood indices should be repeated.

Increased Reticulocyte Count

- Reticulocytosis is increased percentage of reticulocytes
- It is seen in post-hemorrhagic state where the bone marrow is producing more cells to replenish the lost RBCs.
- It is also seen in response to treatment for iron deficiency anemia as the bone marrow starts producing more cells.
- Other causes are pregnancy, leukemia and sickle cell anemia.

Nerve and Muscle Physiology

Chapter 3

3.1 DESCRIBE THE STRUCTURE AND FUNCTIONS OF A NEURON AND NEUROGLIA; DISCUSS NERVE GROWTH FACTOR AND OTHER GROWTH FACTORS/CYTOKINES

SHORT ESSAYS

1. Discuss the structure and functions of a neuron.

Structure of a Neuron

- A neuron or a nerve cell is the structural and functional unit of the nervous system.
- A typical neuron consists of the following structures:
  1. **Cell body or the Soma**
     - It may be stellate, round, fusiform or pyramidal
     - Typically consists of cytoplasm, large nucleus with nuclei but centromeres conspicuously absent.
     - Nissl granules: These are basophilic granules, primarily made of rough endoplasmic reticulum.
     - Neurofibrillae: These are microfilaments and microtubules
     - Pigments like lipofuscin and melanin may be present
  2. **Dendrites**
     - These multiple branch-like structures arising from the cell body
     - They also contain Nissl granules.
  3. **Axon**
     - It is longest process of the neuron
     - It varies in different nerves, sometimes as long as one meter.

– The part between axon and the soma is called the axon hillock. It is followed by the initial segment and is devoid of myelin sheath. It is secreted by the Schwann cell and each cell is responsible for a segment of the axon.

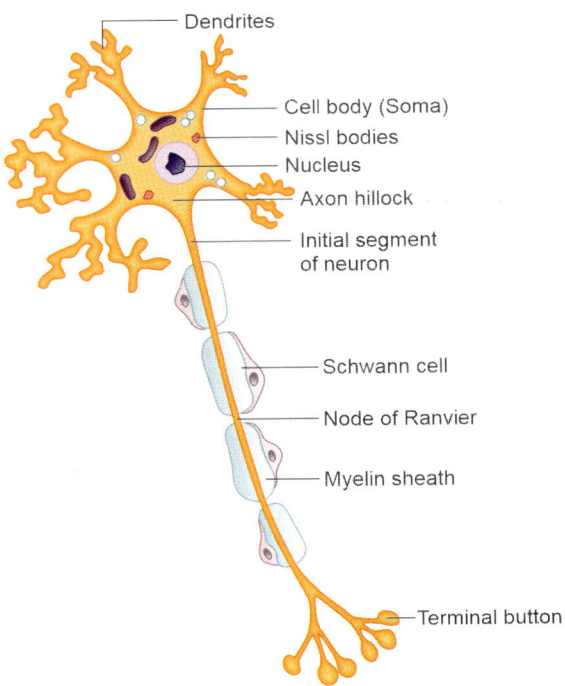

Fig. 3.1

67

– The axon is wrapped by myelin sheath which is absent at regular points called nodes of Ranvier.

– At the end of the axon, there are branch like structures called telodendria which have synaptic knobs at their ends.

Functions of a Neuron

1. Its main function is conduction of impulses
2. It may be from the brain to the periphery or vice versa
3. It may also be from a nerve to a muscle or nerve to another nerve.

2. List types of neuroglia. Explain their structure and functions.

Neuroglia

These are supporting cells present in the brain and the spinal cord.

Types of Neuroglia

Macroglia	Microglia
Large cells of ectodermal origin 1. Astrocytes 2. Oligodendrocytes	Smaller, mesodermal in origin

Astrocytes

Structure	Functions
• These are star-shaped cells • They have multiple processes that envelop the synapse. • They are of two types: Fibrous astrocytes and protoplasmic astrocytes	1. They help in forming the blood–brain barrier around the endothelial cells of the capillaries. 2. They help in providing nutrition to the neurons 3. They help in maintaining ion balance across the cell membrane 4. Help in repair processes following trauma

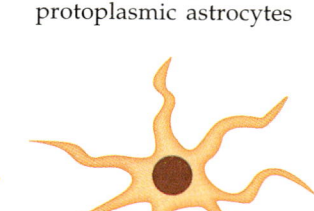

Oligodendrocytes

Structure	Functions
• They are large glial cells. • They have a few dendrons compared to other glia and neurons	1. They are responsible for production of myelin sheath 2. They also provide trophic support to the neurons

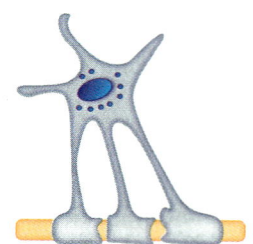

Ependymal Cell

Structure	Functions
• These are ciliated flat cells that line ventricles	1. They line ventricles and spinal canal 2. They secrete CSF (cerebrospinal fluid)

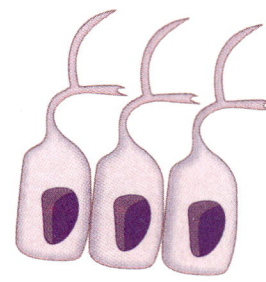

Schwann Cell

Structure	Functions
• The cell wraps around the neuron many layers and nucleus are pushed to one side	1. It helps if formation of myelin sheath 2. Myelin sheath is an important requirement of saltatory conduction

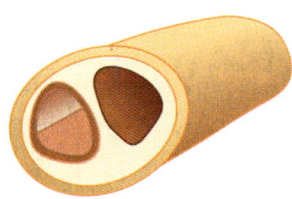

Microglia

Structure	Functions
• They are small cells with multiple dendritic projections	1. They have macrophage like function and thus protect the neurons from external agents. 2. They are constantly scavenging the brain for plaques, damages neurons and microbes. 3. They are also involved in antigen presentation

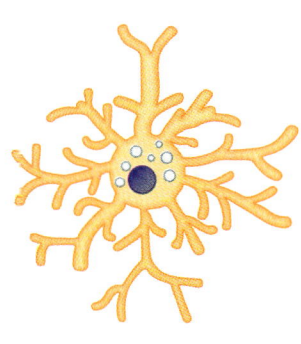

3. What is nerve growth factor?

- It is the first neurotrophin to be discovered.
- Nerve growth factor is a protein which is involved in promoting growth, survival, and maintenance of neurons.
- It is mainly involved in growth of sympathetic nerves and some sensory nerves.
- It is also found in brain and is important for maintenance of cholinergic neurons in the basal forebrain and striatum.

Structure

- NGF is made up of 2α, 2β and 2γ subunits.
- The α subunits have trypsin-like activity.
- The β subunits are similar in structure to insulin and possess all the nerve-growth promoting activities.
- The γ subunits are serine proteases.
- The receptor for NGF is TRK-A (tyrosine kinase activity A).

3.2 DESCRIBE THE TYPES, FUNCTIONS AND PROPERTIES OF NERVE FIBERS

LONG ESSAYS

1. Describe the ionic basis of different phases of nerve action potential with a neat labeled diagram.

Nerve Action Potential

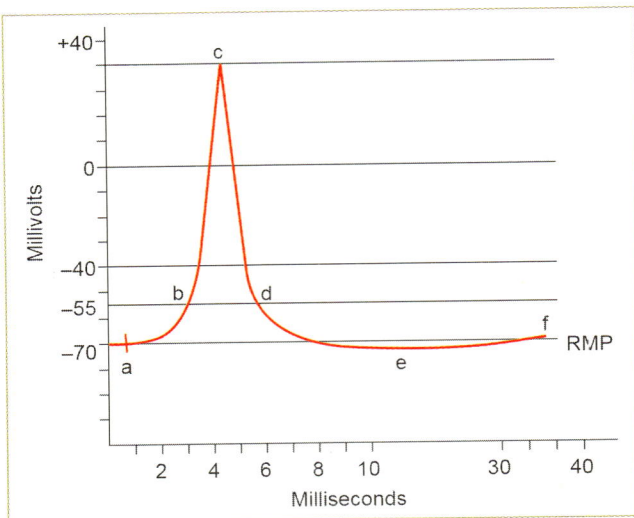

Fig. 3.2

1. **Polarization phase**
   - The resting membrane potential is –70 mV
   - This is due to more cations present in the ECF than ICF
   - This is attributed to NA-K-ATPase which causes efflux of 3 sodium ions in return for influx of 2 potassium ions.
   - Also, there are leaky potassium channels which cause efflux of potassium passively.

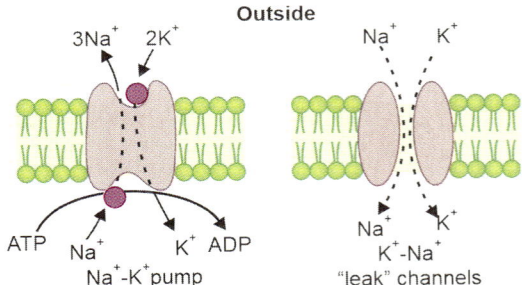

Fig. 3.3

2. **Depolarization**
   - When a threshold stimulus is applied, there is upward deflection of the spike, initially slow. Then rapid.
   - It is due to opening of new sodium channels.
   - After about 15 mV of depolarization, there is an increase in slope of the depolarization wave.
   - Depolarization crosses the isoelectric point (0 mV) and overshoots by +40 mV.

3. **Cessation of depolarization and rapid repolarization**
   - There is a downward deflection of the wave
   - Here the depolarization stops due to excess positivity inside the cell and closure of the sodium channels
   - This is due to opening of potassium channels.
   - This causes efflux of potassium ions and there is closure of sodium channels which prevent influx of sodium

4. **After depolarization**
   - It is a slow repolarization phase, that follows rapid repolarization following spike potential until the attainment of resting membrane potential
   - Slowing down of potassium efflux due to decrease in the electrical gradient

5. **After hyperpolarization**
   - After reaching the resting membrane potential, the hyperpolarization proceeds up to 2 mV more for a prolonged period (35–40 ms)
   - Due to sow efflux of potassium ions

2. Classify nerve fibers based on velocity of conduction of impulse and their diameter. Explain the factors influencing the velocity of conduction of impulse.   (5 + 5 marks)

Factors that Affect Velocity of Conduction

1. **Diameter of the nerve fiber (Fig. 3.4)**
   - Larger the diameter of neuron, faster is its conduction.
   - This is because, larger nerves have a larger surface area and thus more electrons flow on the surface of the nerve.

Classification of nerve fibres			
Erlanger-Gasser classification Based on diameter of nerve fibers and conduction of impulses			
Type	Fiber diameter (µm)	Conduction velocity (m/s)	Function
Aα	12–20	70–120	Proprioception; somatic motor
Aβ	5–12	30–70	Touch, pressure
Aγ	3–6	15–30	Motor to muscle spindles
Aδ	2–5	12–30	Pain, cold, touch
B	<3	3–15	Preganglionic autonomic
C (smallest)			
C-dorsal root	0.4–1.2	0.5–2	Pain, temperature, some mechanoreception, reflex responses
C-sympathetic	0.3–1.3	0.7–2.3	Postganglionic sympathetics

- A and B fibers are myelinated; C fibers are unmyelinated
- Velocity of conduction ∞ thickness of the fibers

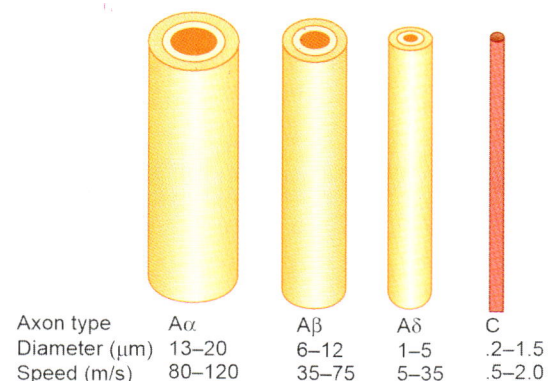

Axon type	Aα	Aβ	Aδ	C
Diameter (µm)	13–20	6–12	1–5	.2–1.5
Speed (m/s)	80–120	35–75	5–35	.5–2.0

Fig. 3.4

2. **Presence or absence of myelination (Fig. 3.9)**

- Myelin sheath produces insulation around the nerve except at nodes of Ranvier. Thus, resistance across membrane increases but capacitance decreases.
- In presence of myelination, the type of conduction is saltatory. The impulse jumps from one to another node of Ranvier. As a result, the velocity of conduction is faster in myelinated nerve fibers.
- In unmyelinated nerves, the conduction is electrotonic and spreads point to point.

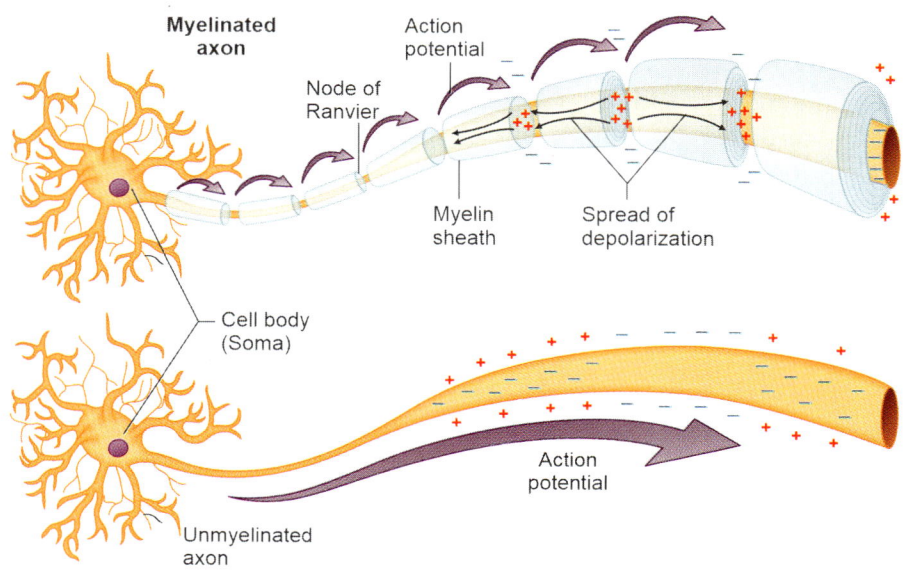

Fig. 3.5

3. **Temperature:** Increase in temperature increases velocity of conduction.

SHORT ESSAYS

1. What is resting membrane potential? Explain its ionic basis.

Resting Membrane Potential

- It is the potential difference across the membrane of a neuron prior to beginning of an action potential and its value is –70 mV. That means the potential inside the nerve fibre is –70 mV lower than its exterior.
- The factors involved in maintaining this potential is the ionic gradient created across the membrane.
- It is mainly maintained through Na-K pump and Na-K leaky channels.

Role of Sodium Potassium Active Pumps

- It is a powerful pump that continuously pumps K^+ ions inside the cell and Na^+ ions outside the cell with the help of ATP
- It is an electrogenic pump, in the sense that, it pumps $3Na^+$ ions out and allows two K^+ ions inside the cell.
- As a result, a negative charge is created. Also, a gradient is created.

Na^+ (extracellular)	142 mEq/L	Ratio: 0.1
Na^+ (intracellular)	14 mEq/L	(inside:outside)
K^+ (extracellular)	4 mEq/L	Ratio: 35
K^+ (intracellular)	140 mEq/L	(inside:outside)

Role of Leak Channels

- These provide leakage of ions across the membrane and are 100 times more permeable to potassium influx.
- As a result, passive influx of sodium ions is much less compared to passive outflux of potassium ions.

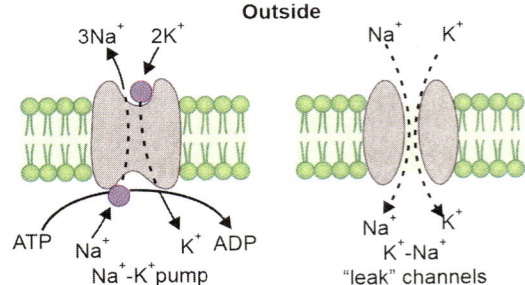

Fig. 3.6

- Further efflux of potassium ions is prevented by relative positivity outside the cell which prevents its efflux and negativity within the cell which keeps the potassium within.

2. Enumerate the properties of nerve fiber. Explain any four of them.

Properties of Nerve Fiber

1. Excitability
2. Conductivity
3. Refractory period
4. Summation
5. Adaptation
6. All-or-none law
7. Infatigability

Excitability

- It is defined as physicochemical changes occurring in the nerve when a stimulus is applied.
- Stimulus is an external agent that produces excitability in a nerve.
- When the nerve is stimulated, depending on the strength of the stimulus applied, two types of potentials are generated.
  1. **Action potential**
     - It develops when a threshold stimulus is applied to a nerve.
     - It is a propagative.
  2. **Electrotonic potential**
     - When the strength of the stimulus is sub-threshold, the potential produced is electrotonic or local potential.
     - It is slight depolarization of around 7 mV.
     - It is nonpropagative and does not obey all-or-none law.

Conductivity

- It is the ability of the nerve to transmit impulse from the area of stimulus to a distal area on the nerve.
- Depolarization occurs at a point on the nerve where stimulus is applied.
- This if followed depolarization of the neighboring area and thus the impulse spreads.
- In an unmyelinated fiber, action potential spreads from point to point.

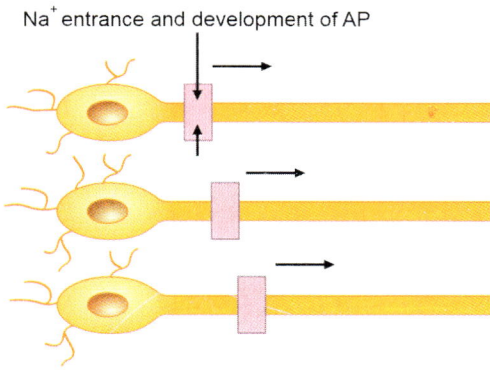

Na$^+$ entrance and development of AP

Fig. 3.7

- In a myelinated nerve, the type of conduction if saltatory.
- As the myelin produces insulation around the nerve, the points at which myelin is absent, form the depolarization points.
- Impulse jumps from one to another node of Ranvier.

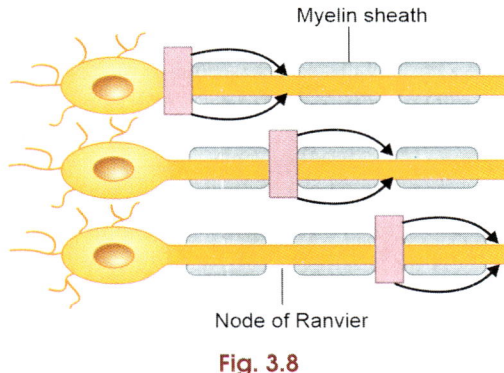

Myelin sheath

Node of Ranvier

Fig. 3.8

Refractory Period

- It is the period of the action potential, during which the nerve cannot respond to another stimulus.
- It is divided as absolute and relative refractory period.
- Absolute refractory period is the period during which the nerve cannot be stimulated by a stimulus of any strength.
- It is the period when the firing level is reached till one-third of repolarization is complete.
- The cause for this is during firing level, fast sodium channels are open. While repolarizing, the sodium channels are closed and potassium channels are not yet open. As a result, the sodium ion channels cannot open till the particular potential is reached.

- Relative refractory period is the period in which the nerve shows response to a suprathreshold of stimulus.
- It extends form the end of absolute refractory period till the beginning of the after depolarization.
- In this phase, sodium ion channels are slowly getting activated and potassium ion channels are open. A supramaximal stimulus can activated more sodium ion channels to open and lead to depolarization.

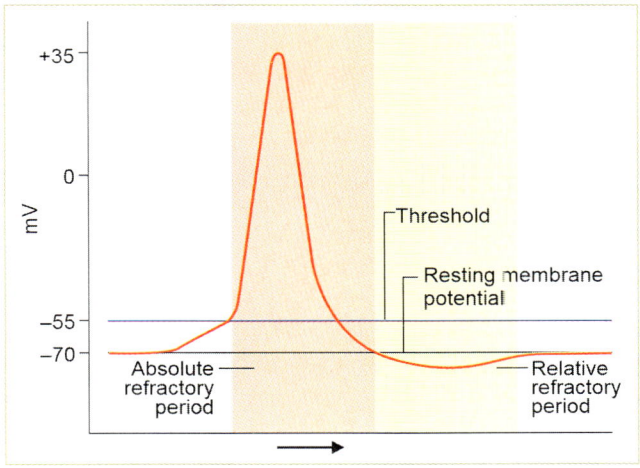

Fig. 3.9

All-or-None Law

- When a nerve is stimulated, it either gives a maximal response or does not give any response depending on the strength of the stimulus.
- When the stimulus is subthreshold, there is no action potential produced (represented by A and B).

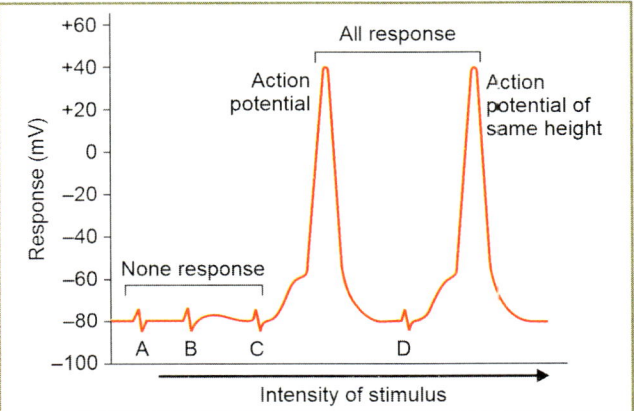

Fig. 3.10

- When the stimulus is threshold, the action potential is produced in full response (represented by C).
- When the stimulus is suprathreshold, same action potential is produced (represented by D).

3. A 6-year-old boy comes to the OPD with a gaping wound in the leg. The doctor who attended the boy had to suture the wound after giving local anesthetics.

A. Explain the mechanism by which local anesthetics block the pain sensation.
                                                                (3 marks)
B. Group the nerve fibers based on their degree of susceptibility to hypoxia, pressure, and local anesthetics.   (2 marks)

A. Mechanism of Local Anesthetics (Fig. 3.11)

- For a nerve to conduct, there should occur depolarization due to entry of sodium ions through sodium channels.
- Local anesthetics like lignocaine and benzocaine bind with these sodium channels.
- This blocks depolarization and blocks conduction of action potential.
- Thus, the sensations of pain are not conducted.

B. Classification of Nerve Fibers

- Letter classification of Erlanger and Gasser is based on the diameter of nerve fibres and their conduction velocity.
- Type A fibres are myelinated, large diameter and conduct fastest. They are most susceptible to pressure and least susceptible to local anesthetics.
- Type B fibers are myelinated, medium diameter and conduct slower than type A. they are most susceptible to hypoxia.

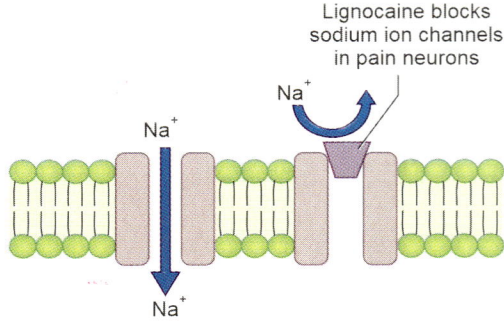

Lignocaine blocks sodium ion channels in pain neurons

Fig. 3.11

- Type C fibres are unmyelinated and have small diameter and thus conduct slowly. They are pain fibers. They are most susceptible to action of local anaesthetics and least susceptible to hypoxia and pressure.

Physio-clinical classification			
Susceptibility to	Most susceptible	Intermediate	Least susceptible
Hypoxia	B	A	C
Pressure	A	B	C
Local anesthetics	C	B	A

A and B fibers are myelinated; C fibers are unmyelinated

4. A patient complained of double vision while looking to the left and some stiffness in the left leg. On examination, while performing leftward gaze her left eye abducts but her right eye does not adduct, though her right eye adduct on convergence of eyeballs. Her left leg is indeed stiff with hyperactive reflexes and a positive Babinski sign. She was diagnosed with multiple sclerosis.   (5 marks)
A. Which property of nerve is disturbed in multiple sclerosis and why?   (2 marks)
B. Mention what type of nerve conduction happening in the otherwise normal nerves affected in this condition.   (1 mark)
C. Describe Erlanger and Gasser classification of nerve fibers.   (2 marks)

A.

- In multiple sclerosis, conduction of the nerve is disturbed.
- Multiple sclerosis is an autoimmune condition characterized by lymphocyte-induced damage to

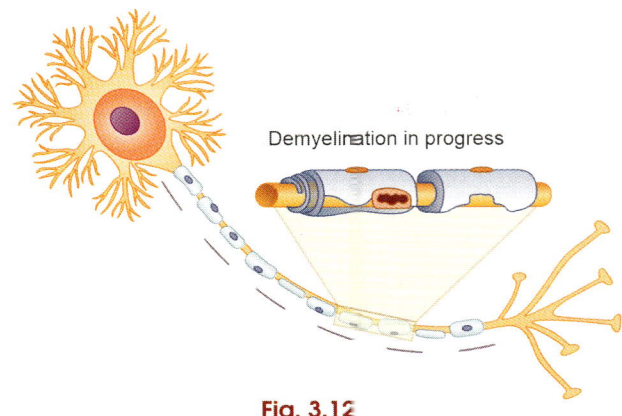

Demyelination in progress

Fig. 3.12

the myelin sheath leading to demyelination of the nerve.

B.

Normally, in myelinated nerves the type of conduction is saltatory conduction.

C Classification of Nerve Fibres

Erlanger-Gasser classification Based on diameter of nerve fibers and conduction of impulses			
Type	Fiber diameter (μm)	Conduction velocity (m/s)	Function
Aα	12–20	70–120	Proprioception; somatic motor
Aβ	5–12	30–70	Touch, pressure
Aγ	3–6	15–30	Motor to muscle spindles
Aδ	2–5	12–30	Pain, cold, touch
B	<3	3–15	Preganglionic autonomic
C (smallest)			
C-dorsal root	0.4–1.2	0.5–2	Pain, temperature, some mechano-reception, reflex responses
C-sympathetic	0.3–1.3	0.7–2.3	Postganglionic sympathetics

- A and B fibers are myelinated; C fibers are unmyelinated
- Velocity of conduction ∞ thickness of the fibers

---

5. A man falls into deep sleep with one arm under his head. This arm is paralyzed when he awakens but it tingles and pain sensation in it is still intact. There is loss of motor function without loss of pain sensation in the nerve to his arm.

A. What sort of nerve injury do you expect in this case? (1 mark)

B. Describe Numerical classification of nerve fiber. (2 marks)

C. Explain the susceptibility of different types of nerve fibers to conduction block produced by various agents. (2 marks)

A

- This nerve injury is called neuropraxia or grade I injury.
- It is characterized by transient loss of function
- Results from mild pressure on the nerve, there is damage to myelin

B. Numerical Classification of Nerve Fiber

Numerical classification		
Number	Origin	Fiber type
Ia	Muscle spindle, annulospiral ending	Aα
Ib	Golgi tendon organ	Aα
II	Muscle spindle, flower-spray ending; touch, pressure	Aβ
III	Pain and cold receptors; some touch receptors	Aδ
IV	Pain, temperature and other receptors	Dorsal root C

C.

- Type A fibres are myelinated, large diameter and conduct fastest. They are most susceptible to pressure and least susceptible to local anesthetics.
- Type B fibers are myelinated, medium diameter and conduct slower than type A. They are most susceptible to hypoxia.
- Type C fibres are unmyelinated and have small diameter and thus conduct slowly. They are pain fibers. They are most susceptible to action of local anaesthetics and least susceptible to hypoxia and pressure.

Susceptibility to	Most susceptible	Intermediate	Least susceptible
Hypoxia	B	A	C
Pressure	A	B	C
Local anesthetics	C	B	A

6. Compare and contrast graded potential with that of action potential.

Parameter	Graded potential	Action potential
Amplitude of the potential	Varies with intensity of the stimulus	Remains constant irrespective of strength of stimulus
Summation	Can get summated	Cannot be summated
Type of polarization	Can be depolarizing or hyperpolarizing	Always depolarizing
Duration	Varies with triggering factor	Always constant
Refractory period	Absent	Present
Generation	Can be generated from spontaneously or by physical or chemical stimulus	Generated only in response to membrane depolarization
Conductivity	Cannot conduct impulses	Can conduct impulses
Examples	Motor endplate potential	Action potential at a nerve fiber

7. Describe transmission of nerve impulse in myelinated and unmyelinated nerve fibers.

Transmission of Nerve Impulse

- When an impulse reaches a nerve, it is propagated. It is called conductivity.
- It differs in a myelinated and a non-myelinated nerve.

Transmission in Myelinated Nerve Fiber: Saltatory Conduction (Fig. 3.13)

- Myelin sheath is like an insulation and thus does not allow flow of current from inside to outside.
- Myelin is absent at points on the nerve called nodes of Ranvier.
- As a result, the local circuit which is generated at these nodes will jump from one node to the other.
- This is 50–100 times faster than electrotonic conduction.

Transmission in Non-myelinated Nerve Fiber: Slow Spread (Fig. 3.14)

- In the resting phase, the axonal membrane is positive on the outside and negative inside.
- When stimulated at the centre of the nerve, impulses are conducted both ways. But if stimulated at one end, it travels to the other direction.

- When stimulated at one point, the exterior of the nerve becomes negative and interior is positive. There is reversal of polarity
- A local circuit is setup between the positive interior and negative exterior.
- This local current moves from the depolarized part of the nerve to the resting part of the nerve.
- The new area is fired up to the level of depolarization and this continues.
- This phenomenon is called electrotonic potential. It is always unidirectional as the previous part of the nerve is in refractory state.

8. What are the types of action potentials? Describe the method of recording.

1. **Monophasic action potential**
   - One electrode is placed within the nerve fiber and the other on the nerve surface. They are connected to a cathode ray oscilloscope.
   - When the nerve is stimulated, an action potential curve is obtained.

2. **Biphasic action potential (Fig. 3.15)**
   - In this, both the electrodes are placed on the surface of the nerve fibre
   - They are connected to a cathode ray tube.
   - When the nerve is stimulated, excitation of one electrode causes a wave in a direction opposite to the other.

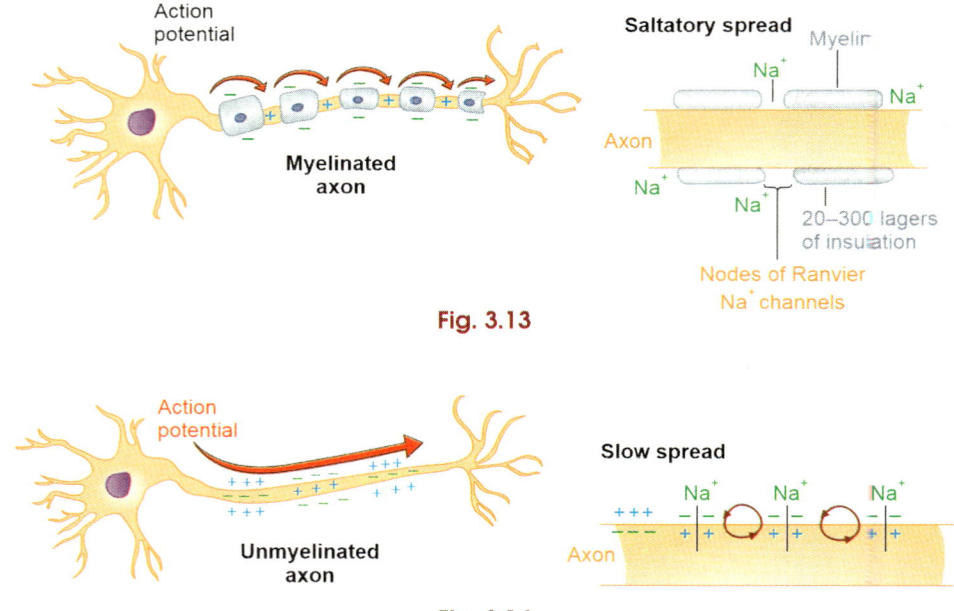

Action potential

Myelinated axon

Saltatory spread Myelin

Na$^+$ Na$^+$

Axon

Na$^+$ Na$^+$

20–300 lagers of insulation

Nodes of Ranvier
Na$^+$ channels

Fig. 3.13

Action potential

Unmyelinated axon

Slow spread

Na$^+$ Na$^+$ Na$^+$

Axon

Fig. 3.14

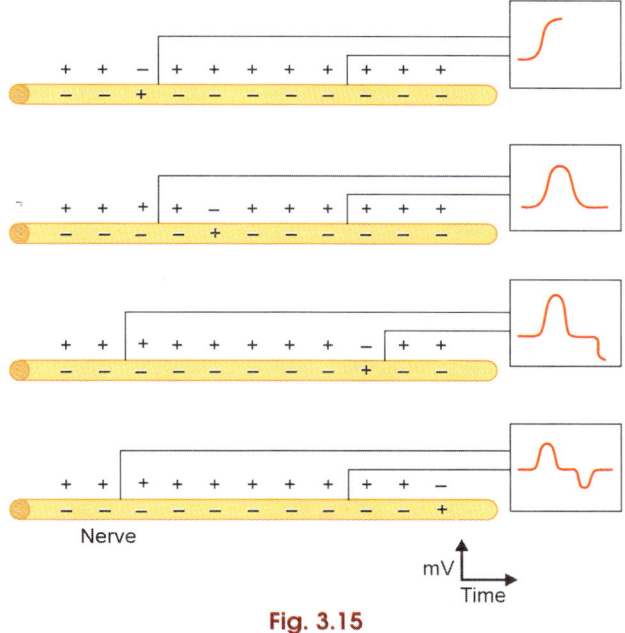

Fig. 3.15

3. Compound action potential (Fig. 3.16)

- It is the monophasic recording of action potential from a mixed nerve which contains different types of nerves with varying diameter.
- The compound action potential is the algebraic sum of action potentials of all neurons.
- This again depends on the threshold for stimulation for every neuron and the distance from the point of application of stimulus.
- When a subthreshold stimulus is applied, none of the neurons conduct due to all-or-none phenomenon.

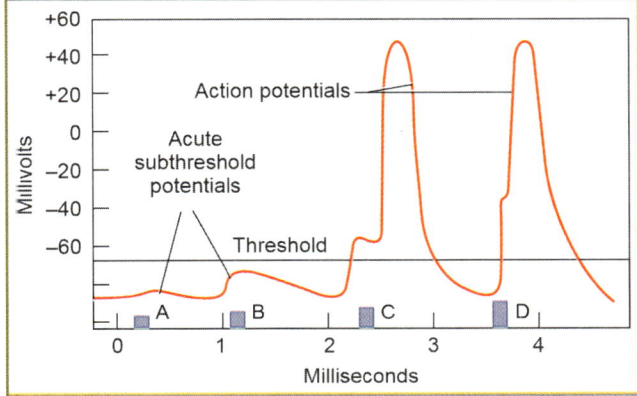

Fig. 3.16

- When the stimulus is slightly increased, neurons whose threshold is lower than the applied stimulus get fired.
- Thus, there is response (represented by A).
- With further increase in threshold, more and more neurons get fired. However, the algebraic sum is not great enough to produce a response. (represented by B).
- Maximal stimulus is the strength of the stimulus which can excite all neurons in a nerve trunk. (represented by C).
- Supramaximal stimulus is the strength of the stimulus which cannot produce any further increase in the action potential (represented by D).

SHORT ANSWERS

1. What is saltatory conduction of impulse?

- It refers to conduction of an action potential in a myelinated nerve.
- Myelin sheath is like an insulation and thus does not allow flow of current from inside to outside.
- Myelin is absent at points on the nerve called nodes of Ranvier.
- As a result, the local circuit which is generated at these nodes will jump from one node to the other.
- This is 50–100 times faster than electrotonic conduction (Fig. 3.17).

2. What is orthodromic and antidromic conduction of nerve impulse?

- Orthodromic conduction is when the impulse travels away from the Soma (Fig. 3.18).
- Antidromic conduction is when the impulse travels towards the Soma.
- This is seen in conduction of a sensory impulse.

3. Describe cathode ray oscilloscope.

Cathode Ray Oscilloscope (Fig. 3.19)

- It is an inertia less instrument used to measure and record live electrical activity in a living tissue.
- It consists of a glass tube with a cathode, fluorescent surface and two sets of electrically charged plates—2 vertical and 2 horizontal.
- Cathode is in the form of a gun. When connected to an anode and electricity passes, the cathode shoots electrons.

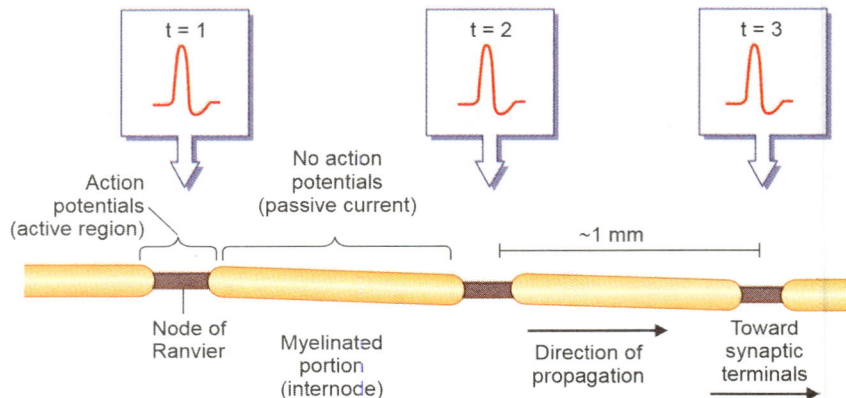

Fig. 3.17

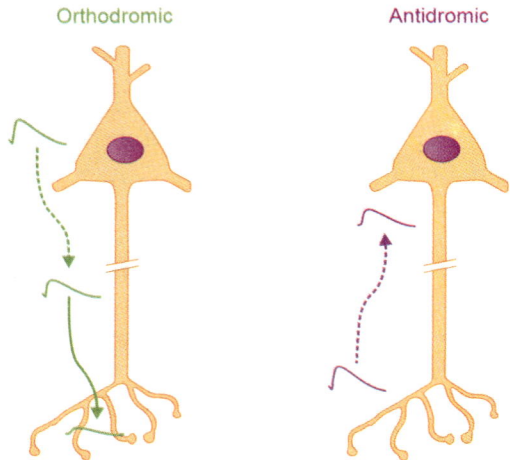

Orthodromic   Antidromic

Fig. 3.18

- The face of the glass tube is coated with fluorescent material and acts as a screen.
- It forms a receptor for the electrons.
- The horizontally oriented plates are placed on either side of the beams and are connected to an electronic sweep generator.
- When a voltage is applied at the plates, the beam of electrons is attracted towards the positively charged plate and is repelled by the negatively charged plate.
- The electron beam is made to sweep the across the fluorescent screen by gradually increasing and suddenly decreasing the voltage across the plates.
- The electrons gradually deflect towards the positively charged plate and then suddenly revert to the centre.

- The vertical deflection plates are placed above and below the electron beam. They are connected to recording electrodes placed on the nerve via an electronic amplifier.
- These plates detect potential changes in the nerve by charging the plates and thus gives a reading on the screen. This helps to record the action potential as vertical deflections.

4. Discuss the implications of the absolute and relative refractory period.

- It is the period of the action potential, during which the nerve cannot respond to another stimulus.
- It is divided as absolute and relative refractory period.

Absolute Refractory Period

- Absolute refractory period is the period during which the nerve cannot be stimulated by a stimulus of any strength.
- It is the period when the firing level is reached till one-third of repolarization is complete.
- The cause for this is during firing level, fast sodium channels are open. While repolarizing, the sodium channels are closed, and potassium channels are not yet open. As a result, the sodium ion channels cannot open till the potential is reached.
- The duration of this period is important in preventing formation of tetanus.
- As absolute refractory period is long in cardiac muscles, tetanus does not occur. However, it is shorter in skeletal muscles and thus there is tetanus when multiple simultaneous stimuli are applied.

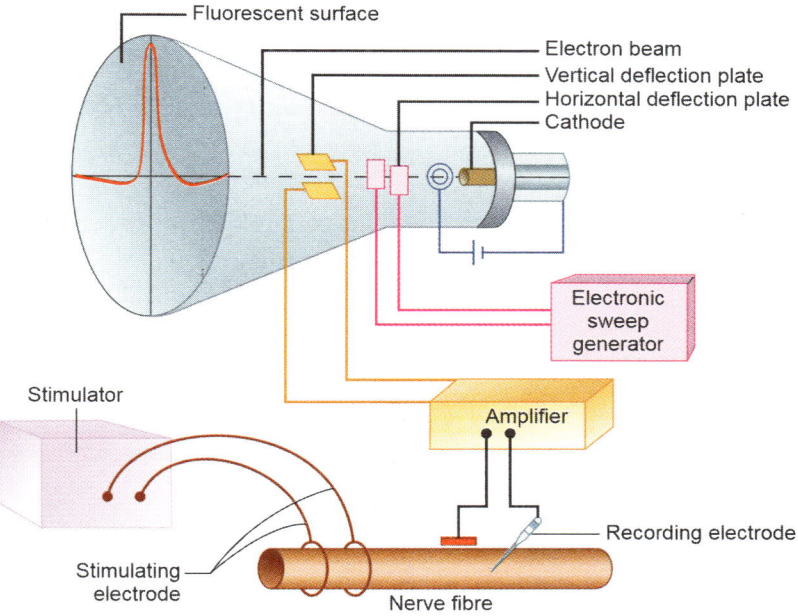

Fig. 3.19

Relative Refractory Period (Fig. 3.20)

- Relative refractory period is the period in which the nerve shows response to a suprathreshold of stimulus.
- It extends from the end of absolute refractory period till the beginning of the after depolarization.
- In this phase, sodium ion channels are slowly getting activated and potassium ion channels are open. A supramaximal stimulus can activate more sodium ion channels to open and lead to depolarization.

5. Explain with the help of a diagram, the concept of 'local currents' in a nerve.

Local Currents (Figs 3.21 and 3.22)

- When a stimulus arrives at a point on the nerve, there is depolarization due to entry of sodium ions.
- As a result, the inside of the nerve in that segment becomes positively charged and the outside becomes negative.
- As a result, electrons move towards positive charge. So, current flows in short segments from the positive depolarized segment to non-depolarized segment adjacent to it.
- This causes a local circuit formation which gets propagated.

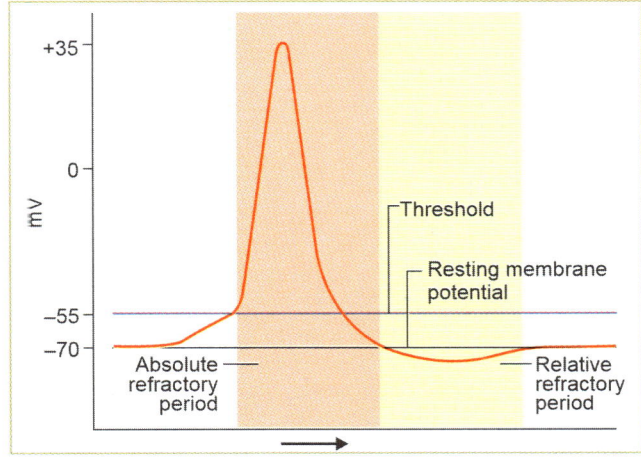

Fig. 3.20

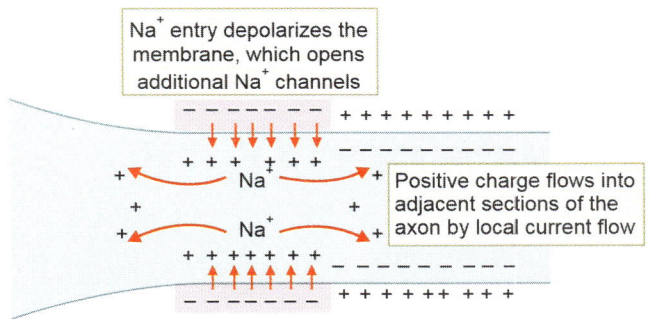

Na$^+$ entry depolarizes the membrane, which opens additional Na$^+$ channels

Positive charge flows into adjacent sections of the axon by local current flow

Fig. 3.21

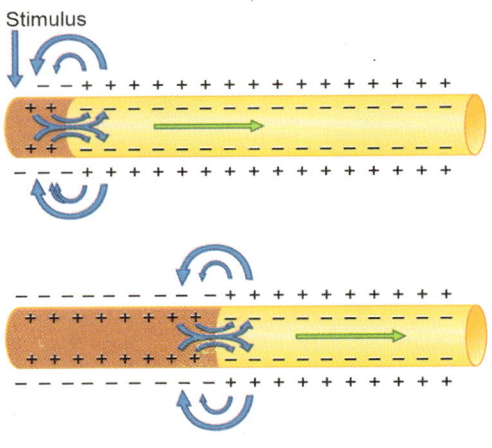

Stimulus

Fig. 3.22

6. List the factors which affect conduction velocity in a nerve.

Factors of the individual

1. Age
2. Temperature

Factors related to the nerve

1. Myelination
2. Diameter
3. Hypoxia

Hormones/drugs

1. Vagal stimulation decreases conduction
2. Adrenergic drugs increase conduction

3.3 DESCRIBE THE DEGENERATION AND REGENERATION IN PERIPHERAL NERVES

LONG ESSAY

1. **A 45-year-old lab technician complains of pain and electric shock like sensation in his left hand at night. He also notices increasing clumsiness and weakness of his left hand. On physical examination, it was noted that there was decreased sensation to light touch, pinprick and temperature on the palmar surface of the thumb and first two fingers on the left hand. The left thumb is weak, and its muscle is atrophied. The right hand is entirely normal in sensation and motor function. The patient is otherwise healthy. He was diagnosed with left-sided carpal tunnel syndrome.**

   A. **Which nerve is affected in this condition?** (1 mark)

   B. **What type of nerve injury do you expect in this condition?** (1 mark)

   C. **Classify different types of nerve injury (3 marks)**

   D. **What is Wallerian degeneration? Describe the changes that happen in the distal segment of the axon when it is sectioned. (3 marks)**

   E. **Describe the regenerative changes that happen following nerve injury** (2 marks)

A. Left Median Nerve is Affected

B. Type of Injury: It is Second Degree Injury or Axonotmesis

C. Different Types of Nerve Injury: Sunderland's Classification

First degree injury	• Transient loss of function • Results from mild pressure on the nerve, there is damage to myelin • Also called neuropraxia • Their function returns within hours or days
Second degree injury	• Severe nerve damage with intact endoneural tube • Results from severe prolonged pressure on the nerve • Also called axonotmesis • There is degeneration of nerve at the site of injury • Regeneration is complete
Third degree injury	• Severely damaged nerve and damage to the endoneural tube • Perineurium and epineurium are intact • Slow regeneration and needs surgical approximation if no recovery
Fourth degree injury	• Severely damaged nerve and disorganized nerve fasciculi • Endoneurium and perineurium disrupted • Perineurium intact • Regeneration only after repair
Fifth degree injury	• Also called neurotmesis • Complete transection and disruption of the whole nerve trunk

D. Wallerian Degeneration

- Changes that occur in the distal part of the nerve following injury is called anterograde degeneration or Wallerian degeneration.
- It starts within 3 hours of injury and regeneration takes about 3 months.
- The changes happen in the distal segment of the axon when sectioned are:
  - The axis cylinder swells up and is broken into pieces. These pieces occupy the space that was occupied by the axis cylinder.
  - The myelin sheath is disintegrated into small droplets of fat. Nissl granules disappear.
  - The neurilemmal sheath is unaffected. Macrophages invade from outside and clear the debris of fat and axonal pieces.
  - Schwann cells multiply steadily. They fill up the cytoplasm of the neurilemmal sheath.

E. Regenerative Changes

Anatomical Regeneration

Stage of fiber formation

- The proximal cut end of the axon gives out around 100 fibrils in all directions.
- These branches grow into the connective tissue at the site of injury.

Stage of entry of fibrils into endoneural tube

- Strands of Schwann cells from the distal end of the nerve guide these fibrils to enter the neuronal tube.
- The fibrils which fail to enter the tube degenerate. The ones within the neuronal tube grow rapidly.

Stage of active growth

- The axonal fibril grows and establishes contact with the peripheral end organ.
- It is bare and devoid of myelin sheath

Stage of myelination

- The Schwann cells slowly form myelin
- It usually takes a year to be complete.

SHORT ESSAYS

1. **A 52-year-old male presented with sever intermittent pain on the left side of the face. Magnetic resonance imaging with contrast revealed a close association of the superior cerebellar artery and the trigeminal nerve on left side of the face. He was diagnosed to have Trigeminal nerve neuralgia.**

   A. What type of nerve injury do you expect in this condition?   (1 mark)

   B. Describe grading of nerve injury. (3 marks)

   C. List any four nerve growth factors (1 mark)

A. This is a First-Degree Nerve Injury or Neuropraxia.

B. Types of Nerve Injuries: Sunderland's Classification

First degree injury	• Transient loss of function • Results from mild pressure on the nerve, there is damage to myelin • Also called neuropraxia • Their function returns within hours or days
Second degree injury	• Severe nerve damage with intact endoneural tube • Results from severe prolonged pressure on the nerve • Also called axonotmesis • There is degeneration of nerve at the site of injury • Regeneration is complete
Third degree injury	• Severely damaged nerve and damage to the endoneural tube • Perineurium and epineurium are intact • Slow regeneration and needs surgical approximation if no recovery

Fourth degree injury	• Severely damaged nerve and disorganized nerve fasciculi • Endoneurium and perineurium disrupted • Perineurium intact • Regeneration only after repair
Fifth degree injury	• Also called neurotmesis • Complete transection and disruption of the whole nerve trunk

C. Neurotrophins

1. Nerve growth factor
2. Brain derived neurotropic factor
3. Neurotrophin 3
4. Neurotrophin 4

2. Describe Wallerian degeneration with the help of a diagram.

- Changes that occur in the distal part of the nerve following injury is called anterograde degeneration or Wallerian degeneration.
- It starts within 3 hours of injury and regeneration takes about 3 months.
- The changes are:
  - The axis cylinder swells up and is broken into pieces. These pieces occupy the space that was occupied by the axis cylinder.
  - The myelin sheath is disintegrated into small droplets of fat. Nissl granules disappear.
  - The neurilemmal sheath is unaffected. Macrophages invade from outside and clear the debris of fat and axonal pieces.

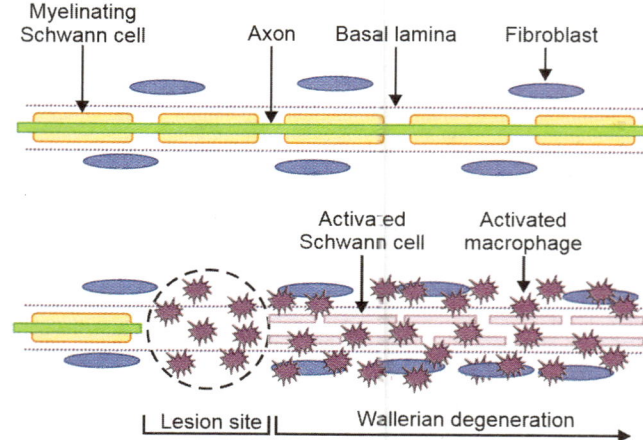

Fig. 3.23

– Schwann cells multiply steadily. They fill up the cytoplasm of the neurilemmal sheath.

SHORT ANSWERS

1. Explain the phenomenon that occurs in the target tissue when a nerve is cut and the distal axon degenerates.

- Changes that occur in the distal part of the nerve following injury is called anterograde degeneration or Wallerian degeneration.
- It starts within 3 hours of injury and regeneration takes about 3 months.
- The changes are:
  - The axis cylinder swells up and is broken into pieces. These pieces occupy the space that was occupied by the axis cylinder.
  - The myelin sheath is disintegrated into small droplets of fat. Nissl granules disappear.
  - The neurilemmal sheath is unaffected. Macrophages invade from outside and clear the debris of fat and axonal pieces.
  - Schwann cells multiply steadily. They fill up the cytoplasm of the neurilemmal sheath.

2. Explain types of nerve injuries.

Types of nerve injuries: Sunderland's classification

First degree injury	• Transient loss of function
	• Results from mild pressure on the nerve, there is damage to myelin
	• Also called neuropraxia
	• Their function returns within hours or days
Second degree injury	• Severe nerve damage with intact endoneural tube
	• Results from severe prolonged pressure on the nerve
	• Also called axonotmesis
	• There is degeneration of nerve at the site of injury
	• Regeneration is complete
Third degree injury	• Severely damaged nerve and damage to the endoneural tube
	• Perineurium and epineurium are intact
	• Slow regeneration and needs surgical approximation if no recovery

Fourth degree injury	• Severely damaged nerve and disorganized nerve fasciculi
	• Endoneurium and perineurium disrupted
	• Perineurium intact
	• Regeneration only after repair
Fifth degree injury	• Also called neurotmesis
	• Complete transection and disruption of the whole nerve trunk

3. List some common causes of neuropathy.

Anatomic
1. Sciatic compression
2. Carpal tunnel syndrome fibular nerve compression in compartment syndrome
3. Traumatic

Systemic
1. HIV infection
2. Paraneoplastic conditions
3. Amyloidosis

Metabolic
1. Diabetes
2. Thyrotoxicosis

Toxic
1. Vitamin B_1, B_6, B_{12} deficiency
2. Heavy metal poisoning
3. Drug induced: Arsenic, mercury, lead

4. Explain the changes during regeneration of a damaged nerve. List the factors affecting nerve regeneration.

Regeneration of a Damage Nerve

Anatomical Regeneration

Stage of fiber formation
- The proximal cut end of the axon gives out around 100 fibrils in all directions.
- These branches grow into the connective tissue at the site of injury.

Stage of entry of fibrils into endoneural tube
- Strands of Schwann cells from the distal end of the nerve guide these fibrils to enter the neuronal tube.
- The fibrils which fail to enter the tube degenerate. The ones within the neuronal tube grow rapidly.

Stage of active growth
- The axonal fibril grows and establishes contact with the peripheral end organ.
- It is bare and devoid of myelin sheath

Stage of myelination

- The Schwann cells slowly form myelin
- It usually takes a year to be complete.

Factors Affecting Nerve Regeneration

1. **Distance between the cut ends:** Should be less than 3 mm

2. **Alignment of the cut ends:** If the cut ends are not aligned, regeneration does not occur.

3. **Presence or absence of neurilemma:** It is integral to regeneration. It is absent in the CNS.

4. **Intactness of the nucleus:** If the nucleus is extruded, regeneration does not occur.

3.4 DESCRIBE THE STRUCTURE OF NEUROMUSCULAR JUNCTION AND TRANSMISSION OF IMPULSES

LONG ESSAY

1. **Describe the structure of neuromuscular junction with the help of a diagram and explain the mechanism of transmission of nerve impulse across it.**

Neuromuscular Junction (Fig. 3.24)

- A neuromuscular junction consists of terminal portion of nerve fibre and muscle fibre.
- Each terminal branch innervates one muscle fibre through neuromuscular junction.
- The nerve fibre loses myelin sheath when it meets the muscle fibre. This portion of the axis cylinder is expanded like a bulb which is called motor endplate.
- It contains mitochondria and synaptic vesicles. These vesicles contain acetylcholine (ACh). The mitochondria synthesize ACh.

Mechanism of Transmission of Nerve Impulse

Release of ACh

- When the action potential reaches the axon terminal, voltage-gated calcium channels open.
- Calcium ions enter the presynaptic membrane, and this leads to rupture of vesicles.
- The ACh that is released is brought out by exocytosis.
- Around 10,000 molecules of ACh are released each time a vesicle bursts and each motor endplate has 300 vesicles that burst.

Action of ACh

- The ACh is released into the presynaptic cleft.
- They bind with the nicotinic receptors on the post-synaptic membrane and form a complex.
- The binding causes opening of the sodium channels.

Development of Endplate Potential

- Influx of sodium decreases the resting membrane potential and generates an endplate potential.
- Its value is around –60 mV. It is nonpropagative in nature but causes formation of action potential.

Development of Miniature Endplate Potential

- It is a minute potential produced during each time during a potential reaches the axon.
- Its magnitude is as low as 0.5 mV.
- It cannot produce action potential by itself. When more and more miniature endplate potentials add up, an action potential is produced.

Destruction of ACh

- Acetylcholinesterase destroys the ACh which is released into the synaptic cleft within a millisecond.
- It is split into acetate and choline which is taken up by the presynaptic membrane and recycled.

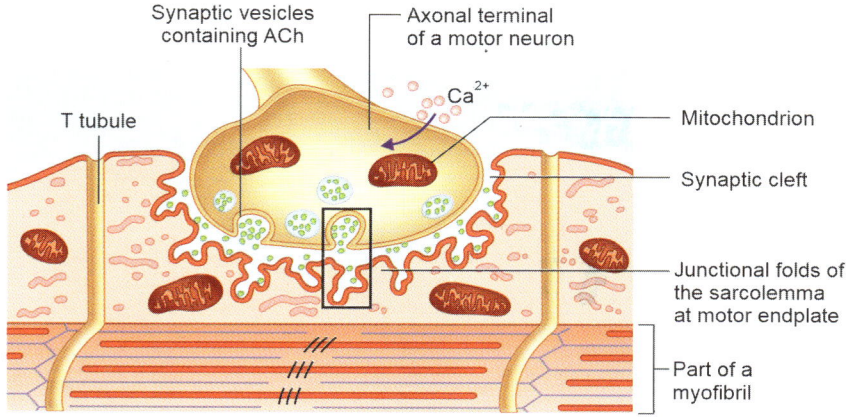

Fig. 3.24

SHORT ESSAYS

1. A middle-aged individual presented with weakness of limbs which is bad at the initiation of the movement and becomes better with repetition. He was diagnosed with Lambert-Eaton myasthenia syndrome.

> **A. What is Lambert-Eaton myasthenia syndrome?** (1 mark)
> **B. Explain why there is improvement in movements with repetition.** (2 marks)
> **C. Enumerate neuromuscular blocking agents with examples.** (2 marks)

A. Lambert-Eaton Syndrome (Fig. 3.25)

- It is a paraneoplastic syndrome usually associated with carcinoma of lung.
- It is seen more in men than women
- In this, there is antibody-mediated destruction of calcium channels on the presynaptic membrane.
- As a result, there is decreased ACh released which decreases myoneural transmission.

B.

- With repetitive exercise, more and more action potentials reach the neuromuscular junction causing increased recruitment of calcium vesicle and their release in the synaptic cleft.
- Thus, due to increased availability of calcium, there is improvement of muscle function.

C. Neuromuscular Blockers

Neuromuscular blocking agents are broadly classified as Depolarizing and Nondepolarizing agents.

1. **Depolarizing agents**
   - The drug which belongs to this category is succinylcholine.
   - It acts by binding to the ACh receptors irreversibly at the postsynaptic membrane.
   - Thereby it causes depolarization. As it is not removed by cholinesterase, it remains attached and cause prolonged depolarization and flaccid paralysis.

2. **Nondepolarizing agents**
   - These agents compete with ACh to bind to the nicotinic receptors on the motor endplate.
   - Thus, they block the action of ACh and thus cannot cause endplate potential.
   - Examples are curare, pancuronium, vecuronium, botulinum toxin, bungarotoxin.

2. What is Lambert-Eaton syndrome?

- It is a paraneoplastic syndrome usually associated with carcinoma of lung (Fig. 3.26).
- It is seen more in men than women
- In this, there is antibody-mediated destruction of calcium channels on the presynaptic membrane.
- As a result, there is decreased ACh released which decreases myoneural transmission.

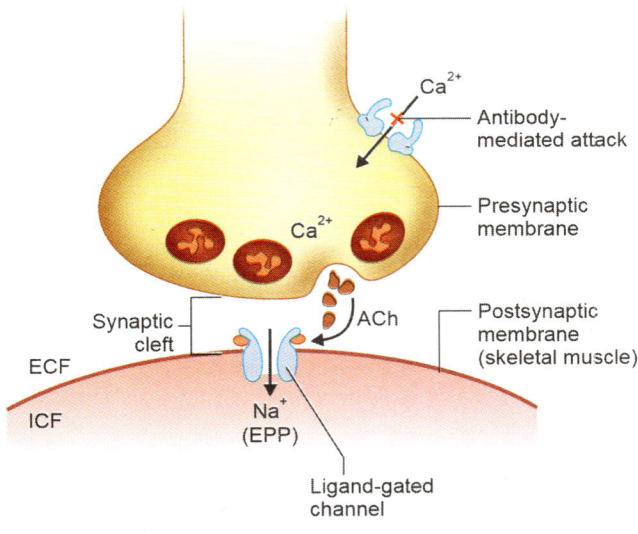

Fig. 3.25

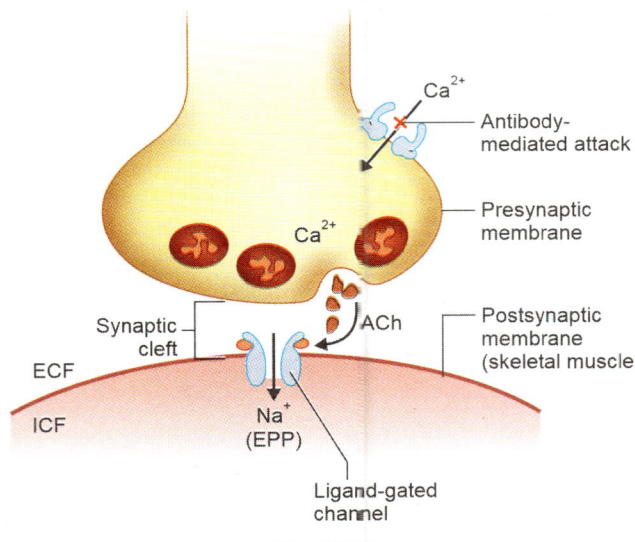

Fig. 3.26

Clinical Features

- There is muscle weakness of legs more than arms and improves on prolonged exercise
- There also may be associated
- Abnormal deep tendon reflexes
- Autonomic disturbances may be present (xerostomia, impotence).

3. List in sequence the events that occur at the neuromuscular junction.

Release of ACh

- When the action potential reaches the axon terminal, voltage-gated calcium channels open.
- Calcium ions enter the presynaptic membrane, and this leads to rupture of vesicles.
- The ACh that is released is brought out by exocytosis.
- Around 10,000 molecules of ACh are released each time a vesicle bursts and each motor endplate has 300 vesicles that burst.

Action of ACh

- The ACh is released into the presynaptic cleft.
- They bind with the nicotinic receptors on the post-synaptic membrane and form a complex.
- The binding causes opening of the sodium channels.

Development of Endplate Potential

- Influx of sodium decreases the resting membrane potential and generates an endplate potential.
- Its value is around –60 mV. It is nonpropagative in nature but causes formation of action potential.

Development of Miniature Endplate Potential

- It is a minute potential produced during each time during a potential reaches the axon.
- Its magnitude is as low as 0.5 mV.

- It cannot produce action potential by itself. When more and more miniature endplate potentials add up, an action potential is produced.

Destruction of ACh

- Acetylcholinesterase destroys the acetyl choline which is released into the synaptic cleft within a millisecond.
- It is split into acetate and choline which is taken up by the presynaptic membrane and recycled.

SHORT ANSWER

1. What is endplate potential?

- It is a local positive change in the resting membrane potential of the skeletal muscle fibre at the neuromuscular junction.
- It occurs due to opening of ACh gated channels for sodium ions which cause influx of sodium ions from ECF and create a positive potential.
- It develops an action potential when 60 mV is reached.

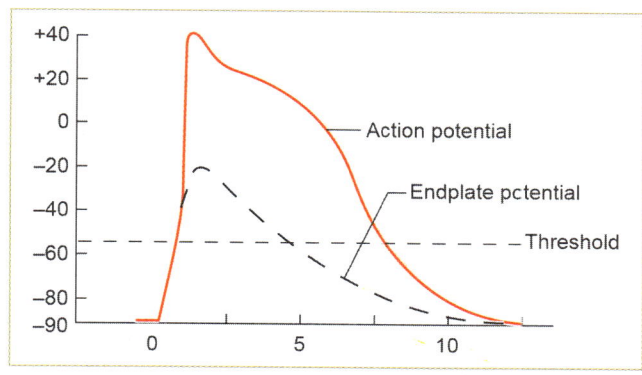

Fig. 3.27

3.5 DISCUSS THE ACTION OF NEUROMUSCULAR BLOCKING AGENTS

SHORT ESSAY

1. **A patient received succinylcholine as muscle relaxant and a general anesthetic for a routine gall bladder surgery. Instead of expected muscle relaxation, massive fasciculation followed by rigidity of muscles developed. It was associated with tachycardia, hypertension, increased respiration, and sudden increase in body temperature to 44°C with decreased blood oxygen and pH. He was diagnosed with malignant hyperthermia, showing hypersensitivity to succinylcholine.**

   A. **What alteration in skeletal muscle metabolism and heat production happens in this condition?** (2 marks)
   B. **Classify neuromuscular blocking agents based on their site and mechanism of action with examples.** (3 marks)

A. Malignant Hyperthermia

- It occurs in susceptible individuals following inhalational anaesthesia or use of succinylcholine.
- They have a defective gene coding for ryanodine receptor located on the sarcoplasmic reticulum.
- Triggers like halothane increase the affinity of the ryanodine receptor to calcium. Thus, they trigger an attack.
- The SERCA (sarcoendoplasmic reticulum Ca^{2+}–ATPase) pumps calcium back into the sarcoplasmic reticulum after cessation of the signal.

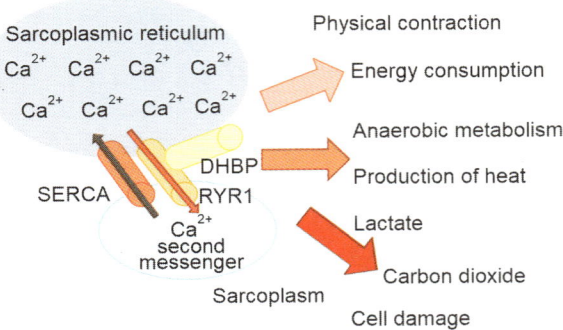

Fig. 3.28

- As a result, excess of calcium ions enters the muscle and cause generalized contraction of muscle and generates enormous heat.
- Also, there is metabolic acidosis as the oxygen may not suffice for muscle contraction and greater amounts of anaerobic metabolism takes place.

B.

Neuromuscular blocking agents are broadly classified as depolarizing and nondepolarizing agents.

1. **Depolarizing agents**
   - The drug which belongs to this category is succinylcholine.
   - It acts by binding to the ACh receptors irreversibly at the postsynaptic membrane.
   - Thereby it causes depolarization. As it is not removed by cholinesterase, it remains attached and cause prolonged depolarization and flaccid paralysis.

2. **Nondepolarizing agents**
   - These agents compete with ACh to bind to the nicotinic receptors on the motor endplate.
   - Thus, they block the action of ACh and thus cannot cause endplate potential.
   - Examples are curare, pancuronium, vecuronium, botulinum toxin, bungarotoxin.

Curare	Bind with ACh receptor on the postsynaptic membrane and prevent the action of ACh → blockage of myoneural transmission → sodium channels not activated → no influx of sodium → no motor end potential
Bungarotoxin Pancuronium	Bind with ACh receptor on the postsynaptic membrane and prevent the action of ACh → blockage of myoneural transmission → sodium channels not activated → no influx of sodium → no motor end potential
Botulinum toxin	It prevents the release of ACh from the vesicles by interfering with the SNARE complex → ACh is not released → no formation motor end potential

SHORT ANSWERS

1. Explain the physiological basis of Botox treatment.

- Botox is an acronym for botulinum toxin.
- It is a product of a bacterium, *Clostridium botulinum.*
- It is responsible for causing botulism—a type of foodborne infection, where there is blockage of neurotransmission across the myoneural junction.

For Normal Myoneural Transmission (Fig. 3.29)

- ACh stored in vesicles fuse with the presynaptic membrane with the help of SNARE proteins and then there is exocytosis of ACh.
- ACh binds with receptors on the post synaptic membrane and lead to influx of calcium due to opening of calcium channels.

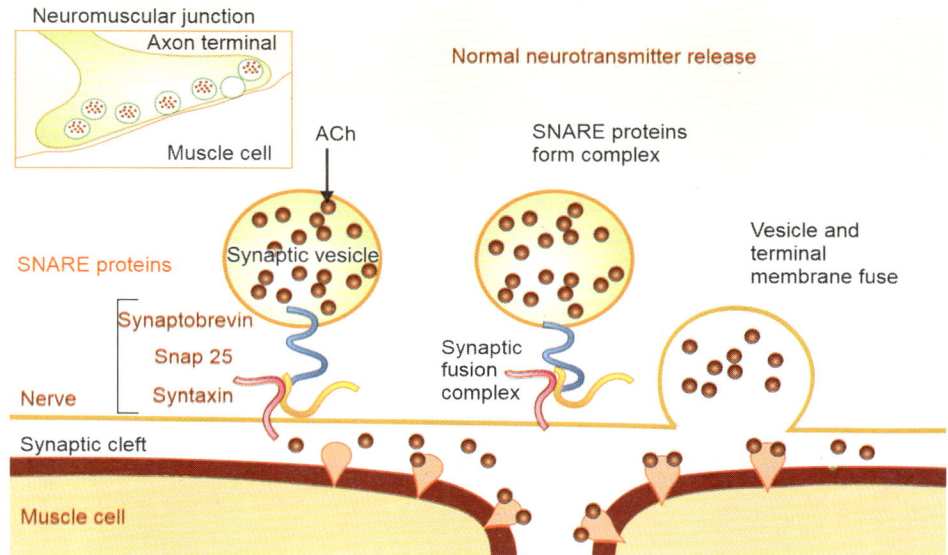

Fig. 3.29

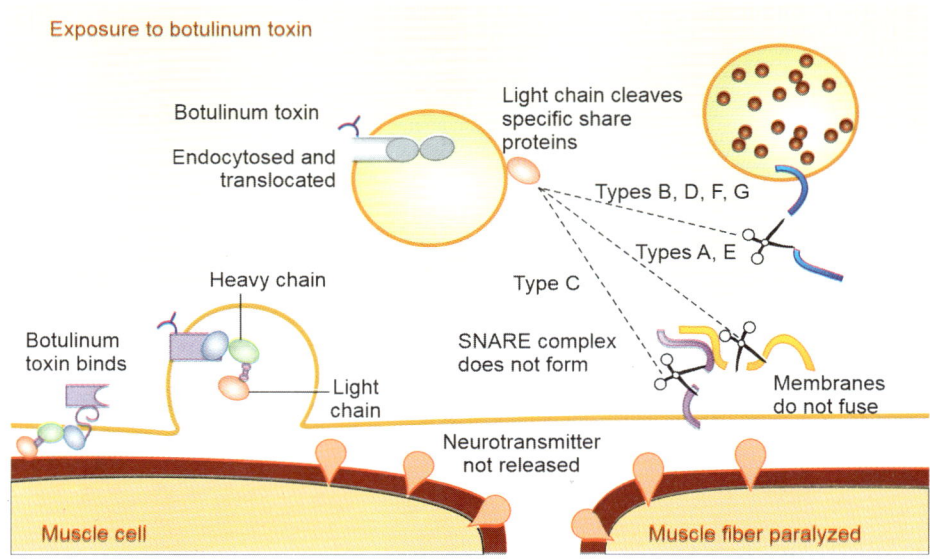

Fig. 3.30

In Botulism (Fig. 3.30)

- The light chain of the botulinum toxin cleaves the SNARE proteins and prevent formation of SNARE complex and thus inhibits release of ACh.
- This causes muscles to not contract excessively.
- This phenomenon is used in various pathologies like treating wrinkles, blepharospasm, spastic squint, overactive bladder, cervical dystonia and relieving sphincteric spasms of the esophagus.

2. Explain the physiological basis of using Curare as arrowhead poison for hunting.

- Curare was a drug used in South America while hunting. It would cause paralysis of the desired animal when shot with an arrow whose head was poisoned with this drug.
- It is a competitive inhibitor of ACh and binds at the nicotinic receptors. As a result, ACh cannot exert its actions.

- This causes sodium channels to remain closed and thus influx of sodium ions does not happen.
- Thus, neuromuscular transmission is blocked.
- Based on this fact, they were introduced as a muscle relaxant in anesthesiology in 1940s.

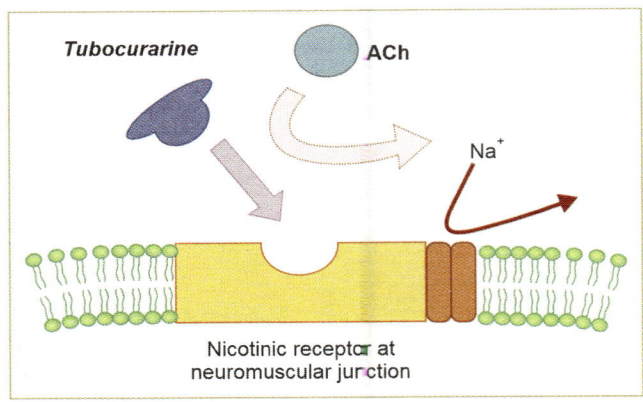

Fig. 3.31

3.6 DESCRIBE THE PATHOPHYSIOLOGY OF MYASTHENIA GRAVIS

SHORT ESSAYS

1. A 32-year-old lady presented with history of ptosis, diplopia, weakness, and easy fatigability, which worsens with repeated movements and as the day progresses, by evening. He was diagnosed with myasthenia gravis.

  A. What is myasthenia gravis? (1 mark)
  B. What is the pathophysiology behind the condition? (1 mark)
  C. How do you treat the condition? Explain its physiological basis. (2 marks)
  D. Name a disorder of transmission across neuromuscular junction in which muscle movements become better with repetition. (1 mark)

A. Myasthenia Gravis

- It is a potentially fatal autoimmune condition in which body develops T cell-mediated immunity against ACh receptors in the postsynaptic membrane in myoneural junction of the skeletal muscles.

B. Pathophysiology

- The activated T cells arise from a thymoma.
- These produce antibodies against the receptors for ACh in the postsynaptic membrane.
- As a result, the ACh that is released, gets destroyed in the synaptic cleft without performing its action.
- In the postsynaptic membrane, there is no activation of sodium channels and formation of potential.
- As a result, the muscles cannot contract.

C. Treatment

- Plasmapheresis to remove antibodies off the plasma
- Thymectomy is another useful treatment to remove the offending immune cells.
- Acetylcholinesterase inhibitors
- These inhibit the action of acetylcholinesterase, an enzyme responsible for destruction of ACh in the synaptic cleft.
- As a result, more ACh is available for myoneural transmission
- Examples: Neostigmine, physostigmine

D. Lambert-Eaton Syndrome

2. What is myasthenia gravis? Explain its Pathophysiology and clinical features. Add a note on its management

Myasthenia Gravis (MG)

It is a potentially fatal autoimmune condition in which body develops T cell-mediated immunity against ACh receptors in the postsynaptic membrane in myoneural junction of the skeletal muscles.

Pathophysiology

- The activated T cells arise from a thymoma.
- These produce antibodies against the receptors for ACh in the postsynaptic membrane.
- As a result, the ACh that is released, gets destroyed in the synaptic cleft without performing its action.

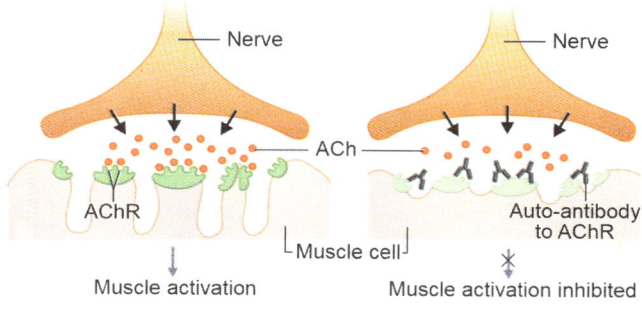

Fig. 3.32

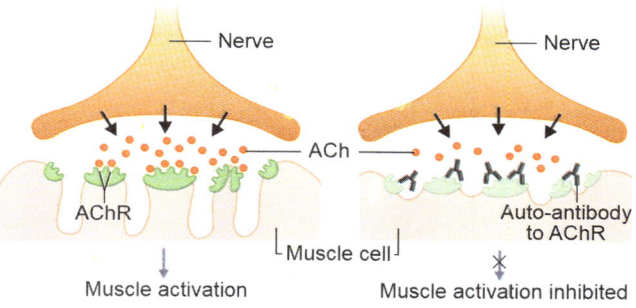

Fig. 3.33

- In the postsynaptic membrane, there is no activation of sodium channels and formation of potential.
- As a result, the muscles cannot contract.

Clinical Features

- MG affects females more.
- The first muscles to be affected are eyelids as they are fast twitch muscles.
- Ocular complaints include ptosis and diplopia due to patchy involvement of extraocular muscles.
- The person also complains of fatigue towards the end of the day.
- The weakness always manifests with increase in activity.
- Respiratory muscle paralysis can prove fatal.

Treatment

- Plasmapheresis to remove antibodies of the plasma

- Thymectomy is another useful treatment to remove the offending immune cells.
- Acetylcholinesterase inhibitors
- These inhibit the action of acetylcholinesterase, an enzyme responsible for destruction of ACh in the synaptic cleft.
- As a result, more ACh is available for myoneural transmission
- Examples: Neostigmine, physostigmine

SHORT ANSWER

1. Compare and contrast the autoimmune disorders of the neuromuscular junction.

The two autoimmune conditions that affect the neuromuscular junction are myasthenia gravis and Lambert-Eaton syndrome.

Common Factors to Both Disorders

- They both cause flaccid paralysis of muscles
- They both affect skeletal muscles only
- Muscles are normal

Differences Between the Two

Parameter	Myasthenia gravis	Lambert-Eaton syndrome
Gender	F>M	M>F
Etiology	Antibodies are developed against the ACh receptors thus block their activity on postsynaptic membrane Usually associated with thymoma	Antibody mediated destruction of calcium channels on the presynaptic membrane. Associated with small cell lung cancer
Pattern of weakness	Worsens on prolonged exercise	Improves on prolonged exercise
Muscles affected	Ocular muscles first to be affected	Legs more than arms
Deep tendon reflexes	Normal	Abnormal
Autonomic dysfunction	Absent	Present (xerostomia, impotence)
Repeated nerve stimulation	Decremental response	Incremental response

3.7 DESCRIBE THE DIFFERENT TYPES OF MUSCLE FIBRES AND THEIR STRUCTURE

SHORT ESSAYS

1. Enumerate different types of skeletal muscle proteins and briefly describe their actions.
(1 + 4 marks)

1. Myosin

- Myosin forms the main muscle associated with contraction of a skeletal muscle.
- It is arranged in the form of sheets with the heads of the myosin molecule on either side.
- The myosin head has two active sites: One for binding with actin and the other with ATP.
- When it binds with actin, in presence of ATP, crossbridges are formed.
- These help in sliding of actin molecules over myosin and subsequent shortening of the muscle.

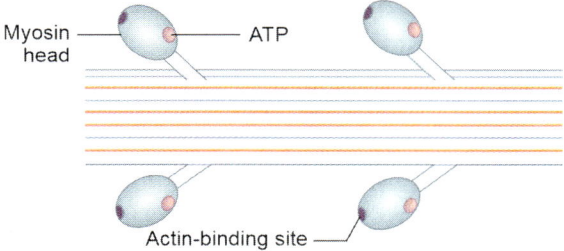

Myosin head — ATP

Actin-binding site —

Fig. 3.34

2 Actin

- These are thin filaments of protein arranged in the form of a double helix.
- They bind with myosin heads and help in decreasing the length of a muscle fiber by sliding over the myosin molecules.

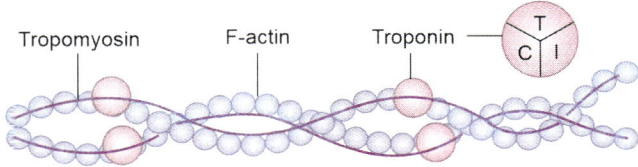

Tropomyosin   F-actin   Troponin — T C I

Fig. 3.35

3. Troponin

- They are small globular proteins which are located at certain points in the tropomyosin molecule.

- They have three parts:
  - Troponin T: It helps in binding of troponin to tropomyosin
  - Troponin C: It helps in binding of calcium and thus initiating the cascade of contraction
  - Troponin I: it inhibits the interaction of active parts of the myosin with actin.

4. Tropomyosin

- These molecules lie in the grove between the actin filaments
- They are regulatory proteins and prevent interaction between the actin and myosin filaments.
- They cover the binding sites on actin for myosin.

5. Other proteins

Actinin	Attached actin filament to Z line
Desmin	Binds Z line with sarcolemma
Nebulin	Runs parallel to actin filaments
Titin	Large protein which connect
Dystrophin	Connects actin to dystroglycan

2. Describe the structure of sarcomere.

- Sarcomere is the segment of the myofibril between two consecutive Z lines.
- It is the structural and functional unit of a muscle.
- It contains half I band, 1 A band and another half I band. A band is the darker portion and I band is the lighter portion.
- It is composed of parallelly arranged thick and thin filaments.
- In the centre of each A band, there is an H zone with no overlap between thick and thin filaments.
- In the centre of each H zone, there is a dark M line which is more pronounced during muscle contraction.
- Z line forms the centre of I bands.
- Each sarcomere is composed of myosin and actin filaments.

Thick Filament

- Myosin molecules are arranged in the form of parallel filaments such that their oblique heads lie on either side.
- As a result, the centre of the myosin filaments are devoid of heads.

Thin Filament

- It is made of actin molecules and regulatory troponin and tropomyosin.
- Actin filaments are arranged in the form of a double helix.
- Tropomyosin filaments are present in the grove between actin molecules.
- Troponin molecules are present at regular intervals on tropomyosin molecules.

Anchoring Proteins

- Alpha actinin link actin filaments to Z line.
- Titin filaments connect Z lines to each other.

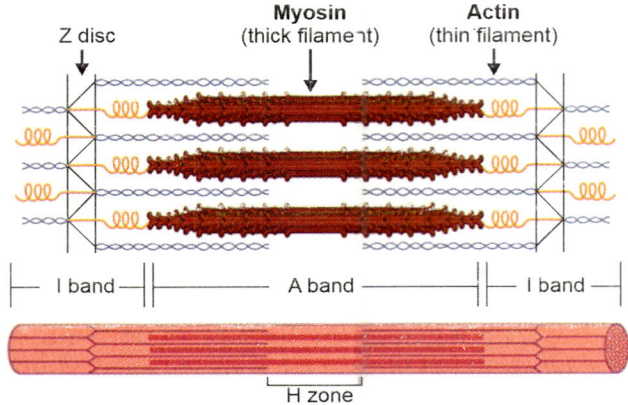

Fig. 3.36

3. Compare and contrast the structure and functions of skeletal, cardiac, and smooth muscle.

Parameter	Skeletal muscle	Cardiac muscle	Smooth muscle
		Structure	
Striations	Present	Present	Absent
Length of fibers	1–40 microns	80–100 microns	50–500 microns
Diameter	50–500 microns	15 microns	2–10 microns
Connection between fibers	No	Yes, gap junctions allow the muscles to function as a syncytium	Yes, in unitary muscles
Nucleus	Single or multiple. Placed at the periphery	Single, central	Single
Thick and thin filaments	Arranged regularly	Arranged regularly	Irregular
Sarcoplasmic reticulum	Very well developed	Less developed as compared to skeletal muscles	Lesser developed
Regulating proteins	Troponin and tropomyosin	Troponin	Calmodulin
Sarcotubular system	Well developed, two triads per sarcomere	One triad per sarcomere	Not well developed
	T tubule present at A-I junction	T tubule present at Z line	
Sodium channels	Fast voltage-gated	Fast voltage-gated	Slow voltage-gated Na-Ca channels
		Functions	
Nerve supply	Somatic motor and afferent	Autonomous	Autonomous, hormonal
Voluntary/involuntary	Voluntary	Involuntary	Involuntary
Actions	Movements of the joints	Pumping action of the heart	Maintaining tone of viscera Movements of viscera

SHORT ANSWERS

1. Draw a neat-labeled diagram of sarcomere.

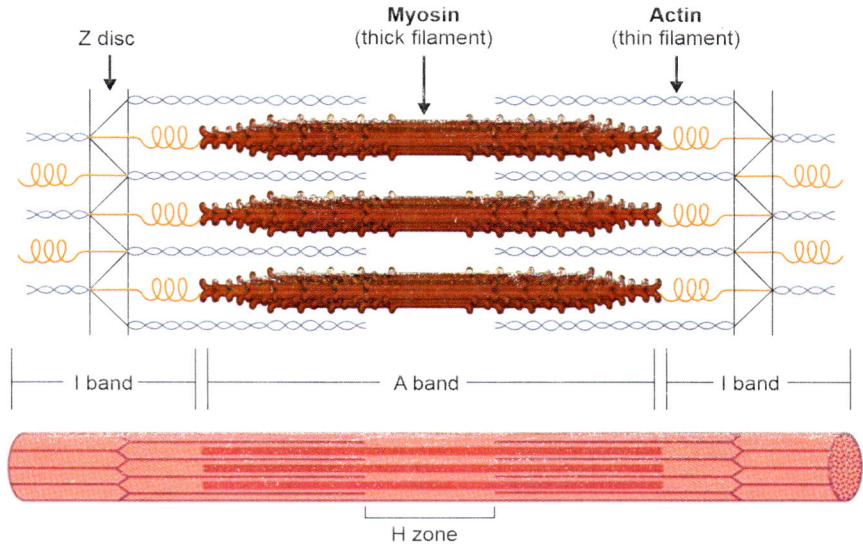

Fig. 3.37

2. Distinguish between slow and fast fibers.

Parameter	Slow fibers	Fast fibers
Muscle fiber type	Red, involved in tonic activity	White and are involved in phasic activity
Sarcoplasmic reticulum	Less	Extensive, thus there is high calcium available for initiation of contraction
Motor unit innervation ratio	120–160 muscle fibers/axon	6 muscle fibers/axon
Metabolism	Aerobic	Anaerobic
Blood supply	High	Normal
Capillary density	High	Low
Glycogen contents	Low	High
Glycolytic enzymes	Lower	Higher
Myoglobin content	High	Low
Diameter of axon	Small	High
Tetanic tension	Small	Large
Type of movements	Mainly involved in posture maintenance	Mainly involved in fine and skilled movements
Fatigability	Resistant to fatigue	Easily fatigable
Twitch duration	Long	Brief

3.8 DESCRIBE ACTION POTENTIAL AND ITS PROPERTIES IN DIFFERENT MUSCLE TYPES
(SKELETAL AND SMOOTH)

LONG ESSAYS

1. Describe action potential, its ionic basis and properties in smooth muscle and compare it with the action potential seen in skeletal muscle.

Action Potential (Fig. 3.38)

- The resisting membrane potential of a smooth muscle is unstable and keeps varying between –50 mV and –75 mV.
- This happens due to intervening pacemaker cells which have varying permeability to calcium and sodium ions.
- Three types of action potentials can be described in a smooth muscle.

1. **Spike potential**
   - Depolarization in a smooth muscle is dependent on the influx of calcium
   - Depolarization is brought about by nervous stimulus, hormones or neurotransmitters.
   - L type of calcium channels on the membrane lead to influx of calcium

2. **Spike potential initiated by slow wave rhythm**
   - This is seen in tissues containing pacemaker cells like the smooth muscles of the gut.

- Spike potentials appear the peak of rhythmic contractions.
- These potentials are self-excitatory due to opening of calcium channels which cause depolarization

3. **Action potential with plateau**
This is due to prolonged exposure of large number of the calcium channels leading to sustained presence of the calcium intracellularly and causes a plateau of depolarization.

Ionic Basis (Fig. 3.39)

Phases of action potential and ionic potential

1. At the beginning of the action potential	Opening of the voltage-gated calcium channels
	Beginning of calcium influx
2. Spike of the action potential	Highest level of calcium level (around isoelectric phase)
3. Repolarization	Opening of calcium dependent potassium channels leading to potassium efflux
4. Slow hyperpolarization	Continued efflux of potassium
5. Slow depolarization	Closure of calcium channels and calcium depended potassium channels

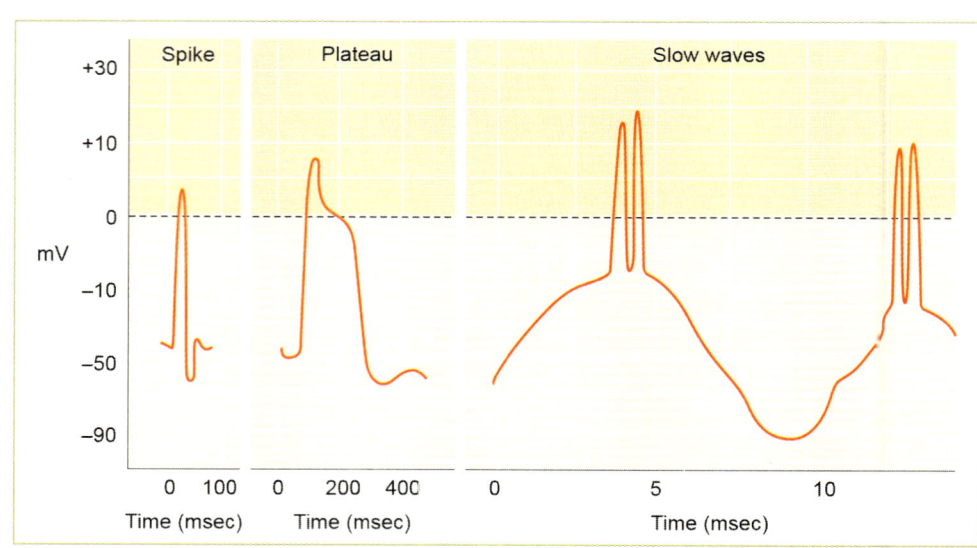

Fig. 3.38

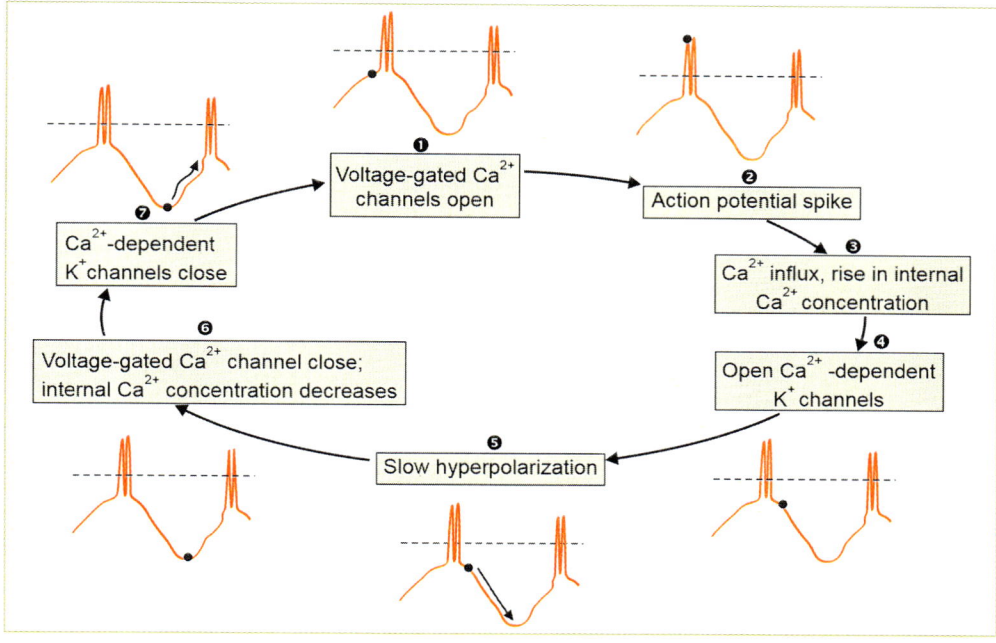

Fig. 3.39

Properties

- The resisting membrane potential of a smooth muscle is unstable and keeps varying between –50 mV and –75 mV.

- This happens due to intervening pacemaker cells which have varying permeability to calcium and sodium ions.

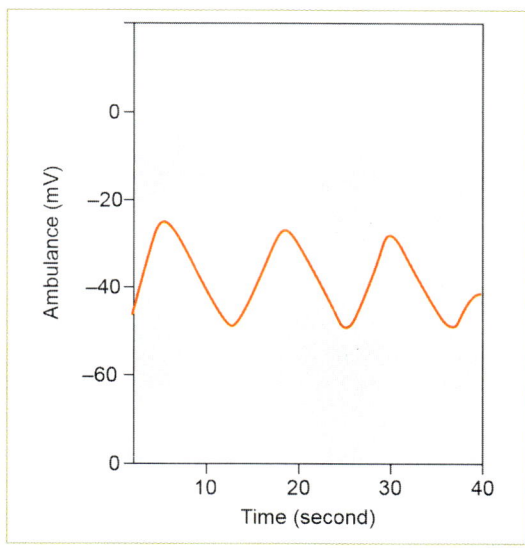

Fig. 3.40

Comparison of Action Potentials

Parameter	Skeletal muscle	Smooth muscle
Resting membrane potential	–90 mV	–55 mV
Duration of action potential	5 ms	100–300 ms
Cause for depolarization	Entry of sodium ions through fast sodium channels	Entry of calcium ions through slow calcium channels
Amplitude of spike	Up to 40 mV	Up to 0 mV
Refractory period	1–3 ms	Not defined

SHORT ESSAYS

1. Compare and contrast type I and type II skeletal muscle fibers.

Parameter	Type I	Type II
Muscle fiber type	Slow, red, involved in tonic activity	Fast, white and are involved in phasic activity
Sarcoplasmic reticulum	Lower compared to type II fibers	Extensive, thus there is high calcium available for initiation of contraction
Motor unit innervation ratio	120–160 muscle fibers/axon	6 muscle fibers/axon
Metabolism	Aerobic	Anaerobic
Blood supply	High	Normal
Capillary density	High	Low
Glycogen contents	Low	High
Glycolytic enzymes	Lower	Higher
Myoglobin content	High	Low
Diameter of axon	Small	High
Tetanic tension	Small	Large
Type of movements	Mainly involved in posture maintenance	Mainly involved in fine and skilled movements
Fatigability	Resistant to fatigue	Easily fatigable
Twitch duration	Long	Brief

2. Explain the physiological basis why skeletal muscle can be tetanized but not the cardiac muscle.

Tetany

- Tetanus is a state of sustained, smooth, and forceful contraction that occurs when the successive stimulus falls from the later part of the latent phase to the contraction phase.
- During tetanus, the tension developed within the muscle is four times the normal.

Ionic Basis

- During a single twitch, calcium ions accumulate in the sarcoplasm of the muscle fiber.
- When a muscle is stimulated successively, more and more calcium ions accumulate in the sarcoplasm and continues to cause recycling of myosin heads.
- This causes the series elastic component to remain in a state of tension and leads to tetanus.
- The skeletal muscles have a short refractory period. In the first half of the latent period, no matter what the strength of the stimulus, the muscle cannot be stimulated. This is the absolute refractory period.
- The second half of the latent period forms the relative refractory period. In this period, stimuli of higher strengths can stimulate the muscles.
- However, in the cardiac muscle, they have a long refractory period.

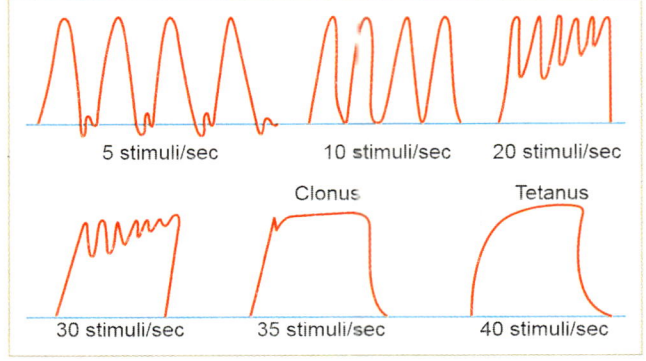

Fig. 3.41

- The total refractory period in a skeletal muscle lasts for 0.1s, whereas in a cardiac muscle it lasts for 0.53s.
- Absolute refractory period extends from phase 0 until halfway of phase 3. In this period, no matter what the strength of the stimulus, the cardiac muscle cannot be stimulated.
- The fast sodium channels are inactivated when the membrane potential approaches the equilibrium for Na^+. As a result, Na^+ ions cannot move out or in. As a result, no impulse can stimulate the cardiac muscle.
- Relative refractory period extends from phase 3 till repolarization is complete. In this phase, a stimulus of greater strength can stimulate a cardiac muscle.

- It is due to the leaking of potassium ions, which makes the membrane potential more negative (i.e. it is hyperpolarised), this resets the sodium channels; opening the inactivation gate, but still leaving the channel closed. Thus, it is possible to initiate an action potential, but a stronger stimulus than normal is required.
- Thus, tetanus is prevented.

3. What is rigor mortis? Explain the molecular mechanism of its occurrence? Mention its clinical significance. (1 + 2 + 2 marks)

Rigor Mortis

- It refers to shortening and rigidity of all muscles of the body after death.
- *Rigor* = stiff, *mortis* = death

Mechanism of Occurrence

- Following death, there is cessation of availability of ATP.
- The cell membranes of skeletal muscles become extremely permeable to calcium ions.
- As a result, many calcium ions enter the muscle and form actomyosin complex and cause contraction of the muscle in the whole body.
- The joints become stiff and locked.
- For relaxation, there is a requirement for ATP and following death, due to lack of oxygen and thus ATP, the complexes of actin and myosin heads which are formed cannot be unlocked.

Clinical Significance

- It begins shortly after death (10 minutes to 3 hours) and is maximum at 24 hours.
- After that due to release of lysosomal enzymes there is degradation of proteins of the muscle leading to resolution of rigor.
- Rigor begins to develop in the facial muscles and then spreads to the rest of the body.
- Based on these facts, the forensic experts can gauge the amount of time elapsed since death occurred.
- Rigor mortis is also influenced by environmental temperature.
- If the person dies of a struggle, then there is excess generation of heat. Thus, in such cases and in hot temperatures, rigor sets in quickly.

Condition of body	Time since death
If body feels warm and flaccid	Dead less than 3 hours
If body feels warm and is stiff	Dead from 3 to 8 hours
If body feels cold and is stiff	Dead from 8 to 36 hours
If body feels cold and flaccid	Dead more than 36 hours

4. Explain denervation hypersensitivity.

- It is a condition that occurs following transection of nerve from a muscle.
- It can occur in a skeletal muscle or a smooth muscle.
- When the motor nerve to a skeletal muscle is severed, the muscle becomes hypersensitive to ACh.
- When the autonomic organ is denervated, the organ becomes hypersensitive to adrenaline.

Reason for Denervation Hypersensitivity

- These effects occur due to increased number of receptors for the specific neurotransmitter.
- There may also be decreased uptake of the neurotransmitter.
- Growth of collaterals from existing neurons.

Example

1. In Horner syndrome, there is oculosympathetic paresis.
   - In a postganglionic lesion, the smooth muscles are devoid of the neurotransmitter-noradrenaline.
   - As a result, when 1% phenylephrine is added, there is dilatation of the involved pupil.
   - It does not happen in a preganglionic lesion, where there is continuous abundance of noradrenaline but no impulse to cause a dilatation.
2. Following transection of spinal cord due to various reasons, there is beginning of reflex activity after some days.
   - At this point a mass reflex may be elicited.
   - In this, when the skin over the lower abdominal wall or inner thighs is scratched, there is a flexor response and evacuation of bowel and bladder.

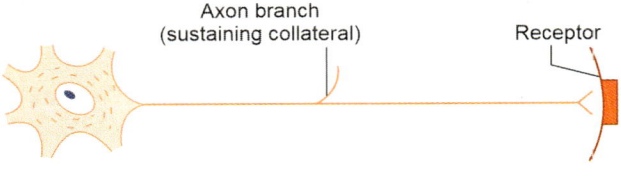

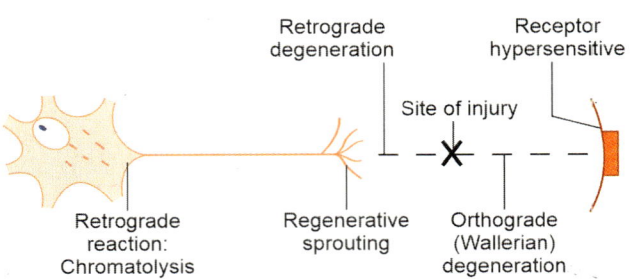

Fig. 3.42

5. Define tone of the muscle. Enumerate abnormal muscle tones with their conditions of occurrence. (1 + 4 marks)

Tone of the Muscle

- It is a state of constant slight contraction of a muscle. It results from low frequency firing of motor units.
- It is present in almost all muscles, more so in extensor muscles.

Abnormal Muscle Tones

Abnormal muscle tone	Condition of occurrence
Hypertonia • Increased muscular tone	Upper motor neuron disease Cerebral palsy
Hypotonia • Decreased muscular tone	Lower motor neuron disease Down syndrome Myasthenia gravis Cerebellar ataxia Muscular dystrophy Botulism Vitamin D deficient rickets
Myotonia • Continuous contraction followed by slow relaxation	Mutation of genes of the channel proteins in sarcolemma • Becker type myotonia • Thomsen type myotonia

6. Enumerate the properties of skeletal muscle fiber. Explain any four of them.

Properties of Skeletal Muscle

Electrical properties	Mechanical properties
1. Excitability 2. Conductivity	1. Contractility 2. Extensibility 3. Elasticity 4. Fatigability

1. Excitability (Fig. 3.43)

- It is a physicochemical change occurring in a skeletal muscle following a mechanical, thermal, chemical or electrical stimulus.
- Responds by production of electrical signals and action potential.
- Subthreshold stimulus produces local potential or endplate potential.
- Application of a threshold stimulus causes a depolarization from –90 mV which is the resting membrane potential.

2. Conductivity

- Propagates nerve impulse in the same manner as an unmyelinated nerve fiber.
- The impulse propagates along the sarcolemma.
- Action potential spreads bidirectionally
- Velocity of conduction is very slow (3–5 m/s)

3. Contractility (Fig. 3.44)

- It is the ability to shorten or contract when stimulated by an action potential.

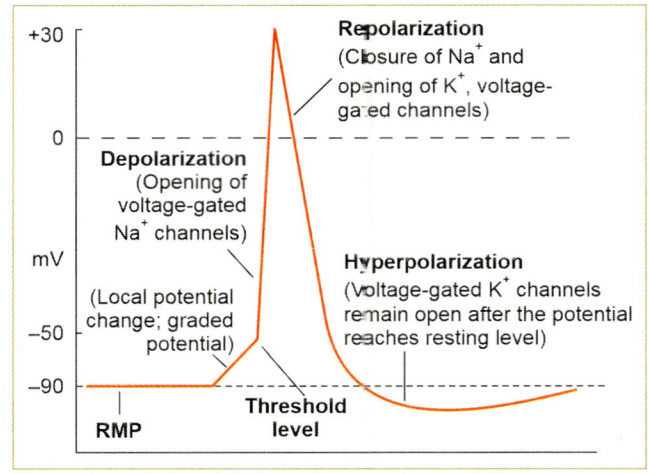

Fig. 3.43

- When a threshold stimulus is applied, the muscle responds by contracting.
- A single action potential causes a contraction followed by relaxation. It is called a simple muscle twitch.
- The depolarization begins at the motor endplate and action potential is conducted and initiates contraction.
- Based on the duration of twitch, muscles are grouped as fast twitch (7 ms) and slow twitch (100 ms).
- Contractility depends on the initial length of the muscle (Starling's law), strength of stimulus, frequency of stimulus, preload and afterload, temperature, and type of muscle.

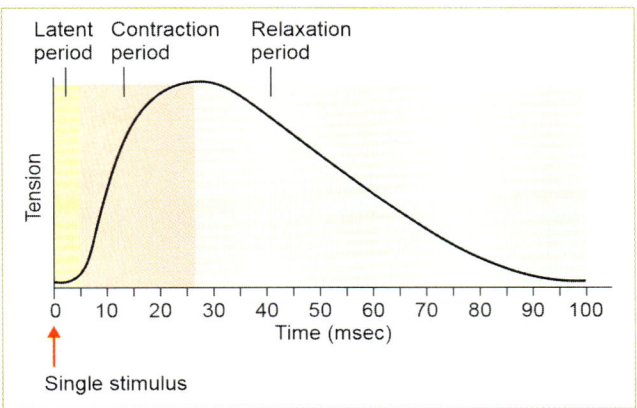

Fig. 3.44

4. **Elasticity**
   - Ability of the muscle to recoil and resume its pre-contraction length is called elasticity.
   - This is due to the presence of parallel elastic component.

7. Describe action potential and its ionic basis in skeletal muscle.

- Action potential is a series of electrical changes that occur in membrane potential when the muscle or nerve is stimulated.
- Voltage-gated sodium and potassium channels play an important role in causing an action potential.
- It has three phases: Latent phase, depolarization and repolarization phases.

1. **Latent period**
   - It is the time taken when no change takes place in the membrane potential after applying a stimulus.

- There is no change in resting membrane potential (–90 mV)
- It is 0.5–1 ms in length.
- Stimulus artefact: It occurs at the time of application of stimulating electrode due to leakage of current from the stimulating electrode to the recording electrode. It occurs prior to latent period.

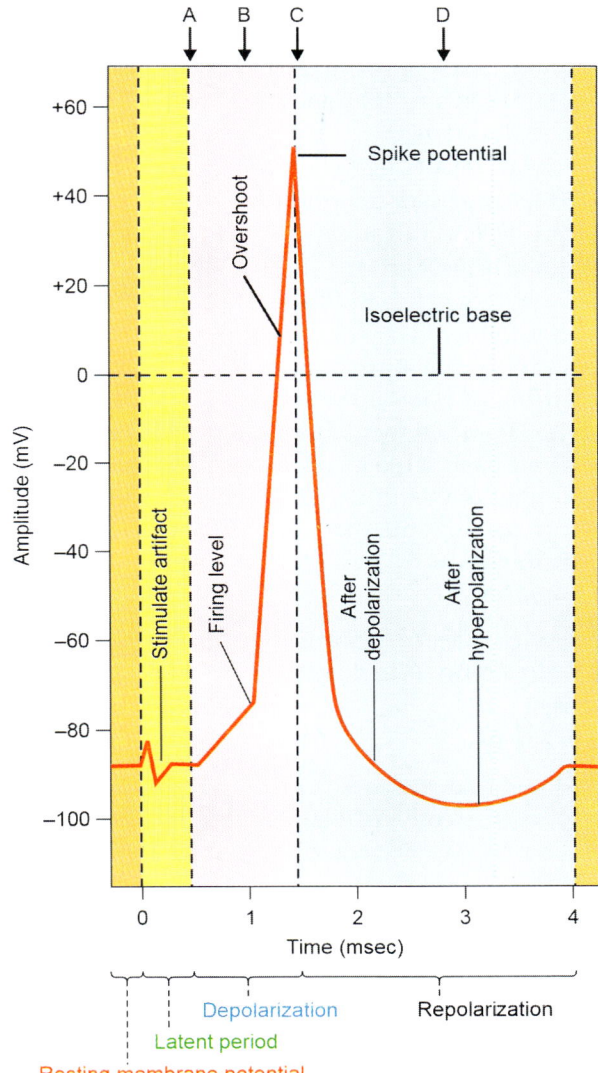

Fig. 3.45

A. Opening of sodium channels leading to influx of sodium ions; B. Opening of more and more sodium channels causing influx of Na⁺; C. Closure of sodium channels and opening of potassium channels leading to efflux of potassium; D. Continued efflux of potassium ions leading to increase in negativity inside the cell

2. Depolarization

- It is a positive wave. For the first 15 mV it is very slow.
- Ionic basis for initial depolarisation: Represented by A in the diagram: It is due to opening of new sodium channels.
- After about 15 mV of depolarization, there is an increase in slope of the depolarization wave. Depolarization crosses the isoelectric point (0 mV) and overshoots by +55 mV.
- Ionic basis for firing level: Opening of more and more sodium channels. It is represented by B in the diagram.

3. Repolarization

- It is marked by reversal of potential from positive to negative.
- Ionic basis: Closure of sodium ions and opening of potassium ions. It is marked C in the diagram.
- It is followed by slow repolarization. Ionic basis: Open potassium ions leading to continuous influx of potassium ions.
- It is then followed by a slow hyperpolarization. Ionic basis: Potassium channels remain open for longer than sodium channels leading to further efflux of sodium ions leading to hyper-polarization. It is represented as D in the diagram.

8. Draw a diagram depicting the length-tension relationship (Starling's law) and explain its basis.

Starling's Law

- It states that the force of contraction of a muscle depends directly on the initial length of the muscle fiber prior to contraction within physiological limits.
- As a result, there is optimum overlapping between actin and myosin.

Physiological Reason Behind Starling's Law

- The reason for this is, when the muscle is stretched, more active binding sites of actin and myosin are exposed.
- So, there is more overlapping of actin and myosin heads and more interaction.
- Thus, the number of crossbridges are more and the strength of contraction increases.

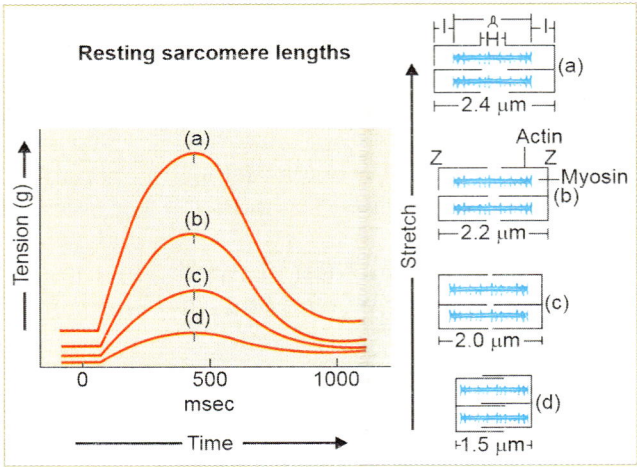

Fig. 3.46

9. Draw a diagram depicting the load–velocity relationship and explain the phenomena.

- Load–velocity relationship graph is obtained by plotting velocity of shortening of a muscle in Y-axis against the increase in load along the X-axis.
- When the load is minimum, the velocity of contraction is highest and is denoted as V_{max}.
- When the load applied increases, the velocity of shortening decreases.
- With increase in the load, a point is reached when the muscle is unable to take the load.

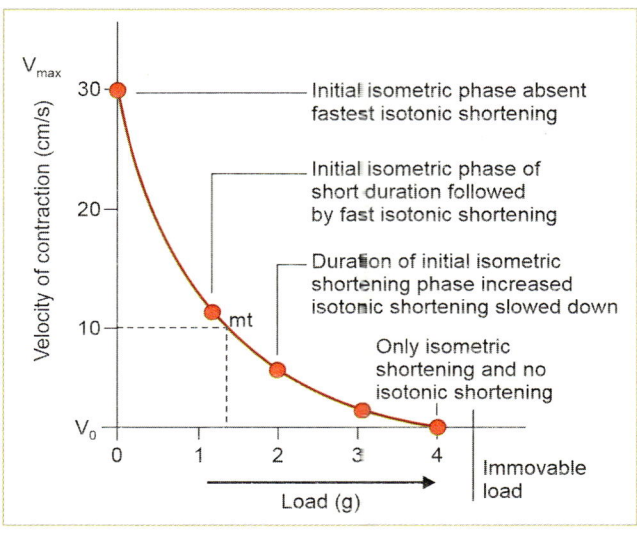

Fig. 3.47

- Thus, between maximum and minimum load, all contractions have variable durations of isometric and isotonic contractions.
- Initially, the contraction is majorly isotonic and then becomes more isometric in nature.
- In this curve, mt is the point of maximum efficiency of the muscle. It lies about 1/3rd of the abscissa and 1/3rd from the ordinate.

10. List the phenomena associated with increasing frequency of stimulation (beneficial effect, treppe, clonus, tetanus) and explain the basis of the phenomena.

1. **Beneficial effect**
   - When stimuli are applied in succession to a motor unit, there is amplitude of first 2–3 contractions increase.
   - Later, the amplitude decreases.

   Physiological basis
   - There is a decrease in the viscosity of the muscle allowing better conductivity
   - There is increase in calcium ions available for contraction of muscles. With each action potential, more calcium arrives into the sarcoplasm.
   - Increase in temperature increases the contractility.

2. **Treppe**
   - Also known as staircase phenomenon
   - Refers to slow increase in force of contraction of muscle when it is stimulated repeatedly with a maximal strength at a low frequency.
   - Treppe is distinct from summation of contractions and tetanus.

   Physiological basis
   - There is a decrease in the viscosity of the muscle allowing better conductivity
   - There is increase in calcium ions available for contraction of muscles. With each action potential, more calcium arrives into the sarcoplasm.
   - Increase in temperature increases the contractility.

3. **Clonus**
   - Refers to a series of rapid and repeated involuntary jerky movements, which occur while eliciting a deep reflex.

- When a deep reflex is elicited in a normal person, the contractions of a muscle or group of muscles are smooth and continuous.

   Physiological basis
   - Clonus occurs when the deep reflexes are exaggerated due to hypertonicity of muscles in pyramidal tract lesion.
   - In pyramidal tract lesions, inhibitory response is removed from the alpha motor neurons.
   - As a result, there is multiple uninhibited stimuli which fire from the spinal cord.

4. **Tetanus**
   - Refers to sustained muscular contraction due to repeated stimuli with high frequency.
   - When the multiple stimuli are applied at a higher frequency in such a way that the successive stimuli fall during contraction period of previous twitch, the muscle remains in state of tetanus.
   - It relaxes only after the stoppage of stimulus or when the muscle is fatigued.

   Physiological basis
   - The Ca^{2+} ions released in the sarcoplasm during single twitch are removed quickly and relaxation occurs.
   - When the muscle is stimulated in rapid succession, there is progressive accumulation of calcium in the sarcoplasm.
   - The longer calcium ions stay in the sarcoplasm, the duration of contraction increases causing tetanus.

SHORT ANSWERS

1. Compare and contrast active tension and passive tension in a muscle.

Active tension	Passive tension
It is the real tension that develops during contractile process.	It is due to stretching of parallel and series electric components of the muscle
It is measured by stretching a muscle between two points.	It is measured by stimulating the muscle which is stretched. This gives total tension. Total tension – passive tension = active tension

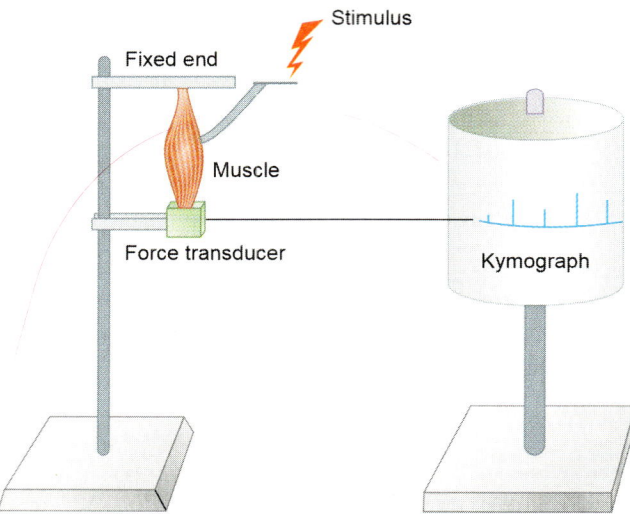

Fig. 3.48

2. Compare and contrast single unit smooth muscle and multiunit smooth muscle.

Single unit smooth muscle/unitary smooth muscle	Multiunit smooth muscle
A unit of many smooth muscle fibers are strongly associated such that they have gap junctions between them.	Each smooth muscle behaves as a single unit. Each smooth muscle fiber is surrounded by a basement membrane like substance
A group of cells function as a single unit.	Each fiber operates as a single unit independent of each other
Stimulated by non-neural stimulus like hormonal influence	Stimulated by a single neuron per fiber and thus, contraction is finer
Pacemaker like tissue may be present.	
Autonomous nervous system can affect the response	No effect of autonomous nervous system
Stretch causes reflex contraction	There is no effect of stretch on contraction
Examples: Smooth muscles of viscera, arterioles	Examples: Smooth muscles of iris, ciliary body

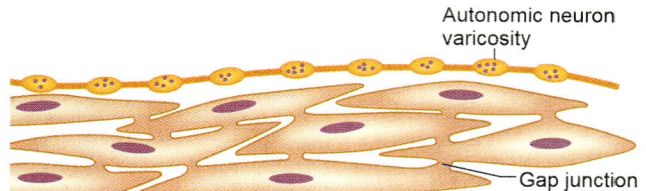

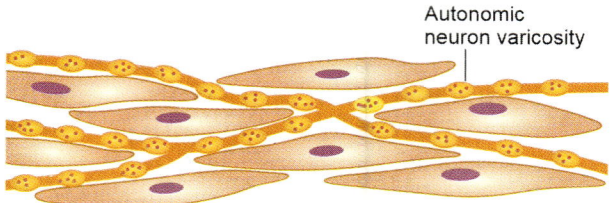

3. Explain why red muscle fibers are resistant to fatigue.

- The fatigability of a muscle depends on its oxidative capacity.
- The features of type 1 fibers which make it resistant to fatigue are:
  - They have low myosin ATPase activity. As a result, they have more ATP to consume.
  - They are slow twitch, thus require less ATP for coupling–uncoupling reactions.
  - They have high oxidative capacity thus there is low amount of lactic acid that gets accumulated.
  - They have low glycolytic capacity. The metabolism is more aerobic.

4. What is beneficial effect? Explain the molecular basis for it.

Beneficial Effect

- When stimuli are applied in succession to a motor unit, there is an increase in amplitude of first 2–3 contractions increase.
- Later, the amplitude decreases.

Molecular Basis

- There is a decrease in the viscosity of the muscle allowing better conductivity
- There is increase in calcium ions available for contraction of muscles. With each action potential, more calcium arrives into the sarcoplasm.
- Increase in temperature increases the contractility.

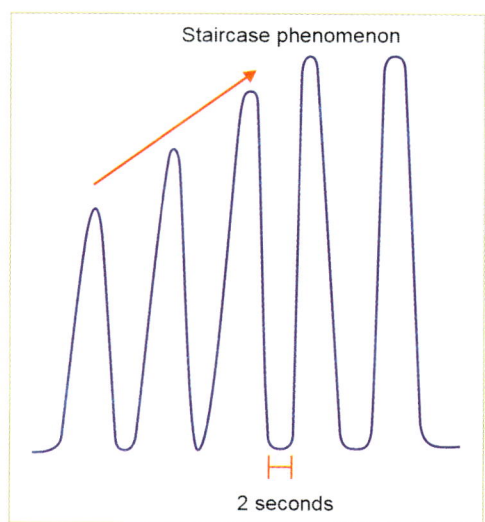

Staircase phenomenon

2 seconds

Fig. 3.49

5. What is all-or-none law? How does it vary in different excitable tissues?

All-or-None Law

- When a nerve is stimulated, it either gives a maximal response or does not give any response depending on the strength of the stimulus.
- When the stimulus is subthreshold, there is no action potential produced (represented by A and B).
- When the stimulus is threshold, the action potential is produced in full response (represented by C).
- When the stimulus is suprathreshold, same action potential is produced (represented by D).

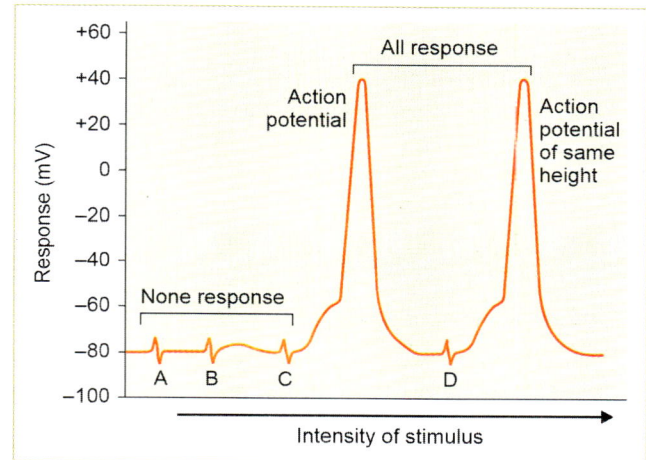

Fig. 3.50

All-or-None Law in Various Excitable Tissues

Neuron	Skeletal muscle	Cardiac muscle	Smooth muscle
Obeyed by all neurons	Obeyed by single muscle fiber	Obeyed by whole muscle	Unitary muscle: Obeyed by whole muscle Multiunit: Obeyed by single muscle fiber

6. Define latent period in a skeletal muscle twitch. What are the factors influencing its duration?

Latent Period

- It is the time duration after which contraction begins a skeletal muscle following application or arrival of stimulus.
- Duration is 0.01 second.

Factors influencing latent period				
At the neuronal end	*At the neuromuscular junction*	*At the muscle*	*External conditions*	*Recording instrument*
Length of the nerve Longer the nerve, longer is the latent period	Any cause for delay in neuromuscular junction can cause increase in latent period	Viscosity of muscle resists travel of impulse	In higher temperature, the latent period is shorter and in lower temperature, the latent period is longer	Inertia of the instrument also may delay the latent period

7. Define the terms (a) resting length, (b) equilibrium length, (c) optimal length

Resting Length

It is the length of the muscle during relaxed state under natural circumstances in the body.

Equilibrium Length

It is the length of the relaxed muscle when cut free from its attachments.

Optimal Length

It is the length of the muscle at which maximum force of contraction is achieved.

8. Define Starling's law of muscle contraction.

- It states that the force of contraction of a muscle depends directly on the initial length of the muscle fiber prior to contraction within physiological limits.

- The reason for this is, when the muscle is stretched, more active binding sites of actin and myosin are exposed.
- As a result, there is optimum overlapping between actin and myosin (Fig. 3.51).

9. Define motor unit.

Motor Unit

- A motor neuron, its axon terminals and the muscle fibers innervated by it are together called motor unit.
- Every motor neuron activates a group of muscle fibers through the axon terminals.
- Stimulation of a motor neuron causes contraction of all the muscle fibers innervated by that neuron.
- The cell bodies of the motor neurons supplying the skeletal muscle fibers lie in the ventral horn of spinal cord (Fig. 3.52).

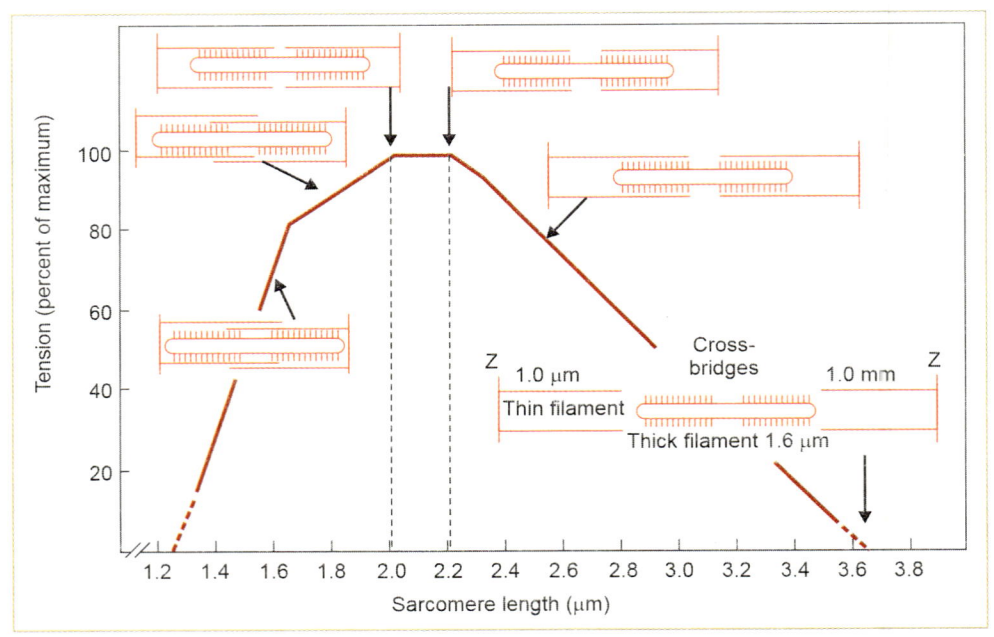

Fig. 3.51

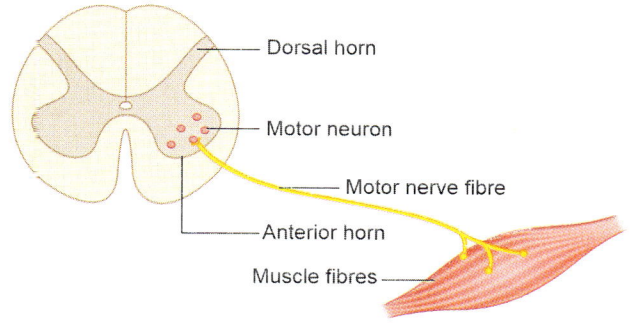

Fig. 3.52

10. Define summation. Enumerate its types.

Summation

- Summation refers to the additive effect of several electrical impulses on a neuromuscular junction, the junction between a nerve cell and a muscle cell.
- Individually the stimuli cannot evoke a response, but collectively they can generate a response.

Types of Summation

1. **Temporal summation:** Successive stimuli on one nerve are called temporal summation.
2. **Spatial summation:** The addition of simultaneous stimuli from several conducting fibres is called spatial summation.

11. Define the terms treppe, clonus and tetanus.

Treppe

- Also known as staircase phenomenon
- Refers to slow increase in force of contraction of muscle when it is stimulated repeatedly with a maximal strength at a low frequency.
- Treppe is distinct from summation of contractions and tetanus.

Clonus

- Refers to a series of rapid and repeated involuntary jerky movements, which occur while eliciting a deep reflex.
- When a deep reflex is elicited in a normal person, the contractions of a muscle or group of muscles are smooth and continuous.
- But clonus occurs when the deep reflexes are exaggerated due to hypertonicity of muscles in pyramidal tract lesion.

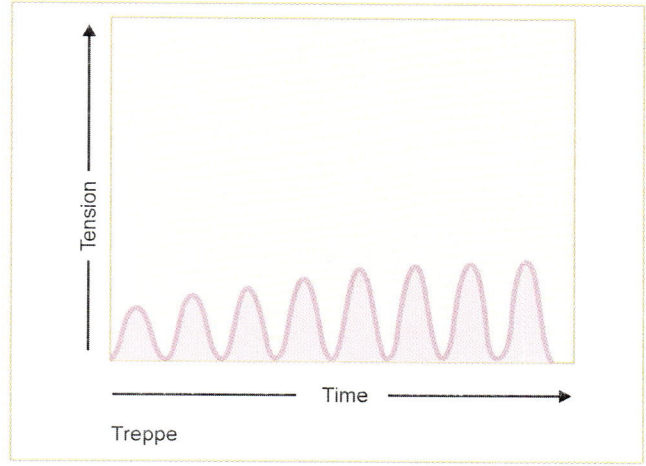

Fig. 3.53

Types of Clonus

1. **Ankle clonus:** Ankle clonus is the repeated rhythmical contractions of calf muscles caused by sudden dorsiflexion of foot (Fig. 3.54).

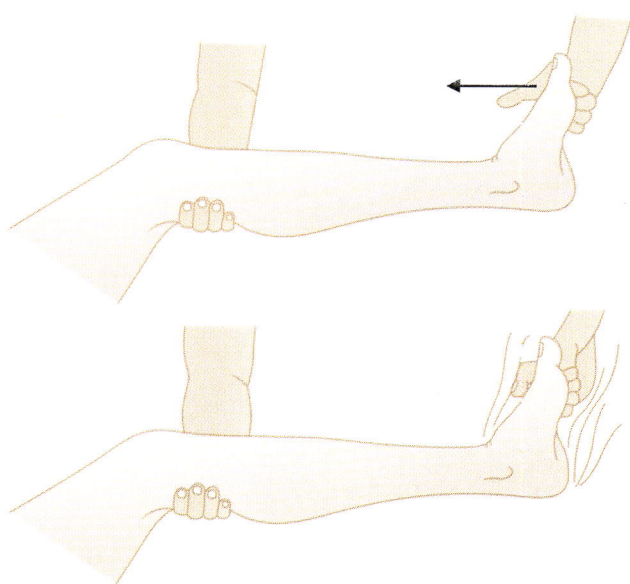

Fig. 3.54

2. **Patellar clonus:** Patellar clonus is the rhythmic jerky movements of patella produced by grasping it between thumb and index finger of the examiner and pushing it down forcibly towards the foot (Fig. 3.55).

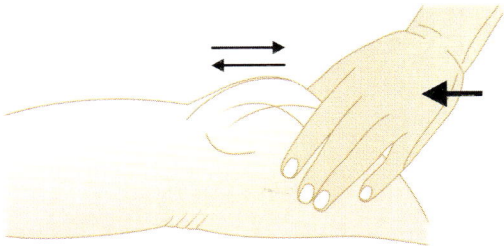

Fig. 3.55

Tetanus

- Refers to sustained muscular contraction due to repeated stimuli with high frequency.
- When the multiple stimuli are applied at a higher frequency in such a way that the successive stimuli fall during contraction period of previous twitch, the muscle remains in state of tetanus.
- It relaxes only after the stoppage of stimulus or when the muscle is fatigued.

Physiological Tetanus

Sustained contraction of muscle due to repeated stimuli of high frequency is called physiological tetanus.

Pathological Tetanus

- Refers to spastic contraction of the different muscle groups in pathological conditions.
- Causative agent is *Clostridium tetani* found in the soil.
- The bacillus enters the body through a cut, wound and manifest their symptoms through their toxin.
- This disease affects the nervous system and its common features are muscle spasm and paralysis.
- Symptoms are spasm of the jaw muscles resulting in locking of jaw.
- Tetanus is also referred to as lockjaw disease.
- If timely treatment is not provided, the condition becomes serious and it may even lead to death.

12. Explain the basis for the phenomenon of quantal summation.

Quantal Summation

- It is also known as recruitment
- It is characterized by increase in the number of cells contracting following increased strength of the stimulus.

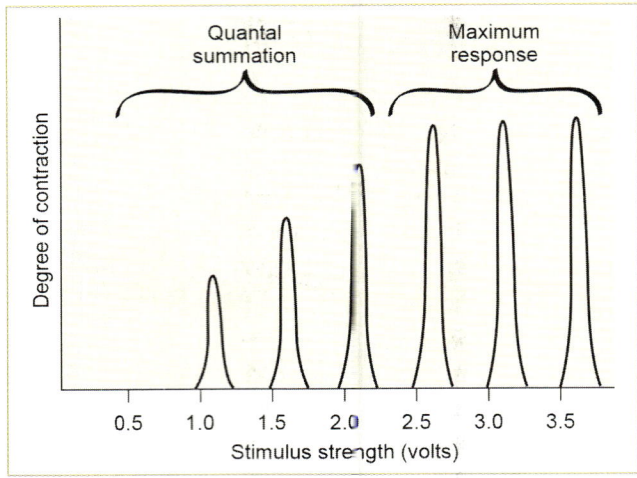

Fig. 3.56

- It can be demonstrated experimentally by increasing the voltage used to stimulate a muscle.
- This is brought about by recruitment of more and more motor units.
- Thus, there is resultant increase in force of contraction with increase in stimulus strength.

13. Define muscle fatigue and explain the mechanisms for it.

Fatigue

- It is defined as decrease in muscle activity due to repeated stimuli.
- When stimuli are continually applied, the muscle does not respond.

Sites of Fatigue

- Neuromuscular junction
- Muscle per se
- Anterior grey horn cells

Causes for Fatigue

- Exhaustion of ACh at the neuromuscular junction causes fatigue. Neuromuscular junction is the first site of fatigue.
- Accumulation of metabolites like lactic acid due to increased work by the muscles.
- Lack of nutrients like calcium and ATP.
- Lack of oxygen: Oxygen is required for aerobic respiration and release of ATP required for muscular contraction.

3.9 DESCRIBE THE MOLECULAR BASIS OF MUSCLE CONTRACTION IN SKELETAL AND IN SMOOTH MUSCLES

LONG ESSAYS

1. Describe the molecular basis of skeletal muscle contraction.

It is explained in the following steps:

1. **Initiation of crossbridge cycling**
   - During resting stage, the myosin binding site on actin is blocked by troponin I and is bound to actin and tropomyosin.
   - Troponin and tropomyosin behave as regulatory proteins as they prevent interaction between actin and myosin.
   - Calcium that is released following an action potential, attach to the troponin C part.
   - This leads to a conformational change in the troponin molecule and causes lateral movement of the tropomyosin molecule. As a result, the active site on the myosin head is exposed.
   - Each molecule of troponin molecule that is bound by calcium is responsible of uncovering of 7 molecules of myosin.

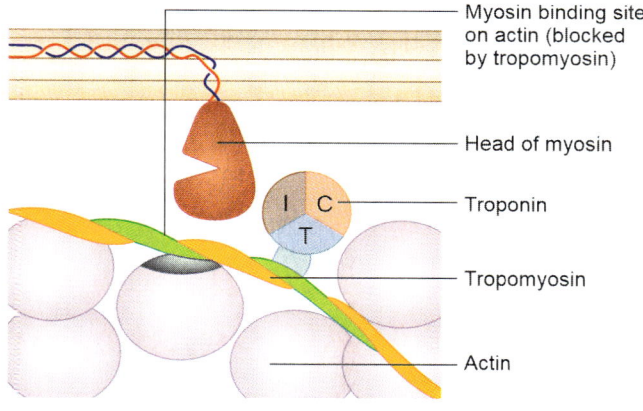

Fig. 3.57

2. **Formation of actin–myosin complex**
   - The head of myosin has two activation sites: One for ATP and another for actin.
   - When ATP attaches to the myosin head, the myosin ATPase enzyme splits ATP to ADP and Pi. This energy is transferred to the myosin head.
   - The activated myosin head bends perpendicularly and moves to meet the actin filament.

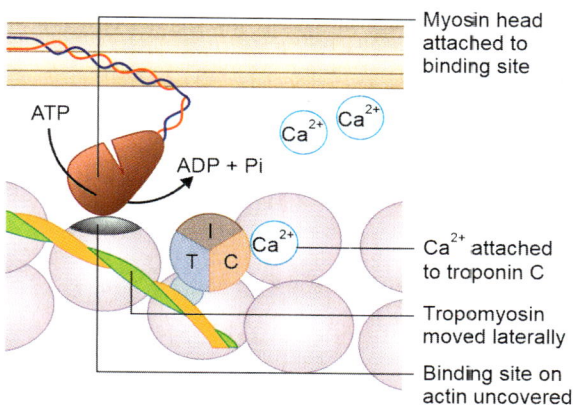

Fig. 3.58

3. **Power stroke**
   - After the release of ADP and Pi from the myosin head, there is a conformational change in the myosin head.
   - There is change in high energy 90° flexion to 45° low energy flexion of the head.
   - As a result, the actin filaments are pulled towards each other.

4. **Detachment of myosin from the actin filament**
   - Once the ADP and Pi are released from the myosin head, a new ATP molecule comes to occupy that position.
   - This myosin ATP has a low affinity for actin and thus gets detached form the actin filament.

5. **Reactivation of the myosin head**
   - The newly bound ATP transfers energy to the myosin head and splits into ADP and Pi.
   - The whole process repeats again.
   - Thus, with cycle, the actin filaments are brought closer and closer.
   - This brings about muscle contraction.

2. Describe the excitation-contraction coupling in a skeletal muscle

Excitation-Contraction Coupling

- When the action potential reaches the tip of a transverse tubule membrane, it activates voltage-gated calcium channels (DHP channels). These undergo conformational change.

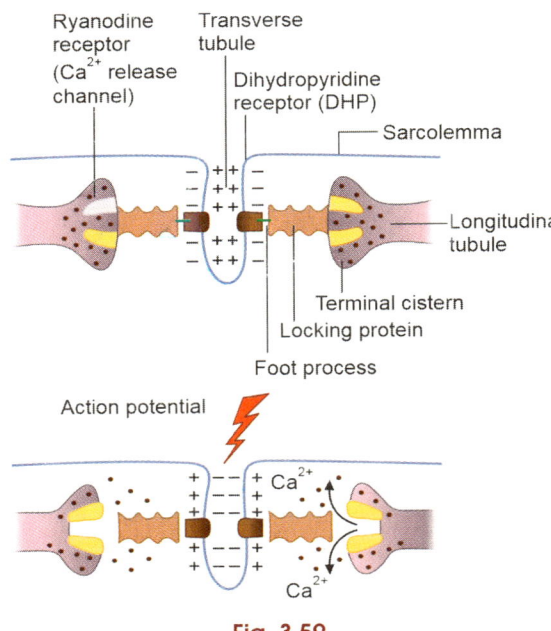

Fig. 3.59

- This leads to opening of calcium release channels located in the terminal cisterns or ryanodine receptor.
- Calcium ions diffuse into the cytoplasm and the concentration of intracellular up to 2000 times.
- The process by which muscle contraction occurs is called sliding theory or rachet theory.
- This is brought about by formation of complexes between actin filaments and myosin heads called crossbridges.

Stages

1. Initiation of crossbridge cycling

- During resting stage, the myosin binding site on actin is blocked by troponin I and is bound to actin and tropomyosin.
- Troponin and tropomyosin behave as regulatory proteins as they prevent interaction between actin and myosin.
- Calcium that is released following an action potential, attach to the troponin C part.
- This leads to a conformational change in the troponin molecule and causes lateral movement of the tropomyosin molecule. As a result, the active site on the myosin head is exposed.
- Each molecule of troponin molecule that is bound by calcium is responsible of uncovering of 7 molecules of myosin.

2. Formation of actin–myosin complex

- The head of myosin has two activation sites: One for ATP and another for actin.
- When ATP attaches to the myosin head, the myosin ATPase enzyme splits ATP to ADP and Pi. This energy is transferred to the myosin head.
- The activated myosin head bends perpendicularly and moves to meet the actin filament.

3. Power stroke

- After the release of ADP and Pi from the myosin head, there is a conformational change in the myosin head.
- There is change in high energy 90° flexion to 45° low energy flexion of the head.
- As a result, the actin filaments are pulled towards each other.

4. Detachment of myosin from the actin filament

- Once the ADP and Pi are released from the myosin head, a new ATP molecule comes to occupy that position.

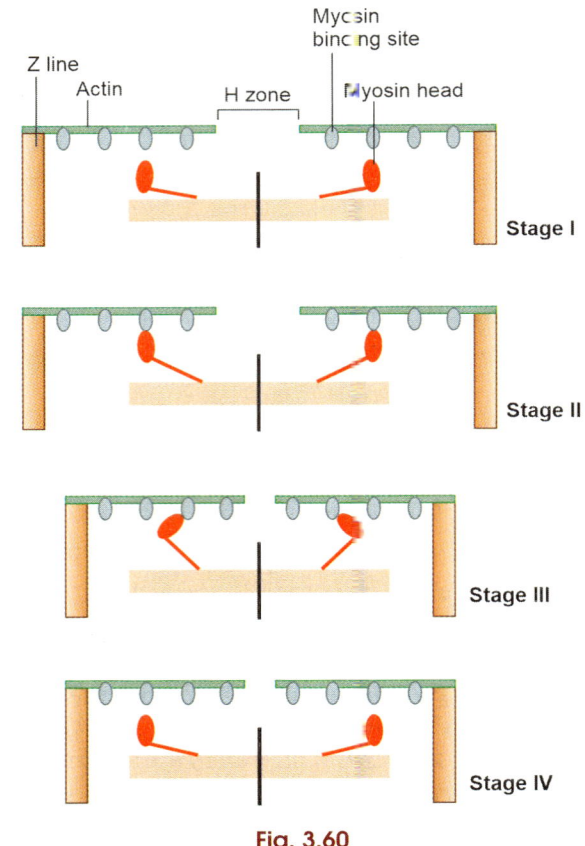

Fig. 3.60

- This myosin ATP has a low affinity for actin and thus gets detached form the actin filament.

5. **Reactivation of the myosin head**
   - The newly bound ATP transfers energy to the myosin head and splits into ADP and Pi.
   - The whole process repeats again.
   - Thus, with cycle, the actin filaments are brought closer and closer.
   - This brings about muscle contraction.

SHORT ESSAYS

1. An individual committed suicide by hanging himself when the body was brought down, all muscles were in the state of sustained contraction.
   A. What is this type of muscle contraction known as? (1 mark)
   B. What is the physiological mechanism behind this? (1 mark)
   C. What is its clinical significance? (1 mark)
   D. Describe the role of ATP in excitation contraction coupling. (2 marks)

A. This is known as rigor mortis.

B. Physiological Mechanism Behind this

- Following death, there is cessation of availability of ATP.
- The cell membranes of skeletal muscles become extremely permeable to calcium ions.
- As a result, many calcium ions enter the muscle and forms actomyosin complex and cause contraction of the muscle in the whole body.
- The position of the joint is determined by the stronger muscle (example, biceps is stronger than triceps, so there is flexion at the elbow)
- The joints become stiff and locked.
- For relaxation, there is a requirement for ATP and following death, due to lack of oxygen and thus ATP, the complexes of actin and myosin heads which are formed cannot be unlocked.

C. Clinical Significance

- It begins shortly after death (10 minutes 3 hours) and is maximum at 24 hours.
- After that due to release of lysosomal enzymes there is degradation of proteins of the muscle leading to resolution of rigor.

- Rigor begins to develop in the facial muscles and then spreads to the rest of the body.
- Based on these facts, the forensic experts can gauge the amount of time elapsed since death occurred.
- Rigor mortis is also influenced by environmental temperature.
- If the person dies of a struggle, then there is excess generation of heat. Thus, in such cases and in hot temperatures, rigor sets in quickly.

D. Role of ATP in Excitation–Contraction Coupling

- The head of myosin has two activation sites: One for ATP and another for actin.
- When ATP attaches to the myosin head, the myosin ATPase enzyme splits ATP to ADP and Pi. This energy is transferred to the myosin head.
- The activated myosin head bends perpendicularly and moves to meet the actin filament.
- After the release of ADP and Pi from the myosin head, there is a conformational change in the myosin head.
- There is change in high energy $90°$ flexion to $45°$ low energy flexion of the head.
- As a result, the actin filaments are pulled towards each other
- This causes muscle contraction

2. Explain the mechanism responsible for tonic contraction in a smooth muscle.

Smooth Muscle Contraction (Fig. 3.61)

Mechanism of Contraction

- In relaxed state, there is actin filament and the head of myosin are not in contact with one another.
- A part of the light chain of myosin serves as a regulatory protein.
- When there is influx of calcium ions, it binds with calmodulin and this complex causes activation of myosin light chain kinase.
- This enzyme causes phosphorylation of myosin regulatory protein.
- Cross-bridging: Following phosphorylation of myosin regulatory protein, the head of the myosin acquires the ability to bind with actin.

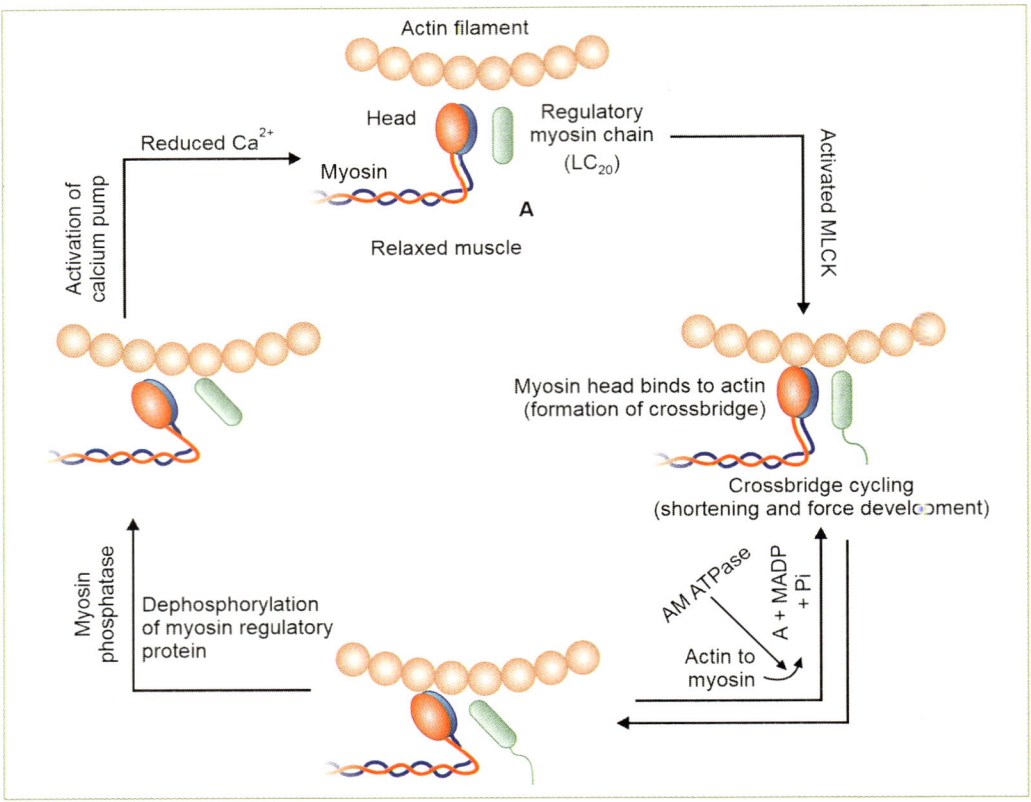

Fig. 3.61

- The binding of actin to myosin in presence of ADP and phosphate ion causes conformational change in the structure of myosin such that the head of myosin bends towards the crossbridge.
- This flexion causes a mechanical force.
- Due to this movement, there is sliding of actin over myosin. Actin is attached to dense bodies which are attached to the plasma membrane. This causes contraction of the muscle fiber.

Tonic Contraction

- Smooth muscles of some visceral organs maintain a tone—a state of partial contraction even in the absence of stimulus.
- This is due to a very slow process of cycling of myosin crossbridges in a smooth muscle. The reason for slow cycling is decreased availability of ATPase activity which causes increased availability of ATP.

- However, the time during which they stay attached is long, thus the force of contraction is very high.
- Also, as a result of less energy requirements, they are able to sustain contraction for a very long time.
- The resting membrane potential is unsteady, it varies between –50 mV and –75 mV.

3. Compare and contrast the mechanism of skeletal muscle contraction and smooth muscle contraction.

Similarities

- Both the muscles contract under the influence of calcium influx and the activator lies within the muscle fiber.
- They both have actin and myosin filaments which slide over each other in presence of ATP.
- Source of calcium: Intracellular stores in the sarcoplasmic reticulum.

Differences between Skeletal Muscle and Smooth Muscle Contraction

Skeletal muscle contraction	Smooth muscle contraction
Rapid contraction and relaxation of muscle	Slow to begin and is sustained
Fast cycling of filament	Slow cycling of filaments (1/10–1/300th that of skeletal muscle)
Greater activity of ATPase	Far less ATPase activity
Duration of contraction is less	Duration of contraction 1–3 seconds
Force of contraction is smaller	Force of contraction is much higher

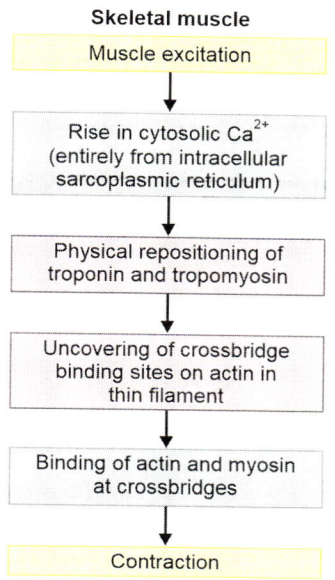

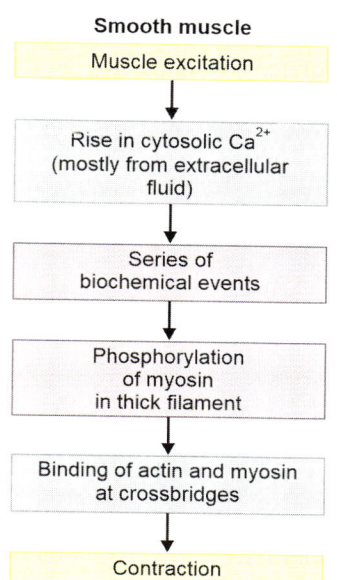

4. Explain why smooth muscle contraction is called latch-bridge mechanism.

Latch Bridge Mechanism (Fig. 3.62)

- In relaxed state, actin filament and the head of myosin are not in contact with one another.
- A part of the light chain of myosin serves as a regulatory protein.
- When there is influx of calcium ions, it binds with calmodulin and this complex causes activation of myosin light chain kinase.
- This enzyme causes phosphorylation of myosin regulatory protein.
- Cross-bridging: Following phosphorylation of myosin regulatory protein, the head of the myosin acquires the ability to bind with actin.
- Latch-bridge is a subset of crossbridges that are involved in keeping actin and myosin together. They have the property of keeping the tone of the muscle without the use of ATP.

- In smooth muscles, they remain attached to each other in a latched form. As a result, smooth muscles have prolonged contractions, sometimes lasting for days.
- The binding of actin to myosin in presence of ADP and phosphate ion causes conformational change in the structure of myosin such that the head of myosin bends towards the crossbridge.
- This flexion causes a mechanical force.

5. Describe the structure and function of Sarcotubular system.

- The cell membrane of the muscle cell—sarcolemma and sarcoplasmic reticulum is known as the sarcotubular system.
- It plays an important role in spreading of depolarization within the muscle.
- It has a transverse and a longitudinal sarcoplasmic reticulum (Fig. 3.63).

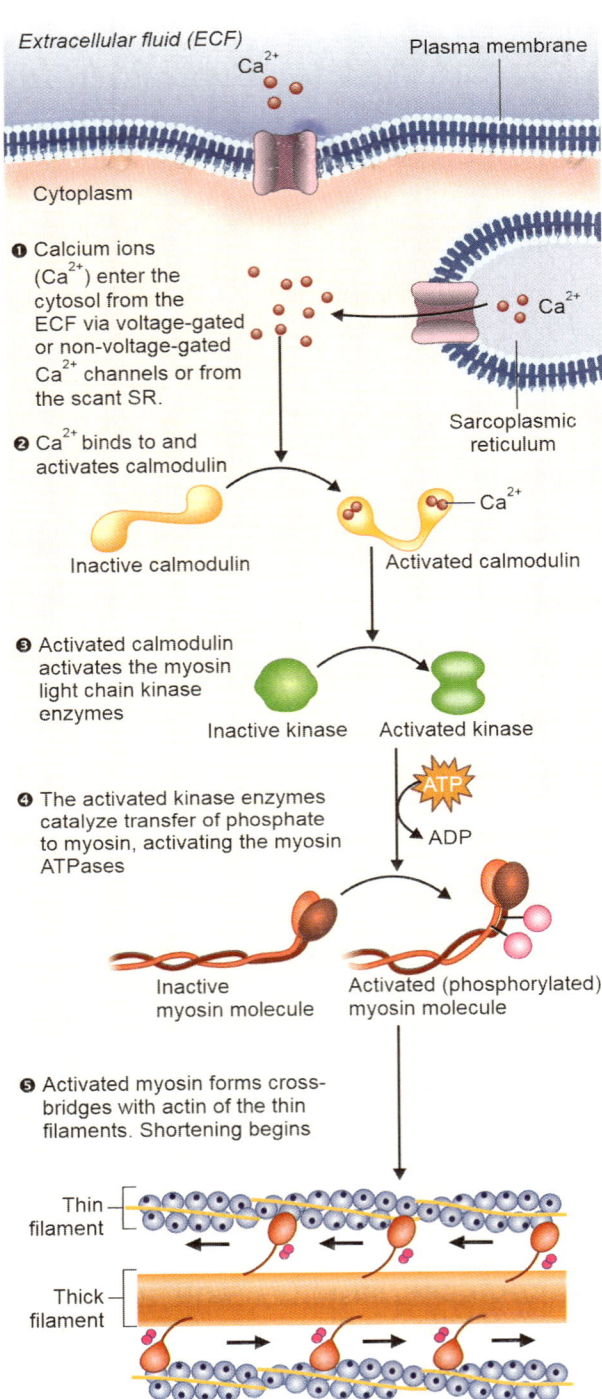

❶ Calcium ions (Ca²⁺) enter the cytosol from the ECF via voltage-gated or non-voltage-gated Ca^{2+} channels or from the scant SR.

❷ Ca^{2+} binds to and activates calmodulin

❸ Activated calmodulin activates the myosin light chain kinase enzymes

❹ The activated kinase enzymes catalyze transfer of phosphate to myosin, activating the myosin ATPases

❺ Activated myosin forms cross-bridges with actin of the thin filaments. Shortening begins

Fig. 3.62

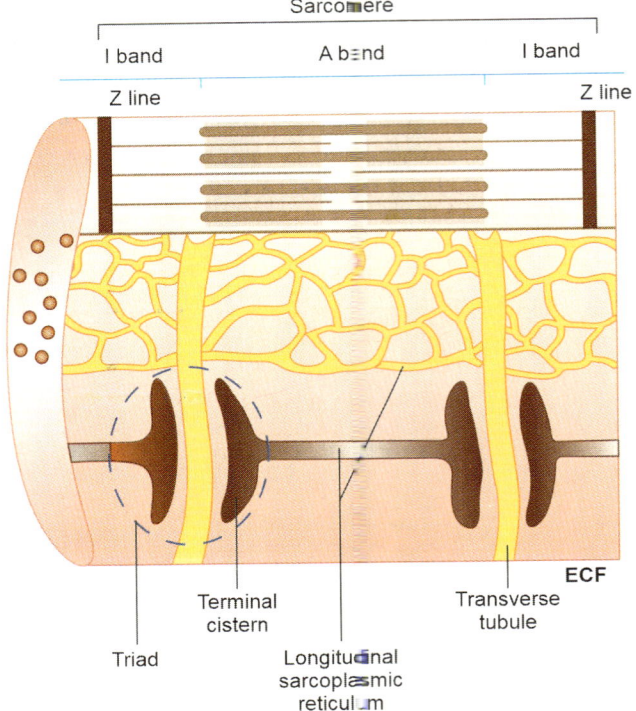

Fig. 3.63

1. Transverse tubular system or T system

– It is formed by through and through invagination of sarcolemma into the muscle in the junction of A and I bands.
– Their lumen contains the ECF.
– The membranes of the T tubules have voltage-gated calcium channels called DHP receptors.

Functions

1. Rapid transmission of impulses from sarcolemma to myofibrils.
2. As T tubules invaginate into the muscle, impulse spreads from exterior to interior very rapidly.

2. Longitudinal tubular system or L system

– These sarcoplasmic tubules run along the length of the muscle
– It forms a close tubular system around each myofibril.
– The longitudinal tubules around T tubules are dilated and are called terminal cistern.
– The T tubule and the cisterns form a triad. There are two such triads in a sarcomere.

Functions
1. These tubules carry lot of calcium ions.
2. When the impulse reaches the cistern, calcium is released the contractile function begins.

6 Describe sliding filament theory.

It is explained in the following steps:

1. Initiation of crossbridge cycling
- During resting stage, the myosin binding site on actin is blocked by troponin I and is bound to actin and tropomyosin.
- Troponin and tropomyosin behave as regulatory proteins as they prevent interaction between actin and myosin.
- Calcium that is released following an action potential, attach to the troponin C part.
- This leads to a conformational change in the troponin molecule and causes lateral movement of the tropomyosin molecule. As a result, the active site on the myosin head is exposed.
- Each molecule of troponin molecule that is bound by calcium is responsible of uncovering of 7 molecules of myosin.

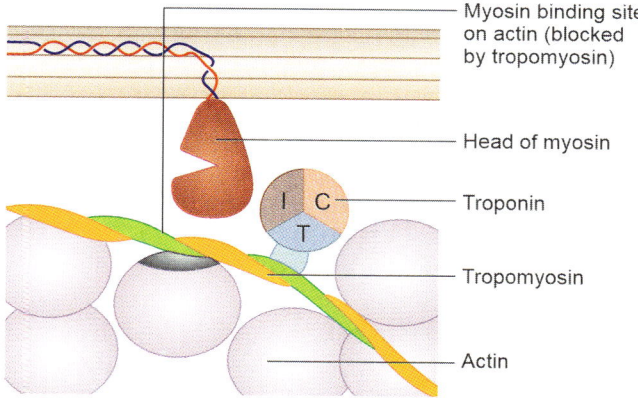

Myosin binding site on actin (blocked by tropomyosin)

Head of myosin

Troponin

Tropomyosin

Actin

Fig. 3.64

2. Formation of actin–myosin complex
- The head of myosin has two activation sites: One for ATP and another for actin.
- When ATP attaches to the myosin head, the myosin ATPase enzyme splits ATP to ADP and Pi. This energy is transferred to the myosin head.
- The activated myosin head bends perpendicularly and moves to come in contact with the actin filament.

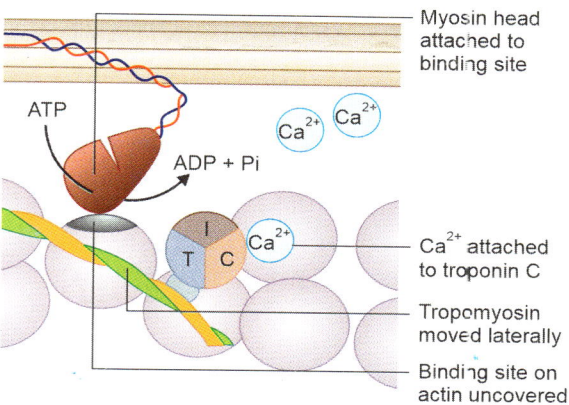

Myosin head attached to binding site

ATP

ADP + Pi

Ca^{2+} attached to troponin C

Tropomyosin moved laterally

Binding site on actin uncovered

Fig. 3.65

3. Power stroke
- After the release of ADP and Pi from the myosin head, there is a conformational change in the myosin head.
- There is change in high energy 90° flexion to 45° low energy flexion of the head.
- As a result, the actin filaments are pulled towards each other.

4. Detachment of myosin from the actin filament
- Once the ADP and Pi are released from the myosin head, a new ATP molecule comes to occupy that position.
- This myosin ATP has a low affinity for actin and thus gets detached form the actin filament.

5. Reactivation of the myosin head
- The newly bound ATP transfers energy to the myosin head and splits into ADP and Pi.
- The whole process repeats again.
- Thus, with cycle, the actin filaments are brought closer and closer.
- This brings about muscle contraction.

7. Explain the molecular basis of smooth muscle contraction.

- In relaxed state, there is actin filament and the head of myosin are not in contact with one another.
- A part of the light chain of myosin serves as a regulatory protein.
- When there is influx of calcium ions, it binds with calmodulin and this complex causes activation of myosin light chain kinase.
- This enzyme causes phosphorylation of myosin regulatory protein (Fig. 3.66).

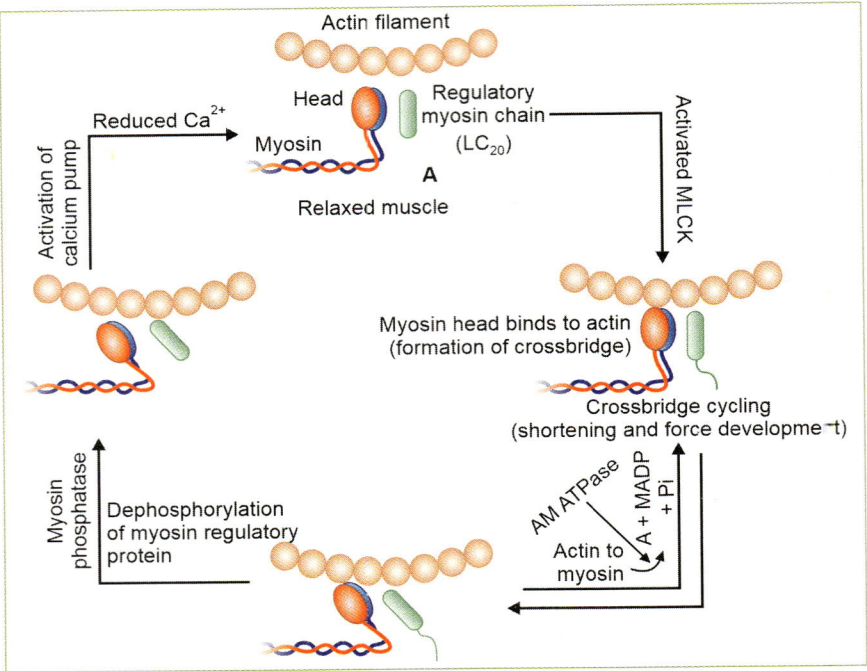

Fig. 3.66

- Cross-bridging: Following phosphorylation of myosin regulatory protein, the head of the myosin acquires the ability to bind with actin.
- The binding of actin to myosin in presence of ADP and phosphate ion causes conformational change in the structure of myosin such that the head of myosin bends towards the crossbridge.
- This flexion causes a mechanical force.
- Due to this movement, there is sliding of actin over myosin. Actin is attached to dense bodies which are attached to the plasma membrane. This causes contraction of the muscle fiber.

8. List the steps involved in excitation–contraction coupling.

or

List the molecular events associated with contraction and relaxation of skeletal muscle.

- Arrival of action potential in the efferent nerve and release of neurotransmitter (ACh).
- Formation of endplate potential and action potential by summation.
- Depolarization of the skeletal muscle caused by entry of sodium ions through fast sodium channels.
- Opening of voltage-gated calcium channels.
- Entry of calcium from sarcoplasmic reticulum into the sarcomere.
- Calcium that is released following an action potential, attach to the troponin C part.
- This leads to a conformational change in the troponin molecule and causes lateral movement of the tropomyosin molecule. As a result, the active site on the myosin head is exposed.
- The head of myosin has two activation sites: One for ATP and another for actin.
- When ATP attaches to the myosin head, the myosin ATPase enzyme splits ATP to ADP and Pi. This energy is transferred to the myosin head.
- The activated myosin head bends perpendicularly and moves to come in contact with the actin filament.
- Once the ADP and Pi are released from the myosin head, a new ATP molecule comes to occupy that position.
- This myosin ATP has a low affinity for actin and thus gets detached form the actin filament.
- The newly bound ATP transfers energy to the myosin head and splits into ADP and Pi.
- The whole process repeats again.

- Thus, with cycle, the actin filaments are brought closer and closer. This brings about muscle contraction.

SHORT ANSWERS

1. Explain the phenomenon of (a) rigor mortis, (b) heat rigor.

Rigor Mortis

- It is a state of contraction of skeletal muscles to cause fixed positions of joints after death of an individual.
- It is due to formation of actin–myosin complexes following calcium entry after death into a muscle.
- As the relaxation requires ATP and ATP is unavailable after death, the muscles remain contracted.

Heat Rigor

- Stiffening of muscles due to denaturation of proteins and shortening of muscle fibers on exposure to extreme high temperatures in a living tissue is called heat rigor.
- The temperature is usually above 65°C.
- This is irreversible

2. Describe the structure and types of smooth muscle.

Structure of a Smooth Muscle

- These are fusiform elongated cells with a size of 2–5 microns
- It has a single, centrally placed elongated nucleus.
- The myofibrils and sarcomere are not very conspicuous
- As there are no striations—they are termed smooth muscles.

Contractile Proteins

- Actin and tropomyosin form thin filaments
- Myosin forms thick filaments
- Dense bodies are specialized structures to which actin and myosin filaments attach
- They are firmly attached to the sarcolemma.

Types of Smooth Muscle

They are mainly of two types: Unitary smooth muscles and multi-unit smooth muscles.

Single unit smooth muscle/ unitary smooth muscle	Multiunit smooth muscle
A unit of many smooth muscle fibers are closely associated such that they have gap junctions between them.	Each smooth muscle behaves as a single unit. Each smooth muscle fiber is surrounded by a basement membrane like substance
A group of cells function as a single unit.	Each fiber operates as a single unit independent of each other

3. Describe the following properties of smooth muscle.
  #### A. Single muscle twitch
  #### B. Latch-bridge mechanism
  #### C. Plasticity

A. Single Muscle Twitch

- The average duration of a spike varies from 25 to 50 ms.
- The amplitude is very less and hardly reaching the isoelectric base.
- It is due to nervous stimuli and leads to contraction of muscle.

B. Latch-bridge Mechanism

- In relaxed state, there is actin filament and the head of myosin are not in contact with one another.
- A part of the light chain of myosin serves as a regulatory protein.

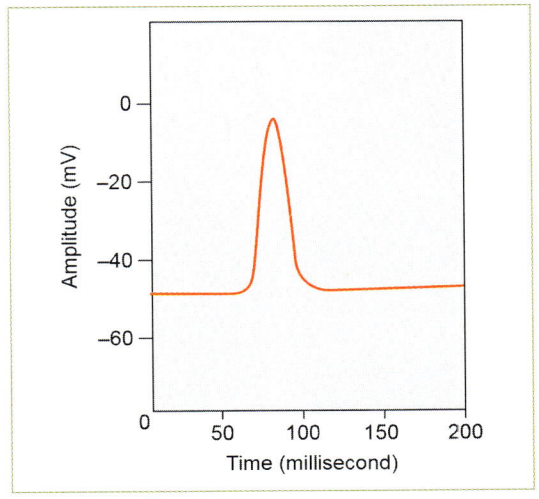

Fig. 3.67

- When there is influx of calcium ions, it binds with calmodulin and this complex causes activation of myosin light chain kinase.
- This enzyme causes phosphorylation of myosin regulatory protein.
- Cross-bridging: Following phosphorylation of myosin regulatory protein, the head of the myosin acquires the ability to bind with actin.
- Latch-bridge is a subset of crossbridges that are involved in keeping actin and myosin together. They have the property of keeping the tone of the muscle without the use of ATP.
- In smooth muscles, they remain attached to each other in a latched form. As a result, smooth muscles have prolonged contractions, sometimes lasting for days.
- This flexion causes a mechanical force.

C. Plasticity

- It is the adaptability of muscle to varying lengths.
- If a smooth muscle is stretched, then it adapts to this new length and contracts only when stimulated.

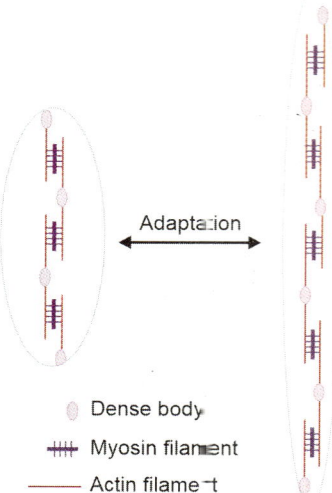

Adaptation

⊙ Dense body
╫╫ Myosin filament
— Actin filament

Fig. 3.68

- As a result, Starling's law does not hold good in a smooth muscle.
- This property is utilized in the GIT. When the volume of food is more, there is increase on the capacity of these hollow organs due to plasticity of the smooth muscles.

3.10 DESCRIBE THE MODE OF MUSCLE CONTRACTION (ISOMETRIC AND ISOTONIC)

SHORT ESSAYS

1. **Mr. X of 34 years was a sprint athlete and Mr. Y of 24 years was a weightlifting champion.**
   A. Compare and contrast the type of muscle contraction that happens in both individuals. (2 marks)
   B. Enumerate different types of heat produced during skeletal muscle contraction.   (3 marks)

A.

- When an individual sprints (Mr. X), it is called isometric contraction of a muscle.
- When an individual lifts the weight (Mr. Y), it is called isotonic contraction of a muscle.

Isometric contraction	*Isotonic contraction*
The length of the muscle fibers does not change	The tension in the muscle fibers remain constant
The tension in the muscle fibers increases during contraction	The length of the muscle fibers decreases during contraction
Mechanism This is produced when the series elastic component of the muscle represented by the tendon provides resistance to the passive stretch of the muscle. Thus, the muscle is able to contract even when length does not decrease.	*Mechanism* This is produced when the parallel elastic component folds upon itself during contraction of a muscle. It also resists against passive stretch Thus, the muscle gains original length after the parallel elastic component unfolds itself.

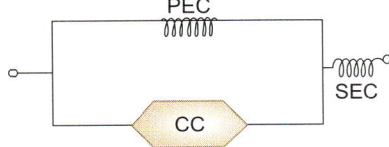

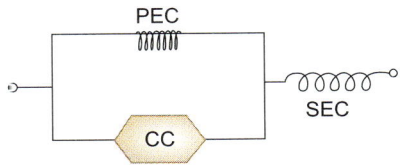

Before and during contraction
CC: Contractile component
PEC: Parallel elastic component
SEC: Series elastic component
Parallel elastic component shortens during contraction

CC: Contractile component
PEC: Parallel elastic component
SEC: Series elastic component

B. Heat Produced during Exercise

During muscular contraction, heat is released in different stages.

1. **Resting heat:** It is the heat produced at resting conditions due to ongoing basal metabolic processes.

2. **Initial heat**
   - It is the heat produced during muscular activity.
   - Heat of activation
     - Before beginning of contraction of muscles
     - It is due to entry of calcium ions into the L tubules.
     - It is also called maintenance heat
   - Heat of shortening
     - Heat produced during contraction of a muscle
     - The heat is produced due to various structural changes (movement of crossbridges, glycolysis, etc).

- Heat of relaxation
  - Heat is produced during contraction of the muscle by use of ATP
  - It is released during relaxation

3. **Recovery heat**
   - It continues for 30 minutes after cessation of exercise.
   - This heat is generated by metabolic processes needed to restore the pre-exercise metabolic state.

2. Compare and contrast types of muscle contraction that happens when an individual tries to push the wall and when he lifts the weight.

- When an individual tries to push the wall, it is called isometric contraction of a muscle.
- When an individual lifts the weight, it is called isotonic contraction of a muscle.

Isometric contraction	Isotonic contraction
The length of the muscle fibers does not change	The tension in the muscle fibers remain constant
The tension in the muscle fibers increases during contraction	The length of the muscle fibers decreases during contraction
Mechanism	*Mechanism*
This is produced when the series elastic component of the muscle represented by the tendon provides resistance to the passive stretch of the muscle. Thus, the muscle is able to contract even when length does not decrease.	This is produced when the parallel elastic component folds upon itself during contraction of a muscle. It also resists against passive stretch. Thus, the muscle gains original length after the parallel elastic component unfolds itself.

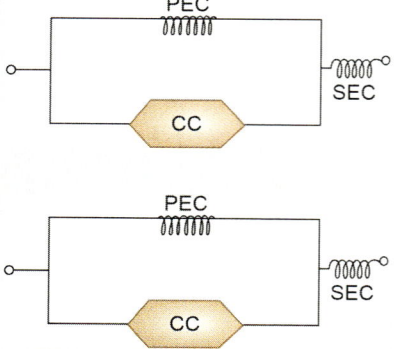

Before and during contraction
CC: Contractile component
PEC: Parallel elastic component
SEC: Series elastic component
Parallel elastic component shortens during contraction

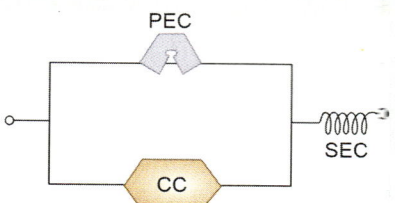

CC: Contractile component
PEC: Parallel elastic component
SEC: Series elastic component

SHORT ANSWERS

1. What is isometric and isotonic muscle contraction. Mention example for each.

Isometric contraction	Isotonic contraction
The length of the muscle fibers does not change	The tension in the muscle fibers remain constant
The tension in the muscle fibers increases during contraction	The length of the muscle fibers decreases during contraction
Example	*Example*
When an individual tries to push the wall, it is called isometric contraction of a muscle.	When an individual lifts up the weight, it is called isotonic contraction of a muscle.

2. List examples of isometric and isotonic muscle contraction.

Isometric contraction	Isotonic contraction
Pushing a wall	Walking
Plank	Yoga
Hand press	Jogging
Chair leg extension	Sprinting
Weightlifting	Cycling
Push-ups and pull-ups	

3.11 EXPLAIN ENERGY SOURCE AND MUSCLE METABOLISM

SHORT ESSAYS

1. Define fatigue. What is the first site of fatigue in nerve muscle preparation and in intact anima? What is the cause for it?   (1 + 2 + 2 marks)

Fatigue

- It is defined as decrease in muscle activity due to repeated stimuli.
- When stimuli are continually applied, the muscle does not respond.

First Site of Fatigue in Nerve Muscle Preparation and in Intact Anima

First site of fatigue in nerve muscle preparation	*First site of fatigue in intact anima*
Neuromuscular junction followed by muscle	Betz cells in the pyramidal cortex followed by: Anterior grey horn cells followed by: Neuromuscular junction followed by: Muscle

Causes for Fatigue

1. Exhaustion of ACh at the neuromuscular junction
2. Accumulation of metabolites like lactic acid
3. Lack of nutrients
4. Lack of oxygen

2. Describe the sources of energy for skeletal muscle.

Muscles require continuous supply of energy which is provided by ATP.

1. Hydrolysis of ATP

- ATP is stored in the skeletal muscles and is used by the myosin kinase when the actin attaches to the myosin head.
- It is hydrolyzed into ADP and phosphate.
- However, all the stored ATP is immediately consumed and thus there is a need for re-synthesis of ATP.

2. Regeneration of ATP (Fig 3.69)

- In resting state, ATP combines with creatine to form creatinine phosphate and APD is released.
- During active contraction of muscle, when ATP needs to be generated, the enzyme creatine kinase provides ATP by cleaving phosphate from the creatine phosphate.

3. Glycolysis (Fig. 3.70)

- After the creatine phosphate has been consumed, glycogen stores are used up.
- In presence of oxygen, the acetyl-CoA enters the Kreb's cycle and in absence of oxygen, the pyruvate is used for conversion into lactic acid.
- In the former, 12 ATP molecules are generated and under anaerobic conditions, only 2 ATP molecules are generated
- Through Cori cycle, the lactic acid is taken up by the liver and re-converted into glucose and returned to blood.

4. Oxidative metabolism (Fig. 3.71)

- It is the final source of energy in a muscle.
- Addition of oxygen to various types of nutrients leads to release of ATP.

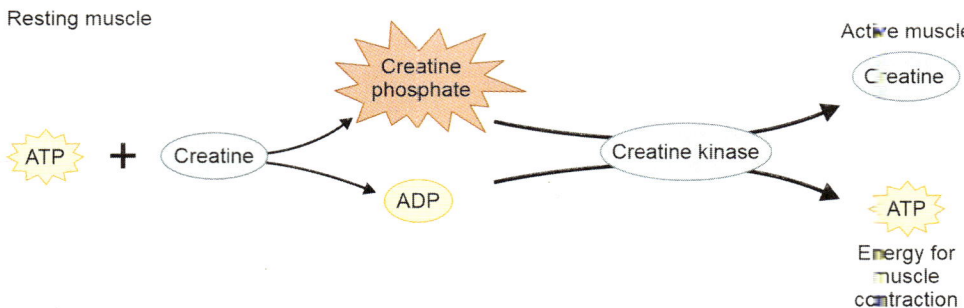

Fig. 3.69

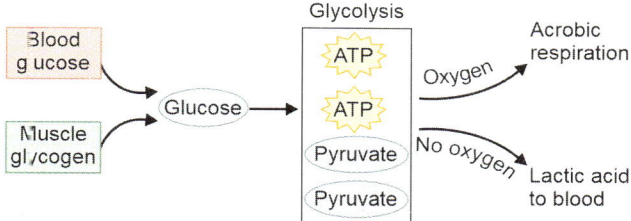

Fig. 3.70

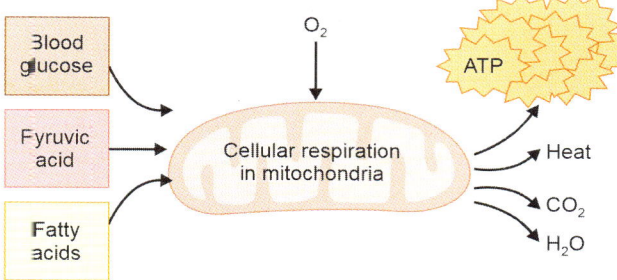

Fig. 3.71

3. Explain different types of heat produced during exercise.

During muscular contraction, heat is released in different stages.

1. **Resting heat:** It is the heat produced at resting conditions due to ongoing basal metabolic processes.
2. **Initial heat**
   - It is the heat produced during muscular activity.
   - Heat of activation
     - Before beginning of contraction of muscles
     - It is due to entry of calcium ions into the L tubules.
     - It is also called maintenance heat
   - Heat of shortening
     - Heat produced during contraction of a muscle
     - The heat is produced due to various structural changes (movement of cross bridges, glycolysis, etc.)
   - Heat of relaxation
     - Heat is produced during contraction of the muscle by use of ATP
     - It is released during relaxation

3. **Recovery heat**
   - It continues for 30 minutes after cessation of exercise.
   - This heat is generated by metabolic processes needed to restore the pre-exercise metabolic state.

SHORT ANSWERS

1. Describe the phenomenon of oxygen debt in skeletal muscle and explain its basis.

- During intense exercise, there is an increased need for oxygen than what is available.
- As a result, glucose is utilized by anaerobic metabolism.
- After the period of exercise, extra oxygen is consumed for a period of 30–45 minutes in the form of hyperventilation.
- This extra oxygen is used to clear up the accumulated lactate, replenish ATP stores ad phosphocreatine stores.
- This extra amount of oxygen consumed to 'repay' the deficit oxygen is called oxygen debt. It is proportional to the oxygen deficit produced during the exercise.

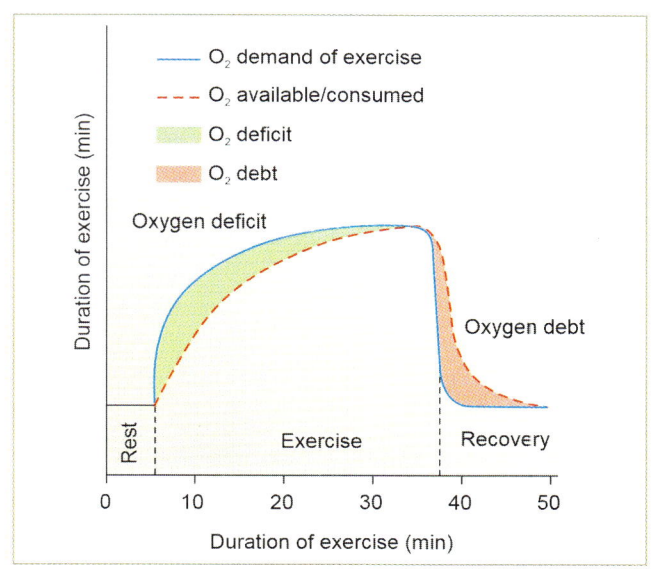

Fig. 3.72

2. Distinguish between muscle hypertrophy and muscle hyperplasia.

Parameter	Hypertrophy	Hyperplasia
Definition	Increase in size of the individual muscle fibres	Increase in the number of muscles fibres
Molecular pathogenesis	Increase in protein synthesis induced by growth factors	Increased proliferation of cells stimulated by growth factors
Morphology	Increased cell number with increase in mitotic figures	Increase in size of the nucleus
Cause	Due to exercise training (mechanical stimulus)	Does not occur following exercise (chemical or hormonal stimulus)

3. List different ways in which performance enhancing drugs act on skeletal muscle.

1. **Anabolic steroids, human growth hormone, IGF-1, insulin**
   - Are modified steroids
   - Increase protein formation (anabolic effect)

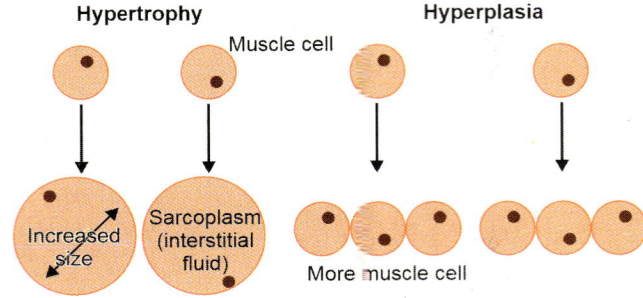

Fig. 3.73

   - Cause hypertrophy of muscles and build the muscles

2. **Nootropics or CNS stimulants**
   - Improve muscle strength
   - Decrease reaction time and decrease fatigue.

3. **Artificial oxygen carriers and erythropoietin**
   - Increase oxygen carrying capacity of blood and thus deliver more oxygen to muscles.
   - More energy is produced when there is excess oxygen and therefore, endurance increases.

3.12 EXPLAIN THE GRADATION OF MUSCULAR ACTIVITY

SHORT ANSWERS

1. Discuss the methods used to grade exercise.

WHO Classification of Exercises

- It is based on heart rate and oxygen consumption
- The oxygen consumption is described in terms of metabolic energy expenditure (MET).
- One MET is around 250 ml of oxygen per minute.

Grade	Level	Heart rate (beats per min)	O_2 consumption (L/min)	Relative load index (RLI) (% of max, O_2 consumption)	METs
I	Light (mild)	<100	0.4–0.8	<25	<3
II	Moderate	100–125	0.8–1.6	25–50	3.1–4.5
III	Heavy	125–150	1.6–2.4	51–75	4.6–7
IV	Severe	>150	>2.4	>75	>7

2. What is VO_2 max? Give its physiological significance.

VO_2 Max

- VO_2 max is the maximal oxygen consumption under aerobic condition that is consumed by a person.
- It is around 75 ml/kg/min.
- It is the level of oxygen consumption beyond which no further increase in O_2 consumption occurs with further increase in the severity of exercise.

Significance

- It is the highest attainable rate of aerobic metabolism for a given maximum of exercise.
- It is a representation of central and peripheral factors.
- Central factors include blood, heart and lungs, and peripheral factors are related to skeletal muscles.
- It is a measure of how well an athlete is trained with respect to his cardiorespiratory adaptations.

3.13 DESCRIBE MUSCULAR DYSTROPHY: MYOPATHIES

SHORT ESSAYS

1. Describe muscular dystrophy.

- It is a congenital disorder of the muscle characterized by inherent defect in the properties of muscle fibers leading to improper functioning and weakness.
- There is primary degeneration of the muscle without involvement of the nerves.
- They do not have the ability to regenerate leading to progressive weakness.
- The most common types are Duchenne's muscular dystrophy and Becker's muscular dystrophy.

1. Duchenne Muscular Dystrophy (Fig. 3.74)

- It is an X-linked recessive disorder characterized by loss of gene called dystrophin on the X chromosome.
- As a result, the sarcolemma becomes unstable. The muscle is more prone to damage due to stress and inflammation.
- This leads to degeneration of the muscle fiber and resultant fibrosis.

2. Becker's Muscular Dystrophy

- It occurs due to decreased production of dystrophin
- It is also X-linked disorder.
- It affects proximal muscles.
- It is characterized by slow progressive weakness of legs and pelvic muscles.
- There is fatigue and difficulty in walking. These children also demonstrate mental retardation.

2. A 12-year-old boy complained of gradual muscle weakness for six months, he was feeling difficulty in getting up from sitting position. What could be the diagnosis? Describe the muscular dystrophies.

Diagnosis

This sign is called Grower sign and is characteristic of a muscular dystrophy (Fig. 3.75).

Muscular Dystrophy

- It is a congenital disorder of the muscle characterized by inherent defect in the properties of muscle fibers leading to improper functioning and weakness.
- There is primary degeneration of the muscle without involvement of the nerves.
- They do not have the ability to regenerate leading to progressive weakness.
- The most common types are Duchenne's muscular dystrophy and Becker's muscular dystrophy.
  1. Duchenne muscular dystrophy (Fig. 3.76)
     - It is an X-linked recessive disorder characterized by loss of gene called dystrophin on the X chromosome.
     - As a result, the sarcolemma becomes unstable. The muscle is more prone to damage due to stress and inflammation.
     - This leads to degeneration of the muscle fiber and resultant fibrosis.

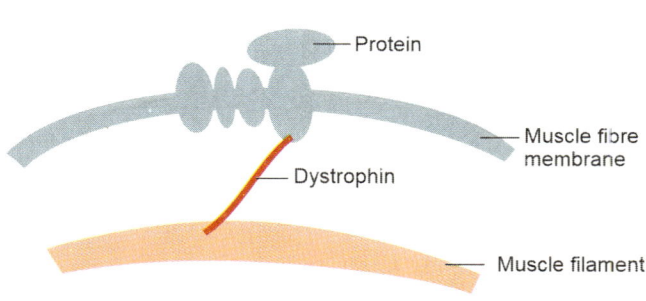

Fig. 3.74

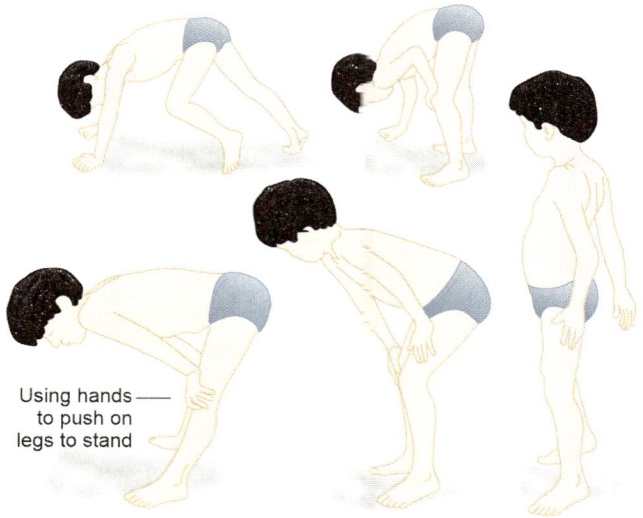

Fig. 3.75

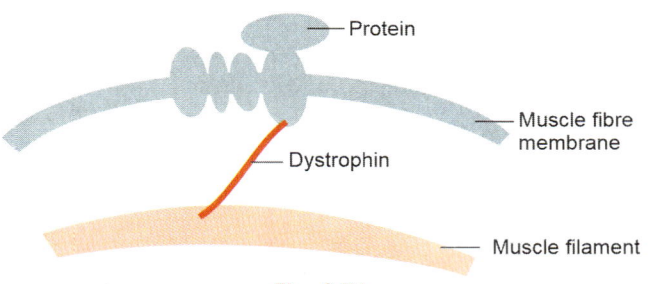

Fig. 3.76

2. **Becker's muscular dystrophy**
    – It occurs due to decreased production of dystrophin
    – It is also X-linked disorder.
    – It affects proximal muscles.
    – It is characterized by slow progressive weakness of legs and pelvic muscles.
    – There is fatigue and difficulty in walking. These children also demonstrate mental retardation.

SHORT ANSWERS

1. List the common causes of myopathies.

Myopathies

* It is dysfunction of a muscle fiber leading to weakness.
* It may be due to several causes

Congenital

* Duchenne's muscular dystrophy
* Becker's muscular dystrophy
* Myotonic dystrophy
* Oculopharyngeal dystrophy

Toxin-induced

* Steroids (Cushing's syndrome)
* Alcohol
* Chloroquine
* Colchicine

Post-inflammation

* Myositis (infectious)
* Polymyositis (autoimmune)

Metabolic

* Glycogen storage disorders
* Lipid storage disorders

Endocrine

* Thyroid abnormalities
* Parathyroid abnormalities

3.14 PERFORM ERGOGRAPHY

SHORT ESSAYS

1. Describe electromyography.

- It is a technique of recording total electrical activity of the motor nerve and the muscle.
- The machine used to study is called electromyograph and the recording is called electromyogram.

Technique (Fig. 3.77)

- Surface electrode: A superficial electrode is placed on the skin overlying the muscle. This helps in studying the overall activity of the muscle.
- Needle electrode: A needle is pierced into a muscle for studying the activity of a single motor unit.

Recordings (Fig. 3.78)

- *In normal relaxed state of muscle:* Normally there is complete electrical silence. There may be insertion activity due to insertion of needle.
- *During voluntary contraction of muscle:* The potential changes recorded during muscle contraction is called MUP (motor unit potential).
  - During minimal voluntary contraction, one or two motor units give off potentials.
  - With moderate voluntary contraction, firing rate of small units increases and recruits more and more muscles. There are still rhythmically appearing MUPs.
  - With maximum contraction, there is overlap of individual MUPs such that they can be differentiated.

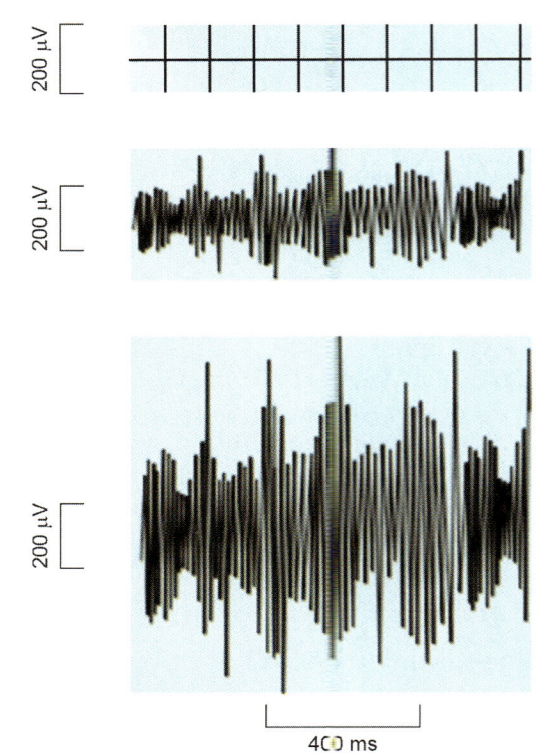

400 ms

Fig. 3.78

Uses

1. To diagnose neuromuscular disorders
2. To diagnose motor neuron lesions
3. To diagnose myopathies

2. What is fatigue? Mention the centers of fatigue.

Fatigue

- It is defined as decrease in muscle activity due to repeated stimuli.
- When stimuli are continually applied, the muscle does not respond.

Centers of Fatigue

Site of fatigue in nerve muscle preparation	Site of fatigue in intact anima
Neuromuscular junction followed by:	Betz cells in the pyramidal cortex followed by:
Muscle	Anterior grey horn cells followed by:
	Neuromuscular junction followed by:
	Muscle

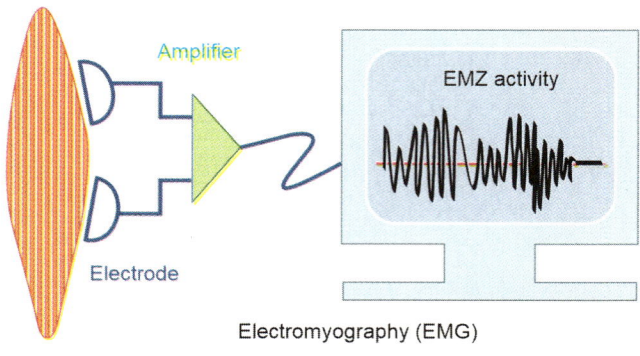

Electromyography (EMG)

Fig. 3.77

3.15 DEMONSTRATE EFFECT OF MILD, MODERATE AND SEVERE EXERCISE AND RECORD CHANGES IN CARDIORESPIRATORY PARAMETERS

SHORT ESSAYS

1. How do you grade exercise? Mention the cardiorespiratory changes during exercise.

WHO Classification of Exercises

- It is based on heart rate and oxygen consumption
- The oxygen consumption is described in terms of metabolic energy expenditure.

Cardiorespiratory Changes during Exercise

Cardiovascular Changes

- Increase in blood flow to the skeletal muscles and increase in pumped venous blood from the skeletal muscles. This is caused by vasodilatation and opening of closed capillaries.
- As a result, there is redistribution of blood flow. More blood is deviated to the coronary vasculature and splanchnic and visceral blood flow is severely diminished. However, cerebral blood flow remains unchanged.

- Due to increased venous return and sympathetic stimulation, there is increased heart rate and increased cardiac output. As a result, there is increased systolic blood pressure.
- Blood volume increases and there is hemoconcentration due to loss of fluid in the capillaries and increased tissue osmotic pressure due to accumulation of metabolites.

Respiratory Changes

- Increase in pulmonary ventilation with increase in the effort of exercise. This is due to neural and chemical mechanisms which detect a need for more oxygen.
- Increase in oxygen uptake by the lungs is brought about by increased pulmonary perfusion, increased alveolar pO_2 gradient and increased pulmonary diffusion capacity.

Grade	Level	Heart rate (beats per min)	O_2 consumption (L/min)	Relative load index (RLI) (% of max, O_2 consumption)	METs
I	Light (mild)	<100	0.4–0.8	<25	<3
II	Moderate	100–125	0.8–1.6	25–50	3.1–4.5
III	Heavy	125–150	1.6–2.4	51–75	4.6–7
IV	Severe	>150	>2.4	>75	>7

3.16 DEMONSTRATE HARVARD STEP TEST AND DESCRIBE THE IMPACT ON INDUCED PHYSIOLOGIC PARAMETERS IN A SIMULATED ENVIRONMENT

SHORT ESSAY

1. What is endurance training? What is maximum heart rate achieved? Explain the effect of Harvard step test on heart rate and blood pressure.   **(1 + 1 + 3 marks)**

Endurance Training

- It is the capacity or the duration till which a muscle can withstand exercise before total exhaustion.
- It is a measure the supply of nutrition of a muscle.
- Endurance training is the act of performing physical exercises to improve endurance.
- Heart rate increases linearly with exercise due to many factors.

Maximum Heart Rate Achieved

It is usually 110–120 beats per minute that is maximally achieved.

Harvard Step Test

- It is used to diagnose cardiovascular diseases,
- It is a stress test.
- There is a small platform of height 50 cm.
- The person performing the test must step up and down every 2 seconds.
- Normally, 30 steps per minute for five seconds can be sustained.

Effect on Heart Rate

- It is an aerobic exercise and thus increases blood flow to the muscles.
- Also, due to pumping action of skeletal muscles, venous return increases.
- As a result, the volume of blood entering the right side of the heart increases.

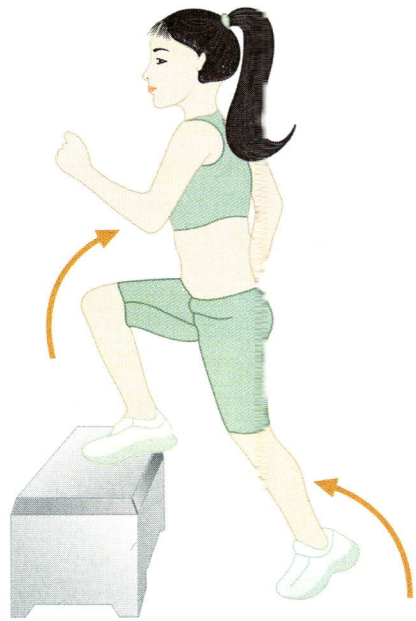

Fig. 3.79

- This causes stimulation of the sinoatrial node and initiates a Bainbridge reflex.
- Hence, there is an increase in heart rate.

Effect on Blood Pressure

- There is an increase in heart rate as explained above
- Also, there is increase in stroke volume following sympathetic stimulation.
- As a result, there is increase in stroke volume and thus increase in systolic blood pressure.
- Due to accumulation of local metabolites in the periphery, there is vasodilatation leading to a fall in the peripheral vascular resistance
- As a result, there is decrease in diastolic blood pressure.

3.17 DESCRIBE STRENGTH-DURATION CURVE

SHORT ANSWER

1. Draw a neat-labeled diagram of strength-duration curve and describe chronaxie, rheobase and utilization time with their importance.

Strength-Duration Curve

It is the relationship between the strength and duration of a stimulus.

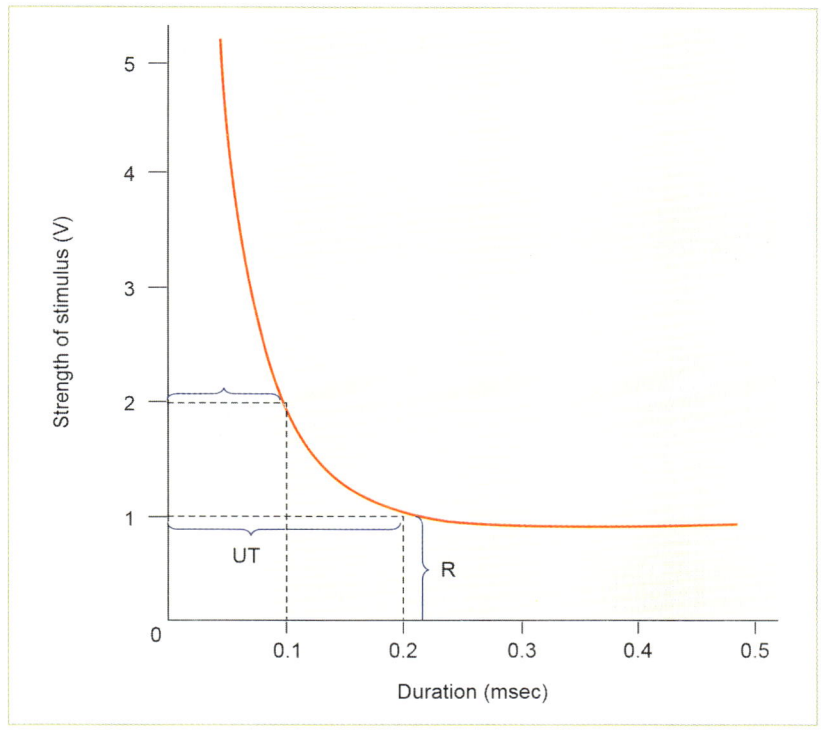

Fig. 3.80

Chronaxie	• It is the minimum time required for a stimulus with double the rheobase stimulus to excite the tissue	• It is an index of excitability of a tissue • Shorter chronaxie value means higher excitability
Rheobase	• It is the minimum strength of stimulus that can excite the tissue	• Lower rheobase values indicate increased excitability • It is lower in sensory nerves than motor nerves
Utilization time	• It is the minimum time for which a rheobase stimulus should act to excite the tissue	• Shorter the utilization time, higher is the excitability of the tissue.

Chapter

4

Gastrointestinal Physiology

4.1 DESCRIBE THE STRUCTURE AND FUNCTIONS OF DIGESTIVE SYSTEM

SHORT ANSWERS

1. What is the function of pyloric glands? Why are gastric ulcers more common in pyloric region?

Function of Pyloric Glands

- Pylorus is the junction between stomach and the duodenum
- It is marked by a sphincter which controls entry of chyme into the duodenum and mainly prevents reflux of alkaline fluid into stomach.
- The pyloric glands secrete mucin which is protective to the mucosa of the stomach.
- They also produce gastrin, a hormone which mediates HCl secretion.

Common Sites of Gastric Ulceration

- Peptic ulcers are more common within one or two centimetres from the pylorus, lesser curvature, gastroesophageal junction and sites of gastrostomy and duodenostomies.
- The prepyloric region is the most common site for ulceration as there are many glands that secrete HCl and there is ulcer formation as a result of their over-secretion.

2. What are Brunner's glands? Where are they present? What is their function?

Brunner's Glands

These are compound tubular mucus producing glands in the intestinal mucosa.

Location

- They are mostly located in the duodenum proximal to sphincter of Oddi.
- They extend from the mucosa into the muscular coat into the submucous coat.

Functions

1. They produce mucous and traces of enzymes.
2. Mucous helps in lubrication
3. The mucous is highly alkaline in nature and is protective against peptic ulcers.
4. Also, the alkaline nature helps in activation of intestinal enzymes.

4.2 DESCRIBE THE COMPOSITION, MECHANISM OF SECRETION, FUNCTIONS, AND REGULATION OF SALIVA, GASTRIC, PANCREATIC, INTESTINAL JUICES AND BILE SECRETION

SHORT ESSAYS

1 Explain the mechanism of gastric acid secretion. What are the factors affecting its secretion? (3 + 2 marks)

Mechanism of Gastric Acid Secretion (Fig. 4.1)

- The cells of the gastric glands secrete about 2500 ml of gastric juices per day.
- The parietal or the oxyntic cells produce gastric acid or HCl, whereas the intrinsic cells or the chief cells produce pepsinogen.
- The secretion of HCl is an active process and happens on the luminal side of the parietal cell.
- The carbon dioxide that is generated within the cell due to metabolic activities combines with water molecules to form H_2CO_3 in the presence of carbonic anhydrase.
- The carbonic acid, being highly unstable, splits into an H^+ ion and HCO_3^-. The chloride ion is actively pumped into the gastric lumen.
- To compensate for the loss of anion, bicarbonate is driven out into the interstitium where it combines with Na^+ and forms sodium bicarbonate.

Factors Affecting Gastric Secretion

Gastric secretion is controlled by the following influences:

1. **Cephalic influences:** Presence of food in mouth, sight, smell and thought of food cause gastric secretion.

2. **Gastric phase**
   - **Local myenteric reflex:** Stimulation of stomach wall by food causes release of acetylcholine which stimulate the gastric glands to secrete HCl.
   - **Vasovagal reflex:** Entry of food into the stomach stimulates the afferents of the vagus nerve which cause secretion of gastric juices.
   - **Hormonal:** Gastrin is a local hormone produced by the G cells in the stomach. It is released when food enters the stomach. It stimulates secretion of pepsinogen and hydrochloric acid.

3. **Intestinal phase:** Entry of chyme into the intestine causes release of gastric secretions. Following this, there is decrease and cessation of gastric acid secretion due to inhibitory effects of somatostatin, cholecystokinin, secretin, gastric inhibitory peptide, vasoactive inhibitory polypeptide and peptide YY.

2. What is Pavlov's pouch? Explain the phase of gastric acid secretion with Pavlov's dog experimental evidence.

A. Pavlov's Pouch (Fig. 4.2)

- Pavlov was a Russian scientist who described his experiments with gastric secretion in a dog
- He separated a small portion of the stomach of his dog, still maintaining its vagal innervation and exteriorized it
- It was used to study gastric secretions.

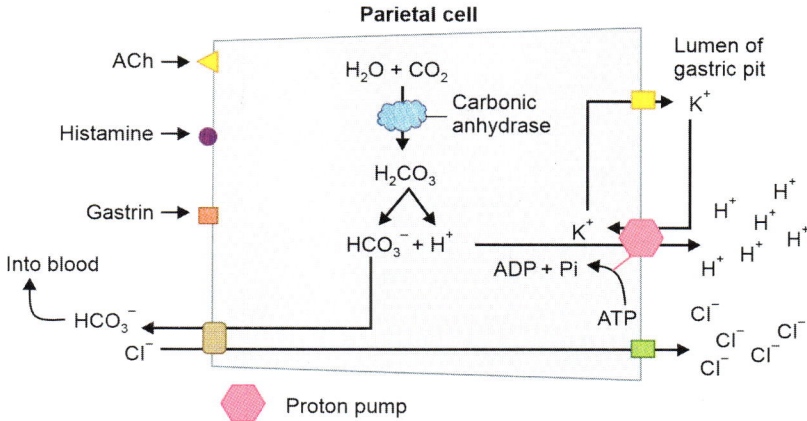

Fig. 4.1

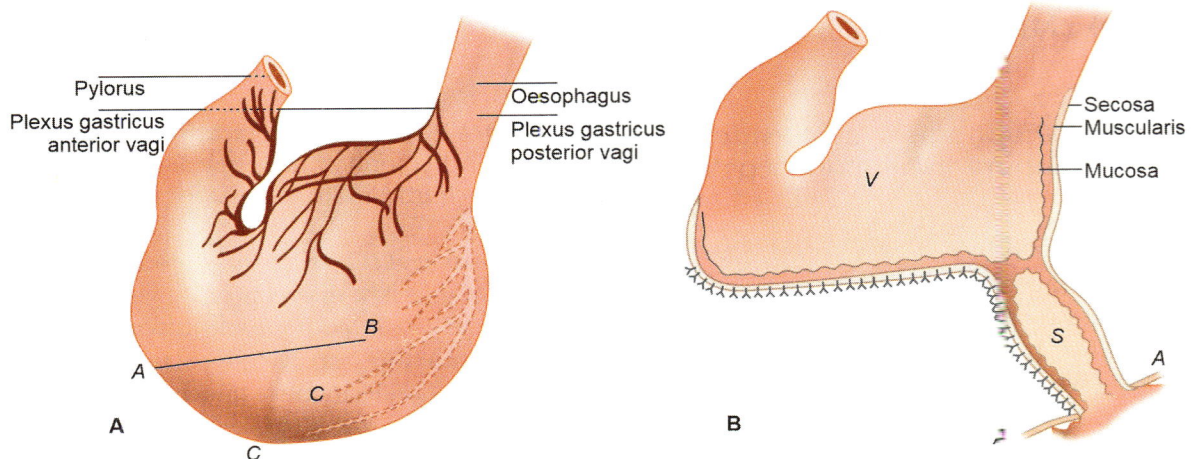

Fig. 4.2A and B

- It was used to describe different phases of gastric secretion and also to explain conditional reflexes.

B. Phases of Gastric Secretion

1. Cephalic phase

- Secretion of gastric juice by nervous stimuli also called appetite juice
- Occurs even without presence of food in mouth

    i. In unconditioned reflex
    - Pavlov gave his dog a piece of meat and the gastric secretions increased
    - It is an inborn reflex
    - It starts when food is placed in mouth, even prior to its entry into the stomach.
    - It is demonstrated by sham feeding following which there is gastric secretion.
    - Pathway for unconditioned reflex
      o Mouth → glossopharyngeal nerve → amygdala and appetite centre (hypothalamus) → dorsal nucleus of vagus → vagal efferent → stomach

    ii. Conditioned reflex
    - Presence of food in mouth is not necessary for this reflex
    - It is initiated by smell, right and thought of food.
    - Pavlov demonstrated this reflex by bringing food into the dog's site
    - The dog starts secreting gastric juices.

    - It is accompanied by a bell ringing
    - The next time, only the bell is rung. This stimulates gastric secretion as there is conditioning of reflex gastric secretion by ringing of bell.

2. Gastric phase

- Secretion of gastric juices upon food entering the stomach
- It is regulated by nervous and hormonal control

    i. Nervous
    - Initiated by local myenteric reflexes
    - Stimulated by stretching of stomach, mechanical stimulation and chemical stimulation by food
    - The local fibres secrete ACh, which stimulate the gastric glands to secrete gastric juices and gastrin
    - Pathway: Vasovagal
      o Afferent vagal nerve endings in the stomach → dorsal nucleus of vagus (medulla) → efferent fiber through vagus nerve → ACh release → gastric juices → it is demonstrated by Pavlov's pouch

    ii. Hormonal mechanism
    - It is mediated through secretion of gastrin by the G cells of the pylorus
    - Mediated by local myenteric and vasovagal reflex
    - gastrin hormone stimulates release of pepsinogen and HCl

3. Intestinal phase

- Secretion of gastric juice when chyme enters the intestine initially
- Later, there is decrease or cessation mediated by enterogastric reflex and gastrointestinal hormones.
- Enterogastric reflex—mediated by Auerbach's plexus
  - Secretin
  - Cholecystokinin
  - Gastroinhibitory peptide
  - Vasoactive peptide
- This phase cannot be explained by Pavlov pouch. But can be demonstrated by Farrell and Ivy pouch.

3. Explain the exocrine pancreatic secretion and its role in digesting different organic components of food.

Exocrine Pancreatic Function

Juices secreted by the pancreas are mainly involved in digesting lipids and proteins.

Digestion of Proteins

1. Trypsin

- It is the most powerful protein digesting enzyme
- It is secreted as inactive trypsinogen and then activated by enteropeptidase which is secreted by the brush border epithelium of the duodenum.
- It is an endopeptidase and breaks inner bonds of the protein into proteoses and polypeptides.
- Also, it activates more trypsinogen and thus there is increased trypsin
- It activates other enzymes like chymotrypsinogen to chymotrypsin, procarboxypeptidase to carboxypeptidase, caseinogen to casein, prolipase to lipase and proelastase to elastase.
- Other actions are activation of collagenase, phospholipases A and B.

2. Chymotrypsin

- It is also an endopeptidase and breaks proteins into proteoses and polypeptides.
- It also activates caseinogen to casein helping in digestion of milk.

3. Others: Carboxypeptidase, nuclease, elastase and collagenase

- Procarboxypeptidase A → carboxypeptidase A (breaks proteins with aliphatic or aromatic compounds)
- Procarboxypeptidase B → carboxypeptidase B (breaks proteins with basic compounds)
- These are exopeptidases which act on the terminal bond of proteins are release aminoacids.
- Nucleases digest RNA and DNA into mononucleotides
- Elastase digests elastic fibres
- Collagenase digests collagen

Digestion of Lipids

Pancreatic secretion plays an important role in digestion of lipids. Bile juice helps in the same.

Pancreatic Lipase

- It is a powerful enzyme involved in digestion of lipids.
- Bile salts help in micelle formation of the lipids
- Colipase is a coenzyme to lipase which breaks down the triglycerides into monoacyl glycerol molecules.

Other Enzymes

Cholesterol ester hydrolase	Cholesterol ester into free cholesterol and fatty acid by hydrolysis
Phospholipase A	Converts phospholipids into lysophospholipids Lecithin → lysolecithin Cephalin → lysocephalin
Phospholipase B	Lysophospholipids into phosphoryl choline and free fatty acids
Cholesterol esterase or bile salt activated lipase	Hydrolyses cholesterol ester, phospholipids and triglycerides

Digestion of Carbohydrates

- Pancreatic amylase breaks down starch into dextrin and maltose.
- It is similar to salivary amylase.
- It serves as a marker for pancreatic inflammation

4. What is the composition of salivary secretion? What are the functions of saliva? Explain the modification of salivary secretion in the ducts.

Composition of Saliva

- It is majorly formed by water (99.5%).
- The remaining 0.5% is formed by solids.
- Organic substances are salivary amylase, lipase, maltase, lysozyme, phosphatase, carbonic anhydrase, IgA, mucin, albumin and free amino acids.
- Inorganic substances include ions of Na, K, Ca, Mg, Br and gases like oxygen, nitrogen and CO_2.

Functions of Saliva

1. Helps in chewing of food, mixing and preparation of bolus.
2. Moistens the mucous membrane of the mouth and keeps it healthy.
3. Saliva digests various solutes in food and helps in appreciation of taste.
   - Saliva has three important enzymes: Amylase, lipase and maltase.
     - Amylase helps in digestion of starch into dextrin and maltose.
     - Maltase converts maltose into glucose
     - Lingual lipase converts triglycerides into free fatty acids.
4. Due to its rinsing action, it keeps teeth clean off the debris of food.
5. Lysozyme is a protective enzyme and has bactericidal effect.
6. Lactoferrin also has bactericidal effects.
7. Lactoferrin helps in building tooth enamel.
8. It helps in articulation of speech
9. Many organic and inorganic substances are excreted into the saliva.

Modification of Salivary Secretion

- Salivary secretion is a two-step process. The first happens in the acini and the second in the ducts.
- The acini secrete a primary saliva rich in amylase and mucin. Its concentration of ions is akin to the ECF.
- En route the duct, sodium ions are actively reabsorbed from the duct and potassium ions are introduced into the saliva. As a result, the concentration of Na^+ in the saliva decreases and potassium increases.

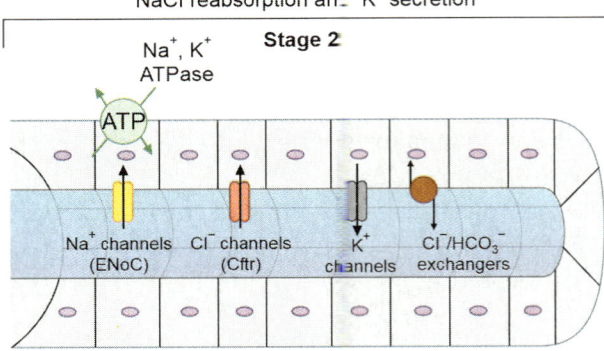

Fig. 4.3

- The reabsorption of sodium exceeds the secretion of potassium creating a potential of −70 mV
- As a result, chloride ions are also reabsorbed leading to a decrease in chloride concentration.
- Lastly, bicarbonate is secreted into the duct by both active and passive processes.
- As a result, the concentration of Na^+ and Cl^- ions are greatly decreased, whereas K^+ and HCO_3^- ions are greatly increased compared to the plasma.

5. Describe conditioned and unconditioned reflexes that stimulate salivary secretion.

Conditioned Reflex

- It is an automatic response established by training to an ordinarily neutral stimulus.
- Pavlov rang a bell when he showed the dog his food. The dog was conditioned to the sight of food

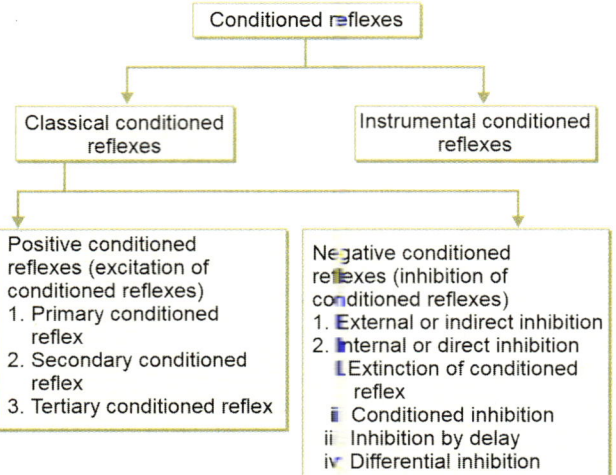

Fig. 4.4

to the ring of the bell. Next time, when Pavlov rang a bell, there was increased salivation by the dog. This is conditioned reflex.

- It is the one that is acquired by experience and it needs previous experience
- Presence of food in the mouth is not necessary to elicit this reflex.
- The stimuli for this reflex are the sight, smell, hearing or thought of food.

Unconditioned Reflex (Fig. 4.5)

- It is an unconditioned reflex present since birth.
- When there is a thought, smell or sight of food, there is increase in salivation.
- It is mediated from the cortex which stimulate the salivatory nuclei.
- The appetite area is in close proximity to the anterior hypothalamus which cause parasympathetic discharge.
- Pavlov conducted experiments with his dog. There was increased salivation when he showed food to the dog. This is an unconditioned reflex.

Conditioned reflex	Unconditioned reflex
Acquired reflex	Present since birth
Requires previous experience	Does not require previous experience
Requires learning	Does not require learning

6. Explain various phases of salivary secretion. What is conditioned reflex?

Phases of Salivary Secretion

1. **Cephalic phase**
   - It is an unconditioned reflex present since birth.
   - When there is a thought, smell or sight of food, there is increase in salivation.
   - It is mediated from the cortex which stimulates the salivatory nuclei.
   - The appetite area is in close proximity to the anterior hypothalamus which causes parasympathetic discharge.
   - Pavlov conducted experiments with his dog. There was increased salivation when he showed food to the dog. This is an unconditioned reflex.
   - Pavlov rang a bell when he showed the dog his food. The dog was conditioned to the sight of food to the ring of the bell. Next time, when Pavlov rang a bell, there was increased salivation by the dog. This is conditioned reflex.

2. **Oral phase**
   - Presence of food in the mouth stimulates the salivary glands by contact.
   - The taste and tactile stimuli from tongue, pharynx and mouth send impulses to the salivatory nuclei in the pontomedullary junction.
   - After taking origin from this nucleus, the preganglionic fibers run through nervus

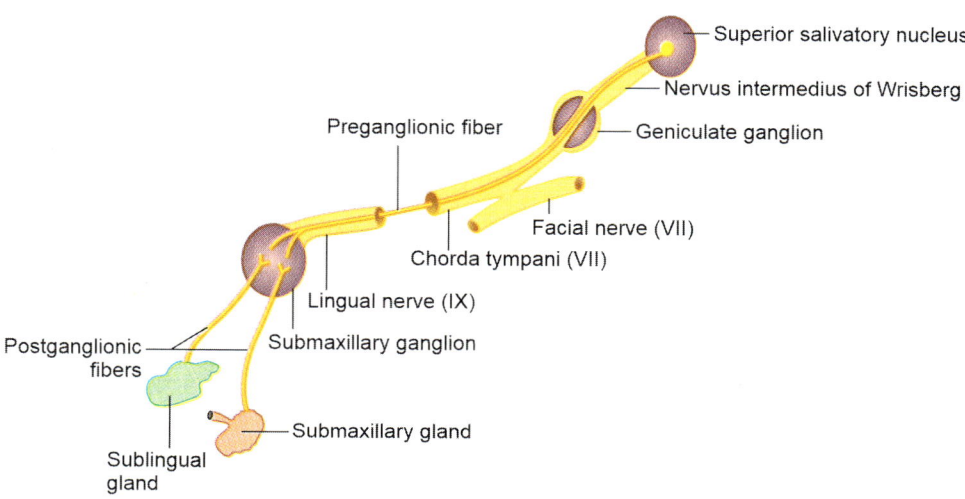

Fig. 4.5

intermedius of Wrisberg, geniculate ganglion, the motor fibers of facial nerve, chorda tympani branch of facial nerve and lingual branch of trigeminal nerve and finally reach the submaxillary ganglion.

3. **Gastric and intestinal phase**

- When there is irritation of the stomach and small intestine by irritant foods, there is increase in reflex salivation.
- This is a protective response to protect the mucosa from irritants.
- Also, there is increase in salivation due to irritants to gastric mucosa during gastroenteritis which causes increased saliva production.

Conditioned Reflex

- It is an automatic response established by training to an ordinarily neutral stimulus.
- Pavlov rang a bell when he showed the dog his food. The dog was conditioned to the sight of food to the ring of the bell. Next time, when Pavlov rang a bell, there was increased salivation by the dog. This is conditioned reflex.
- It is the one that is acquired by experience and it needs previous experience.
- Presence of food in the mouth is not necessary to elicit this reflex.
- The stimuli for this reflex are the sight, smell, hearing or thought of food.

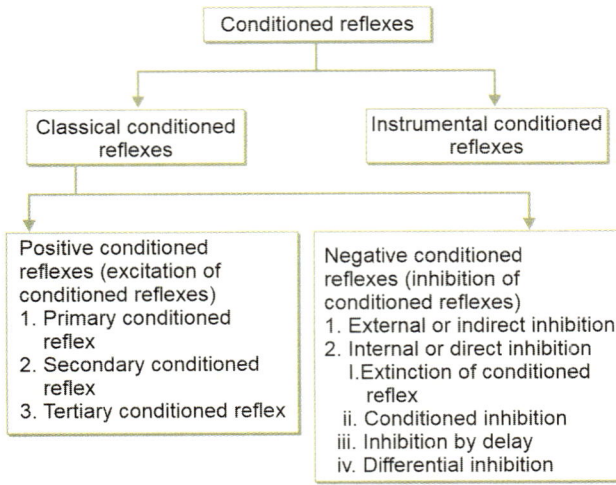

Fig. 4.5a

7. Explain the cephalic phase of gastric secretion with sham feeding experiment.

Cephalic Phase of Gastric Secretion

- Secretion of gastric juice by nervous stimuli also called appetite juice
- Occurs even without presence of food in mouth

In Unconditioned Reflex

- Pavlov gave his dog a piece of meat and the gastric secretions increased
- It is an inborn reflex
- It starts when food is placed in mouth, even prior to its entry into the stomach.
- It is demonstrated by sham feeding following which there is gastric secretion.
- Sham feeding means false feeding. In this, esophagus is transected and brought out through the neck. When food is given through mouth, it comes out through the esophagostomy. Thus, it does not enter the stomach.
- Pathway for unconditioned reflex
  Mouth → glossopharyngeal nerve → amygdala and appetite centre (hypothalamus) → dorsal nucleus of vagus → vagal efferents → stomach

Conditioned Reflex

- Presence of food in mouth is not necessary for this reflex.
- It is initiated by smell, sight and thought of food.
- Pavlov demonstrated this reflex by bringing food into the dog's site
- The dog starts secreting gastric juices.
- It is accompanied by a bell ringing
- The next time, only the bell is rung. This stimulates gastric secretion as there is conditioning of reflex gastric secretion by ringing of bell.

SHORT ANSWER

1. Enumerate the functions of bile juice.

1. **Emulsification of fats:** Emulsification of fat globules into minute droplets by the action of bile salts. Following this, lipids can be digested by the lipolytic enzymes.
2. **Fat absorption:** Bile salts combine with fats and make micelles.
3. **Choleretic action:** Bile salts stimulate the secretion of bile from the hepatocytes.

4. **Cholagogue action:** Bile salts stimulate the excretion of bile form the gall bladder.

5. **Laxative action:** Stimulates defecation by stimulation of peristalsis.

6. **Prevent formation of gall stones:** Bile salts prevent formation of gall stones by keeping cholesterol and lecithin in solution.

7. **Excretory function:** Chemicals like cholesterol, heavy metals like copper and iron, some bacteria like typhoid, lecithin.

8. **Maintenance of pH:** As bile is alkaline, it neutralizes the acidic chyme.

9. **Antiseptic action:** Bile inhibits the growth of some bacteria in the intestinal lumen.

4.3 DESCRIBE GIT MOVEMENTS, REGULATION AND FUNCTIONS. DESCRIBE DEFECATION REFLEX. EXPLAIN ROLE OF DIETARY FIBRE

LONG ESSAYS

1. Explain the different types of small intestinal mobility. What is paralytic ileus explain.

(8 + 2 marks)

Different Types of Intestinal Motility

Movements of Small Intestine

- It is necessary for mixing chyme with various digestive juices secreted by the pancreas, liver and the small intestine.
- There are four types of small intestinal movements

1. **Mixing movements**
   - *Segmental contractions*
     - Commonly occurring, rhythmic.
     - They occur at regular intervals along the length of the intestine, each segment of 1–5 cm length.
     - There are alternating segments of contraction and relaxation.
     - This is followed by relaxation of the contracted segments and vice versa
   - *Pendular movements:* Small segments of the small intestine sweep forward and backward like a pendulum.

2. **Propulsive movements**
   - These movements are responsible for movement of chyme towards the anus
   - It is of two types:
     i. *Peristaltic movements*
        - A wave of contraction is followed by a wave of relaxation of muscles.
        - Entry of chyme acts as a point stimulus.
        - The peristalsis starts from that point and moves forward.
        - Starling's law: According to this, the response of small intestines for a local stimulus is caused by contraction of smooth muscles proximal to the point of stimulus and relaxation of smooth muscles distal to it.
        - As a result, the chyme is propelled forwards/aborally.
        - Stimulus is caused by food entering the stomach mediated by the gastroenteric reflex.

   ii. *Peristaltic rush*
       - Caused by extreme distension
       - Characterized by a powerful peristaltic wave.
       - It traverses the whole length of the SI within a span of minutes.

3. **Migrating motor complex**
   - Occurs during periods of prolonged fasting
   - It involves large portion of small intestine around 20–30 cm, peristalsis occurs every 11/2–2 hours
   - It is necessary for sweeping away the digestive juices into colon

4. **Movements of villi**
   - As the smooth muscles extend into the villi, they also move along with movements of the small intestine.
   - They elongate and shorten alternatingly.
   - Elongation helps in increasing the surface area to increase absorption
   - Villikinin is a local hormone which causes movements of these villi.

Movements of Large Intestine

- Sluggish compared to those of small intestine
- Mainly mixing and propulsive
- *Mixing movements:* Large segmental contractions occur at regularly placed intervals (around 2.5 cm)
- *Propulsive movements*
  - Helps push feces along the length of the colon towards the anus
  - Usually is in the morning, 10 minutes prior to or following breakfast.

Electrical Activity of Intestinal Smooth Muscles

Slow Waves

Small undulating variations in the membrane potential, between 5 and 15 mV, occurs 3–12 per minute.

Stomach	3
Duodenum	12
Ileum	9

Spike Potentials

- Actual action potentials, –50 to –60 mV amplitude is the normal resting potential.
- When there is a positive spike, it reduces to around –40 mV
- Depolarization of muscle fibres causes hyperexcitability. Hyperpolarization of muscle causes reduced excitability.
- Factors which cause hyperexcitability: Stretching of muscle fibers, specific hormone, ACh.
- Factors which cause reduced excitability are sympathetic stimulation.

Paralytic Ileus

- It is also called adynamic intestinal obstruction.
- The intestines fail to transmit peristalsis due to failure of neuromuscular transmission through Auerbach and Meissner's plexus.
- Most common cause is postoperative ileus. Others are hypokalemia, sepsis and retroperitoneal hemorrhage.
- They present with constipation and failure to pass feces or flatus.
- Treatment depends on the cause.
- Flatus tube may be inserted aborally to relieve bloating.

SHORT ESSAYS

1. Explain the phases of deglutition. Write a note on achalasia cardia. (3 + 2 marks)

Or

A 9-month-old female infant was admitted to the hospital for vomiting of every meal. On investigations she was diagnosed to have achalasia cardia. Describe various stages of deglutition. What is the cause of achalasia cardia? (3 + 2 marks)

Phases of Deglutition

- Deglutition or swallowing is an active process by which the ingested food bolus enters the stomach from mouth via the oesophagus.
- There are three stages

1. **Oral stage**
   - Voluntary stage
   - The food ingested in created into a bolus by the action of teeth and tongue and is placed in the posterior aspect of the tongue. This is called the preparatory phase.
   - The anterior portion of the tongue is depressed and retracted followed by elevation of the posterior part of the tongue which propels the bolus posteriorly into the pharynx.

2. **Pharyngeal stage**
   - Involuntary stage
   - In this, pharynx forms a common passage for air and food and thus a complex mechanism exists so that the food enters the esophagus and air enters the larynx. It communicates to the oral cavity, nasal cavity superiorly through nasopharynx, larynx downward and anteriorly and esophagus downward and posteriorly. The direction of bolus always is unidirectional from mouth to the esophagus.
   - The backward movement of bolus into the mouth is blocked by the tongue and positive pressure created by the tongue in the mouth.
   - Elevation of soft palate and uvula prevent the passage of bolus into the nasopharynx.
   - During swallowing, the vocal cords approximate, larynx moves higher and anteriorly, and the epiglottis seals the laryngeal opening thus preventing entry of bolus into the larynx.
   - The upward movement of larynx opens the esophagus, the cricopharyngeal muscle (upper esophageal sphincter) relaxes and peristalsis of the pharynx = x drives the bolus into the esophagus.

3. **Oesophageal stage**
   - Involuntary stage
   - The movements of the esophagus are designed such that the bolus reaches the stomach.
   - A wave of contraction is followed by a wave of relaxation of the esophageal muscles.
   - When the bolus arrives the oral end of the esophagus, primary peristalsis begins. The pressure becomes negative due to relaxation of muscles and then suddenly increases due to contraction.
   - Secondary peristalsis is set in when the primary contractions cannot pass the bolus downward.
   - Relaxation of the lower esophageal sphincter leads to entry of the bolus into the stomach. As soon as the bolus reaches the stomach, the sphincter closes.

Achalasia Cardia

- Achalasia is dis-coordinated smooth muscle relaxation of the lower esophageal sphincter.
- It causes pain in the chest, and hence the name.
- It is a neuromuscular disease of genetic etiology where there is increased tone of the lower esophageal sphincter on entry of the bolus—be it solid or liquid. The myenteric plexus does not respond to inhibitory impulses.
- As a result, the patient develops dysphagia—inability to swallow and regurgitation of food. Also, there is increased chances of aspiration of food into the lower airways and the patient develops weight loss.
- It is diagnosed by typical history, imaging studies (barium swallow) and endoscopy. Barium swallow shows severely narrowed lumen of the lower esophagus and widened upper esophagus.

2. Explain the following: (2.5 + 2.5 marks)
   A. Mass movements
   B. Defecation reflex

A. Mass Movements

- These are the movements of the large intestine
- It causes propulsion of feces from colon towards anus.
- Usually, this movement occurs only a few times every day.
- The timing of mass movement is round 10 minutes in the morning prior to or following breakfast.
- It occurs just prior to defecation and is controlled by neurogenic factors.
- Other factors are gastrocolic reflex, duodenocolic reflex which can lead to a mass peristalsis.

B. Defecation Reflex

> When feces reach the rectum, it distends and thereby stimulates the local myenteric plexus

> This causes peristalsis of colon, sigmoid colon and rectum

> As the peristalsis reaches the anus, the internal anal sphincter is relaxed due to inhibitory signals by the myenteric plexus. It is supplemented by efferent from the sacral segments in the form of parasympathetic outflow, which strengthen the peristalsis

> If accompanied by voluntary relaxation of the anal sphincter, then defecation occurs

Fig. 4.6

Other Changes during Defecation

- Deep inspiration
- Closure of glottis
- Diaphragm moves down
- Contraction of muscles of the abdominal wall

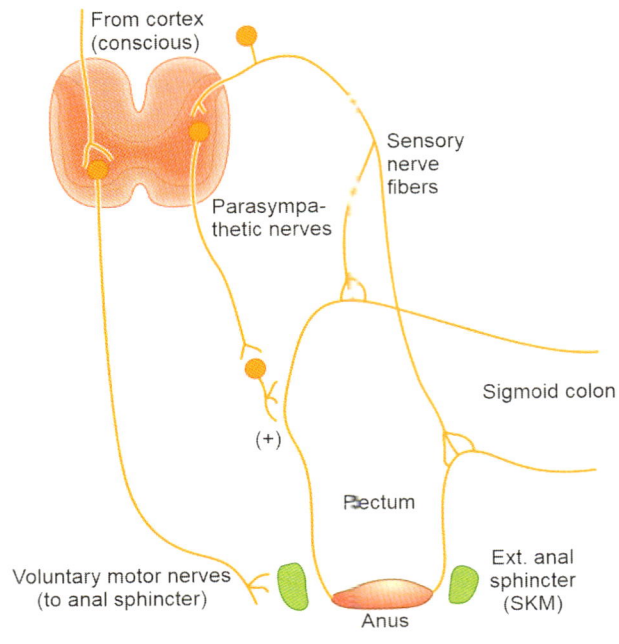

Fig. 4.7

3. Describe
   A. Hunger contractions
   B. Basic electrical rhythm
   C. Haustral contractions

A. Hunger Contractions

- Hunger contractions are the movements of empty stomach and are related to the sensations of hunger.
- By nature, they are peristaltic waves superimposed over the contractions of gastric smooth muscle.
- Hunger contractions differ from normal peristaltic waves in a manner that they involve the whole stomach, whereas the latter involves only body and pyloric parts of the stomach.
- They are of three types:

1. **Type I hunger contractions**
   - These are the first to appear in the empty stomach, when the tone of the gastric muscles is low.

- Each contraction lasts for about 20 seconds and the interval between the next is about 3 to 4 seconds.
- Pressure produced by these contractions is about 5 cm of H_2O.

2. Type II hunger contractions

- They appear when the tone of stomach is stronger.
- This happens when food intake is postponed, even after the appearance of the type I contractions.
- Each of the type II contractions lasts for 20 seconds
- Pressure produced by these contractions is 10–15 cm of H_2O.

3. Type III hunger contractions

- These contractions appear when the hunger becomes severe and the tone increases to a great extent.
- Type III hunger contractions are rare in man as the food is taken usually before the appearance of these contractions.
- These contractions last for 1–5 minutes.
- The pressure produced by these contractions increases to 10–20 cm of H_2O.
- When the stomach is empty: Sequence of contractions
- The type I contractions occur first, followed by type II contractions.
- If food intake is still postponed, then type III contractions appear and as soon as food is consumed, hunger contractions disappear.

B. Basic Electrical Rhythm

- Some of the muscles of the stomach wall exhibit tonic contractions and also called electrical control activity.
- These are called pacemaker cells of the gut or interstitial cells of Cajal.
- These are slow waves which last for several minutes and even hours.
- *Mechanism of production*
  - The details are not clear as of how these potentials are generated.
  - These waves are produced by continuous repetitive spikes.
  - There is cyclic depolarization followed by repolarization in the cells of Cajal.

- These cells are in connection with smooth muscles of the stomach through gap junctions.
  - The potential fluctuates between –65 mV and –45 mV.
  - The frequency of these spikes of potential also is dependent on hormones.
  - It is also caused by continuous influx of calcium ions.
- Frequency
  - In stomach: 3/minute
  - Duodenum: 11–12/minute
  - Ileum: 9/minute
  - Colon: 2–13/minute

C. Haustral Contractions

- These are nothing but mixing movements in the large intestine
- Large constriction rings occur at frequent intervals in the large intestine.
- They are around 2.5 cm wide and the circular muscles contract and can constrict the lumen in that segment. Whereas the longitudinal muscles arranged in the form of three linear bands, contract such that the adjacent unstimulated portions of the large intestine to form bag-like sacculation called haustrations.
- They form strong contractions about 30 seconds and then relax for about 60 seconds.
- Functions
  1. Mainly, mixing movements
  2. Mild propulsive movements—when consistent for around 8–12 hours, the chyme is propelled towards the sigmoid colon.

SHORT ANSWERS

1. How does dietary fiber help in maintaining get health?

Or

What is the therapeutic role of dietary fibers?

Dietary Fibers

- Food rich in dietary fibers are fruits, vegetables, cereals, bread and wheat grain.
- Health benefits of dietary fiber
  1. It increases the bulk of feces and thereby helps in easy defecation
  2. It helps in maintaining a good BMI by reducing excess binge eating as it requires more chewing

and promotes satiety by prolonging the gastric transit time thus giving the person a sense of fullness of stomach.

3. Diet with high fiber content are low in absorbable and metabolizable carbohydrates and help in weight loss.

4. It contains some useful substances such as antioxidants

5. They form complexes with cholesterol and are removed in the feces. Thus, it decreases hyperlipidemia.

6. They help in treating constipation, irritable bowel syndrome, diabetics and ulcer.

7. They delay colon cancer.

2. Explain the mechanism of defecation.

Defecation

- Voiding of feces is known as defecation
- The feces are stored in the sigmoid colon and voided through the anus upon arrival of a stimulus.
- The rectum is usually empty as there is a sharp angulation between the rectum and the sigmoid colon.
- When the feces reach the rectum, a desire to defecate occurs. There is contraction of the rectum and relaxation of anal sphincters.

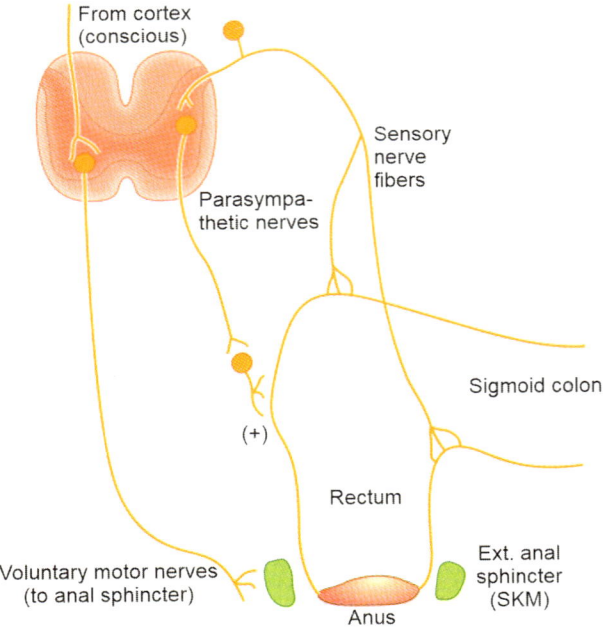

Fig. 4.7a

- Continuous dribbling of feces is prevented by two sphincters—an internal sphincter which is formed by several centimeters of the muscular layer of the anus consisting of smooth muscles and an external sphincter which is formed by striated voluntary muscles which is distal to the internal sphincter.

Defecation Reflex

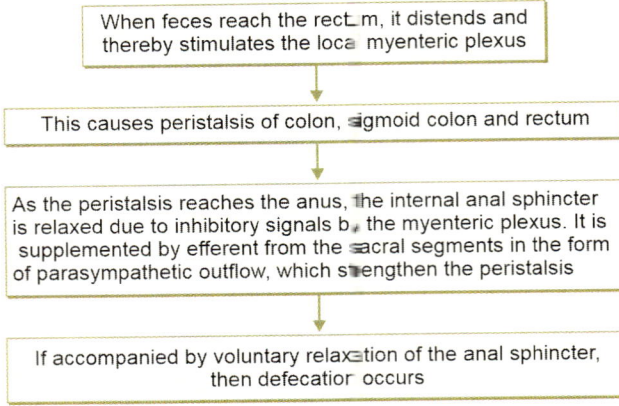

When feces reach the rectum, it distends and thereby stimulates the local myenteric plexus

This causes peristalsis of colon, sigmoid colon and rectum

As the peristalsis reaches the anus, the internal anal sphincter is relaxed due to inhibitory signals by the myenteric plexus. It is supplemented by efferent from the sacral segments in the form of parasympathetic outflow, which strengthen the peristalsis

If accompanied by voluntary relaxation of the anal sphincter, then defecation occurs

Fig. 4.7b

Other Changes during Defecation

- Deep inspiration
- Closure of glottis
- Diaphragm moves down
- Contraction of muscles of the abdominal wall

3. Define
A. Mass reflex
B. Gastrocolic reflex

A. Mass Reflex

- These are the movements of the large intestine
- It causes propulsion of feces from colon towards anus.
- Usually, this movement occurs only a few times every day.
- Duration of mass movement is about 10 minutes in the morning before or after breakfast.
- It occurs just prior to defecation and is controlled by neurogenic factors.
- Other factors are gastrocolic reflex, duodenocolic reflex which can lead to a mass peristalsis

B. Gastrocolic Reflex

- It is a reflex of the large intestine following intake of food.
- There is increased motility of the large intestine following stretching of the stomach.

Pathway

- Several chemical neuropeptides have been suspected to cause this reflex—cholecystokinin, gastrin, serotonin, and neurotensin.
- As a result, there is increased impulses in the myenteric plexus.
- Sigmoid colon is greatly stimulated by this reflex.
- As a result, there are cyclic periods of contraction followed by relaxation and propel the food aborally.
- The rectum gets filled with feces and there is an urge to defecate.

Purpose

Makes space for accommodating more food.

Pathology

Increased gastrocolic response is seen in patients with irritable bowel syndrome.

4. Explain chewing or mastication reflex.

Mastication Reflex

- Ingestion of food involves three main steps—prehension (grasping or introducing food into mouth), mastication (chewing) and deglutition (swallowing).
- Mastication reflex is majorly involuntary, although it can be controlled voluntarily.
- Teeth are well designed for mastication. The incisors are mainly for incising or cutting food and molars are designed to grind the food.

Innervation

- Most of the muscles of mastication are supplied by the motor branch of fifth cranial nerve.
- The chewing is controlled by brainstem

Pathway for Mastication Reflex

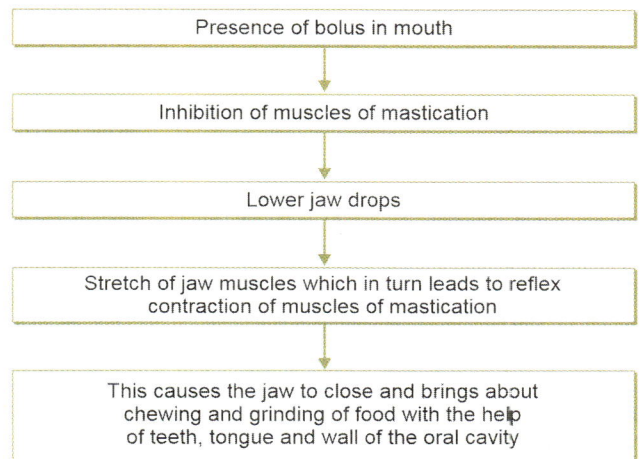

Fig. 4.8

5. What is motilin? What is its role in GIT? What is its clinical significance?

Motilin

- Motilin is a gastrointestinal; hormone secreted by Mo cells of the stomach and intestine.
- It is also believed to be secreted by enterochromaffin cells of intestine.
- Chyme entering the duodenum is a strong stimulant of rots secretion.

Role of Motilin in Gastrointestinal Tract

Its main action improving motility of the gut towards the aboral end.
1. Shortens gastric transit time
2. Increases the mixing and propulsive movements of small intestine
3. Increases the peristalsis in colon.

Clinical significance

- Motilin acts on the movement of the gastrointestinal tract by regulating the migrating motor complex, called hunger contraction.
- The migrating motor complex occurs in the fasting, interdigestive periods.
- The migrating motor complex occurs at 90-minute intervals. The migrating motor complexes facilitate the transportation of the undigested foods, aids

bacterial transport forms the small intestine into the large intestine, and inhibit the bacterial migration from the large intestine into the terminal ileum.

The migrating motor complexes consist of four phases.

- Phase I is when the smooth muscle of the gastrointestinal tract is quiescent.
- Phase II is when peristalsis of the smooth muscle of the digestive tract is getting started.
- Phase III, which is the most characteristic phase of the migrating motor complex, is when the smooth muscle of the gastrointestinal tract rapidly contracts.

- In phase III, the pylorus of the stomach remains open, allowing undigested food to move into the small intestine.
- Phase IV is the transition phase between the contraction of phase III and the inactive state of phase I.
- Motilin's primary function is to increase the migrating motor complex.
- Motilin raises pepsin output and the acid secretion in the stomach.
- The motilin effect in the lower oesophageal sphincter is the contraction of the sphincter and increased resting pressure of the sphincter.
- Motilin causes contraction of the stomach and the lower esophageal sphincter.

4.4 DESCRIBE THE PHYSIOLOGY OF DIGESTION AND ABSORPTION OF NUTRIENTS

LONG ESSAY

1. What is succus entericus? Explain the digestion of carbohydrates, lipids and proteins with respect to these GI secretions.

Answer:

Succus entericus: The secretion of digestive juices from small intestine is called succus entericus.

Digestion of carbohydrates

- Enzymes that are involved in carbohydrate digestion are sucrase, maltase, lactase, dextrinase and trehalase.
- These act on disaccharides and convert into monosaccharides.

  Maltose $\longrightarrow$ glucose + glucose

  Lactose $\longrightarrow$ glucose + galactose

  Sucrose $\longrightarrow$ glucose + fructose

Digestion of lipids

Intestinal lipase converts triglycerides into fatty acids.

Digestion of proteins

The juices secreted by small intestine cause final break down of proteoses and polypeptides into amino acids by the action of aminopeptidases, tripeptidases and dipeptidases.

SHORT ESSAY

1. What are the different protein digesting enzymes present in our body? How is it absorbed?

Digestion of Proteins

Stomach

- Digestion of proteins begins in the stomach.
- It contains pepsin which breaks down complex proteins into proteoses, peptones and large polypeptides.

Small intestine

Most of the proteins are digested by the pancreatic juice and succus entericus.

Pancreatic Enzymes

1 **Trypsin**
   - It is the most powerful protein digesting enzyme

   - It is secreted as inactive trypsinogen and then activated by enteropepetidase which is secreted by the brush border epithelium of the duodenum.
   - It is an endopeptidase and breaks inner bonds of the protein into proteoses and polypeptides.
   - Also, it activates more trypsinogen and thus there is increased trypsin.
   - It activates other enzymes like chymotrypsinogen to chymotrypsin, procarboxypeptidase to carboxypeptidase, caseinogen to casein, prolipase to lipase and proelastase to elastase.
   - Other actions are activation of collagenase, phospholipases A and B.

2. **Chymotrypsin**
   - It is also an endopeptidase and breaks proteins into proteoses and polypeptides.
   - It also activates caseinogen to casein helping in digestion of milk.

3. **Others—carboxypeptidase, nuclease, elastase, and collagenase**
   - Procarboxypeptidase A $\rightarrow$ carboxypeptidase A (breaks proteins with aliphatic or aromatic compounds)
   - Procarboxypeptidase B $\rightarrow$ carboxypeptidase B (breaks proteins with basic compounds)
   - These are exopeptidases which act on the terminal bond of proteins are release aminoacids.

Succus Entericus

The juices secreted by small intestine cause final break down into amino acids by the action of aminopeptidases, tripeptidases and dipeptidases.

Absorption of Proteins

- Proteins are absorbed in the form of amino acids from small intestine, mainly in the duodenum and jejunum.
- The levo-amino acids are actively absorbed by means of sodium cotransport.
- The dextro-amino acids are absorbed by means of facilitated diffusion.

SHORT ANSWERS

1. What is intrinsic factor? What is the role of GIT in the absorption of Vit B$_{12}$? Define achlorhydria.

Intrinsic Factor

It is secreted by the parietal cells of the stomach. It is required for absorption of extrinsic factor or vitamin B$_{12}$.

Absorption of Vitamin B$_{12}$

- Vitamin B$_{12}$ is ingested in the food binds with R binder or cobalophilin that is secreted in saliva.
- After entering stomach, the intrinsic factor of Castle is secreted by the P cells of the stomach. Pepsin cleaves B$_{12}$ from the proteins of the food.
- In the duodenum, trypsin acts on the cobalophilin and cleaves B$_{12}$ from it. now, B$_{12}$ combines with intrinsic factor.
- One molecule of intrinsic factor combines with 2 molecules of B$_{12}$. The whole IF-B$_{12}$ complex is internalized. It may be noted that B$_{12}$ is absorbed from ileum, while folic acid is from jejunum.
- The whole IF-B$_{12}$ complex gets internalized by the mucosa of the ileum. From the intestine, it is transported along with transcobalamin and stored in liver.
- In absence of intrinsic factor, B$_{12}$ is excreted out of the intestine unabsorbed.
- As most of the B$_{12}$ is stored in liver, it takes at least 2–3 years to manifest following decrease in intrinsic factor.

Achlorhydria

- It is a condition in which there is decreased production of hydrochloric acid in the stomach.
- It is invariably associated with vitamin B$_{12}$ deficiency as a result of decreased production of intrinsic factor.

Causes

1. Pernicious anemia: Antibodies are directed against parietal cells of the stomach.
2. Infection with *Helicobacter pylori* which decreases hydrochloric acid secretion.
3. Overuse of antacids
4. Hypothyroidism
5. Sjögren's syndrome

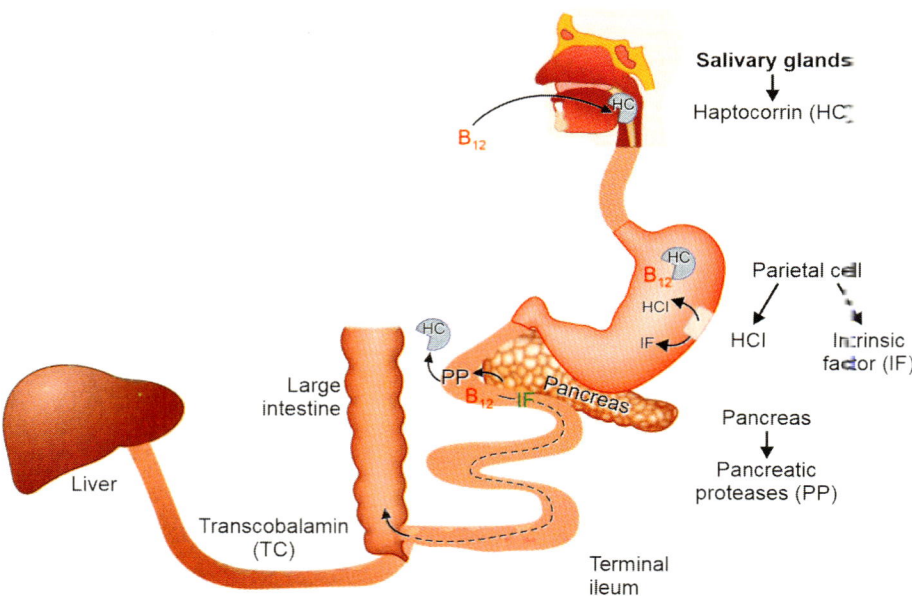

Fig. 4.9

4.5 DESCRIBE THE SOURCE OF GIT HORMONES, THEIR REGULATION AND FUNCTIONS

SHORT ESSAYS

1. Explain the functions of following GI hormones.
  A. Gastrin
  B. Secretin
  C. Cholecystokinin

A. Gastrin

Source

- Gastrin is a gastrointestinal hormone secreted by G cells of the stomach.
- It is also secreted in small quantities by intestinal mucosa.
- Food entering stomach in the form of bolus is a stimulant of gastrin secretion.
- Mechanism of gastrin release is vasovagal or local myenteric reflex.

Actions

1. It stimulates the secretion of hydrochloric acid and pepsinogen by the gastric glands.
2. It also stimulates the secretion and release of pancreatic juice when it enters the pancreas.
3. It stimulates growth of gastric mucosa.

B. Secretin

Source

- It is secreted by S cells of the small intestine—especially duodenum and jejunum.
- It is secreted as prosecretin and the activated by acidic chyme entering the duodenum.

Actions

1. It causes release of pancreatic juice by acting on the pancreatic ductules by increase in cyclic AMP.
2. It causes bicarbonate rich juice to be secreted by small intestine.
3. It causes constriction of pyloric sphincter and inhibits motility of stomach.
4. It also inhibits gastrin secretion.
5. It increases potency of cholecystokinin.

C. Cholecystokinin

Source

- Also called pancreozymin
- It is secreted by I cells of the duodenum and jejunum

- Chyme which is acidic and rich in fatty acids stimulate secretion of cholecystokinin.

Actions

1. As the name goes it causes contraction of gall bladder and pancreatic duct to cause emptying of its contents into duodenum.
2. It causes pancreatic secretion rich in pancreatic enzymes.
3. It inhibits gastric motility
4. It stimulates the secretion of enterokinase
5. It increases motility of intestine
6. It contracts pyloric sphincter
7. It suppresses hunger

2. Explain the following gastrointestinal hormones—CCK-PZ, somatostatin, motilin.

Cholecystokinin Pancreozymin (CCK-PZ)

Also called pancreozymin

Source of Secretion

- It is secreted by I cells of the duodenum and jejunum.
- Chyme which is acidic and rich in fatty acids stimulate secretion of cholecystokinin.

Actions

1. As the name goes it causes contraction of gall bladder and pancreatic duct to cause emptying of its contents into duodenum.
2. It causes pancreatic secretion rich in pancreatic enzymes.
3. It stimulates the secretion of enterokinase
4. It inhibits gastric motility
5. It increases motility of intestine
6. It contracts pyloric sphincter
7. It suppresses hunger

Somatostatin

Source of Secretion

- It is an endocrine secretion of the delta cells of pancreas
- It is also secreted by the hypothalamus

- It is also secreted by the D cells of the stomach and duodenum.
- It is secreted as prosomatostatin and activated by the D cells of the pancreas. It is then degraded in the liver.

Functions

1. It inhibits both insulin and glucagon secretion
2. It decreases the motility of stomach, small intestine and gall bladder.
3. Hypothalamic somatostatin inhibits growth hormone secretion and thus is helpful in gigantism.
4. It also inhibits secretion of gastrin, VIP, GIP and CCK-PZ and hence used in treatment of gastrinoma.

Motilin

- Motilin is a gastrointestinal hormone secreted by Mo cells of the stomach and intestine.
- It is also believed to be secreted by enterochromaffin cells of intestine.
- Chyme entering the duodenum is a strong stimulant of rots secretion.

Role of Motilin in Gastrointestinal Tract

Its main action improving motility of the gut towards the aboral end.

1. Shortens gastric transit time
2. Increases the mixing and propulsive movements of small intestine
3. Increases the peristalsis in colon.

Clinical Significance

- Motilin acts on the movement of the gastrointestinal tract by regulating the migrating motor complex, called hunger contraction.
- They occur in the fasting, interdigestive periods and recur every 90 minutes.
- They are responsible for transportation of the undigested foods, aids bacterial transport forms the small intestine into the large intestine, and inhibit the bacterial migration backwards from the large intestine into the terminal ileum.
- Motilin causes constriction of the lower esophageal sphincter and increases its resting pressure.

SHORT ANSWERS

1. Explain the gastrointestinal hormone secretin.

Secretin

- Peptide hormone secreted by the S cells of small intestine—duodenum, jejunum and ileum.
- It is secreted in the inactive form and activated by chyme.

Actions

1. It stimulates pancreatic juice secretion by acting in the cells of the pancreatic duct and releases exocrine secretion rich in bicarbonate.
2. It inhibits gastric acid secretion.
3. It inhibits motility of stomach.
4. It causes constriction of pyloric sphincter.
5. It increases the potency of cholecystokinin on pancreatic secretion.

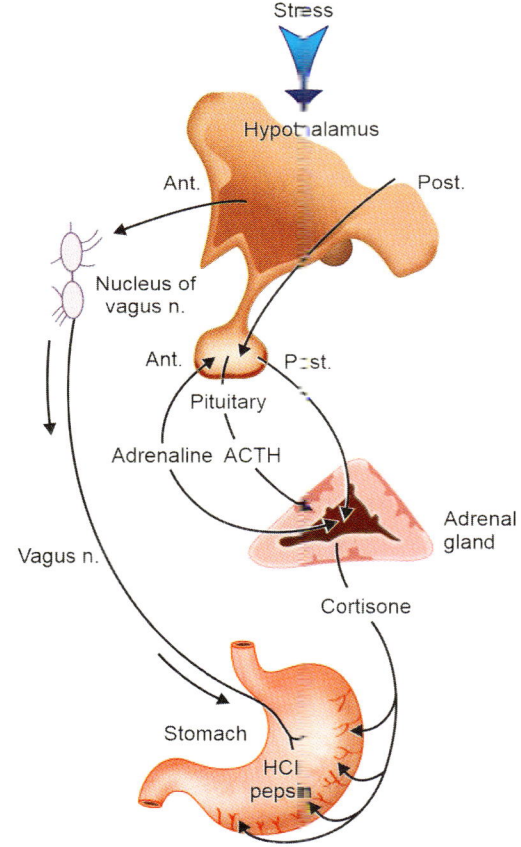

Fig. 4.10

2. Explain the GI hormones gastrin. What is the effect of emotions on its secretion?

Source

- Gastrin is a gastrointestinal hormone secreted by G cells of the stomach.
- It is also secreted in small quantities by intestinal mucosa.
- It is released when food enters the stomach
- Mechanism of gastrin release is vasovagal or local myenteric reflex.

Actions

1. It stimulates the secretion of pepsinogen and hydrochloric acid by the gastric glands.
2. It also stimulates the secretion and release of pancreatic juice when it enters the pancreas.
3. It stimulates growth of gastric mucosa

Effect of Emotions (Fig. 4.10)

- Increased stress due to emotions causes increased release of gastrin hormone by increasing ACTH and cortisone secretion.
- This is explained by stress-induced gastritis.
- Stress → stimulation of posterior pituitary → ACTH release → cortisone production by adrenal → stimulates G cells to produce gastrin.
- Stress → stimulation of anterior pituitary → stimulation of vagus nerve → gastrin production.

4.6 DESCRIBE THE GUT-BRAIN AXIS

SHORT ESSAYS

1. Explain gut-brain axis.

- Gut-brain axis (GBA) is a bidirectional communication between the central and enteric nervous system, linking emotional and cognitive centres of the peripheral functions of the intestine.
- The gut flora plays an important role in biochemical signalling that takes place between the gut and the CNS.
- The GBA involves the HPA axis, neuroendocrine and neuroimmune system, sympathetic and parasympathetic nervous system, enteric nervous system, and gut microbiota.
- Early discovery of the GBA was explained by cephalic phase of gastric secretion by Pavlov.

Gut Flora

- Gut contains the most numerous and varied types of microorganism compared to the whole body.
- The gut flora produces several chemicals by metabolism of carbohydrates like ACh, catecholamines, gamma aminobutyric acid, histamine, melatonin, and serotonin.
- These chemicals help in promoting peristalsis and sensation of gut.
- These chemicals activate the vagus nerve that process information to the brain about intestines.

- Also, under stressful situations, there is a change in the gut flora mediated through the HPA.

Clinical Applications

- Probiotics have been tried for treating some central nervous disorders.
- Gut flora have also been implicated in some anxiety and mood disorders.
- Many children with autism develop gastrointestinal disorders. As autism develops pretty much at the same time as does gut flora, they both have thought to have a connection.

2. Write a note on intrinsic nervous system in gut.

- It is also called the enteric nervous system and consists of about 100 million neurons (Fig. 4.11).
- It is a highly developed nervous system

Extent

- It extends from the beginning of the esophagus till the anus
- The enteric nervous system consists of two layers:

1. **Myenteric or outer layer**
   - It is also called Auerbach's plexus
   - Lies within the muscular layer—thus the name (*myo*—muscle, *enteron*—gut)
   - Its main function is associated with gastrointestinal movements

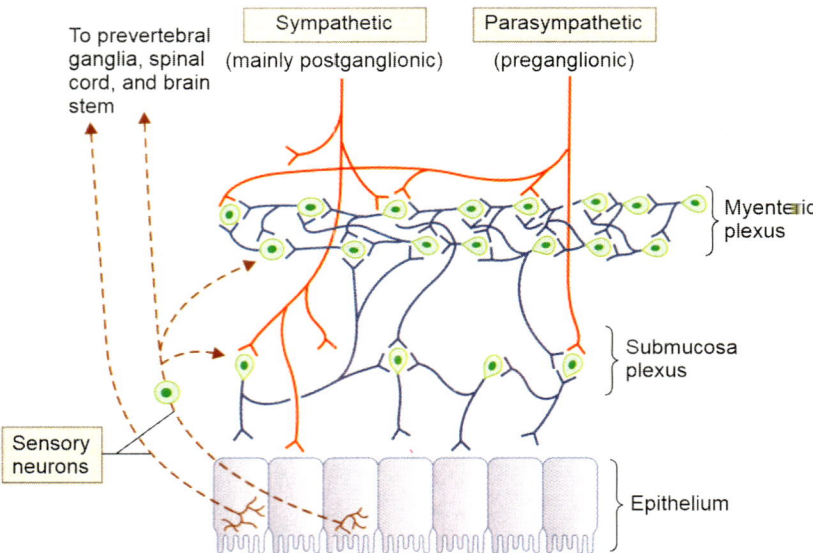

Fig. 4.11

- When these plexuses are stimulated, there is tonic contraction of the gut wall, increased intensity of tonic contractions, increased rate, and intensity of the contractions.
- Not all neurons in the myenteric plexus are excitatory: Some secrete VIP and are inhibitory. This is exemplified in some sphincters like pyloric sphincter and ileocecal sphincter.

2. **Submucosal or inner layer**
   - It is also called Meissner's plexus
   - It lies just below the mucosa
   - Functions are associated with secretion of various glands in the gut mucosa
   - They are involved in local control of secretion following stimuli originating in the mucosa.

Connections

- Sympathetic and parasympathetic fibres supply both the plexus
- There are connections between both types of plexus.
- Sensory connections are to the prevertebral ganglia of the sympathetic nervous system, various segments of the spinal cord and via the vagus nerve to the brain stem.

Neurotransmitters Involved in Enteric Nervous System

Excitatory	Inhibitory
ACh	Norepinephrine
Cholecystokinin (excitatory to bile duct)	Epinephrine
Dopamine (excitatory to lower GIT)	Vasoactive intestinal polypeptide
	Cholecystokinin (inhibitory to stomach)
	Dopamine (to upper GI)

4.7 DESCRIBE AND DISCUSS THE STRUCTURE AND FUNCTIONS OF LIVER AND GALL BLADDER

SHORT ESSAYS

1. Explain enterohepatic circulation. Write a note on obstructive jaundice.

Enterohepatic Circulation

- Enterohepatic circulation is circulation of a substance from the intestine to the liver.
- A lot of substances undergo enterohepatic circulation—bile salts are the most important of all. Others are drugs and bilirubin.
- More than 90% of the bile salts secreted in bile are reabsorbed into the blood from the small intestine
- In this, 50% diffuse through mucosa in duodenum and early part of jejunum, whereas the remainder is absorbed by an active transport process through the intestinal mucosa in the distal ileum.
- They then enter the portal circulation and are circulated back to the liver hepatocytes.
- As a result, there is recycling of substances.

Result of Recycling

- These bile salts are transported to hepatic cells via the sinusoids.

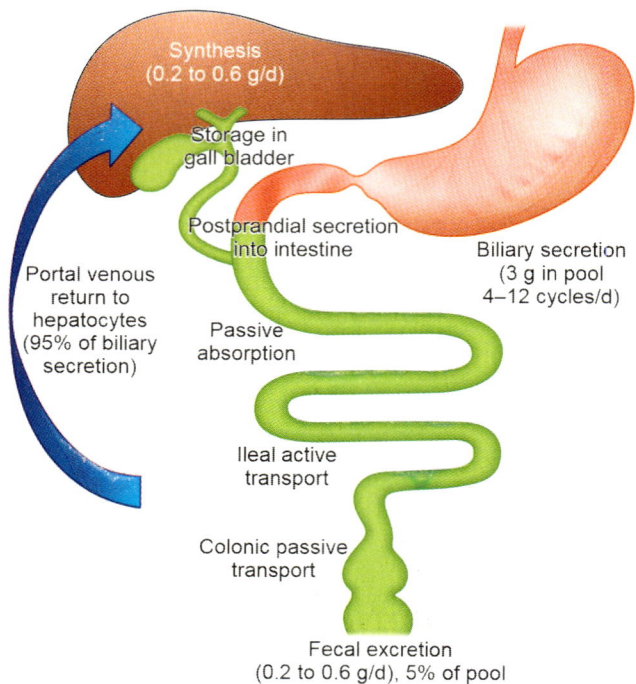

Fig. 4.12

- They are resecreted as bile from the hepatic cells.
- On an average, these salts make the entire circuit around 17 times before being thrown out in the feces.
- The small quantities of bile salts lost into the feces are replaced by new amounts formed continually by the liver cells. Also, the amount of bile salts newly produced is dependent on the bile salts that are circulated back to the liver. If less bile reaches the liver, more *de novo* synthesis happens.
- This is known as enterohepatic circulation of bile.

Importance

- Some lipid soluble and bile soluble drugs' bioavailability is increased due to enterohepatic circulation. If they are excreted in bile, due to enterohepatic circulation, they are brought back to liver and are metabolized.
- When enterohepatic circulation is hampered by ileal disease or resection, more bile salts are lost in feces causing fatty diarrhea or steatorrhea. It is almost always associated with malabsorption of fats and fat-soluble vitamins. They also have an increased propensity to gall stone formation due to decreased solubility of cholesterol.
- Some toxins enter the liver again and cause increased liver damage by enterohepatic circulation.

Obstructive Jaundice

It refers to jaundice due to obstruction of bile outflow or due to sluggish bile flow.

Causes

- Extrinsic causes
  - Gall stones are the main cause for obstructive jaundice. They cause obstruction when they block the opening of the common bile duct.
  - Carcinoma of the head of pancreas and ampulla of Vater
- Intraluminal causes include worm infestations
- Mural causes: Cholangiocarcinoma, sclerosing cholangitis
- Primary biliary cirrhosis

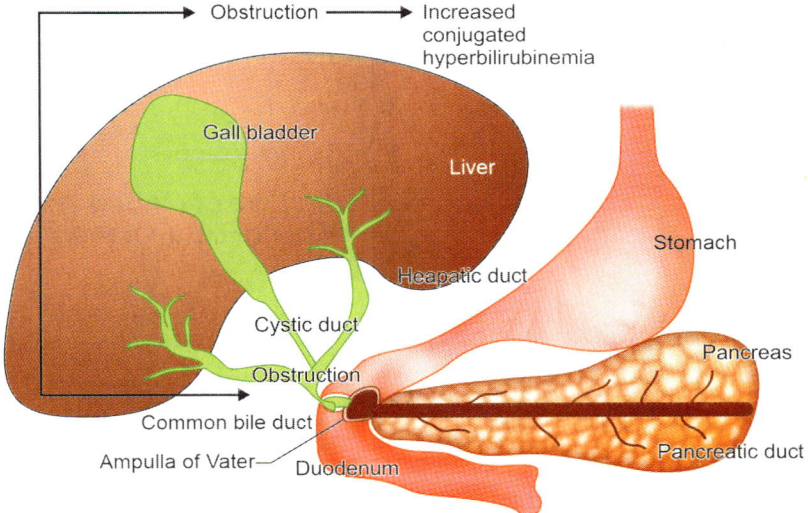

Fig. 4.13

Pathophysiology (Fig. 4.13)

- Increase in conjugated bilirubin causes its back pressure into hepatocytes. Conjugated bilirubin diffuses into the circulation.
- As a result, there is increased bilirubin in blood.
- There is no bilirubin that reaches the intestine. As a result, stercobilinogen is not formed.

Clinical Features

- Jaundice is apparent in form of icterus, yellowish discoloration of skin
- Discoloration of urine
- Pale slate colored stools due to absence of stercobilinogen
- Generalised itching due to bilirubin irritating the skin.

2. What is the role of bile salts and bile acids in lipid digestion and absorption?

Role of Bile Acids

- Triglycerides form the majority of the fats present in our food.
- A very small quantity of lipids is digested in stomach by the action of lingual lipase secreted by the lingual glands in the mouth.
- Rest of the fat digestion takes place in the following manner.

Emulsification of Fats by Bile Acids and Bile Salts

- This is the first step in digestion of lipids (Fig. 4.14)
- Emulsification is a process by which the fat is broken down into minute micelles by the soap-like action of lecithin, which is present in the bile.

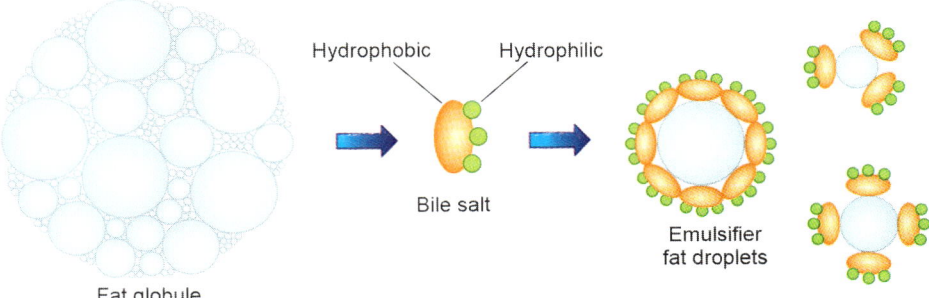

Fig. 4.14

- The bile salts and lecithin have a polar and a non-polar surface.
- As a result, the lipids attach to the non-polar surface and the polar surface of the bile salts project out in a micelle.
- As a result of decrease in the size and formation of multiple micelles, the surface area is greatly increased.
- This is extremely important for the enzyme lipase to act as it acts only on the surface of the fats. Also, lipase is a water-soluble enzyme.
- Lipase acts on these emulsified droplets and fragments triglycerides into monoacyl and diacyl glycerols.
- The importance of bile is demonstrated by the fact that obstruction of bile duct due to many diseases cause steatorrhea: Fatty stools. Also, these patients are severely malnourished due to malabsorption of fats and develop deficiencies of water insoluble vitamins (A, D, E and K)
- Also, the bile salts have an additive effect. The splitting of TG into monoacyl glycerol and free fatty acids is a highly reversible process. Thus, when bile salts are present in the vicinity of these products, they quickly form a micelle with free fatty acids and block the reversal and re-formation of triglycerides.

Role of Bile Salts (Fig. 4.15a)

- Bile salts minute micelles with free fatty acids and ferry them to the brush border epithelium of the small intestine.
- These micelles migrate near the intervillous recesses due to the movement of the microvilli.

- Due to high solubility of lipids in the membrane of the epithelium, the fatty acids, sterols and mono-acyl glycerol get absorbed into the intestinal mucosa.

SHORT ANSWERS

1. What are cholagogues? Give its physiological importance in digestion and absorption.

Cholagogues

- These are substances which cause contraction of the gall bladder to empty its contents into the small intestine.
- Bile salts are the most abundant cholagogues. They have cholagogue action by indirectly causing secretion of cholecystokinin. Other cholagogues are calcium, amino acids and fatty acids.

Physiological Importance

Role of Bile Acids in Lipid Digestion (Fig. 4.15b)

- Emulsification is a process by which the fat is broken down into minute micelles by the soap-like action of lecithin, which is present in the bile.
- The bile salts and lecithin have a polar and a non-polar surface.
- As a result, the lipids attach to the non-polar surface and the polar surface of the bile salts project out in a micelle.
- The surface area is greatly increased.
- This is extremely important for the enzyme lipase to act as it acts only on the surface of the fats. Also, lipase is a water-soluble enzyme.
- Lipase acts on these emulsified droplets and fragments triglycerides into monoacyl and diacyl glycerols.

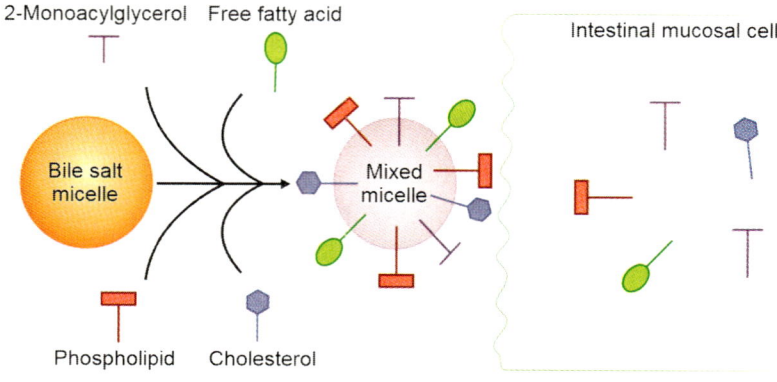

Fig. 4.15a

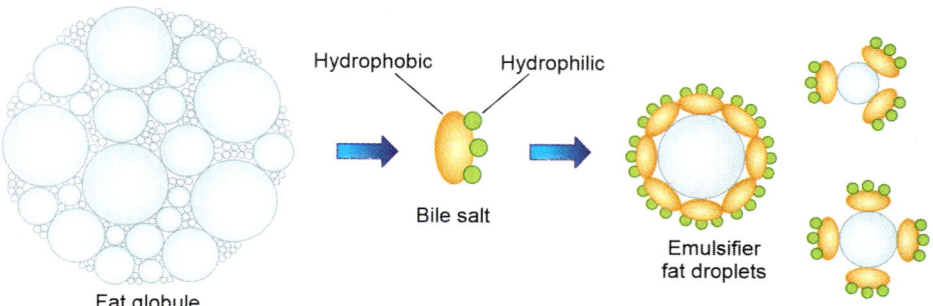

Hydrophobic   Hydrophilic

Bile salt

Emulsifier
fat droplets

Fat globule

Fig. 4.15b

Role of Bile Salts in Absorption of Fats

- Bile salts minute micelles with free fatty acids and ferry them to the brush border epithelium of the small intestine.
- These micelles migrate near the intervillous recesses due to the movement of the microvilli.
- Due to high solubility of lipids in the membrane of the epithelium, the fatty acids, sterols and mono-acylglycerol get absorbed into the intestinal mucosa.

2. What are cholagogue and choleretic agents? Give two examples of each.

Cholagogues

These are substances which cause contraction of the gall bladder to empty its contents into the small intestine.

Examples

- Bile salts are the most abundant cholagogues. They have cholagogue action by indirectly causing secretion of cholecystokinin.
- Other cholagogues are calcium, amino acids and fatty acids.

Choleretics

- These are substances which cause secretion of bile from liver into the gall bladder
- They are mainly used as therapeutic agents in cholestasis.

Examples

Ursodeoxycholic acid, ursodiol

4.8 DESCRIBE AND DISCUSS GASTRIC FUNCTION TESTS, PANCREATIC EXOCRINE FUNCTION TESTS AND LIVER FUNCTION TESTS

SHORT ANSWERS

1. Mention 4 gastric function tests.

Fractional test meal	Collection of stomach contents by Ryle's tube at frequent interval following a test meal
Alcohol stimulation test	After an overnight fast, 100 ml alcohol is administered via a Ryle's tube and gastric secretions are analyzed for free acid, total acidity and presence of bile.
Pentagastrin stimulation test	Synthetic peptide of gastrin, is given subcutaneously and gastric secretion is studied for acid concentration
Augmented histamine test	Histalog is used to stimulate gastric secretion
Insulin stimulation test	Measurement of free acid and total acidity in the gastric secretions following intravenous injection of 25 units of insulin

2. Explain synthetic functions of liver.

- Liver is a major organ in the body and is responsible for many functions.
- It is involved in metabolism and excretion of many substances

1. **Bile production**
   - Bile is produced by the hepatocytes.
   - It contains large quantities of bile acids, salts, cholesterol and lecithin.
   - From the hepatocytes, bile is released into the ductules which join to form the bile duct.

2. **Synthesis of glucose**
   - In states of starvation, fatty acids are used to form glucose by gluconeogenesis.
   - Also, glucogenic amino acids are used to form glucose for supply of energy.
   - It takes place in the mitochondria of the hepatocytes.

3. **Synthesis of plasma proteins**
   - Almost all proteins in plasma are produced by liver.
   - Albumin is the main plasma protein produced by liver and serum albumin is used.

- Others are hormone binding proteins and complement factors.
- The proteins which are not synthesized in liver are immunoglobulins

4. **Synthesis of clotting factors**
   - Most of the clotting factors are synthesized in liver.
   - Fibrinogen, factor V, VII, IX, X, XI, XII, are produced by hepatocytes.
   - The sinusoidal endothelium produces factor VIII and von Willebrand factor.

5. Synthesis of hormones like somatostatin, anticoagulants like heparin also take place in liver.

3. Give 4 tests to assess pancreatic functions.

Pancreatic function can be analyzed by noninvasive and invasive tests.

Non-invasive Tests

Serum amylase	It is an enzyme secreted by exocrine pancreas for carbohydrate digestion	Normal values: <140 U/L High in pancreatitis
Serum lipase	It is an enzyme secreted by exocrine pancreas for lipid digestion	Normal values: 12–70 U/L High in pancreatitis Enzyme spills into circulation during inflammation
Fecal elastase	It is an enzyme secreted by the exocrine pancreas and remains unchanged through its transit in the intestine	Normal values: 200–500 microgram/g of stool It is decreased in pancreatic insufficiency and obstruction to the opening of the pancreatic duct
Serum trypsinogen	It is a proenzyme which is responsible for protein digestion	Low levels are seen in chronic pancreatic insufficiency

Invasive Tests

- ERCP—endoscopic retrograde cholangiopancreatography
- MRCP—magnetic resonance cholangiopancreatography
- In these techniques, the structure of the pancreas and its ductular system is studied after injecting a dye and studying by using fluoroscopy or magnetic resonance imaging

4.9 DISCUSS THE PHYSIOLOGY ASPECTS OF: PEPTIC ULCER, GASTROESOPHAGEAL REFLUX DISEASE, VOMITING, DIARRHOEA, CONSTIPATION, ADYNAMIC ILEUS, HIRSCHSPRUNG'S DISEASE

SHORT ANSWERS

1. Explain Hirschsprung's disease.

- It is also called congenital megacolon
- It is a congenital condition resulting from poor development of Auerbach and Meissner's plexus in the anorectum which may extend proximally to involve the whole colon.
- It is characterized by narrow spasmodic non-relaxing segment of the terminal part of colon and anorectum.
- The segment proximal to the diseased part has normal ganglions. They undergo hypertrophy to push the feces out.
- As a result, the child is not able to defecate normally.
- It passes goat-like pellet like stools. There is abdominal distension.
- Treatment is use of proximal colon to create an opening just below the anal sphincter.

2. Explain the pathophysiology of peptic ulcer disease.

Peptic ulcer is an area of loss of mucosa of the esophagus, stomach or duodenum due to erosive action of gastric secretions.

Common Sites of Peptic Ulceration (Fig. 4.16)

- 1 cm proximal to pyloric sphincter on the lesser curvature is the most common site for ulceration
- Others are first part of duodenum, lower end of esophagus and opening of a gastrostomy.

Pathophysiology

- Peptic secretion and a protective mucosal response maintain a balance and prevent ulceration.
- Normally, ulcer formation is prevented by some protective mechanisms
- Gastroduodenal mucosal barrier
- Ample amounts of mucosal glands
- Alkaline mucus secreted by the Brunner's glands in the first part of duodenum
- Alkaline pancreatic secretion and bile with high concentration of bicarbonate ions
- Also, there is reflex inhibition of gastrin secretion when acidic chyme enters the duodenum
- Presence of acidic chyme in small intestine causes secretion of secretin which causes pancreas to secrete alkaline fluid.

Ulcerogenic Factors (Fig. 4.17)

- Infection with *Helicobacter pylori*:
  - This is perhaps the most important factor for ulcerogenesis
  - It is a lifelong infection unless eradicated by antimicrobial therapy
  - These microorganisms have an ability to penetrate layers of mucosa and break the mucosal barrier
  - This increase the propensity of the gastric juices to cause ulceration.
- Intake of hot and spicy food
- Abuse of non-steroidal anti-inflammatory drugs: Can break the mucosal barrier

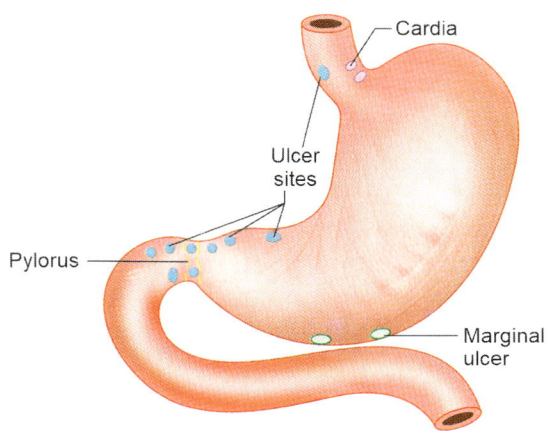

Fig. 4.16

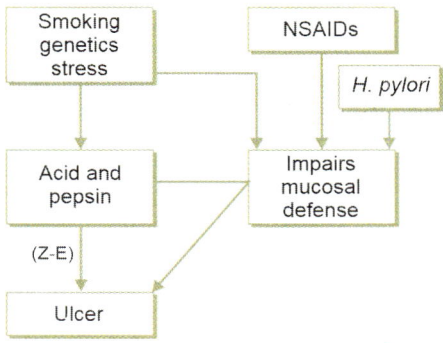

Fig. 4.17

- Smoking: Increased nervous stimulation of the stomach
- Alcohol ingestion
- Severe emotional and physical stress

3. A female 24 weeks of pregnancy complains of heart burn after food, and at night. What are the factors that lead to gastroesophageal reflux disease?

- Gastroesophageal reflux is reflux of contents of the stomach into the distal part of the oesophagus
- Normally, this is prevented by a tight lower esophageal sphincter, caused by a tight band of circular muscles (Fig. 4.18).
- Factors which lead to reflux are:

1. **Sphincter related**
   - Lax sphincter causes reflux of acid from stomach to enter the esophagus
   - Causes are:
     o Diaphragmatic hernia where the esophagus and a part of stomach herniates through the diaphragmatic hiatus into the thorax
     o Increased progesterone causes smooth muscle relaxation leading to a lax sphincter. This is the reason why reflux is common in pregnant ladies
     o Obesity: It causes the sphincter to be lax and allows contents of the stomach to regurgitate.

2. **Stomach related**
   - An overdistended stomach is the most common cause. The sphincter is just a tight band of muscles which gives way when the stomach is over distended. Also, lying down after a heavy meal causes the contents to spill into the esophagus
   - Decreased space in the abdomen in presence of ascites or a gravid uterus, pushes the gastric contents into the esophagus due to increase in intra-abdominal pressure.
   - Increased gastric secretion can be induced by a lot of causes like aspirin overuse, smoking, alcohol ingestion, hot and spicy food intake.

4. What is motilin? How does cholera cause diarrhoea?

Motilin is a hormone built by 22 amino acid residues.

Source

- It is secreted by Mo cells, which are present in stomach and intestine.
- It is also believed to be secreted by entero-chromaffin cells of intestine.

Stimulant for Secretion

Motilin is secreted when the chyme from stomach enters the duodenum.

Functions

1. Accelerates gastric emptying
2. Increases the mixing and propulsive movements of small intestine
3. Increases the peristalsis in colon.

Pathophysiology of Diarrhea in Cholera

To understand this, normal absorption of ions in the mucosa of the intestine must be understood.

Absorption of Sodium, Chloride and Bicarbonate

- The basolateral surface of the mucosal cells has Na-K-ATPase which actively pump out sodium into the interstitium, creating a low concentration of intracellular sodium to about 50 mEq (Fig. 4.19).
- As a result, Na is drawn from the luminal surface into the cell by diffusion. And water follows due to the osmotic gradient.
- Following absorption of Na^+ ions there is a negativity created in the chyme which causes Cl^- ions to diffuse into the mucosal cell. This happens mainly in the duodenum and jejunum.
- The bicarbonate ions are secreted by the microvilli of the ileum.

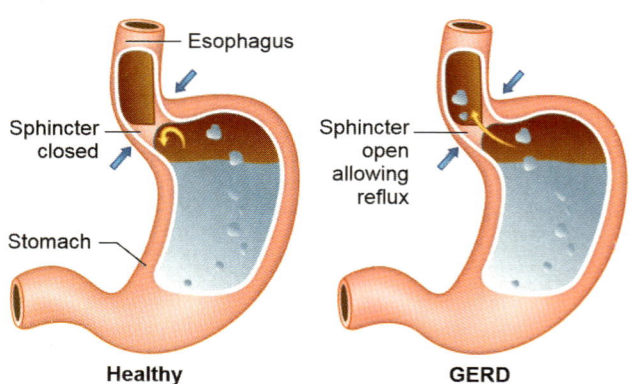

Esophagus

Sphincter closed

Sphincter open allowing reflux

Stomach

Healthy   GERD

Fig. 4.18

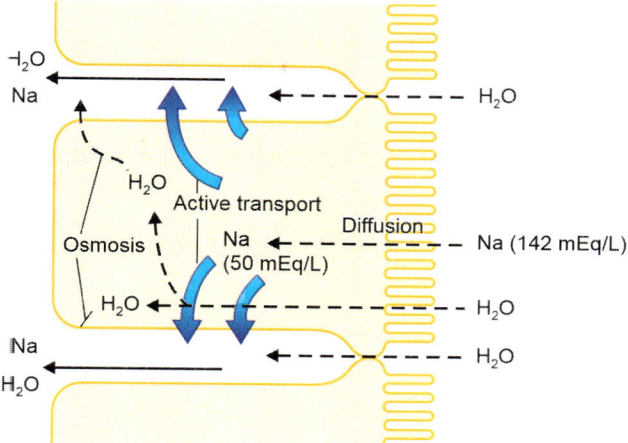

Fig. 4.19

Pathophysiology of Diarrhea in Cholera (Fig. 4.20)

- *V. cholerae* secretes a toxin which activates the G protein leading to activation of the cyclic AMP.
- The beta subunit binds to the glycoclipids on the surface of the host cell and alpha subunit penetrates inside.
- This leads to secretion of all types of ions—Cl⁻ and bicarbonate by the cell.
- There is also increased water secretion.
- As a result, severe watery diarrhea results.
- Death may occur due to hypovolemic shock.

5. Explain the pathophysiology of constipation.

Constipation is defined as a decrease in frequency or increase in consistency of stools. It happens due to slow movement of the colon. As a result, more and more fluids are absorbed.

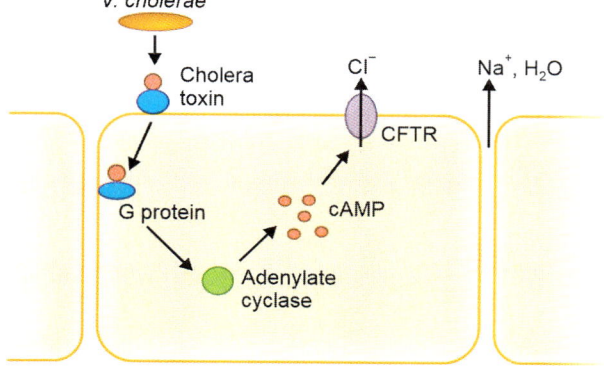

Fig. 4.20

Normal colonic function—absorption and motility

- Normally the colon receives around 1400 ml of fluid from the small intestine. The faeces contain only 200–400 ml of water. Thus, the large amount of water absorption that takes place is a slow and meticulous time bound function of the colon.
- There is an active sodium pump which causes sodium absorption and then water follows.
- The longer the stools stay in colon, more water is absorbed.
- The colon has mainly mixing and propulsive movements.
- Mass movements of the colon are responsible for defecation and are very active in the morning. They are also called high amplitude propagated contractions. (HAPCs)
- A number of factors can be involved in a normal motility of the intestine as it is a complex process.
- Gut motility is controlled by the enteric nervous system and influenced by serum electrolytes and hormones.
- It is also dependent on the contents of the colon.

Constipation

- In spite of ruling out all other organic disorders associated with constipation, there may be functional disorders too.
- The tonicity of the colon is also decreased in cases of laxative abuse and when defecation is controlled when its reflexes are excited over a long period of time. A daily routine of timely meals and regular bowel habits is required to have a timely mass reflex.
- Features of constipation are abnormally hard stools, straining for defecation, bloating, feeling of inadequate emptying of the rectum.

Causes

Primary causes (they have normal colonic transit time)	Irritable bowel syndrome It is a functional disorder of the GIT characterized abnormal bowel movements where no structural cause can be found. Irregular bowel habits Decreased fluid intake, decreased fiber intake Fasting Dyssynergic defecation It occurs due to improper innervation of the pelvic floor muscles

Secondary causes	Electrolyte and hormone related • Hypercalcemia • Hypothyroidism Structural problems • Strictures • Congenital megacolon • Intestinal obstruction due to worms or tumour Neurological disorders • Diabetes mellitus • Parkinson's disease • Spinal cord disease Medications • Anticholinergics • Opioids • Calcium channel blockers

6. A 56-year male patient underwent abdominal surgery under spinal anaesthesia. He was asked not to have food or water for 6 hours. What could be the reason? Explain the others causes of adynamic ileus.

Parasympathetic Supply

- Stomach, duodenum, jejunum, ileum, pancreas, proximal half of colon: Vagus nerve
- Distal colon, rectum and anus: S2, S3, S4

Sympathetic Supply

- The whole of the GIT is supplied by sympathetic supply from T5 to L2.

- These preganglionic fibres synapse in coeliac ganglion and mesenteric ganglia.

Spinal Anaesthesia

- It is mainly used for obstetric and gynaecological procedures, orthopaedic and plastic surgeries of the lower limbs and urological procedures
- It is injection of an anaesthetic into the sub-arachnoid space between L3 and L4.
- As a result, the sympathetic outflow is blocked.
- Parasympathetic outflow is increased. This causes overactivity of the intestine with relaxed sphincters.
- When food is ingested within 6 hours, (gastric emptying time), it may enter the esophagus and cause aspiration into the respiratory tract and lead to aspiration pneumonia—a potentially lethal condition.

Causes for Adynamic Ileus

- It is also known as paralytic ileus
- The intestines fail to transmit peristalsis due to failure of neuromuscular transmission through Auerbach and Meissner's plexus
- Most common cause is post-operative ileus.
- Others are hypokalaemia, sepsis and retro-peritoneal hemorrhage.

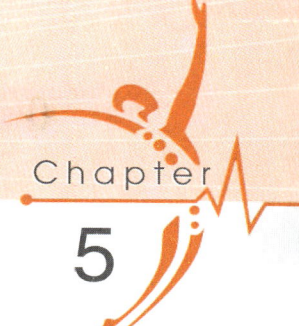

Cardiovascular Physiology (CVS)

5.1 DESCRIBE THE FUNCTIONAL ANATOMY OF HEART INCLUDING CHAMBERS, SOUNDS; AND PACEMAKER TISSUE AND CONDUCTING SYSTEM

SHORT ESSAYS

1. Explain the conducting system of the heart with a neat labelled diagram. What is the physiological significance of AV nodal delay?
(4 + 1 marks)

Conductive System of the Heart

- It is formed by a specialized system of cardiac fibers.

- The components are:
  1. **Sino-atrial node or the SA node**
     - It is called pacemaker of the heart
     - It is situated in the right atrium just inferior to the opening of the superior vena cava.
     - It sends out spontaneous impulses at regular intervals and impulses are conducted to both atria.

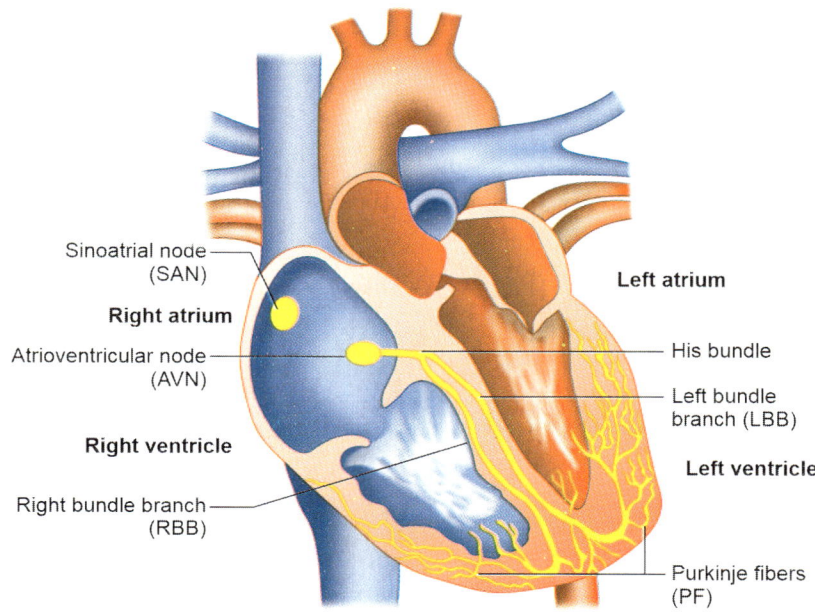

Sinoatrial node (SAN)

Right atrium

Atrioventricular node (AVN)

Right ventricle

Right bundle branch (RBB)

Left atrium

His bundle

Left bundle branch (LBB)

Left ventricle

Purkinje fibers (PF)

Fig. 5.1

– Through internodal fibers, impulses reach the AV node. There are three types: Anterior (Bachman), intermediate (Wenckebach) and posterior internodal fibers (Thorel)

2. **Atrioventricular node or the AV Node**
   – It receives from impulses from the SA node through the internodal fibres.
   – It is situated immediately below the right atrium and anterior to the leaflet of the tricuspid valve.

3. **Bundle of His**
   – It continues from the AV node and conducts impulses along the interventricular septum.
   – Midway, it divides into right and left bundle branches

4. **Right and left bundle branches and Purkinje fibres:** The bundle branches run along the respective sides of interventricular septum and culminate as Purkinje fibres which innervate the myocardium.

AV Nodal Delay Physiological Significance

- After firing of impulses in the SA node, a delay of 0.12 seconds is noticed prior to activation of the AV node.
- It is the time taken for impulses to travel from SA node to AV node.
- It is seen as PR interval on ECG
- This delay in the cardiac pulse is extremely important as it ensures that the atria of the heart have ejected their blood into the ventricles of the heart first before the ventricles contract.

2. Write briefly on Korotkoff sounds

- These are the sounds heard while measuring blood pressure by auscultatory method.
- The bell of stethoscope is placed over the antecubital fossa and the cuff is inflated.

- When the pressure is as high as the systolic pressure of the heart or the maximum pressure, the artery is occluded. This leads to collapse of the brachial artery and there are no sounds heard.
- When the cuff is slowly released, the sounds that heard over the antecubital fossa are called Korotkoff sounds.
- The exact cause of the production of Korotkoff sounds is not clearly known but is thought to be blood jetting through the partially occluded vessel.

Zero phase	No sound	Pressure equal to more than systolic BP
First phase	Tapping sound	Pressure is just below the systolic blood pressure—taken as systolic BP
Second phase	Louder tapping, followed by a murmur	Pressure around 15 mm below systolic BP
Third phase	Gong follows murmur	Pressure around 25–30 mm below systolic BP
Fourth sound	Muffled character	Pressure around 35 mm below systolic BP
Fifth phase	Disappearance of sound	Marks diastolic blood pressure

SHORT ANSWER

1. Name the different heart sounds and how are they produced?

Different Heart Sounds

First heart sound—lub	Produced by closure of mitral and tricuspid valves
Second heart sound—dub	Produced by closure of semi-lunar valves
Third heart sound—low pitched	Produced by filling of the ventricle with blood during diastole
Fourth heart sound—inaudible	Produced by contraction of atrial muscles

5.2 DESCRIBE THE PROPERTIES OF CARDIAC MUSCLE INCLUDING ITS MORPHOLOGY, ELECTRICAL, MECHANICAL AND METABOLIC FUNCTIONS

SHORT ESSAYS

1. Explain the properties of cardiac muscle.

Cardiac muscles have these four important properties:

1. **Excitability**
   - It is defined as the ability of a cardiac cell to respond to a stimulus.
   - The initial response is in the form of electrical activity followed by mechanical which is seen as contraction of muscle fibre.
   - The resting membrane potential of a cardiac muscle is –90 mV. Followed by a stimulus, there is initial rapid depolarization up to around +10 mV followed by transient initial repolarization, plateau stage and late slow repolarization.
   - This is due to a sequence of opening of fast sodium channels, potassium channels, calcium channels and finally potassium channels, respectively.
   - Action potential spreads through all muscles of atria and ventricles through gap junctions. The fibres act as a syncytium.

2. **Rhythmicity**
   - It is a specialized feature of all cardiac muscle fibers only.
   - They can maintain rhythmicity and auto-generation of impulses.
   - Sinoatrial node has the property of automatic rhythmicity of highest order. It generates most frequent and powerful impulses. Therefore, it is called the pacemaker
   - If the SA node is diseased, its work is taken up by the AV node.

3. **Conductivity**
   - It is formed by a specialized system of cardiac fibers.
   - The components are:
     i. *Sino-atrial node or the SA node*
        - It is called pacemaker of the heart
        - It is situated in the right atrium just inferior to the opening of the superior vena cava.
        - It sends out spontaneous impulses at regular intervals and impulses are conducted to both atria.
        - Through internodal fibers, impulses reach the AV node. There are three types: Anterior (Bachman), intermediate (Wenckebach) and posterior internodal fibers (Thorel)
     ii. *Atrioventricular node or the AV node*
        - It receives from impulses from the SA node through the internodal fibres.
        - It is situated immediately below the right atrium and anterior to the leaflet of the tricuspid valve.
     iii. *Bundle of His*
        - It continues from the AV node and conducts impulses along the interventricular septum.
        - Midway, it divides into right and left bundle branches
     iv. *Right and left bundle branches and Purkinje fibres:* The bundle branches run along the respective sides of interventricular septum and the culminate as Purkinje fibres which innervate the myocardium.

4. **Contractility**
   - It is the ability of the cardiac muscle fiber to shorten in length in response to a stimulus.
   - These fibers have some laws with respect to contractility.
     i. *All-or-none phenomenon:* In response to a stimulus, irrespective of its strength, the cardiac muscle responds either maximally or does not respond at all
     ii. *Staircase phenomenon*
        - When stimuli arrive at shorter intervals, there is incremental response by the cardiac muscle as in a staircase.
        - This is especially helpful in increasing the cardiac output by repeated stimuli provided by the sympathetic system in times of need.
     iii. *Refractory period*
        - The total refractory period in a skeletal muscle lasts for 0.1s, whereas in a cardiac muscle it lasts for 0.53s.

– Cardiac cells have two refractory periods.

a. Absolute refractory period extends from phase 0 until halfway of phase 3. In this period, no matter what the strength of the stimulus, the cardiac muscle cannot be stimulated.

Cause: the fast sodium channels get inactivated when the membrane potential approaches the equilibrium for Na^+. As a result, Na^+ ions cannot move out or in. As a result, no impulse can stimulate the cardiac muscle.

b. Relative refractory period extends from phase 3 till repolarization is complete. In this phase, a stimulus of greater strength can stimulate a cardiac muscle.

Cause: It is due to the leaking of potassium ions, which makes the membrane potential more negative (i.e. it is hyperpolarized), this resets the sodium channels; opening the inactivation gate, but still leaving the channel closed. Thus, it is possible to initiate an action potential, but a stronger stimulus than normal is required

– Significance of prolonged refractory period in cardiac muscle

o Prevents tetany

o Summation of contraction does not occur

o Fatigue does not occur

2. Explain cardiac ventricular action potential. Why is the refractory period of ventricular action potential prolonged? (4 + 1 marks)

Or

With a neat graph explain the electrical events of ventricular muscle. What is the cause and importance of its long refractory period?

Cardiac Ventricular Action Potential

- Action potential in the cardiac muscles are a little different from other types of muscle fibres.
- The duration lasts for 200–250 m seconds.
- The resting membrane potential is –90 mV

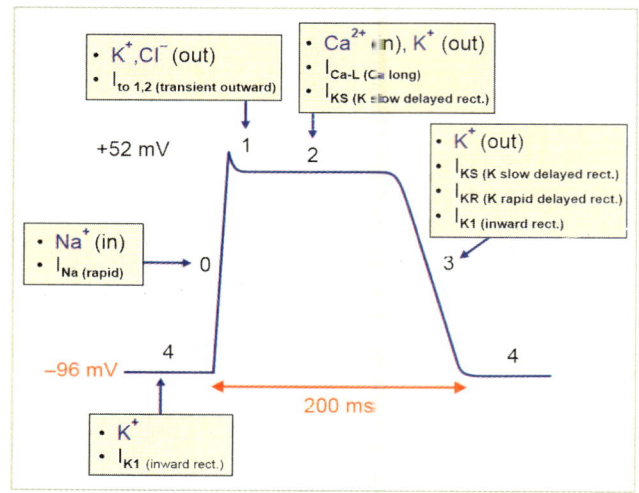

Fig. 5.2

Phase 0 Depolarization	Caused by opening of fast sodium channels which last for 1/10000 of a second and lead to influx of sodium within the cell	Causes the membrane potential to rise up to around 40 mV which leads to inactivation of these channels
Phase 1 Initial rapid repolarization	Due to outflux of K^+ Closure of fast sodium channels and opening of slow sodium channels	There is mild decrease in the membrane potential
Phase 2 Plateau	Balance between outflux of potassium and influx of calcium maintains a plateau	Last for around 200 m seconds in atrial muscle and 300 m seconds in ventricular muscles
Phase 3 Prolonged repolarization	Due to efflux of potassium ions	Lasts for 60–70 milliseconds
Phase 4	Restoration of RMP	Due to the sodium potassium pump, Na^+ ions are pumped back out and K^+ ions are pumped back in

Significance of Prolonged Refractory Period in Cardiac Muscle

- Prevents tetany
- Summation of contraction does not occur
- Fatigue does not occur

3. Explain the following properties of heart:
   #### A. Automaticity
   #### B. Refractory period

A. Automaticity

- It is the ability of a tissue to produce its own impulses regularly.
- All fibres of the cardiac muscle have property of automatic rhythmicity
- Sinoatrial node has the property of automatic rhythmicity of highest order. It generates most frequent and powerful impulses. Therefore, it is called the pacemaker.
- If the SA node is diseased, its work is taken up by the AV node.

Mechanism of Electrical Activity in SA Node

- The resting membrane potential of the pacemaker cells is –40 mV to –55 mV, much higher compared to ventricular muscle fiber. This is known as pacemaker potential.
- The cause for this is leaky cell membrane to sodium and calcium channels.
- Due to the higher resting membrane potential, the fast sodium channels are in inactivated

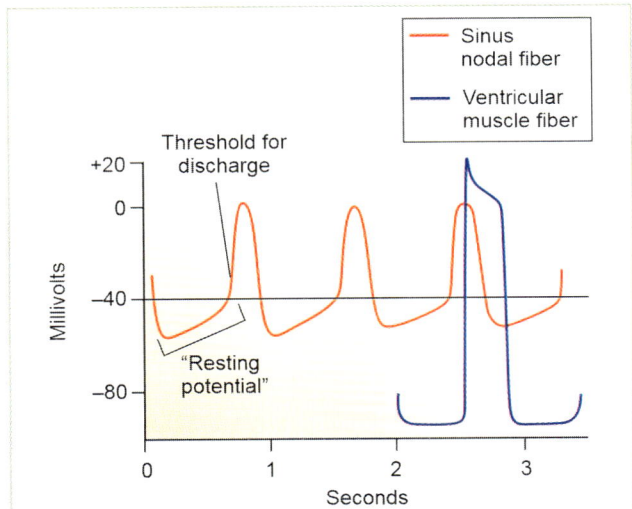

Fig. 5.3

state. Therefore, electrical activity depends on slow sodium and calcium channels. Thus, the depolarisation is slow and less.
- There is abundance of sodium ions in the extra-cellular fluid which constantly leak into the cell to cause depolarisation.
- When the membrane potential reaches –40 mV, then the sodium–calcium channels get activated. There is slow influx of calcium and sodium ions.
- After about 100–150 ms, these channels get inactivated and the potassium channels open leading to efflux of potassium channels.
- As a result, the potential drops to –55 mV when the sequence repeats itself.
- Thus, automaticity is established.

B. Refractory Period

- The total refractory period in a skeletal muscle lasts for 0.1 s, whereas in a cardiac muscle it lasts for 0.53 s.
- Cardiac cells have two refractory periods.
   1. **Absolute refractory period:** Extends from phase 0 until halfway of phase 3. In this period, no matter what the strength of the stimulus, the cardiac muscle cannot be stimulated.
   Cause: The fast sodium channels get inactivated when the membrane potential approaches the equilibrium for Na$^+$, as a result, Na$^+$ ions cannot move out or in. As a result, no impulse can stimulate the cardiac muscle.
   2. **Relative refractory period:** Extends from phase 3 till repolarization is complete. In this phase, a stimulus of greater strength can stimulate a cardiac muscle.
   Cause: It is due to the leaking of potassium ions, which makes the membrane potential more negative (i.e. it is hyperpolarized), this resets the sodium channels; opening the inactivation gate, but still leaving the channel closed. Thus, it is possible to initiate an action potential, but a stronger stimulus than normal is required.

4. Explain preload and afterload in cardiac muscle. What is Frank-Starling's law?

Preload

- Preload is the stretching of the cardiac muscle just prior to systole.
- It depends on the venous return to the heart.

- Preload is an important determinant of cardiac output. As the amount of blood filling in the ventricles causes stretching of the cardia fibres, there is increase in length of the fibers.
- This causes increased contractility as described by Frank-Starling's law.
- Thus, force of contraction and cardiac output depend directly on the preload

Afterload

- It is the force against which the ventricles must pump the blood
- It is determined by the systemic arterial resistance. It is governed by the caliber of the vessels.
- After load determines the diastolic blood pressure.
- The cardiac output is inversely proportional to the peripheral arterial resistance.

Frank-Starling's Law

- It is based on the relationship between initial length of the cardiac muscle and its contractility.
- Cardiac output depends on the force of contractility.
- According to the Frank-Starling's law, the force of contraction of the cardiac muscle is directly proportional to the initial length of the muscle fiber prior to the onset of contraction.
- The force of contractility thus depends on the preload or the end-diastolic volume. During diastole, the ventricular pressure rises due to filling of blood and thus length of the ventricular musle fibres increases due to stretching.

SHORT ANSWER

1. Explain Frank-Starling's law.

- It is based on the relationship between initial length of the cardiac muscle and its contractility.
- Cardiac output depends on the force of contractility.
- According to the Frank-Starling's law, the force of contraction of the cardiac muscle is directly proportional to the initial length of the muscle fiber prior to the onset of contraction.
- The force of contractility thus depends on the preload or the end-diastolic volume. During diastole, the ventricular pressure rises due to filling of blood and thus length of the ventricular musle fibres increases due to stretching.

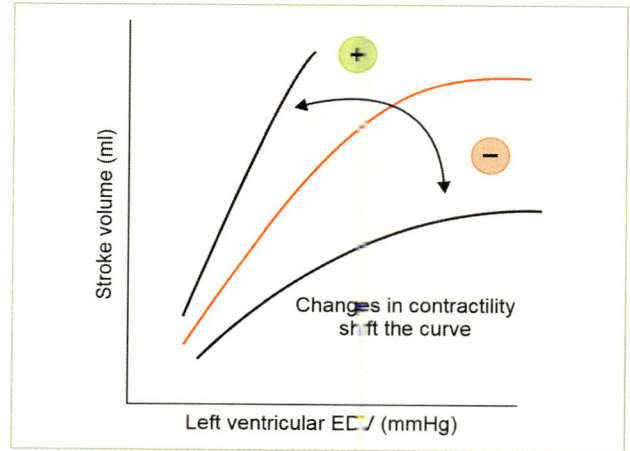

Fig. 5.4

5.3 DISCUSS THE EVENTS OCCURRING DURING THE CARDIAC CYCLE

LONG ESSAY

1. **Explain different phases of cardiac cycle. Write the hysteresis loop and explain the pressure and volume relationship in a cardiac cycle**
(6 + 4 marks)

Cardiac Cycle

- Cardiac cycle encompasses the cardiac events occurring from the beginning of one heartbeat till the beginning of the next heartbeat.
- Each cycle is initiated by an impulse generated at the sinoatrial node.
- The main components of cardiac cycle are diastole (relaxation of the muscles and hence the chambers) and systole (contraction of the chambers).
- During systole, there is contraction of the heart muscles leading the blood to be pumped forwards into the arteries and during diastole, the chambers relax and receive blood from the venous end.

Duration and Timing

Total duration of the cardiac cycle	0.8 second
Atrial systole	0.1 second
Atrial diastole	0.7 second
Ventricular systole	0.3 second
Ventricular diastole	0.5 second

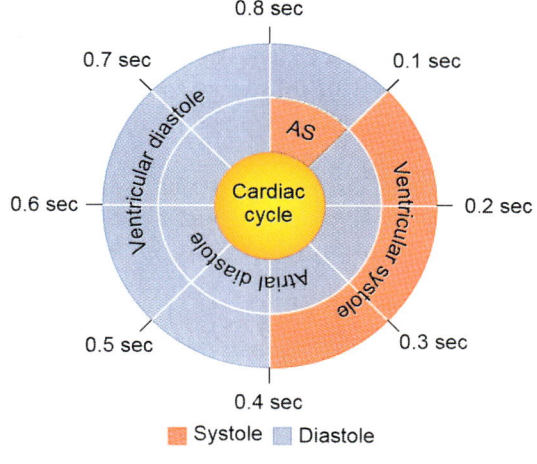

Fig. 5.5

Events of Atria

1. **Atrial systole**
   - Also called the last rapid filling stage
   - Lasts for 0.11 second
   - It overlaps the final phase of ventricular diastole
   - During this phase, blood is forced from atria to ventricles.
   - Contraction of atria causes the fourth heart sound.

2. **Atrial diastole**
   - It follows atrial diastole.
   - It lasts for 0.69 and overlaps ventricular systole.
   - The atria get filled during this phase; the vena-cavae empties deoxygenated blood into the right atrium and left atrium receives oxygenated blood through the pulmonary veins.

Events of Ventricles

Since ventricular phase determines the output, systole always refers to ventricular systole and diastole refers to ventricular diastole.

1. **Ventricular systole:** It consists of two phases—isometric contraction (0.05 second) and ejection period (0.22 second).

   i. *Isometric contraction*
      - First phase of ventricular systole, lasts for about 0.05 second
      - There is increase in the tension within the heart muscles without a change in their length.
      - At this phase, the AV valves are shut and the tension in the fibres increase without a change in the volume of the ventricles.
      - As a result, there is sharp rise in the pressure. This sharp rise in pressure iis required to overcome that in the pulmonary artery and aorta, thus causing opening of the semilunar valves.
      - Due to closure of AV valves at the beginning of the systole, there is first heart sound.

   ii. *Ejection period*
      - Lasts for 0.22 second
      - Isotonic contraction of the muscles of the ventricles leads to gush of blood from ventricles into the aorta and the pulmonary artery.

- The initial part of the ejection is rapid and lasts for 0.13 second
- The late part of the ejection is slow and lasts for 0.09 second.
- At the end of ejection, some blood remains within the ventricles—it is called end systolic volume and is around 60–80 ml.
- The percentage of amount of blood pumped out during ejection phase to the amount of the blood that enters the ventricles during diastole is measured as ejection fraction and is around 65%.

2. **Ventricular diastole**
   i. *Protodiastole*
      - It marks the beginning of diastole, the pressure in the ventricle falls following ejection and the semilunar valves close.
      - It lasts for 0.04 second.
      - No other events occur in this phase
   ii. *Isometric relaxation*
      - The tension within the cardiac muscles comes down without decrease in the length of the muscle fibres
      - As a result, the pressure within the ventricles drop
      - It lasts for 0.08 second
      - This steep drop in the ventricular pressure causes the semilunar valves to open
   iii. *Rapid filling phase*
      - In this period, the AV valves are now open and there is gush of blood from the atria into the ventricles
      - It lasts for 0.11 second
      - The filling of the ventricles causes the third heart sound. This phase contributes to 70% of the blood filling.
   iv. *Slow filling phase*
      - Lasts for 0.19 second
      - 20% of blood fills in this stage
   v. *Last rapid filling*
      - Occurs due to atrial systole
      - 10% ventricular filling takes place in this phase.

Hysteresis Loop

- It represents changes in volume with change in pressure of the left ventricle
- Time is not represented in this plot.

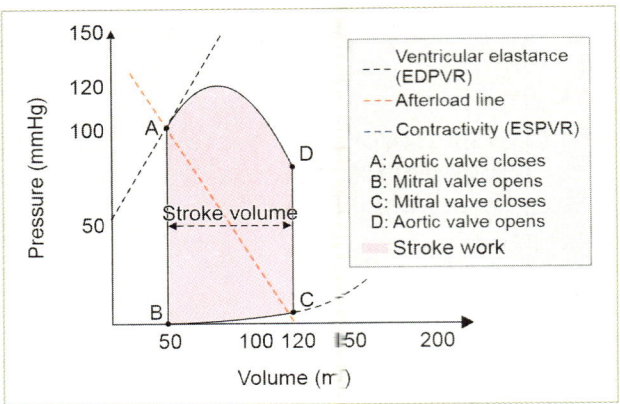

Fig. 5.6

- ABC represents ventricular diastole and CDA represents ventricular systole
- AB represents isovolumetric relaxation—there is a sharp dip in pressure with no change in volume. At the end of this, mitral valve opens.
- BC represents three phases of ventricular filling: Rapid filling, slow filling, and last rapid filling. At the end of this, mitral valve closes.
- C represents end diastolic volume and pressure.
- CD represents isovolumetric contraction of the ventricles leading to a steep rise in pressure and at the end of this phase, the aortic valve opens.
- The DA represents ejection phase. It is seen that volume decreases and there is a rise in pressure followed a slow dip.
- A represents end systolic pressure or volume at a point of time.

Inference of the Hysteresis Loop

- The distance between B and C in the loop represents the stroke volume
- The slope BC gives the elastance of the left ventricle. Increased elastance is seen in diastolic dysfunction like restrictive pericarditis. This is seen as increased slope of BC.
- The ejection fraction also can be calculated from this curve (stroke volume/end diastolic volume)
- The difference of pressure between D and A gives pulse pressure.
- Preload is given by the end of diastolic volume
- Afterload is given by the slope CA as it represents
- The shape of the loop and the values help in understanding various valvular heart diseases.
  Example: In aortic stenosis, the afterload slope is increased. In mitral stenosis, slope of BC is increased.

SHORT ESSAYS

1 A 50-year-old male patient comes with the history of dyspnea. His JVP was raised. What is JVP? Explain the waves. What does raise in JVP signify? Give the types of heart failure.

Jugular Venous Pulse (JVP)

- Jugular venous pulse is a measurement of the venous pulsation in the internal jugular vein.
- It is a measure of pressure changes in the atrium.
- The parts of the normal JVP are:
  1. **a wave**
     - It is the first positive wave
     - Represents atrial systole
     - Normally, the pressure in right atrium is 5 mm Hg and left atrium is 7 mm during systole
  2. **x wave**
     - First negative wave
     - Occurs due to relaxation of atria just prior to diastole
  3. **c wave**
     - It is the second positive wave
     - Due to isometric contraction
     - Closure of AV valves causes rise in pressure
  4. **x1 wave**
     - It is the second negative wave
     - It is the caused during ejection phase due to indrawing of AV valves leading to fall in pressure
  5. **v wave**
     - It is the third positive wave, gradual rise in amplitude
     - Occurs during atrial diastole due to filling

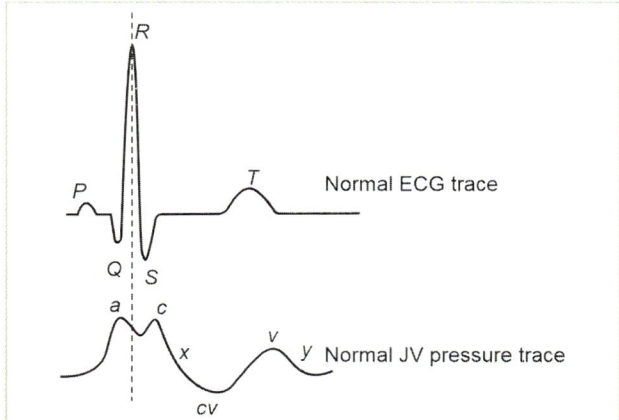

Fig. 5.7a

  6. **y wave**
     - It is the third negative wave
     - It occurs due blood emptying into the ventricles with AV valves open.

Significance of Raised JVP

- It is increased in hyperdynamic states like volume overload or renal dysfunction.
- Also, when there is increased pressure on the right side of heart.
- It can be caused by:
  - Tricuspid stenosis
  - Pulmonary hypertension
  - Congestive cardiac failure
  - Constrictive pericarditis
  - Superior vena caval obstruction

Types of Heart Failure

1. **Systolic heart failure**
   - It is due to decreased pumping capacity of the heart.
   - It may be left sided or right sided
2. **Diastolic failure**
   - It is due to decreased ability of the ventricles to relax and accumulate blood in ventricles.
   - It can be seen in cardiac tamponade and constrictive pericarditis.
3. **Right-sided heart failure**
   - The right ventricle's ability to pump blood is decreased leading to backpressure on the parenchymal organs causing liver congestion, pedal edema and ascites.
   - It is seen in pulmonary hypertension following long standing COPD or asthma, pulmonary stenosis.
4. **Left-sided heart failure**
   - It is due to diseased left ventricle
   - As a result of pump failure, blood accumulates in lungs causing pulmonary edema.

2. Define cardiac cycle. Explain its duration. Which phase of cardiac cycle is compromised when heart rate increases?

A. Definition of Cardiac Cycle

- The succession of coordinated events taking place in the heart during each beat.
- Each heartbeat consists of two major periods called systole and diastole.

- During systole, there is contraction of the heart muscles leading to pumping of the blood through arteries.
- During diastole, heart relaxes, and blood gets filled within the chambers of the heart.
- These sequences of events are repeated during every heartbeat, in a cyclic manner.

B. Duration of Cardiac Cycle

- Events of cardiac cycle
  1. Atrial events
  2. Ventricular events.
- When the heart beats at a normal rate of 72/minute, duration of each cardiac cycle is about 0.8 second.
- Atrial events are divided into two divisions:
  1. Atrial systole = 0.11 (0.1) sec
  2. Atrial diastole = 0.69 (0.7) sec.
- Ventricular events are divided into two divisions:
  1. Ventricular systole = 0.27 (0.3) sec
  2. Ventricular diastole = 0.53 (0.5) sec.
- Ventricular systole is divided into two subdivisions and ventricular diastole is divided into five subdivisions.

- *Ventricular systole*

		Time (second)
Isometric contraction	=	0.05
Ejection period	=	0.22
Total	=	0.27

- *Ventricular diastole*

		Time (second)
Protodiastole	=	0.04
Isometric relaxation	=	0.08
Rapid filling	=	0.11
Slow filling	=	0.19
Last rapid filling	=	0.11
Total	=	0.53

C. Phase of Cardiac Cycle which is Compromised During Increased Heart Rate

Diastole

SHORT ANSWER

1. Describe the waves of JVP.

Jugular Venous Pulse

- Jugular venous pulse is a measurement of the venous pulsation in the internal jugular vein.

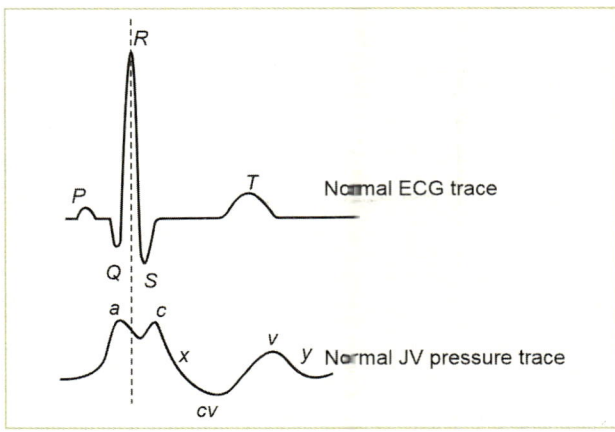

Fig. 5.7b

- It is a measure of pressure changes in the atrium.
- The parts of the normal JVP are:
  1. **a wave**
     - It is the first positive wave in JVP
     - Represents atrial systole
     - Normally, the right atrial pressure is 5 mm Hg and left atrium is 7 mm during systole
  2. **x wave**
     - First negative wave
     - Occurs due to relaxation of atria just prior to diastole
  3. **c wave**
     - It is the second positive wave
     - Due to isometric contraction
     - Closure of AV valves causes rise in pressure
  4. **x1 wave**
     - It is the second negative wave
     - It is caused during ejection phase due to indrawing of AV valves leading to fall in pressure
  5. **v wave**
     - It is the third positive wave, gradual rise in amplitude
     - Occurs during atrial diastole due to filling
  6. **y wave**
     - It is the third negative wave
     - It occurs due blood emptying into the ventricles with AV valves open.

5.4 DESCRIBE GENERATION, CONDUCTION OF CARDIAC IMPULSE

SHORT ESSAY

1. Draw a neat-labelled diagram of conduction system of heart and explain the conducting mechanism. Explain type II heart blocks.

(3 + 2 marks)

Conductive System of Heart

- It is formed by a specialized system of cardiac fibers.
- The components are:
  1. **Sinoatrial node or the SA node**
     - It is called pacemaker of the heart
     - It is situated in the right atrium just inferior to the opening of the superior vena cava.
     - It sends out spontaneous impulses at regular intervals and impulses are conducted to both atria.
     - Through internodal fibers, impulses reach the AV node. There are three types: Anterior (Bachman), intermediate (Wenckebach) and posterior internodal fibers (Thorel)
  2. **Atrioventricular node or the AV node**
     - It receives from impulses from the SA node through the internodal fibres.
     - It is situated immediately below the right atrium and anterior to the leaflet of the tricuspid valve.

3. **Bundle of His**
   - It continues from the AV node and conducts impulses along the interventricular septum.
   - Midway, it divides into right and left bundle branches
4. **Right and left bundle branches and Purkinje fibres:** The bundle branches run along the respective sides of interventricular septum and the culminate as Purkinje fibres which innervate the myocardium.

Type II Heart Block

- II degree heart block is a type of incomplete heart block.
- Some impulses produced by the SA node fail to reach the ventricles.
- One impulse is conducted for every 2, 3 or 4 impulses generated in the SA node.
- Thus, in ECG, QRS interval occurs after 2, 3 or 4 P waves

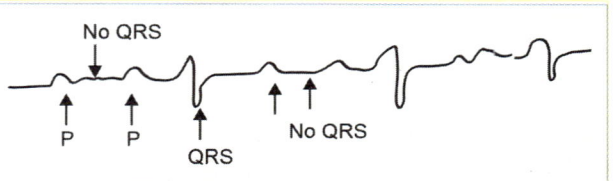

Fig. 5.8

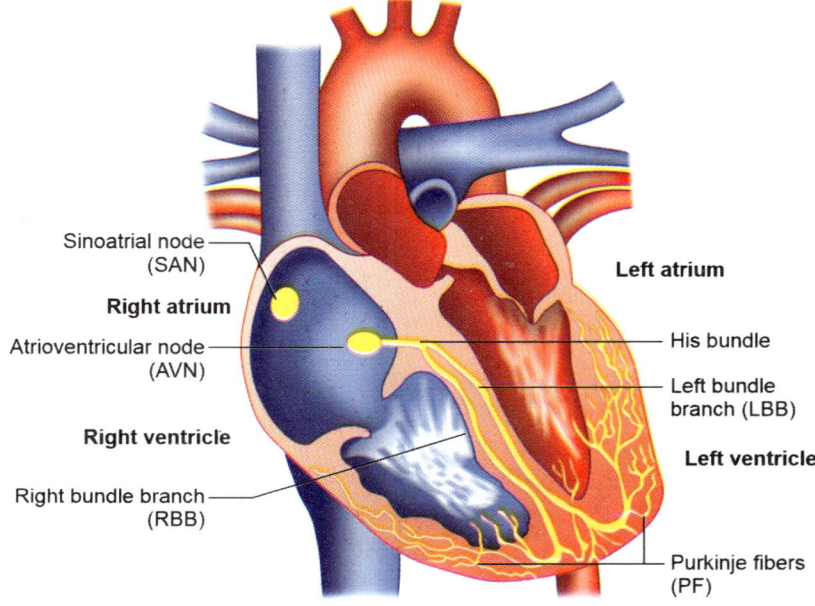

Fig. 5.9

5.5 DESCRIBE THE PHYSIOLOGY OF ELECTROCARDIOGRAM (ECG), ITS APPLICATIONS AND THE CARDIAC AXIS

SHORT ESSAY

1. What is the PR interval in ECG? Give its normal value. What is its clinical importance? Write a note on heart blocks.

PR Interval

It is the time interval between the onset of P wave and the onset of Q wave.

Normal Value

0.12 to 0.2 seconds

Clinical Importance

- After firing of impulses in the SA node, a delay of 0.12 seconds is noticed prior to activation of the AV node.
- It is the time taken for impulses to travel from SA node to AV node. It is seen as PR interval on ECG.
- This delay in the cardiac pulse is extremely important as it ensures that the atria of the heart have ejected their blood into the ventricles of the heart first before the ventricles contract.

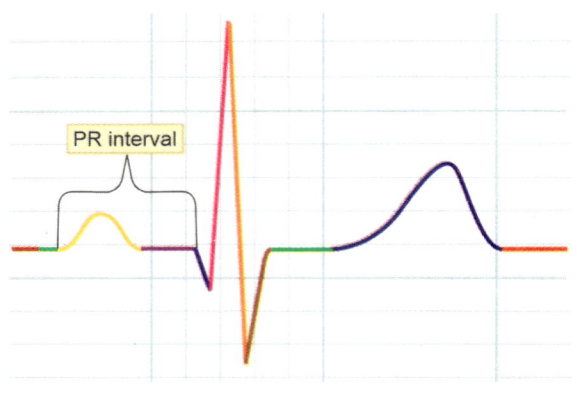

Fig. 5.10

- Increased PR interval is seen in bradycardia and first-degree heart block.
- Decreased PR interval is seen in tachycardia, Wolff-Parkinson-White syndrome, Lown-Ganong-Levine syndrome.

Heart Blocks

- It is an interruption in conduction of impulses in the conductive system of the heart.
- Normally, impulses are generated at the SA node and then conducted through AV node, bundle of His and Purkinje fibres into the ventricular musculature.
- In heart block, the impulses cannot be conducted from one point to other. As a result, ectopic (other than SA node) take part in generating impulses.
- Based on the area affected, it is classified as:

1. **Sinoatrial block**
   - Also called sinus block. There is failure of transmission from SA node to AV node.
   - Since the SA node cannot generate an impulse, the AV node takes up the pacemaker function. However, the rate is slower and is around 40–60/minute.
   - There is break in fibers conducting impulses from SA node to AV node.
   - It is of three types depending on the site in the AV node of origin of impulses

2. **Atrioventricular block**
   - In this block, the impulses are not conducted from AV node further.
   - It is of two types—incomplete and complete heart block

Upper nodal rhythm	Middle nodal rhythm	Lower nodal rhythm
• Impulses are discharged from upper part of AV node	• All chambers of the heart contract simultaneous	• Ventricles contract prior to atria
• P wave in inverse and the rest of the ECG is normal	• P waves merge with QRS complex	• As a result, the QRS precedes P wave
		• It is also called reverse heart block

Incomplete heart block	Complete heart block

• Impulses from AV node are slowed, but not blocked.
• It is of four types
  1. Type 1 heart block
  2. Type 2 heart block
  3. Wenckebach phenomenon
  4. Bundle branch block
	• The impulses do not reach ventricles at all.
	• Also called third degree heart block
	• As a result, ventricles beta at their own rhythm which is much slower. It is also called idioventricular rhythm.
	• It is of two types:
	  1. AV nodal block: The effected part of the AV node does not conduct.
	  2. Infranodal block: The distal part of conducting system, Purkinje fibres, conduct impulse at 35/min.

Type 1 Heart Block

- It is characterised by prolonged PR interval
- Characteristically seen in athletes.
- They are usually asymptomatic

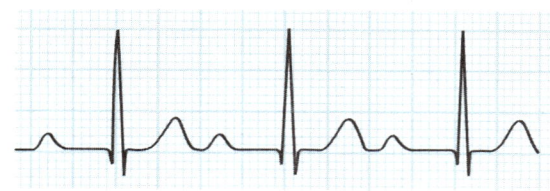

Fig. 5.11

Type 2 Heart Block

- Only one of 2, 3 or 4 impulses is conducted.
- As a result, QRS complex appears once in 2, 3 or 4 beats.

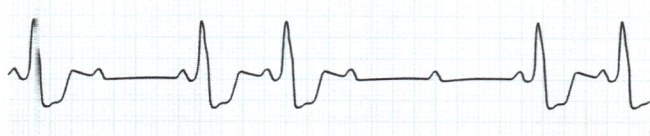

Fig. 5.12

Wenckebach Phenomenon

- It is characterised by progressively increasing AV nodal delay followed by skipping of beat
- Following this, there is a normal beat with increased PR interval.

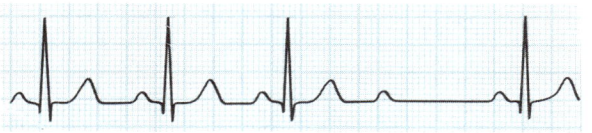

Fig. 5.13

Bundle Branch Block

- As there is block of conduction to one side, the impulse travels to the normal side first and then to the affected ventricle.
- QRS complex is delayed or distorted.

SHORT ANSWER

1. Explain His bundle electrocardiogram.

- It is an invasive electrophysiological test that records electrical activity of the bundle of His. This specialized fibrous tissue is responsible for maintaining the interval between atrial and ventricular contractions.
- Bundle of His is a specialized tissue present at the anterior inferior end of the interatrial septum.
- This test is performed by inserting an electrode catheter in the femoral vein and advancing into the right atrium through the inferior vena cava. This is done under fluoroscopy.
- Through the right atrium, the electrode is further advanced into the right ventricle and pulled back such that the continuous ECG recording shows a spike between P wave and the QRS complex. This is the recording of the Bundle of His.
- It can also be performed by noninvasive surface methods.

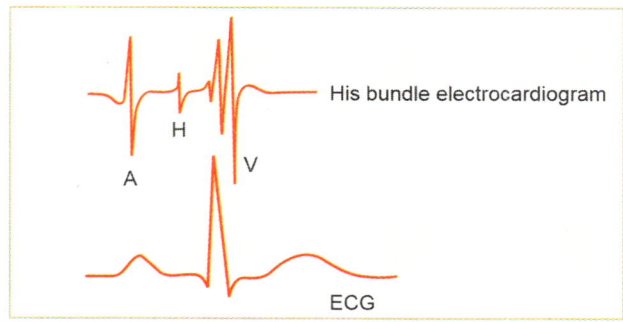

Fig. 5.14

Components of His Bundle ECG

- A wave: Represents activation of the AV node. Coincides at the midportion of p wave
- H wave: Signifies activation of the bundle of His, during PR segment, rapid and biphasic
- V wave: Signifies the ventricular contraction.
- The His bundle ECG and standard three lead ECG helps to divide the PR interval into three segments
  - *PA interval:* It represents interatrial conduction, i.e., from SA node to AV node. Normal duration is 135–150 milliseconds.
  - *AH interval:* It is the time from beginning of the onset of His bundle activity. It approximates AV nodal conduction, can be used to measure the AV nodal delay.
  - *HV interval:* Onset of His bundle activity to beginning of V wave
- They reveal important findings in relation to various arrhythmias like first, second- and third-degree heart blocks.

5.6 DESCRIBE ABNORMAL ECG, ARRHYTHMIAS, HEART BLOCK AND MYOCARDIAL INFARCTION

SHORT ESSAYS

1. A 20-year-old male athlete during his regular check-up revealed splitting of second heart sound. A2 followed by P2 during deep inspiration. During expiration there was no splitting. His blood pressure was normal. Explain the origin of 4 heart sounds. What is physiological splitting of second heart sound? What is gallop rhythm?

Heart Sounds

First heart sound—lub	Produced by closure of mitral and tricuspid valves
Second heart sound—dub	Produced by closure of semilunar valves
Third heart sound—low pitched	Produced by filling of the ventricle with blood during diastole
Fourth heart sound—inaudible	Produced by contraction of atrial muscles

Splitting of S2

It occurs due to asynchronous closure of semilunar valves.

Physiological Splitting

- It occurs during deep inspiration due to the aortic valve closing prior to the closure of pulmonary valve.
- This happens because, during deep inspiration, there is increased venous return to the right atrium. But there is a decrease in blood entering the left atrium. As a result, the pulmonary valve stays open for slightly longer time than the aortic valve.
- This interval between the two valves widens during inspiration and narrows during expiration.

Pathological Splitting

- It is seen in pulmonary stenosis, right bundle branch block and right ventricular hypertrophy.
- Reverse splitting: Here, the aortic valve closes prior to pulmonary valve. Reverse splitting is common in left bundle-branch block, aortic stenosis and left ventricular hypertrophy.

Gallop Rhythm

- It is an abnormal rhythm of heart characterised by three clear heart sounds during each heartbeat.
- It is due to an abnormal third or fourth heart sound seen in some cardiovascular diseases like myocardial infarction and severe hypertension.

2. What are heart blocks? Classify heart blocks. What are the respective ECG changes?

Heart Blocks

- It is an interruption in conduction of impulses in the conductive system of the heart.
- Normally, impulses are generated at the SA node and then conducted through AV node, bundle of His and Purkinje fibres into the ventricular musculature.
- In heart block, the impulses cannot be conducted from one point to other. As a result, ectopic (other than SA node) take part in generating impulses.

Classification

Based on the Area Affected

1. **Sinoatrial block**
   - Also called sinus block. There is failure of transmission from SA node to AV node.
   - Since the SA node cannot generate an impulse, the AV node takes up the pacemaker function. However, the rate is slower and is around 40–60/minute.
   - There is break in fibers conducting impulses from SA node to AV node.
   - It is of three types depending on the site in the AV node of origin of impulses.

Upper nodal rhythm	Middle nodal rhythm	Lower nodal rhythm
• Impulses are discharged from upper part of AV node	• All chambers of the heart contract simultaneously	• Ventricles contract prior to atria
• P wave in inverse and the rest of the ECG is normal	• P waves merge with QRS complex	• As a result, the QRS precedes P wave • It is also called reverse heart block

2. **Atrioventricular block**
   - In this block, the impulses are not conducted from AV node further.
   - It is of two types—incomplete and complete heart block

Incomplete heart block	Complete heart block
• Impulses from AV node are slowed, but not blocked. • It is of four types 　1. Type 1 heart block 　2. Type 2 heart block 　3. Wenckebach phenomenon 　4. Bundle branch block	• The impulses do not reach ventricles at all. • Also called third degree heart block • As a result, ventricles beta at their own rhythm which is much slower. It is also called idioventricular rhythm. • It is of two types 　1. AV nodal block: The effected part of the AV node does not conduct. 　2. Infranodal block: The distal part of conducting system, Purkinje fibres, conduct impulse at 35/min.

Type 1 Heart Block

- It is characterised by prolonged PR interval
- Characteristically seen in athletes.
- They are usually asymptomatic

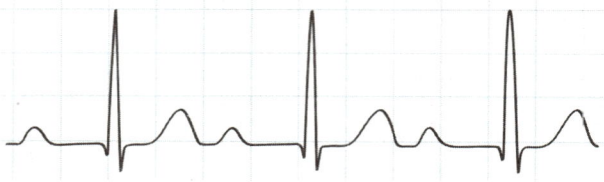

Fig. 5.15

Type 2 Heart Block

- Only one of 2, 3 or 4 impulses is conducted.
- As a result, QRS complex appears once in 2, 3 or 4 beats.

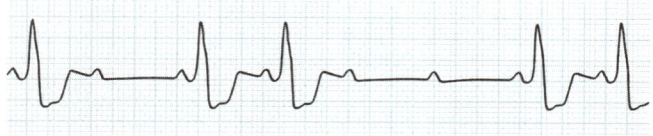

Fig. 5.16

Wenckebach Phenomenon

- It is characterised by progressively increasing AV nodal delay followed by skipping of beat
- Following this, there is a normal beat with increased PR interval.

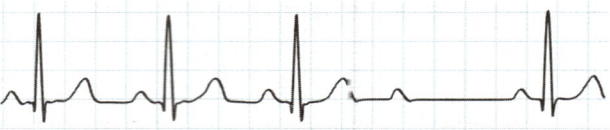

Fig. 5.17

Bundle Branch Block

- As there is block of conduction to one side, the impulse travels to the normal side first and then to the affected ventricle.
- QRS complex is delayed or distorted.

3. A 33-year-old male patient is brought to the emergency, unconscious after electrocution. His pulse rate was thready and ECG showed the following pattern.

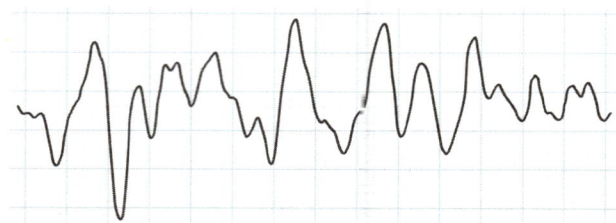

Fig. 5.18

What is the diagnosis? What are the causes? Why is it fatal? How is it treated?   (1+1+2+1)

- This patient has ventricular fibrillation.
- It is a potentially fatal arrhythmia characterized by rapid and irregular twitching of the ventricles at the rate of 400–500/minute.

Causes for Ventricular Fibrillation

1. Electrocution
2. Coronary occlusion
3. Chloroform and cyclopropane inhalation

Physiological Effects of Ventricular Fibrillation

- When the ventricles are beating at a rate of 400–500/minute, there is no actual diastole.
- The ventricles are just flickering or twitching.
- As a result, the ventricles are not able to fill (preload becomes practically zero).
- So automatically, cardiac output becomes minimal
- This presents as very low blood pressure (unmeasurable) and a thready pulse.
- It is a fatal condition and required immediate treatment

Treatment

- Electroshock defibrillation is a technique by which a transient alternating current of high voltage (110V) is passed directly through the ventricles.
- It throws all the ventricular muscles into a period of refractoriness. Thus, fibrillation stops.
- The heart becomes quiescent for 3–5 seconds and then starts to beat again.
- It should be done within 1 minute, otherwise there is permanent damage due to absence of blood flow to the coronary musculature.
- In the absence of defibrillator, intermittent chest thrusts should be given to keep the heart beating. This is called cardiopulmonary resuscitation.

4. Explain the following:

A. Paroxysmal tachycardia
B. Torsades des pointes
C. Bundle of Kent
D. Stokes-Adams syndrome
E. Wolff-Parkinson-White syndrome

A. Paroxysmal Tachycardia

- Also called Bouveret-Hoffmann syndrome
- It is characterized by sudden attacks of increased heart rate arising from the ectopic which are in atria, AV node or ventricles.
- The heart rate prior to and after the attack is normal.
- It is classified into atrial, AV nodal and ventricular tachycardia.

B. Torsades de Pointes

- It literally means torsion at the points
- It is a description of ECG of a potentially fatal polymorphic ventricular tachycardia.
- It can be congenital or acquired by usage of certain drugs which cause increase in the QT interval (amiodarone, chlroquine).
- Hypokalemia, hypocalcemia and hypomagnese-mia also can cause this condition.
- In ECG, there is twisting and prolongation of the QRS complex due to prolongation of the repolarization.
- In some cases, it may revert to normal rhythm and in some may degenerate to ventricular fibrillation leading to death.

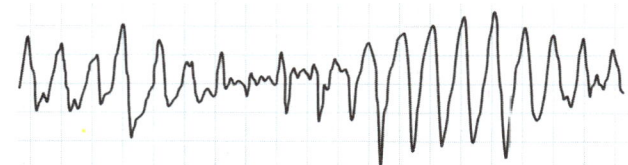

Fig. 5.19

C. Bundle of Kent

- It is a system of abnormal junctional tissues which conduct impulses directly from atria to ventricles when there is a conduction block in the normal conduction system
- It is fasted than the normal conduction process.
- It forms a pathway for reentrant circuit in cases of AV nodal block.

D. Stokes-Adams Syndrome

- It is a sudden attack of dizziness and loss of consciousness.
- It occurs due to a third-degree heart block.
- The impulse from the SA node is not conducted to the ventricles leading to sudden fall in blood pressure.
- Ectopic pacemaker starts functioning at a slower rate after 5–15 seconds.
- If ectopic does not discharge impulses even after 30 seconds, death results.

E. Wolff-Parkinson-White Syndrome

- It is a type of AV nodal paroxysmal tachycardia
- In this condition, there is a block of conduction at the AV node.

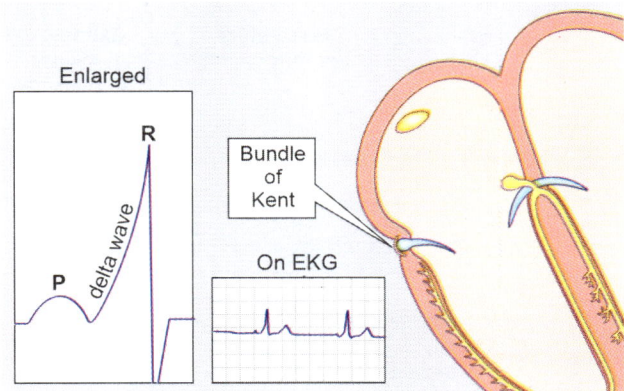

Fig. 5.20

- As a result, the impulses travel to ventricle through the bundle of Kent causing a delta wave on the ECG.
- When the block is cleared, the impulse travels in the reverse direction from ventricle to the AV node, this is called circus rhythm. It causes atria to beat again.

SHORT ANSWERS

1. Write a note on myocardial ischemia. What are the ECG changes in myocardial infarction?

Normal Blood Supply of the Heart Muscles

- Coronary circulation is unique by its outside-in fashion. The vessels are epicardial and pierce the muscle and provide branches.
- Also, there are natural bypasses between arteries without intervening capillaries. These provide an alternate oxygen pathway for myocardium following coronary stenosis.
- Coronary autoregulation is described as the ability of the blood vessels to maintain a relatively constant blood flow across a wide range of perfusion pressure. Coronary blood flow remains constant between arterial pressures 60–140 mmHg.

- Blood flow is regulated through coronary vessels in response to increased contractility by local need for increased nutrition.

Causes for Decrease in Myocardial Perfusion

- In hyperlipidemic states, atherosclerotic plaques are formed within the coronary vasculature—this leads to progressive narrowing of the coronary vessels.
- During rest, the perfusion may be sufficient and the patient remains asymptomatic.
- During exertion, there is an increase in myocardial oxygen demand.
- Other causes are emboli which are released from a distant site and occlude the coronary vessels. Sudden vasospasm due to sympathetic over-activity can also decrease perfusion.
- The left ventricle is more vulnerable to ischemia due to its increased work load and thickness when compared to the tight ventricle.
- When there is a decrease in myocardial perfusion, the pumping ability of the heart decreases and there is exertional dyspnea associated by chest pain. This is known as angina pectoris.

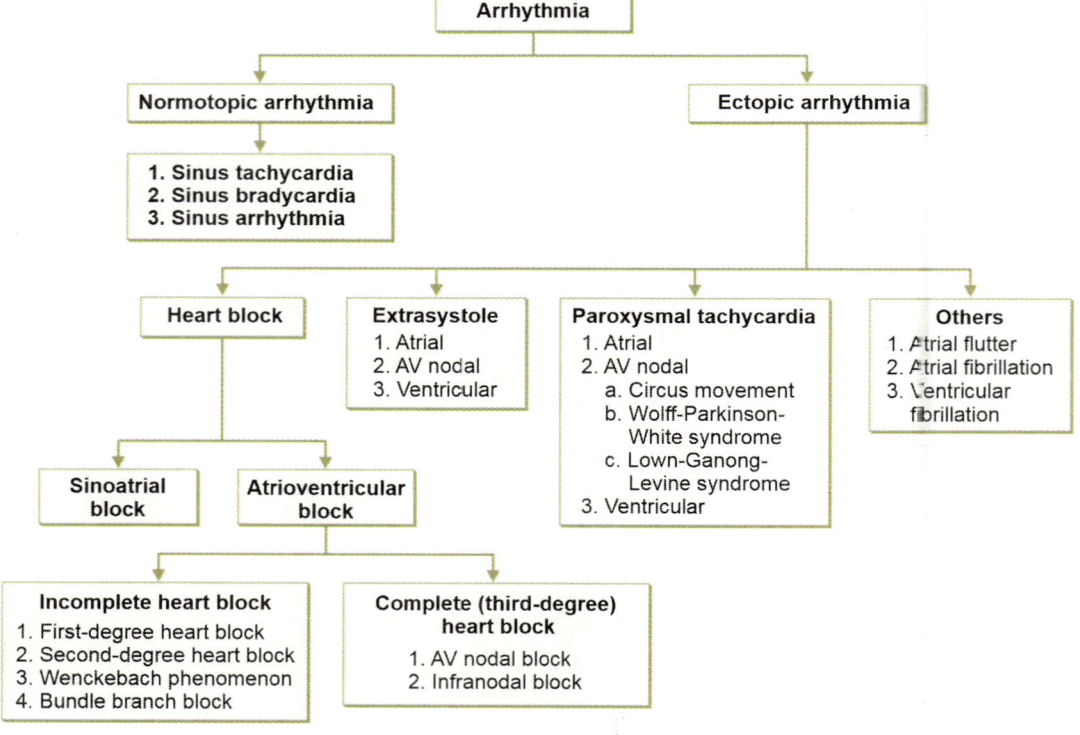

Fig. 5.21

Myocardial Infarction

- It is the next step in ischemia
- When a part of the muscle is not supplied by either collateral become infarcted. Or dead. They heal by fibrosis and thus cannot take part in pumping.
- The subendocardial tissue is most vulnerable to infarction.
- If the patient survives, there is a gradual decrease in ejection fraction of the heart leading to chronic left ventricular failure.

ECG Changes

- Large peaked T waves are earliest changes
- ST segment elevation, negative T waves develop later
- Pathologic Q waves in old MI

2. Define arrhythmia. How are they classified?

Definition

Arrhythmias are defined as abnormal or irregular heart rate.

Classification (Fig. 5.21)

Arrhythmias are broadly classified based on the origin of the impulse.

3. What is sinus arrhythmia? Explain the physiological basis for the same.

Definition

Sinus arrhythmia is a physiological irregularity of the heart rate with phases of respiratory cycle.

Pattern (Fig. 5.22)

- During inspiration, there is an increase in heart rate.
- During expiration, there is a decrease in heart rate.
- In ECG, RR interval (inter-beat interval) varies during various phases of respiration.
- RR interval shortens during inspiration and lengthen during expiration.

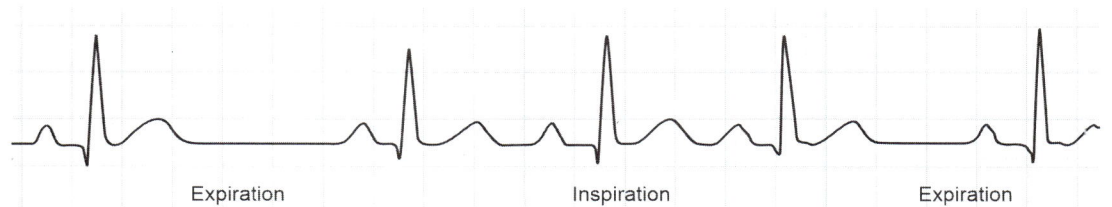

| Expiration | Inspiration | Expiration |

Fig. 5.22

Physiological Basis of Sinus Arrhythmia (Fig. 5.23)

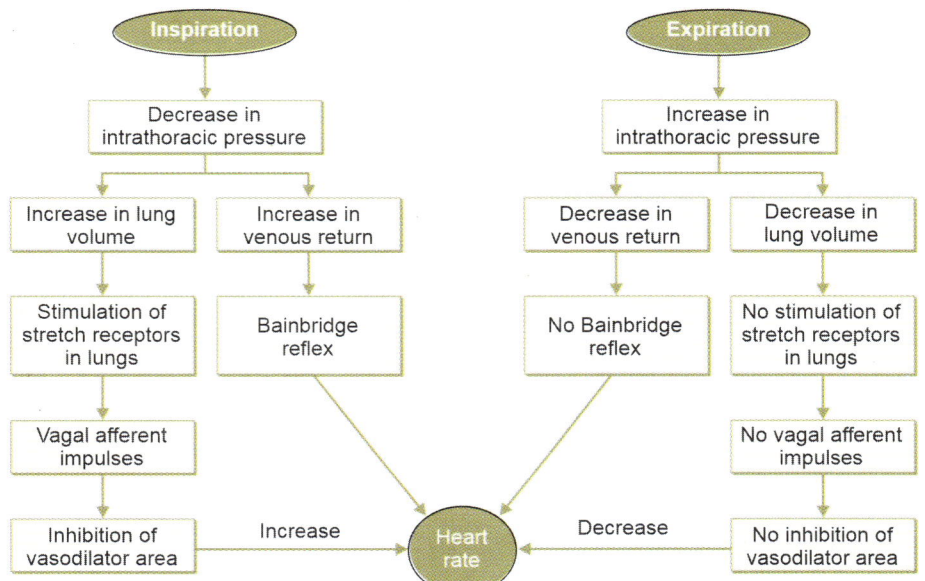

Fig. 5.23

4. Mention the effects of electrolytes on ECG.

Changes in Sodium Concentration

- Hyponatremia decreases the electrical activity of the cardiac muscles
- ECG shows low voltage waves.

Changes in Potassium Concentration

- Hyperkalemia decreases the resting membrane potential of the myocyte
- It increases the excitability of the muscle

K⁺ concentration	ECG changes
6–7 mEq/L	Tall T wave, P wave and QRS are normal
7–8 mEq/L	PR interval I prolonged, QRS complex is widened. There is decrease in heart rate
>9 mEq/L	Atrial muscle cannot be excited. Ventricular fibrillation

- Hypokalemia decreases the excitability of the myocytes.

K⁺ concentration	ECG changes
Up to 2 mEq/L	Depression of ST segment. T wave is small, flat or inverted. Appearance of U wave
Below 2 mEq/L	Severe depression of ST segment below isoelectric line. T wave inversion. Prolongation of PR interval

Changes in Calcium Concentration

- Normal serum calcium is 4.5–5.5 mEq/L
- Hypercalcemia causes increased contractility of the heart.
- ECG changes: Short ST segment, QT interval and appearance of U wave
- Hypocalcemia reduces the excitability of the heart
- ECG changes: Prolongation of ST segment, prolongation of QT interval and prominent U wave

5.7 DESCRIBE AND DISCUSS HAEMODYNAMICS OF CIRCULATORY SYSTEM

SHORT ESSAY

1. Write a note on microcirculation.

Microcirculation

It refers to flow of blood in minute vessels—arterioles, capillaries and venules.

Structure

- Each artery divides 6–8 times to become arterioles, which have a diameter of 10–15 micrometers. These further branches 2–5 times to from meta-arterioles.
- These meta-arterioles do not have a continuous muscular coat like arterioles but are intermittently placed.
- Capillaries arise from the ends of meta arterioles. At the point at which capillaries emerge from the meta arteriole, a smooth muscle encircles the meta arteriole. This is called precapillary sphincter.
- This sphincter controls the entry of blood into the capillaries.
- The capillaries converge to form venules. Venules are larger than arterioles and do not have a muscular coat.
- There exists a pathway between arteriole and venule which are not involved in exchange of gases or nutrients. It is called a vascular or anatomical or non-nutritional shunt.
- They are the pathway of blood during resting conditions.
- Preferential capillaries: They have same diameter as the meta arterioles and are a continuous connection between the arterial and venous system.

- True capillaries: They are involved in nutrient exchange.
- The microcirculation of each organ is specially designed to serve the functions of the organ.

Structure of Capillaries

- There are around 10 billion capillaries in the human body with a surface area of 500–700 m^2.
- They are formed by a single layer of endothelial cells and are wrapped by pericytes.

Endothelium

- The endothelial cells are flattened polygonal, which are joined through tight junctions
- They are sensitive to chemical messengers and hormones and can modify the diameter and porosity of the capillaries.
- They have intervening fenestrations which provide leakage of necessary molecules and substances.

Pericytes

- Also called rouget cells or mural cells.
- They are perivascular mesenchyme like cells with long extensions which embrace the endothelial cells.
- They have contractile properties and themselves secrete some vasoactive substances.
- They are involved in controlling the fenestrations between the endothelium.

Features of Capillary Circulation

- The blood flow is not continuous. The precapillary sphincters alternately close and open
- Blood flows as a single row of cells.

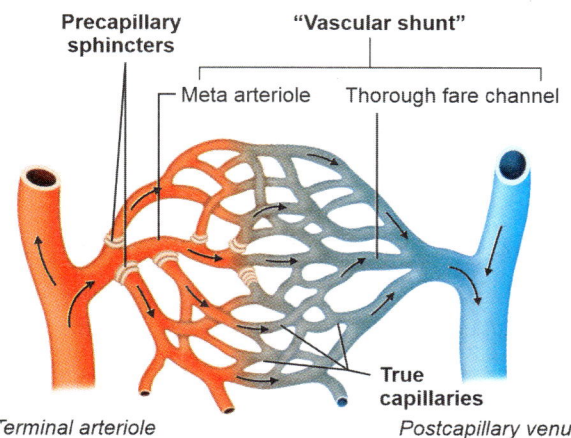

Fig. 5.24

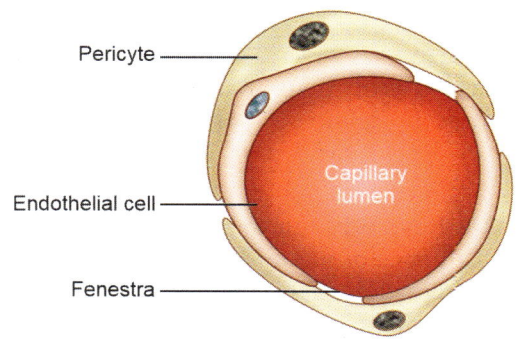

Fig. 5.25

- Velocity of blood is least: 0.05 cm/second. As a result, the amount of blood flowing through the capillary system is 150 ml/min
- In resting state, the capillaries are closed. Only during activity, they open.

Functions of capillaries

Diffusion

- Most important function of capillaries
- Helps in two-way exchange of gases, water, glucose, urea and other substances between the tissues and blood.
- These substances diffuse through the intercellular clefts

Filtration

- Filtration occurs through slit pores between the endothelial cells.
- The force is determined by Starling's forces.
- Main feature in kidney, intestinal mucosa, cardiac muscles, and skeletal muscles.

Pinocytosis

The endothelium engulfs larger molecules and form vesicles which are transported to tissue by the process of pinocytosis.

SHORT ANSWERS

1. Explain the following:

A. Reynolds' number
B. Capacitance vessels

A. Reynolds' Number

- Blood flow in a blood vessel is usually smooth and streamline.
- When there is increased heart rate (physiological or pathological), or there is an obstruction within the vessel, there is turbulence.
- As a result, whorl-like currents are set up called eddy currents
- These currents offer severe resistance to blood flow
- The measure of this turbulence to blood flow is measured in Reynolds' number.

$$Re = \frac{v \cdot d \cdot \rho}{\eta}$$

Re is the Reynolds' number, a measure of tendency for turbulence of blood flow
    v is the mean velocity of blood velocity (cm/s)
    d is the diameter of the vessel
    ρ is the density
    η is the viscosity of blood

- When Reynolds' number is 200–400, the turbulence dies off in a smooth portion of the vessel.
- If it is more than 2000, turbulence is present even in a straight smooth vessel.
- Physiological variations: In aorta it is in several thousands, in larger arteries it is between 200–400 and very minimal in smaller arterioles.

B. Capacitance Vessels

- Blood circulates in a closed system—aorta → arteries → arterioles → capillaries → venules → veins → vena cava → right atrium
- Capacitance is defined as the ability of a vessel to store certain amount of blood per unit rise in pressure.
- Veins hold 60% of the total blood volume
- Capacitance is increase in volume divided by increase in pressure. It depends on distensibility but does not equal distensibility.
- Veins have more capacitance than arteries.
- Capacitance vessels are defined as a part of the circulation that can contain most amount of blood and can readily accommodate changes in blood volume.

Causes for Increased Capacitance of Veins and Venule

- Due to increased diameter
- Poor muscular coat which does not offer resistance and rather accommodates blood.

2. Describe the functions of arterioles, capillaries, and veins.

Functions of Arterioles, Capillaries, and Veins

Arterioles

- Arterioles are continuation of arteries and have more muscular tissue than fibrous content.
- They are mainly involved in regulating peripheral resistance.
- They are muscular and sensitive to action of noradrenaline.

Capillaries

- These are fenestrated part of the circulatory system
- They are involved in the exchange of substances

Veins

- Veins carry blood from organs towards the heart
- They are called capacitance vessels as they hold around 60% of the total blood.

5.8 DESCRIBE AND DISCUSS LOCAL AND SYSTEMIC CARDIOVASCULAR REGULATORY MECHANISMS

LONG ESSAY

1. **A 60-year-old man, who is a known case of diabetes mellitus on treatment for 10 years, presents with dizziness as soon as he wakes from the bed early in the morning. His BP was 150/90 mm Hg in supine position and on standing immediately his BP is 126/80 mm Hg.**
   A. **What is the clinical condition the patient is suffering from?** (2 marks)
   B. **What is the normal range of blood pressure?** (2 marks)
   C. **What is the neural regulation/short-term regulation of BP?** (6 marks)

A.

The clinical condition is known as orthostatic hypotension. It is clinically defined as a fall of more than 20 mm Hg of systolic blood pressure or a decrease in more than 10 mm Hg of diastolic blood pressure within 3 minutes of standing from a supine or sitting position. It is usually caused due to hypovolemia due to decreased fluid intake or increased fluid (water or blood) loss.

B.

Normal blood pressure in an adult is 120/80 mm Hg (systolic/diastolic). It ranges from: Systolic: 110–140 mm Hg/diastolic: 60–80 mm Hg. In children, it depends on age.

C.

Regulation of blood pressure is done by 4 mechanisms: Nervous or short-term, renal or long-term, hormonal and local.

Short-term Mechanism

- It begins quick and ends quick
- Operates via vasomotor system
- The vasomotor system has three operational areas: Vasomotor centre, vasoconstrictor fibres and vasodilator fibres.

1. **Vasomotor centre**
   - Located in reticular formation of medulla oblongata and lower part of pons.
   - It consists of a vasoconstrictor area, vasodilator area and a sensory area.
   - The vasoconstrictor area is also called pressor area. It sends impulses to blood vessels through sympathetic fibres. It forms the lateral part of vasomotor region.
   - Vasodilator area is also called depressor area. It suppresses the vasoconstrictor zone and brings about vasodilatation. It forms the medial part of the vasomotor region.
   - Sensory area is in the nucleus solitarius. It is situated in posterolateral part of medulla. It receives signals from baroreceptors through glossopharyngeal and vagus nerves. It controls the vasoconstrictor and vasodilator areas.

2. **Vasoconstrictor fibres**
   - Sympathetic fibres
   - They discharge a continuous set of impulses and maintain vasomotor tone
   - Cause vasoconstriction through discharge of adrenaline group of drugs (adrenaline and noradrenaline) and act at alpha receptors of smooth muscles

3. **Vasodilator fibres**
   - Parasympathetic fibres cause vasodilatation by releasing acetylcholine
   - Sympathetic vasodilator fibres cause vasodilatation in skeletal muscles and improve blood flow to skeletal muscles during exercise.
   - Antidromic fibres are associated with cutaneous receptors and produce vasodilatation.

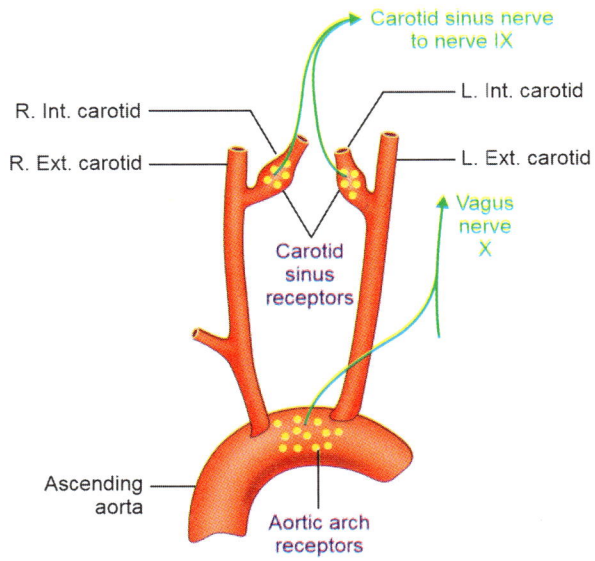

Fig. 5.26

Mechanism of Action (Fig. 5.26)

There are two main receptors involved in short-term neuro-regulation of blood pressure.

1. Baroreceptor mechanism

- These are pressure sensors
- They are situated in aorta wall and carotid sinuses.

Response to Increase in Blood Pressure

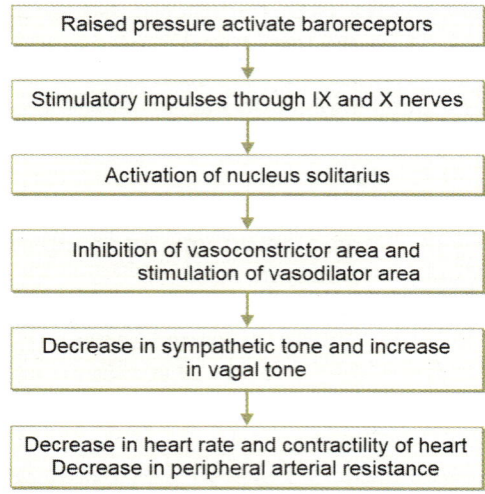

Fig. 5.27

Response to Decrease in Blood Pressure

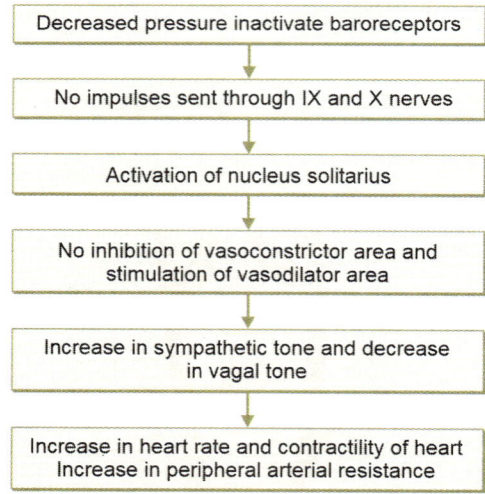

Fig. 5.28

2. Chemoreceptor mechanism

- They give information regarding the composition of blood

- They are situated in the carotid body and aortic body.
- They are sensitive to hypoxia and hypercapnia and relay in respiratory centres.
- They bring about increased oxygen by bringing about changes in respiration.
- It increases venous return by causing pressure changes in thoracic cavity.

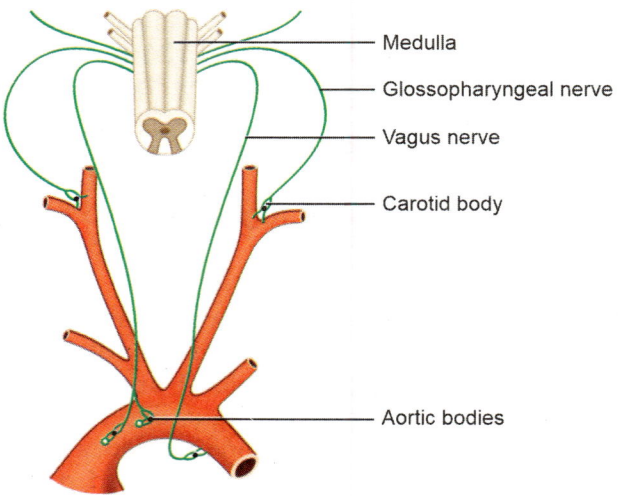

- Medulla
- Glossopharyngeal nerve
- Vagus nerve
- Carotid body
- Aortic bodies

Fig. 5.29

SHORT ESSAYS

1. Explain the hormonal mechanisms of BP regulation

Hormones that cause increase in blood pressure:

1. Adrenaline

- Secreted into the blood stream from the adrenal medulla.
- It has ionotropic effect on heart muscles and increases cardiac output and thus systolic BP. Also, it decreases peripheral vascular resistance by vasodilatation and decreases diastolic blood pressure.

2. Noradrenaline

- It is also secreted by the adrenal medulla.
- It increases diastolic blood pressure by increasing the total peripheral resistance. Its action is more marked on diastolic BP.
- It has mild inotropic effect.

3. Thyroxine

- It increases systolic blood pressure and decreases diastolic blood pressure.

- The fall in peripheral resistance is due to metabolites produced due to increased metabolic activity due to thyroxine.

4. Aldosterone
- It is secreted by the adrenal cortex.
- It causes retention of sodium and water, thereby increasing ECF volume and blood pressure.

5. Vasopressin
- It is also called antidiuretic hormone
- It is secreted by posterior pituitary in response to increased osmolarity in blood.
- It causes vasoconstriction of all blood vessels. Also, it increases water reabsorption at the distal tubules and increases the volume of ECF.

6. Angiotensin
- It is produced from renin. It causes constriction of afferent arteriole of the glomerulus leading to decrease in GFR and increase in ECF volume and thus BP.
- It also causes generalized constriction of arterioles leading to increase in peripheral resistance and diastolic BP.
- Angiotensin II increases water intake by stimulating the thirst center.
- It increases the release of ADH from posterior pituitary

7. Serotonin
- It also causes generalized vasoconstriction and thus increases diastolic blood pressure.

Hormones that cause decrease in blood pressure

Vasoactive intestinal peptide	Causes vasodilatation and brings about decrease in diastolic blood pressure.
Bradykinin	Released during inflammatory conditions, causes vasodilatation
Prostaglandins	Causes drop in blood pressure by vasodilatation
Histamine	Released in response to allergy Causes drop in blood pressure by vasodilatation
Atrial natriuretic peptide Brain natriuretic peptide C type natriuretic peptide	Causes drop in blood pressure by vasodilatation Causes drop in blood pressure by vasodilatation

2. A 70-year-old male comes to medical OPD for regular check-up for hypertension. His BP was 170/100 mm of Hg. He says he has no symptoms of increase BP like giddiness, sweating. What are baroreceptors? What is baroreceptor set point? Explain baroreceptor mechanism of BP regulation.

Baroreceptors

- These are specialized sensors present in the walls of arteries which can sense a change in blood pressure.
- They are present in carotid sinus and wall of aorta.

Set Point

- The carotid sinus baroreceptros are activated at a blood pressure above 60 mm Hg and are highest activated above 180 mm Hg.
- The aortic barorecptors are activated at pressure levels 30 mm Hg above that of carotid sinus baroreceptors.

Mechanism of Blood Pressure Regulation

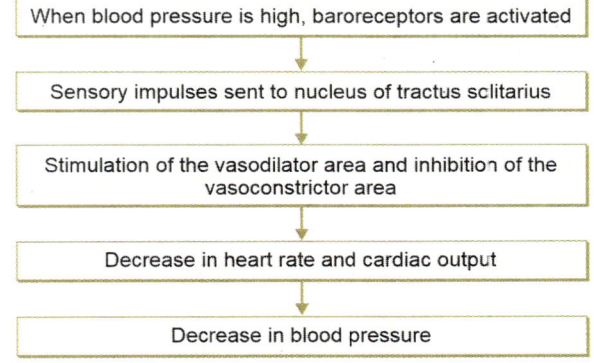

Fig. 5.30

When there is decrease in blood pressure, the receptors are not stimulated. As a result, the above-mentioned changes do not occur. There is increase in blood pressure.

5.9 DESCRIBE THE FACTORS AFFECTING HEART RATE, REGULATION OF CARDIAC OUTPUT AND BLOOD PRESSURE

SHORT ESSAYS

1. Define cardiac output. What are the factors that affect cardiac output? What is the effect of regular excessive training on cardiac output?
(3 + 2 marks)

Cardiac Output

- The volume of blood pumped by the left ventricle is called cardiac output.
- Cardiac output in one minute is called minute volume. Its value is 5 liters.
- Cardiac output per beat is called stroke volume and its value is 60–70 ml.

Factors Affecting Cardiac Output

1. **Venous return**
   - It is the amount of blood that return the right atrium from different parts of the body
   - Cardiac output directly depends on the venous return
2. **Force of contraction**
   - Cardiac output varies proportional to the force of contraction of the ventricle.
   - It depends on the preload (amount of stretching of the cardiac fibres due to distension with blood) and afterload (pressure in the aorta and the pulmonary artery)
3. **Heart rate:** Cardiac output is a direct function of the heart rate. Hence, it increases with increase in heart rate or positive chronotropic effect.
4. **Peripheral resistance:** Cardiac output is inversely proportional to peripheral arterial resistance

Physiological variations occur in cardiac output due to variations in:

- Age
- Sex
- Body built
- Environmental temperature
- Emotional conditions
- Exercise
- High altitude
- Pregnancy
- Sleep

Effect of Regular Exercise on Cardiac Output

- During exercise, the heart rate increases and increases the cardiac output.
- This is to meet the metabolic demands of the skeletal muscles and to lose heat through skin by vasodilatation.
- However, when a person is regularly exercising, the heart muscles undergo hypertrophy
- Thus, the contractility is better and thus, a higher cardiac output at lower heart rates is maintained.

2. Explain venous return. How is cardiac output measured through Fick's principle?

Venous Return (Fig. 5.31)

- It is the amount of blood that reaches the right atrium from different parts of the body.
- The superior vena cava bring blood from upper part of the body, whereas the inferior vena cava brings blood from the lower part of the body.
- The amount of venous return is a determinant for cardiac output. The higher the venous return, the more is the cardiac output. This is due to Frank-Starling law, according to which, the force of contraction depends on the initial length of the fibre prior to contraction—venous return.
- The factors that help in venous return are negative thoracic pressure during inspiration that cause blood to flow into the heart, the peripheral muscle pumps which cause pumping of blood when they contract, transmitted pressure from the arterial bed and sympathetic tone.
- The venous return curve is shown below. It shows a correlation between venous return and right atrial pressure. With increase in right atrial

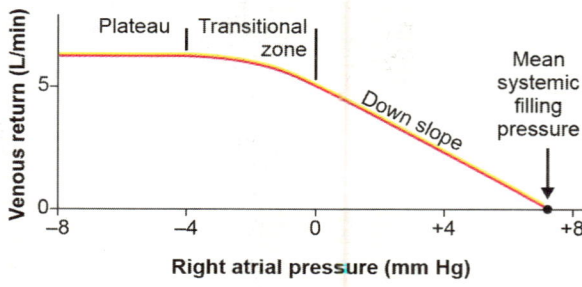

Fig. 5.31

pressure due to ventricular pump failure, there is transmission of force backwards leading to a decrease in venous return. It is seen that, when the right atrial pressure is around 7 mm Hg, the venous return becomes zero. Also, due to decreased venous return, cardiac output also becomes zero.

- This pressure at which venous return and cardiac output are in equilibrium is called systemic filling pressure.
- This is the physiological basis for pedal edema in congestive cardiac failure.

Measurement of Cardiac Output

- It can be done by direct and indirect methods:
  - Direct methods involve use of cardiometer and flowmeter.
  - Indirect methods include Fick's principle, ink dilution method, thermodilution technique, ultrasound Doppler transducer technique and echocardiography.

Fick's Principle (Fig. 5.32)

- According to this principle, the amount of blood flowing through an organ or coming out of it equals the product of the amount of blood flowing through the organ and arteriovenous difference across the organ.
- Cardiac output is calculated as amount of substance taken or given by the organ in one minute divided by the arteriovenous difference of the substance across the organ.
- It can be calculated based on oxygen consumption or carbon dioxide that is given out.

Measurement of Cardiac Output Based on Oxygen Consumption

- The amount of oxygen consumed by an organ is measured and calculated by using a respirometer or a Benedict Roth apparatus.

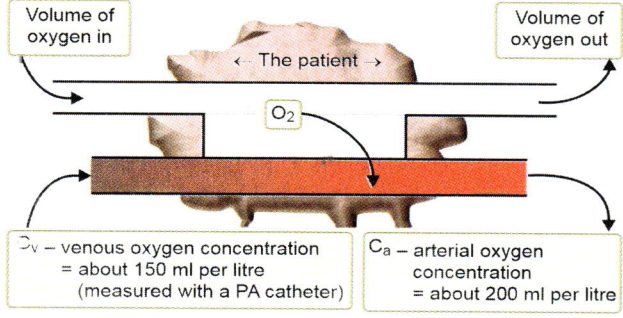

Fig. 5.32

- Arterial blood is collected from any artery to calculate oxygen content and venous blood is calculated from pulmonary artery or right atrium.
- It is collected by introducing a catheter through the basilar vein of forearm.
  The blood flowing through the lungs is calculated as:

$$\frac{\text{Oxygen consumption in one minute}}{\text{Oxygen content in arterial blood} - \text{oxygen content in venous blood}}$$

Example:
- Oxygen consumption in one minute = 250 ml/min
- Oxygen content in arterial blood = 20 ml/100 ml of blood
- Oxygen content in venous blood = 15 ml/100 ml of blood
- Cardiac output = 250/20–15 ml/100 ml = 250/5 × 100 = 5000 ml or 5 litre

Calculation of Cardiac Output Using Carbon Dioxide

- It is measured in the similar way as with oxygen consumption.
- The blood flowing through the lungs is calculated as:

$$\frac{\text{Carbon dioxide produced by lungs in one minute}}{\text{CO}_2 \text{ content in venous blood} - \text{CO}_2 \text{ content in arterial blood}}$$

Example:
- CO_2 consumption in one minute = 200 ml/min
- CO_2 content in arterial blood = 56 ml/100 ml of blood
- CO_2 content in venous blood = 60 ml/100 ml of blood
- Cardiac output = 200/60–56 ml/100 ml =200/4 × 100 = 5000 ml or 5 litre

3. Name the different heart sounds. How are they produced?

Different Heart Sounds

First heart sound—lub	Produced by closure of mitral and tricuspid valves
Second heart sound—dub	Produced by closure of semilunar valves
Third heart sound—low pitched	Produced by filling of the ventricle with blood during diastole
Fourth heart sound—inaudible	Produced by contraction of atrial muscles

4. What is meant arterial pressure? What is its physiological importance?

Mean Arterial Pressure

- It gives an average blood pressure throughout all arteries. It is not mathematical average of systolic and diastolic BP as the average arterial pressure is more towards diastolic BP.
- It is calculated by adding diastolic blood pressure and one-third of pulse pressure
- It can also be calculated by 40% of systolic + 60% diastolic BP
- It is normally 93 mm Hg

Example:
- Systolic blood pressure = 120 mm Hg
- Diastolic blood pressure = 80 mm Hg
- Therefore, pulse pressure = 40 mm Hg
- Mean arterial pressure is 80 + 1/3 (40) = 80 + 13 = 93 mm Hg

Physiological Importance

- Mean arterial pressure gives an idea of the average existing pressure in all arteries.
- Thus, it gives a better idea about the perfusion of organs.
- The normal range is 70–100 mm Hg
- A minimum of 60 mm Hg is required to perfuse kidneys, coronary arteries and brain.
- High MAP leads to increased cardiac load and can lead to cardiovascular disorders.
- Low MAP is an indicator of shock.

SHORT ANSWERS

1. What is the role of furosemide diuretic in reducing the blood pressure?

- A diuretic is a substance that increases urine output.

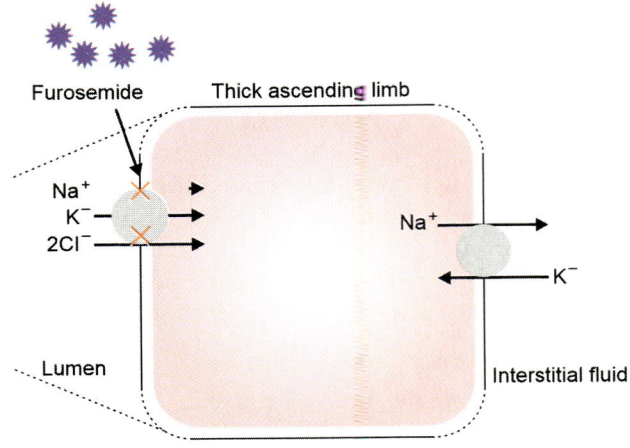

Fig. 5.33

- Most diuretics act by decreasing Na⁺ reabsorption and causing natriuresis (escape of sodium in urine) and thus leading to diuresis.
- Loop diuretics like furosemide block active Na⁺ absorption from the thick ascending loop of Henle by blocking the 1 sodium, 2 chloride, 1 potassium cotransporter on the luminal side of the tubular epithelium.
- As a result, the tubular fluid is rich in Na⁺ ions and hence more sodium reaches the distal part of the nephron. As a result, more water is retained within the tubules.
- Also, they disrupt the countercurrent multiplier system by decreasing the absorption of ions from the loop of Henle into the medullary interstitium. As a result, a huge volume of extracellular fluid is lost.
- Thus, it decreases the blood pressure in a rapid fashion.

2. Define the terms and give its normal values.
   A. Stroke volume
   B. Cardiac output
   C. Cardiac index

Sl. No	Parameter	Definition	Normal value
A	Stroke volume	It is the volume of blood pumped by the left ventricle during each contraction.	60–80 ml when the heart rate is 72/min
B	Cardiac output	The amount of blood pumps through the circulatory system in one minute	5000 ml/min
C	Cardiac index	It is the minute volume (blood pumped in one minute) per square meter of body surface area	2.8 +/–0.3 L/m² body surface area/min

3 Write briefly on Korotkoff sounds.

- These are the sounds heard while measuring blood pressure by auscultatory method.
- The bell of stethoscope is placed over the antecubital fossa and the cuff is inflated.
- When the pressure is as high as the systolic pressure of the heart or the maximum pressure, the artery is occluded. This leads to collapse of the brachial artery and there are no sounds heard.
- When the cuff is slowly released, the sounds that heard over the antecubital fossa are called Korotkoff sounds.
- The exact cause of the production of Korotkoff sounds is not clearly known but is thought to be blood jetting through the partially occluded vessel.

Zero phase	No sound	Pressure equal to more than systolic BP
First phase	Tapping sound	Pressure is just below the systolic blood pressure—taken as systolic BP
Second phase	Louder tapping, followed by a murmur	Pressure around 15 mm below systolic BP
Third phase	Gong follows murmur	Pressure around 25–30 mm below systolic BP
Fourth phase	Muffled character	Pressure around 35 mm below systolic BP
Fifth phase	Disappearance of sound	Marks diastolic blood pressure

4. Explain the role of renin in BP homeostasis.

- Renin is a hormone secreted by juxtaglomerular cells.
- It is secreted when there is a decrease in blood pressure or decreased Na^+ concentration in the thick ascending limb. Sympathetic stimulation also causes renin release.
- Most of the actions are produced due to formation of angiotensin II.

Action on Blood Vessels

- Renin acts on blood vessels via angiotensin II and causes vasoconstriction. Thereby, it increases peripheral arterial resistance and BP.
- It also increases noradrenaline release from the adrenal gland to bring about increase in blood pressure.

Action on Adrenal Cortex

- Renin stimulates the adrenal cortex to produce aldosterone
- Aldosterone is a mineralocorticoid and increases sodium retention and thus increases blood pressure.

Action on Glomerular Apparatus

- It constricts the afferent arteriole and decreases the blood flowing into the glomerulus and thus decreases glomerular filtration. This increases the ECF volume.
- It leads to contraction of the glomerular mesangial cells, thereby decreasing the surface area of glomerulus.
- It increases sodium reabsorption from the proximal tubules.

Action on Brain

- Renin causes inhibition of the baroreceptors through angiotensin II.
- Angiotensin II increases water intake by stimulating the thirst center.
- It increases the release of ADH from posterior pituitary.
- It increases the release of CRH from hypothalamus. This in turn leads to increased release of corticosteroids.

5. Define the following and give the normal values.

A. End diastolic volume
B. End systolic volume
C. Cardiac index

Definition	Normal values
End diastolic volume It is the amount of blood in the ventricle (left or right), just prior to systole or at the end of diastole	130–150 ml per ventricle
End systolic volume It is the amount of blood that remains in each ventricle at the end of each ejection	60–80 ml per ventricle
Cardiac index It is the amount of blood pumped out of each ventricle in every minute per square meter area of body surface	2.8 ± 0.3 L/m^2 of body surface area/minute (in an adult with average body surface area of 1.734 m^2 and normal minute volume of 5 L/minute)

6. Explain the determinants of mean arterial pressure.

- It gives an average blood pressure throughout all arteries. It is not mathematical average of systolic and diastolic BP as the average arterial pressure is more towards diastolic BP.
- It is calculated by adding diastolic blood pressure and one-third of pulse pressure. It can also be calculated by 40% of systolic + 60% diastolic BP. It is normally 93 mm Hg.
- It is determined by three factors: Cardiac output (CO), peripheral arterial pressure (PAR) and central venous pressure (CVP).
- MAP = (CO × PAR) + CVP. As CVP is negligible, MAP is determined by CO and PAR.
- MAP is directly proportional to cardiac output. Increase in cardiac output causes increased blood flowing into the aorta and the arterial system and thus increases systolic pressure.
- MAP is also directly proportional to peripheral arterial resistance, provided cardiac output does

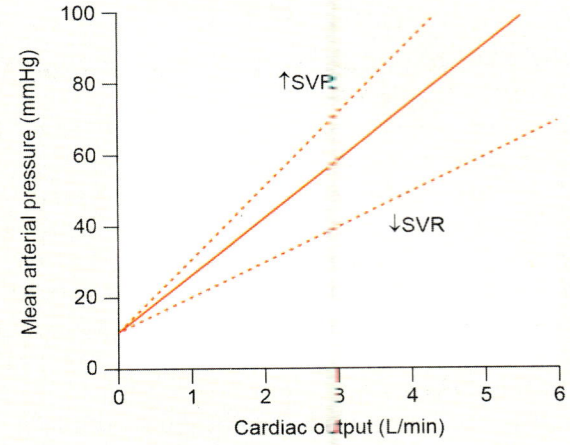

Fig. 5.3

not change. Increase in peripheral arterial resistance causes an increase in diastolic pressure and thus increase in MAP.

- If cardiac output increases, peripheral arterial resistance has to decrease to keep MAP constant.

5.10 DESCRIBE AND DISCUSS REGIONAL CIRCULATION INCLUDING MICROCIRCULATION, LYMPHATIC CIRCULATION, CORONARY, CEREBRAL, CAPILLARY, SKIN, FOETAL, PULMONARY AND SPLANCHNIC CIRCULATION

SHORT ESSAYS

1. Explain the blood flow in coronary circulation. Which region of cardiac muscle is prone for myocardial infarction?   (4 + 1 marks)

A. Phasic Blood Flow in Coronary Circulation

- The myocardium receives its nutrition through the coronary circulation. It is so-called as the arteries resemble a 'corona' or a crown.
- The main trunks lie on the surface of the heart and the smaller vessels then penetrate the muscle to perfuse the muscles. The inner 1/10th mm of endocardium receives oxygen from the blood within the chambers.
- The blood flow in the coronary vessels is not constant. It decreases during systole and increases during diastole. This happens due to the structure of blood vessels that are laid perpendicular to the cardiac muscles. When the cardiac muscles contract, the vessels constrict, and the blood flow

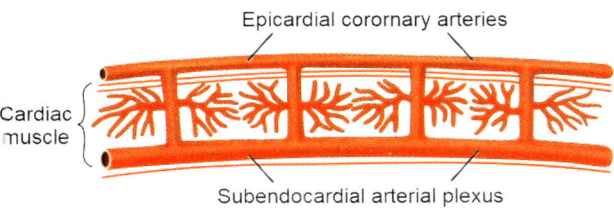

Fig. 5.35

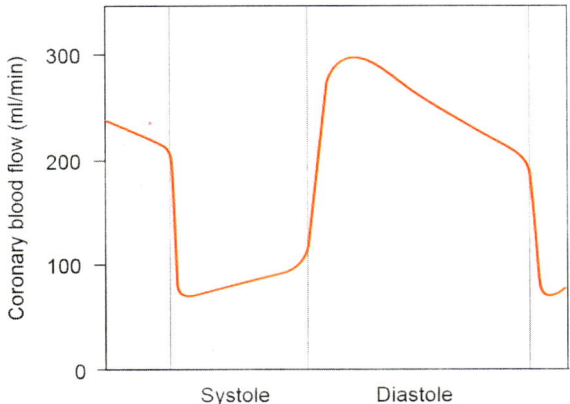

Fig. 5.36

decreases. The reverse happens in diastole—when the muscle fibres relax, vessels also dilate leading to increase in blood flow. During systole, the subendocardial vessels are greatly compressed.

- These changes are more pronounced in the left ventricle due to the thickness of muscles being highest.

Systole	Diastole
• During isometric contraction, the blood flow declines sharply due to increased contraction of myocardial fibres and decreased pressure in the aorta.	• In the initial stages, there is sharp increase in perfusion through coronary vessels.
• During ejection phase, it improves slightly due to increased pressure in the aorta. Nevertheless, perfusion is less.	• In the later stages of diastole, the perfusion pressure falls as the pressure in the aorta also drops.

B.

- During myocardial infarction, the subendocardial muscles are the ones that get most severely affected, more so of the left ventricle.
- This is because the subendocardial vessels are greatly compressed during systole and these muscles have higher oxygen demand than the rest in the heart.

2. Describe how cerebral blood flow is regulated.

- Normal blood flow to brain is 50–65 ml/100 g of brain tissue/minute.
- Three regulatory parameters:
  1. Metabolic parameters
  2. Autoregulation
  3. Nervous factors

Metabolic Parameters

Three metabolic parameters are associated with regulation of cerebral blood flow.

1. **Carbon dioxide concentration**
   - Increase the concentration of carbon dioxide in blood that perfuses the brain increases blood flow.

- 70% of increase in $PaCO_2$ doubles the cerebral blood flow.
- The excess CO_2 combines with water and forms the unstable carbonic acid. It splits into H^+ and HCO_3^-. H^+ ions cause vasodilatation.

2. **Hydrogen ion concentration:** Increased hydrogen ions in the blood causes vasodilatation and helps in removal of excess hydrogen ions.

3. **Oxygen concentration**
   - A PaO_2 around 30 mm Hg causes preferential flow of blood to brain compared to other organs
   - It is a protective response
   - This mechanism fails for PaO_2 <20 mmHg

Autoregulation (Fig. 5.37)

- It is the main mechanism of regulation of cerebral blood flow and acts even in absence of sympathetic supply
- Effective perfusion pressure is the balance between arterial and venous pressure. Since venous pressure in the brain is zero, arterial pressure determines autoregulation
- Cerebral blood flow is autoregulated for systolic BP from 60 mm Hg to 140 mm Hg.
- Vascular resistance is offered by the CSF pressure. Increase in CSF pressure increases the arterial pressure. This is called Cushing reflex. It is a protective response.
- Autoregulatory mechanisms are decreased in conditions of the white matter called posterior reversible encephalopathy syndrome (PRES) and is associated with many anti-cancer drugs and eclampsia.

Nervous Factors

- Under normal conditions, sympathetic supply does not play a role in altering the cerebral blood flow.

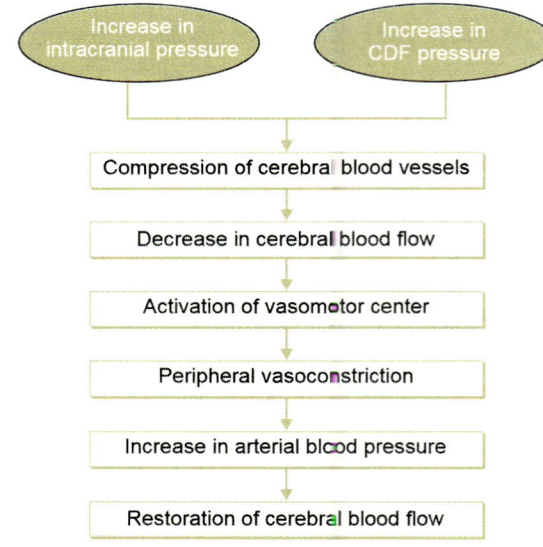

Fig. 5.37

- In severe hypertension, there is constriction of the precapillary arterioles leading to decreased blood flowing to the capillaries leading to protection of the brain tissues

3. Explain triple response.

- Triple response is a type of vascular response of stem, which occurs in dermis vasculature in response to surface mechanical stimuli.
- Also called Lewis triple response, as it was discovered by Sir Lewis Thomas.
- Following a mechanical stimulus, reaction by skin occurs in 3 consecutive stages.
- When a pointed stimulus is drawn over skin, a red line appears along the course of the stimulus.

	Characteristics	Duration	Cause
Red reaction	Appearance in red line	15 seconds	Dilatation of capillaries due to release of substance
Flare: If stroke is applied with higher force	Redness surrounding the red line	Lasts 30 seconds	One to axonal reflex, is arteriolar dilation
Wheal: If stroke is applied with severe force	The skin surrounding the stroke is raised up to 2 mm	Appears in 3 minutes and replaces the red line. Takes hours to disappear	Due to leakage of fluid from capillaries. It does not depend on nervous mechanism

4. Explain the changes that occur in the fetal circulation immediately after birth. What is ASD? Explain.

Changes in Fetal Circulation After Birth

1. **First breath of the child**
   - The lungs start functioning immediately after birth
   - As there is sudden cessation of oxygen delivery through the placental vessels, there is sudden hypoxia and hypercapnia.
   - It leads to strong stimulation of respiratory centres leading to expansion of lungs and beginning of respiration.

2. **Flow of blood to lungs**
   - Due to expansion of lungs, there is reduction of pulmonary vascular resistance leading to entry of blood into the lungs.
   - Blood flows to the lungs from the right ventricle through pulmonary artery.

3. **Closure of foramen ovale**
   - Due to closure of placental blood vessels, there is sudden decrease in pressure in the inferior vena cava.
   - As a result, the pressure in the right atrium falls.
   - Also, due to return of blood from the lungs, there is increase in the pressure in the left atrium.
   - As a result, there is closure of the foramen ovale. It then fuses with atrial valve.

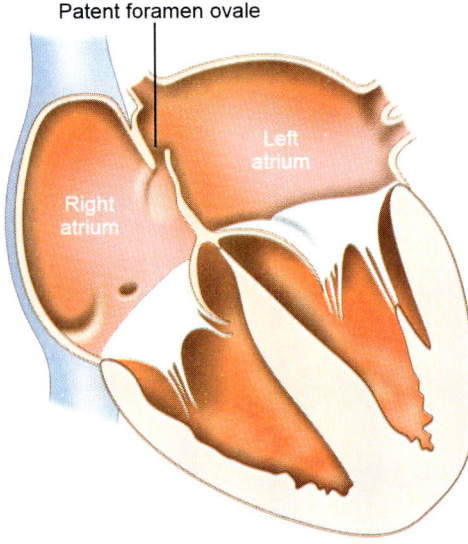

Patent foramen ovale

Left atrium

Right atrium

Fig. 5.38

4. **Reversal of flow in the ductus arteriosus**
   - It connects the pulmonary artery to the aorta.
   - In the fetus, there is high pulmonary artery pressure and thus blood flows from pulmonary artery to the aorta.
   - However, in the fetus, due to increase in pressure in the aorta, the flow is reversed.
   - It is heard as a continuous murmur in infants.

5. **Closure of ductus venosus**
   - In fetus, the ductus venosus collects blood form the fetal abdomen and joins the umbilical vein to empty into the inferior venacava.
   - Within few hours of blood, there is closure of umbilical vein.
   - Also, the smooth muscles of the ductus venosus also contract leading to increase in pressure of blood to about 10 mm Hg. This forces blood to flow into the liver sinusoids.

6. **Closure of ductus arteriosus**
   - Closure begins immediately after birth and is completed within 2 days.
   - Rarely, it can be patent and is pathological.

Atrial Septal Defect

- It occurs due to failure of the foramen ovale to close completely.
- It is an acyanotic congenital heart disease and most common variety.
- As a result of patency, there is flow of oxygenated blood from left atrium to right atrium.
- There is hypertrophy of the right atrium to pump blood against the pressure gradient.
- This is followed by right ventricular enlargement.
- Usually, there are asymptomatic. A small proportion of patients develop pulmonary hypertension and recurrent LRTIs due to pulmonary congestion.
- It is managed by correction of the defect surgically.

5. Describe how coronary blood flow is regulated by coronary autoregulation.

Coronary Autoregulation

- In human body, brain, kidney and coronary circulation have autoregulatory mechanism when it comes to vasculature.
- Coronary circulation is unique by its outside-in fashion. The vessels are epicardial and pierce the muscle and provide branches.

- Also, there are natural bypasses between arteries without intervening capillaries. These provide an alternate oxygen pathway for myocardium following coronary stenosis.
- Coronary autoregulation is described as the ability of the blood vessels to maintain a relatively constant blood flow across a wide range of perfusion pressure. Coronary blood flow remains constant between arterial pressures 60–140 mmHg.
- Blood flow is regulated through coronary vessels in response to increased contractility by local need for increased nutrition.

Mechanisms of Autoregulation

1. **Oxygen concentration**
   - When there is a decrease in oxygen concentration in the blood being delivered to the tissue, there is release of certain vasodilator chemicals (adenosine, potassium, hydrogen, CO_2, bradykinin) which cause vasodilatation and increase blood supply.
   - When oxygen concentration falls, ATP gets converted into AMP and adenosine is released by further degradation of AMP.
   - Adenosine causes vasodilatation.
   - This forms a progressive cycle: Increased blood supply brings more metabolites and there is increase in vasodilatation.

2. **Metabolic demand**
   - When there is increase in metabolism due to increased exercise, the oxygen is insufficient

- 95% of the energy in the heart muscle is dependent on aerobic respiration and thus, ATP. When ATP is insufficient, adenosine is formed.
- The muscle fibers are semipermeable to adenosine, due to which adenosine leaks into blood and causes vasodilation.
- As a result, there is accumulation of metabolites as described above which cause vasodilatation and restore blood supply to the myocardium.

3. **Coronary perfusion pressure**
   - It is the difference between the pressure in the aorta and the right atrium.
   - As the pressure in right atrium is low, perfusion is maintained well.

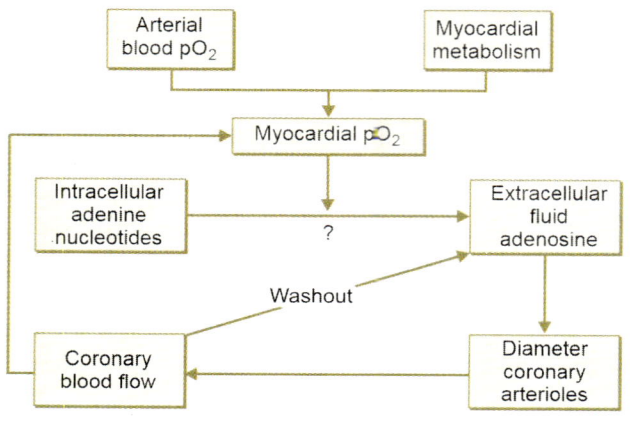

Fig. 5.39

5.11 DESCRIBE THE PATHOPHYSIOLOGY OF SHOCK, SYNCOPE AND HEART FAILURE

LONG ESSAY

1. A 30-year-old male met with a road traffic accident. He had severe blood loss. He was immediately shifted to hospital where his BP was recorded to be 60/40 mm of Hg, pulse was feeble and thready. What type of shock is he suffering from? Explain the different types of shock and give its physiological basis of treatment.

This patient is suffering from hypovolemic shock due to uncontrolled hemorrhage.

Different Types of Shock

- Shock represents a state of systemic dysfunction of one or many organs.
- Clinically, shock represents circulatory shock.
- Shock is a state of systemic hypoperfusion which may be caused due to varied etiologies, but usually culminates in death if not treated aggressively.
- It is of four major types:
  1. **Hypovolemic shock**
     - It is due to decrease in blood volume in the intravascular compartment leading to inability to perfuse body tissues.
     - It is characterized by tachycardia, low blood pressure, cold clammy extremities, confusion and finally death.
     - Causes are due to excess loss of blood or hemorrhage or fluids or due to burns.
     - It is the most commonly encountered type of shock.
  2. **Vasogenic shock**
     - In this type of shock, the blood volume is normal.
     - But due to vascular abnormalities, they are not able to maintain the ECF volume.

- It is seen in neurogenic shock, which can be caused by extreme fear, anaesthesia and drugs, vasovagal attack, snakebites leading to capillary failure and anaphylaxis. Other important cause is sepsis. The inflammatory mediators due to sepsis cause a sudden drop in the vasomotor tone and shock ensues.
  3. **Cardiogenic shock**
     - Shock resulting due to primary cardiac abnormality.
     - It can be due to left ventricular failure, cardiac tamponade or myocarditis or ventricular fibrillation.
  4. **Obstructive shock:** Due to obstruction to blood flow in the circulatory system like pulmonary embolism.

Principles of Treatment for Shock

A cause underlying the shock must be diagnosed prior to administration of treatment.

1. **Hypovolemic shock**
   - Stabilize the patient with inhalational oxygen
   - Elevate limb to increase venous return
   - Increase the ECF volume
   - Since the cause is decreased intravascular fluid or blood, it has to be restored.
   - Administration of crystalloids, plasma and blood is done in necessary situations.
   - Hypovolemia due to incessant diarrhea are treated with fluid correction
   - Hypovolemia due to loss of plasma as in burns are treated with plasma infusion
   - Hypovolemia due to uncontrolled hemorrhage is corrected with blood transfusion

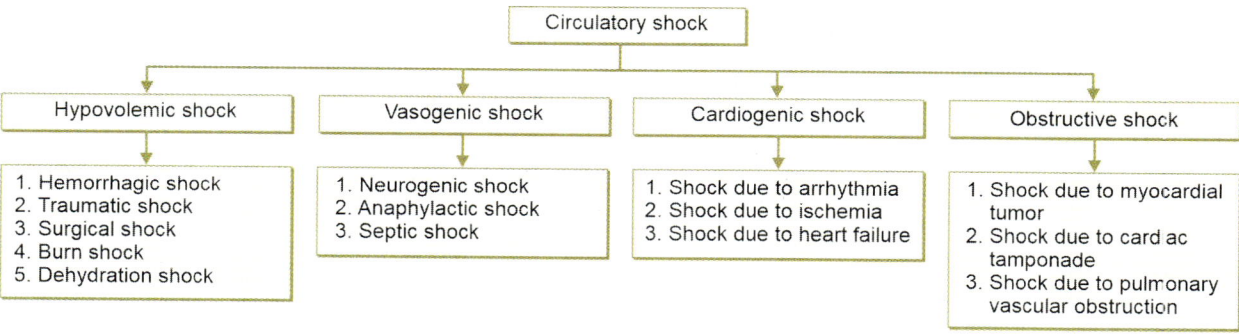

Fig. 5.40a

- Treat the underlying cause
  - Anti-diarrheal drugs for diarrhea
  - Surgical correction of the bleeding site
- Increase the sympathetic effect by giving sympathomimetics like dopamine and nor-adrenaline to increase peripheral arterial resistance and increase cardiac output.

2. **Vasogenic shock**

Neurogenic shock Postural	Lie the patient supine
Anaphylactic shock	Intramuscular epinephrine Intravenous hydrocortisone
Septic shock	Antimicrobial agents Life support

3. **Cardiogenic shock:** Recognize the type of heart disease leading to cardiogenic shock and then treat it

Ischemic heart disease—acute myocardial infarction	Intravenous streptokinase Anxiolytics Intracoronary stent or streptokinase
Arrhythmias	Anti-arrhythmic drugs Pacemakers, Defibrillators
Congestive heart failure	Decrease the preload by administering diuretics
Left ventricular failure	Diuretics to decrease the preload Intracardiac adrenaline

4. **Obstructive shock**
   - Treatment of underlying cause.
   - *Pulmonary embolism:* Intravenous anticoagulants, intra-arterial embolectomy

SHORT ANSWERS

1. Describe briefly different types of shock.

- Shock represents a state of systemic dysfunction of one or many organs.

- Clinically, shock represents circulatory shock.
- Shock is a state of systemic hypoperfusion which may be caused due to varied etiologies, but usually culminates in death if not treated aggressively.
- It is of four major types:
  1. **Hypovolemic shock**
     - It is due to decrease in blood volume in the intravascular compartment leading to inability to perfuse body tissues.
     - It is characterized by tachycardia, low blood pressure, cold clammy extremities, confusion and finally death.
     - Causes are due to excess loss of blood or hemorrhage or fluids or due to burns.
     - It is the most commonly encountered type of shock.
  2. **Vasogenic shock**
     - In this type of shock, the blood volume is normal.
     - But due to vascular abnormalities, they are not able to maintain the ECF volume.
     - It is seen in neurogenic shock, which can be caused by extreme fear, anaesthesia and drugs, vasovagal attack, snakebites leading to capillary failure and anaphylaxis. Other important cause is sepsis. The inflammatory mediators due to sepsis cause a sudden drop in the vasomotor tone and shock ensues.
  3. **Cardiogenic shock**
     - Shock resulting due to primary cardiac abnormality.
     - It can be due to left ventricular failure, cardiac tamponade or myocarditis or ventricular fibrillation.
  4. **Obstructive shock:** Due to obstruction to blood flow in the circulatory system like pulmonary embolism.

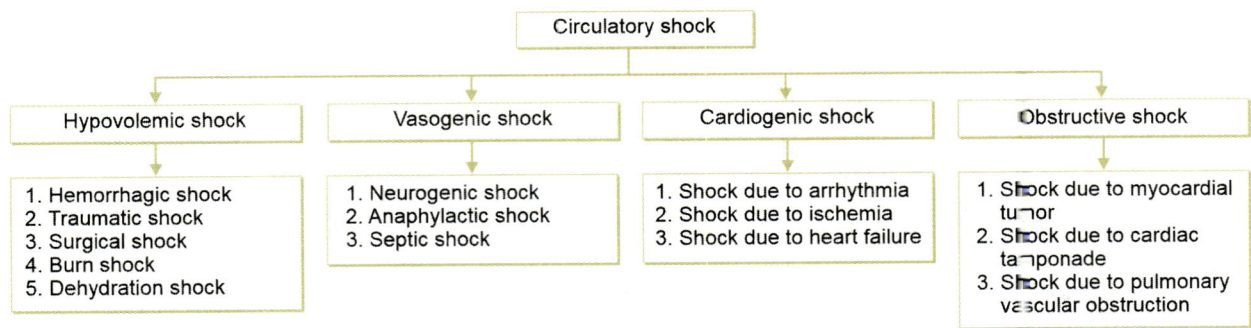

Fig. 5.40b

5.12 RECORD BLOOD PRESSURE AND PULSE AT REST AND IN DIFFERENT GRADES OF EXERCISE AND POSTURES IN A VOLUNTEER OR SIMULATED ENVIRONMENT

LONG ESSAYS

1. A 25-year-old male athlete who is on training for a marathon run, runs better than an untrained individual   (4 + 4 + 2 marks)
   A. What are the cardiorespiratory changes that occur with exercise training?
   B. What are the different types of exercises? compare and contrast.
   C. What is sudden cardiac arrest that occur in athlete training? Why does it happen so?

A. Cardiorespiratory Changes that Occur with Exercise Training

Cardiac Changes

- Marathoners have a 40% more cardiac output than untrained individuals due to hypertrophy of cardiac muscles.
- However, resting cardiac output is same.

Respiratory Changes

- With exercise, the oxygen consumption and pulmonary ventilation increase at rest and during exercise in a well-trained athlete.
- The maximal breathing capacity is at least 50% better in a trained athlete than an untrained person.
- The rate of oxygen usage under maximum aerobic conditions (VO_2 max) in a trained athlete is 45% greater than an untrained person.
- Oxygen diffusing capacity also increases in well-trained athletes.

B. Different Types of Exercises

Static exercises	Dynamic exercises
• Also called isometric exercises	• Also called isotonic exercises
• There is no change in length of the muscle but there is increase in tone. Examples include pushing against a wall	• There is change in length of the muscle, i.e. the joints are in motion
• There is increase in diastolic BP as the peripheral resistance increases.	• In this type of exercise, there is increase in cardiac output, stroke volume, heart rate and systolic BP. However, diastolic BP is unaltered.
• Cardiac output, stroke volume heart rate and systolic blood pressure also increase.	

Other classification is

Aerobic exercise	Anaerobic exercise
Low intensity, performed over long time	High intensity, short period
The energy is derived in the presence of oxygen. It is obtained from glycogen in the beginning and later from fat.	The energy is derived in the absence of oxygen, therefore there is accumulation of lactic acid. This causes fatigue.
Requires large amounts of oxygen	Leads to increase in muscle strength
	Also called 'body-building'
Examples include fast walking, jogging, running, bicycling, swimming, rowing	Examples include pull ups, push-ups, sprinting, weight lifting

C. Sudden Cardiac Arrest During Athlete Training

- Death during an athletic event resulting due to cardiac causes within 6 hours of onset of symptoms is called sudden cardiac death.
- Most important causes are hypertrophic obstructive cardiomyopathy, anomalous origin of left coronary artery, ruptured aortic aneurysm, myocarditis and others
- In HOCM, the heart muscles are so hypertrophied that they block the ventricular filling by causing obstruction and leads to death during a highly strenuous moment.

2. Define cardiac output. What are the factors that affect cardiac output? What is the effect of regular excessive training on cardiac output?
   (2 + 5 + 3 marks)

Cardiac Output

- The volume of blood pumped by the left ventricle is called cardiac output.
- Cardiac output in one minute is called minute volume. Its value is 5 liters
- Cardiac output per beat is called stroke volume and its value is 60–70 ml.

Factors Affecting Cardiac Output

Venous Return

- It is the amount of blood that return the right atrium from different parts of the body
- Cardiac output directly depends on the venous return

Force of Contraction

- Cardiac output is directly proportional to the force of contraction of the ventricle.
- It depends on the preload (amount of stretching of the cardiac fibres due to distension with blood) and afterload (pressure in the aorta and the pulmonary artery)

Heart Rate

Higher the heart rate, more is the cardiac output.

Peripheral Resistance

- Cardiac output is inversely proportional to peripheral arterial resistance
- Physiological variations occur in cardiac output due to variations in:
  1. Age
  2. Sex
  3. Body built
  4. Environmental temperature
  5. Emotional conditions
  6. Exercise
  7. High altitude
  8. Pregnancy
  9. Sleep

Effect of Regular Exercise on Cardiac Output

- During exercise, the heart rate increases and increases the cardiac output.
- This is to meet the metabolic demands of the skeletal muscles and to lose heat through skin by vasodilatation.
- However, when a person is regularly exercising, the heart muscles undergo hypertrophy and maintain a higher cardiac output at lower heart rates.

SHORT ESSAY

1. A healthy 32-year-old woman undergoes a training regimen in preparation for her first marathon. Explain the cardio-respiratory changes that occur due to moderate aerobic exercise training. Explain doping.

Cardiorespiratory Changes

- Aerobic exercises are isotonic exercises, that is, there is movement along joints and there is change in length of the muscle.

- With aerobic exercises, there is increased requirement of oxygen.
- Moderate aerobic exercise requires 50–74% of $VO_{2\,max}$
- Based on the time and usage of $VO_{2\,max}$, aerobic exercises are categorised as:

Light	30–49% of $VO_{2\,max}$
Moderate	50–74% of $VO_{2\,max}$
Submaximal	60–85% of $VO_{2\,max}$

- Based on time duration, short term is 5–10 min and long term is more than 30 minutes of exercise.

Effect of Moderate Exercise

- At the beginning of exercise, there is initial increase in stroke volume and heart rate. This is due to increase in venous return from the contracting muscles. Hence, there is an increase in preload.
- Thus, there is increase in cardiac output to a plateau state for about the next 30 minutes. Cardiac output steadies in about 2 minutes and reflects the fact that cardiac output is sufficient to meet the metabolic demands of the activity.
- As a result, systolic blood pressure also increases. It also plateaus like cardiac output.
- Due to increase in local lactate and potassium, there is vasodilatation. As a result, there is decrease in diastolic blood pressure. Mean arterial pressure also remains constant.
- When long-term exercise is over a long period, there is hypertrophy of the ventricles. As a result, there is increased efficiency of muscles.

Respiratory Changes

- With exercise, the oxygen consumption and pulmonary ventilation increase at rest and during exercise in a well-trained athlete.
- The maximal breathing capacity is at least 50% better in a trained athlete than an untrained person.
- The rate of oxygen usage under maximum aerobic conditions ($VO_{2\,max}$) in a trained athlete is 45% greater than an untrained person.
- During a moderate exercise, 40–50% $VO_{2\,max}$ is achieved within 30 minutes.
- Oxygen diffusing capacity also increases in well-trained athletes.

Doping

- It refers to illegal use of performance enhancing drugs in sports by athletes.
- These drugs are banned.
- Commonly used drugs are corticosteroids, anabolic steroids, and psychological stimulants. These are amphetamine, caffeine, cocaine and ephedrine.

Mechanisms

1. **Increasing muscle mass:** Anabolic steroids are used to increase muscle mass and physical strength.
2. **Increasing oxygen carrying capacity of blood**
   - Some athletes even use erythropoietin to increase RBCs to increase oxygen carrying capacity of blood. This enhances $VO_{2\,max}$.

- Others are hypoxia inducible factor, blood transfusion, hemoglobin-based oxygen carriers and perfluorocarbons.

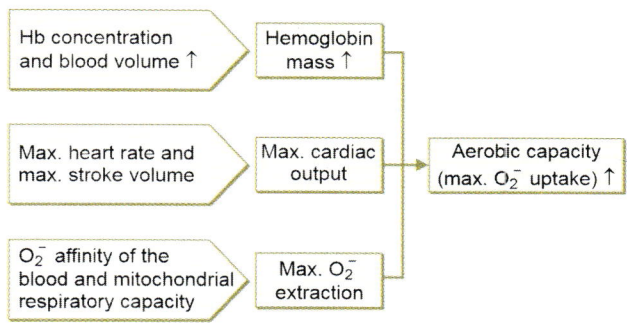

Fig. 5.41: Achieving maximum aerobic capacity

5.13 RECORD AND INTERPRET NORMAL ECG IN A VOLUNTEER OR SIMULATED ENVIRONMENT

SHORT ANSWER

1. Draw a lead II electrocardiogram and explain its waves.

Lead II Electrocardiogram

- It is obtained by connecting right arm and left leg.
- It is also called the rhythm strip

1. **P wave**
   - It is the first positive wave in the ECG.
   - It is also called the atrial wave.

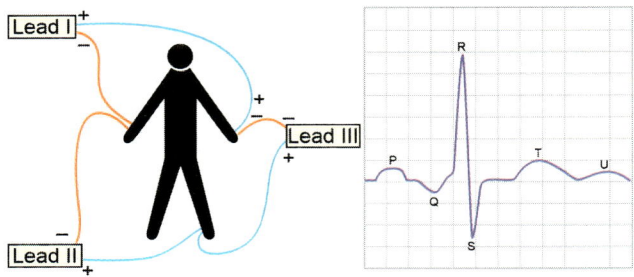

Fig. 5.42

- Produced due to depolarization of atria
- Its duration is 0.1s and amplitude is 0.1–0.2 mV

2. **QRS complex**
   - Represents ventricular complex
   - It has q—a negative wave, R—a positive wave and S—a negative wave
   - Q wave is generated due to depolarization of the basal portion of the interventricular septum, of amplitude 0.1–0.2 mV
   - R wave is generated due to depolarization of the apical portion of the interventricular septum, of amplitude 1 mV
   - S wave is generated due to depolarization of the basal portion of the ventricular muscle
   - Its normal duration is 0.08–0.1 second

3. **T wave**
   - It is the final ventricular wave due to repolarization of the ventricles
   - It is positive in lead II
   - Normal duration is 0.2 s
   - Amplitude is 0.3 mV

5.14 OBSERVE CARDIOVASCULAR AUTONOMIC FUNCTION TESTS IN A VOLUNTEER OR SIMULATED ENVIRONMENT

SHORT ESSAY

1. Describe the effects of Autonomic nervous system on Heart and Blood vessels.

Autonomic Nervous System

- The sympathetic fibres run along the subepicardial space, more on in the ventricles.
- The parasympathetic fibers through vagal nerve run subendocardial, more in the atrial musculature

Effect of Sympathetic

- Sympathetic discharge flows from the left stellate ganglion and reach the left ventricle and lead to increase in contractile strength and increased cardiac output. (positive inotropic effect)
- Thus, there is increase in systolic blood pressure.
- Norepinephrine released from the right stellate ganglion supplies the SAN and AVN. It causes increased heart rate and shortens the AV conduction (positive chronotropic effect).
- Epinephrine is released into circulation by the adrenal cortex and exerts effects on both the myocardium and peripheral vessels. It increases the contractility of myocardium.
- These actions are mediated through beta 1 receptors.
- It also has a positive dromotropic effect.

Effect of Parasympathetic

- The right vagus innervates the SA node and the left vagus innervates the AV node. Also, atrial musculature is innervated by the right vagus, but the ventricles have minimal vagal innervation.
- As a result, it causes decrease in heart rate (negative chronotropic effect).
- It also has a negative dromotropic effect.

Autonomic Nervous System and Blood Vessels

Effect of Sympathetic

- Circulating norepinephrine and epinephrine cause increased constriction of peripheral vasculature causing increased resistance and increased diastolic pressure. Sympathetic supply also increases tone of the veins and increases venous return.
- These changes are mediated through alpha1 and beta 2 receptors.
- Norepinephrine is secreted at the postganglionic nerve fibers causing vasoconstriction.

Effect of Parasympathetic

Acetylcholine is released at the postganglionic parasympathetic nerve endings and cause contraction of smooth muscles. This causes vasoconstriction.

5.15 DEMONSTRATE THE CORRECT CLINICAL EXAMINATION OF THE CARDIOVASCULAR SYSTEM IN A NORMAL VOLUNTEER OR SIMULATED ENVIRONMENT

SHORT ESSAY

1. Perform the clinical examination of cardio-vascular system in the given subject. Write the normal JVP.

Cardiovascular system examination involves the following

A. Examination of the Arterial Pulse

- The radial artery is chosen as it is convenient and is present in the exposed part of the body.
- It is palpated against the head of the radius in semi-pronated position of the right hand.
- Three fingers of the examiner are used to palpate the radial artery. The index finger exerts pressure on the artery, the middle finger feels the pulsations and the ring finger prevents transmission of pulsations from the palmar arch.
- The pulse is examined for the following characteristics.

Rate	The normal rate is 60–100 beats per minute
	If <60/min, it is termed bradycardia
	If >100/min, it is termed tachycardia
Rhythm	The regularity of the pulse is tested
	If there is irregularity in the pulse, it should be classified as regularly irregular or irregularly irregular
Volume	The volume is decreased in hypo-volemic conditions
	Increased in hyperkinetic circulation—pregnancy, anemia, thyrotoxicosis
Character	This is clearly seen in a recording
	Various types of pulse should be assessed—pulsus parvus, alternans, paradoxus, water hammer pulse
Vessel wall	It is felt by rolling the vessel against the underlying bone
	In young individuals, it is compliant and hence cannot be felt separately.
	Thickening is felt in arteriosclerosis and increases with age
Equality on both sides	It should be equal in either radial arteries
Examination of peripheral pulses	Carotid, brachial, femoral, posterior tibial and dorsalis pedis are commonly examined.

B. Examination of the Neck Veins

- Internal jugular vein examination is the most important as it is a direct extension of the right atrium
- It extends from the angle of the jaw, passes medial to the clavicular head of the sternocleidomastoid.
- This test is performed by asking the patient to lie in semi-recumbent position (45 degree) with the face turned slightly to the left
- In a normal individual, the JVP should be at the level of angle of Lewis in 45 degree position.
- It is around 2–3 cm of water.
- Anything more than is recorded as increased JVP.

C. Examination of the Heart

Inspection

- Precordium is the part of the chest wall lying anterior to the heart.
- Look for deformities, bulging of chest wall
- Apex beat is the most prominent, outermost and lowest definite cardiac pulsation and is usually located in the fifth intercostal space medial to the left mid-clavicular line.
- It may not be visible in fat individuals and in ladies.
- Look for other pulsations.

Palpation

- Locate the apex beat with ulnar border of the hand as it is more sensitive
- The 5th intercostal space is calculated by counting downwards from the sternal angle which marks the second intercostal space.
- Look for change in the position of apex beat with change in posture. Normally, it does not change.

Percussion

- It is done by striking the middle finger of the left hand while placing it in the intercostal space.
- Percussion is begun at the second intercostal space in the right till the liver dullness if found.
- Then it is done from laterally inwards till dullness is appreciated. Normally right border of the heart lies behind the sternum.
- Left border of the heart is calculated by percussing upwards from the apex beat.

- Area of cardiac dullness increases in pleural effusion and decreases in emphysema and pneumothorax.

Auscultation

- Mitral area: Corresponds to the apex beat
- Tricuspid area: Immediately left of the left lower border of the sternum
- Aortic area: Immediately right of the right upper border of the sternum
- Pulmonary area: It lies on the left of the left upper border of the sternum
- Auscultation is done with the diaphragm of the stethoscope
- S_1 and S_2 are normally heard as lub-dub.
- Added sounds should be looked for.

Normal Jugular Venous Pulse

- Jugular venous pulse is a measurement of the venous pulsation in the internal jugular vein.
- It is a measure of pressure changes in the atrium.
- The parts of the normal JVP are:
  1. **a wave**
     - It is the first positive wave
     - Represents atrial systole
     - Normally, the pressure in right atrium is 5 mm Hg and left atrium is 7 mm during systole.
  2. **x wave**
     - First negative wave
     - Occurs due to relaxation of atria just prior to diastole
  3. **c wave**
     - It is the second positive wave

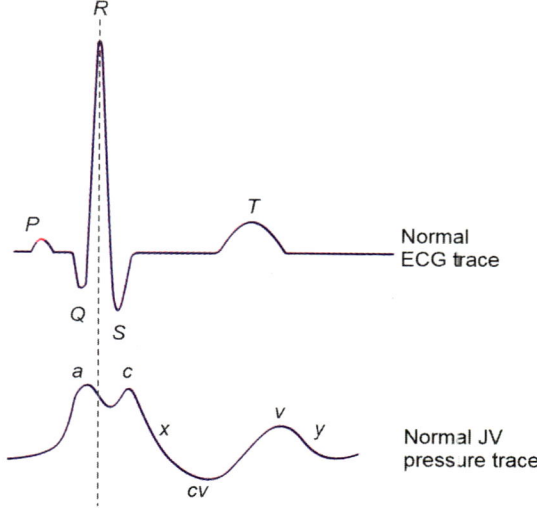

Fig. 5.43

     - Due to isometric contraction
     - Closure of AV valves causes rise in pressure
  4. **x_1 wave**
     - It is the second negative wave
     - It is caused during ejection phase due to indrawing of AV valves leading to fall in pressure
  5. **v wave**
     - It is the third positive wave, gradual rise in amplitude
     - Occurs during atrial diastole due to filling
  6. **y wave**
     - It is the third negative wave
     - It occurs due blood emptying into the ventricles with AV valves open.

5.16 RECORD ARTERIAL PULSE TRACING USING FINGER PLETHYSMOGRAPHY IN A VOLUNTEER OR SIMULATED ENVIRONMENT

SHORT ESSAY

1. Explain the waves of radial artery pulse tracing.

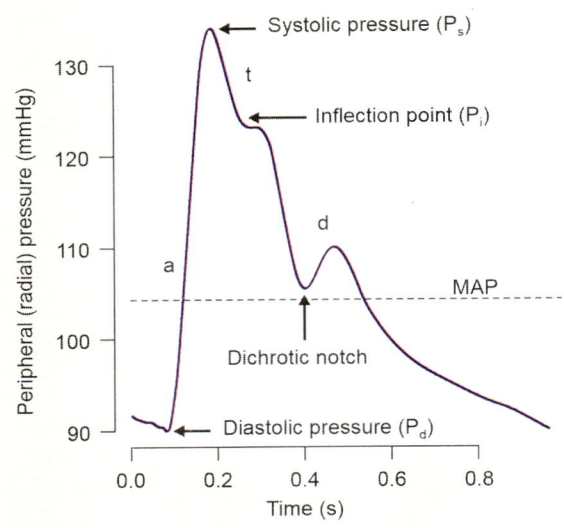

Fig. 5.44

Anacrotic Wave or Limb (a)

- The radial artery wave has a steep ascending limb called the anacrotic wave (a).
- It is formed due to expansion if the vessel wall due to ejection phase.
- The peak of this wave gives the value of systolic blood pressure.

Tidal Wave (t)

- A downward wave following systolic peak (t)
- It is formed by the elasticity of the aorta, there is a small decrease in pressure.

Dicrotic Notch and Dicrotic Wave (d)

- A notch is formed due to the elastic recoil of the aorta causing blood to recede back into the heart for a transient amount of time
- When the aortic valves close, there is a rebound increase in pressure causing a positive dicrotic wave (d).
- *Systole*—lasts from the upstroke of the anacrotic limb till the dicrotic notch.

- *Diastole*—lasts from the dicrotic notch till the beginning of the anacrotic wave.

2. Explain pulsus bisferiens, pulsus alternans and water hammer pulse.

Pulsus Bisferiens (Fig. 5.45)

- It has two peaks in the systole. It is a recording of the ascending aorta, arch of aorta and carotid artery.
- Also known as biphasic pulse
- It is seen hypertrophic cardiomyopathy as the anterior motion of mitral leaflet is blocked from re-entering the left ventricle.

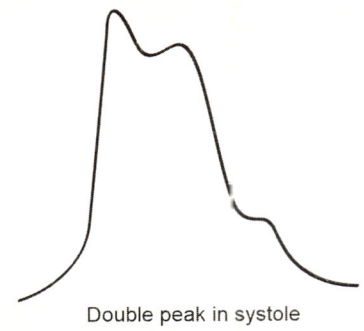

Double peak in systole

Fig. 5.45

Pulsus Alternans (Fig. 5.46)

- It is an alternating pulse
- It is characterized by regular but alternating large and small pulse waves.
- It is seen in a failing pump (left ventricular failure)

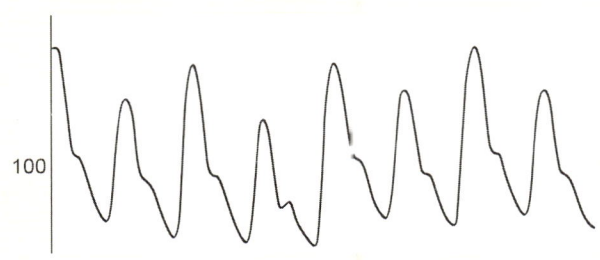

Fig. 5.46

Water Hammer Pulse (Fig. 5.47)

- Also called Corrigan's water hammer pulse
- It is characterized by abrupt rise and sudden fall in pulse wave.
- This is due to very high systolic pressure and a very low diastolic pressure. The fall is due to diastolic run off into the ventricle. The upstroke is due to increased stroke volume which stretches the carotid sinus and decreases the peripheral arterial resistance.
- It is seen in aortic regurgitation.

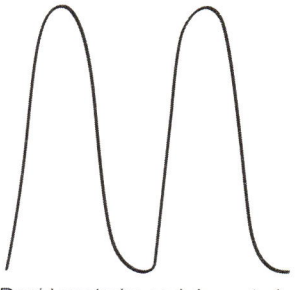

Rapid upstroke and downstroke

Fig. 5.47

Respiratory Physiology

6.1 DESCRIBE THE FUNCTIONAL ANATOMY OF RESPIRATORY TRACT

SHORT ESSAY

1. Explain the non-respiratory functions of lung.

Respiration or gas exchange is the main function of the lung other than that it has several other functions which are listed below.

1. **Acid–base balance**
   - It is a short-term regulation of the acid–base balance
   - When pH of the blood falls, there is an increase in hydrogen ions.
   - It combines with bicarbonate in blood to form, H_2O and CO_2.
   - CO_2 is easily blown out by hyperventilation by the lungs. Hyperventilation is caused by chemoreceptors which are triggered by hydrogen excess.

2. **Immune response against inhaled antigens**
   - The inhaled air may contain a lot of allergens and antigens.
   - They are filtered by the upper respiratory tract. The ones which reach the alveoli are phagocytosed by the pulmonary alveolar macrophage, also called the dust cell.
   - It is present in the alveolar wall along the pneumocytes.
   - They are also involved in phagocytosis of necrotic cells and apoptotic cells.
   - They are highly effective against bacteria.

   - Once engulfed, they deposit the debris along the mucociliary escalator or drain along the lymph or the blood.

3. **Drug metabolism**
   - It is an important site for extrahepatic drug metabolism
   - The endothelium forms an important site for binding and metabolism of drugs.

4. **Vascular reservoir**
   - The volume of blood in the pulmonary capillaries is almost equal to the right ventricular output which is 70–100 ml.
   - The vessels are highly distensible and accommodate an increase or decrease in the pressure.
   - There is also a phenomenon of recruitment of vessels in times of increased cardiac output. Some vessels which were not being perfused during resting conditions, get perfused.

5. **Secretion of hormones**
   - Pulmonary neuroendocrine cells secrete small amounts of serotonin.
   - They also play a role in cell growth and differentiation.
   - It activates angiotensin I when it passes through the pulmonary circulation.
   - Some hormones like bradykinin, ANP, prostaglandins get deactivated.

6. Secretion of heparin
- Lungs are a rich source of heparin and thromboplastin.
- Also, lungs behave as a chemical filter—the endothelium secretes fibrinolysin activator which is capable of degrading clots.

7. Temperature regulation
- Loss of humidified air as it leaves the lung from an important way of losing water and heat along with it.

SHORT ANSWERS

1. Write a note on type II alveolar cells of lungs and its physiological importance.

Type II Alveolar Cells
- Alveolar epithelium consists of two types of cells: Type I and type II.
- Type I cells (95%) are associated with gas exchange.
- Type II cells (5%) are associated with surfactant production. They are cuboidal in shape and are also called granular cells. They secrete alveolar fluid and produce surfactant.

Physiological Importance
- The type II pneumocytes are rich in lipid, which is secreted in the form of surfactant.
- Surfactant is a complex mixture of phospholipids, proteins, and ions. The most important is a phospholipid→dipalmitoyl phosphor→phosphatidyl choline.
- It reduces the surface tension of water by dissolving unevenly in water.

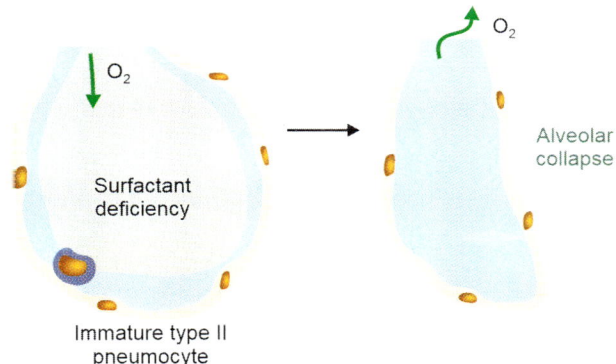

Fig. 6.1

- Normal surface tension in the alveolus is 50 dynes/cm but is reduced to 5–10 dynes/cm due to the action of surfactant.
- In the absence of air, the alveoli tend to shut because of negative intra-alveolar pressure and a positive surface tension. In the presence of surfactant, this collapse is prevented.
- Its clinical implication is understood in respiratory distress syndrome of the newborn, especially premature, who are born without surfactant. They are therapeutically administered surfactant into the lungs.

2. Explain the different zones of respiratory tract.

The respiratory tract is mainly divided into a conducting zone and a respiratory zone.

1. Conducting zone
- It consists of nose, pharynx, larynx, trachea, bronchi and the bronchioles.
- They take part in conduction of oxygen towards the alveoli and transport of carbon dioxide towards the nose.
- They do not take part in respiration.
- Other function is mechanical filtration of the air.
- The trachea divides into two major bronchi
- Bronchi divide into lobar bronchi → segmental bronchus → subsegmental bronchus → conducting bronchiole → terminal bronchiole

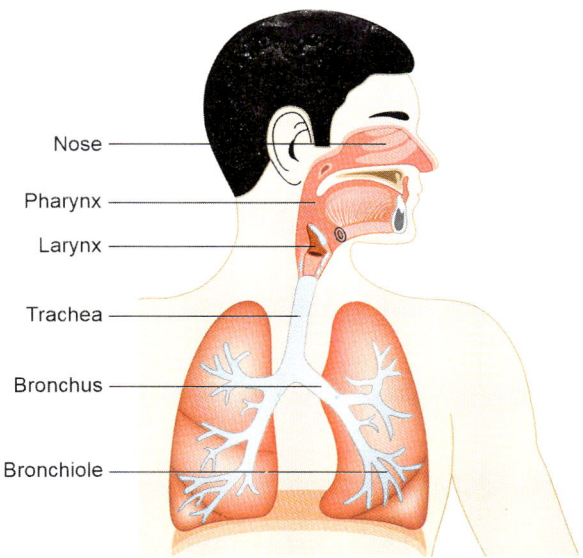

Fig. 6.2: Conducting zone

2. **Respiratory zone**
   - It includes the respiratory bronchioles, alveolar ducts and alveoli.
   - It is the site of exchange of gases with the blood.
   - Each respiratory bronchiole divides into alveolar duct, which further enters an alveolar sac.
   - The alveolar sac contains a set of alveoli.
   - Alveoli is lined by endothelium and pneumocytes.

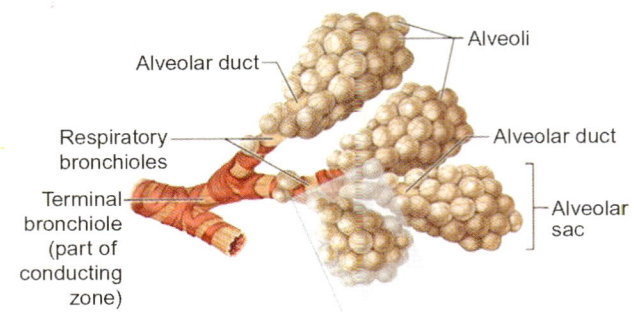

Fig. 6.3

6.2 DESCRIBE THE MECHANICS OF NORMAL RESPIRATION, PRESSURE CHANGES DURING VENTILATION, LUNG VOLUME AND CAPACITIES, ALVEOLAR SURFACE TENSION, COMPLIANCE, AIRWAY RESISTANCE, VENTILATION, V/P RATIO, DIFFUSION CAPACITY OF LUNGS

LONG ESSAYS

1 A 70 years old male patient comes to medical OPD with wheeze. His history reveals that he is a known case of COPD.

   A. What are the different types of lung disorders broadly classified as? **(2 marks)**

   B. What are state and dynamic lung volumes? Give their normal values. **(6 marks)**

   C. Define FEV. Give its physiological importance and its normal value. **(2 marks)**

A. Classification of Diseases of Respiration

Diseases of the respiratory tract are mainly classified as restrictive and obstructive respiratory disease. It is based on lung function test and particularly FEV.

	Obstructive	Restrictive
Component of breathing affected	Expiration is affected	Inspiration is affected
Examples	Laryngotracheitis Epiglottitis Asthma COPD Emphysema Cystic fibrosis	Myasthenia gravis Flail chest Interstitial fibrosis Pleural effusion Pleural effusion Paralysis of diaphragm

B Static Lung Volumes

Volumes of air breathed by an individual

1. **Tidal volume**
   - Volume of air inhaled and exhaled out of lungs in a single normal quiet respiration
   - Normal value: 500 ml

2. **Inspiratory reserve volume**
   - It is the additional volume of air that can be inhaled forcefully after the end of a normal quiet inspiration
   - Normal value: 3,300 ml

3. **Expiratory reserve volume**
   - It is the additional volume of air that can be exhaled out forcefully after normal expiration
   - Normal value: 1,000 ml

4. **Residual volume**
   - It is the volume of air remaining within the airways even after forced expiration (which cannot be emptied)
   - Normal value: 1,200 ml

Dynamic Lung Volume

1. **Forced vital capacity**
   - It is the volume of air in ml that can be brought out through forceful rapid expiration after a maximal and deep inspiration.
   - Normal value = 4,800 ml (same as vital capacity)
   - It may be less in certain pulmonary conditions.

2. **Forced expiratory volume**
   - It is the volume of air that can be expired fully in each unit of time.
   - FEV1 = FEV in one second
   - FEV2 = FEV in 2 seconds
   - FEV3 = FEV in 3 seconds

C. FEV

- Forced expiratory volume is the volume of air that can be expelled forcefully in each unit of time (after deep inspiration)
- It is also called timed vital capacity
- Normal values
  - FEV1= 83% of total vital capacity
  - FEV2= 94% of total vital capacity
  - FEV3= 97% of total vital capacity
  - After 3 seconds = 100% of TVC
- Importance (Fig. 6.4)
  - It helps to distinguish obstructive from restrictive lung disorders. It is significantly decreased in obstructive diseases.
  - Also, it helps to differentiate asthma from emphysema. There is 20% improvement in FEV1 following inhalation of short acting bronchodilators in asthma, but not in emphysema.

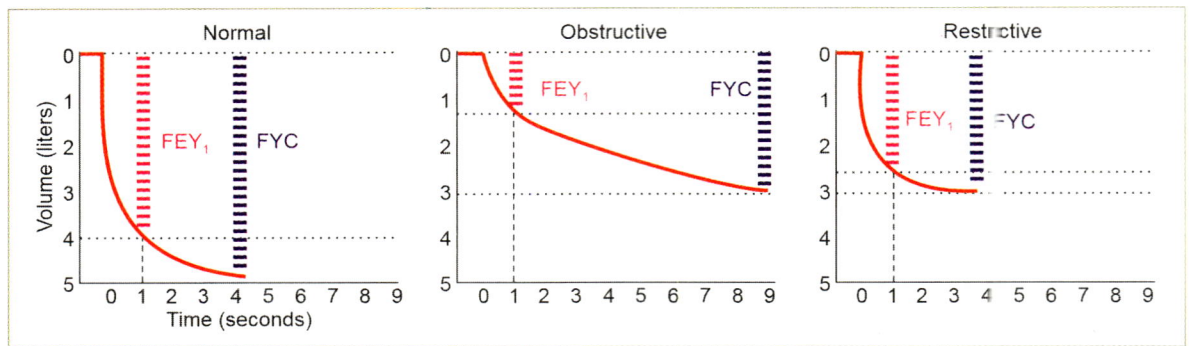

Fig. 6.4

2. Explain the following: (4 + 4 + 2 marks)
A. Concept of hysteresis with the pressure-volume curve.
B. Compliance of lung and factors affecting it.
C. Intrapleural pressure and transpulmonary pressure.

A. Hysteresis with pressure–volume curve

- It is a study of pressure–volume relationship of the lung.
- It is the ability of the lung to regain its original volume when pressure decreases.
- The curve is plotted by keeping the changes in lung volume with respect to changes in intrapleural pressure changes during inspiration and expiration.
- It describes the behavior of the chest wall and the lungs during inspiration and expiration.

B. Compliance of Lung

- It is defined as the capacity of the lungs and thorax to distend or expand.
- It is a measure of stiffness of lungs and is measured in change in volume per unit change in pressure (ml/cm of H_2O).
- Normal value is 0.1–0.4 L/cm of water.
- It is of two types

Static compliance	Dynamic compliance
It is measured under static conditions, i.e. when breathing does not take place.	It is measured during breathing.
It is the pressure required to overcome the elastic recoil of the airway for a given volume of air.	It is decreased in pathological conditions.

- Factors affecting compliance
  1. **Elasticity of tissues of lung**
     - It decreases physiologically in old age
     - Pathological conditions like fibrosis, emphysema of lung decrease the compliance of lung.
     - Thoracic cage abnormalities like kyphoscoliosis can affect compliance
     - Paralysis of extraocular muscles decreases compliance
  2. **Surface tension at air–water interface:** Decreased action of surfactant due to ARDS can decrease compliance.

C. Intrapleural pressure and transpulmonary pressure

- Intrapleural pressure is the pressure existing between the parietal and visceral pleura.
- It is always negative (–2 mmHg) and increases with inspiration (–6 mmHg)
- Intraalveolar or intrapulmonary pressure is the pressure within the alveoli
- Normal value is equal to atmospheric pressure that is 760 mmHg. During inspiration, –1 mm decreases.

3. Explain the respiratory centers and neural regulation of respiration. Write a note on Ondine's curse.   (4 + 4 + 2 marks)

Respiratory Centres

- The respiratory centre is located bilaterally in the medulla oblongata and pons.
- It consists of three group of neurons—dorsal, ventral and pneumotaxic centre.

a. **Dorsal group of neurons**
   - Associated with inspiration
   - Present in the dorsal part of the brainstem, throughout the length of the brainstem
   - It discharges rhythmic impulses and maintains rhythmic basic rhythm of respiration
   - Most of the neurons are in the nucleus of tractus solitarius, which forms the sensory termination of glossopharyngeal nerve and vagus nerve. These nerves collect sensory information through peripheral chemoreceptors, baroreceptors, and numerous other receptors in the lung.
   - The basic cause for this discharge is unknown and continues even when the medulla is transected above and below this level.
   - It produces impulses that are conducted to the diaphragm in a ramp-like fashion and hence named inspiratory ramp signals. It begins slowly and increases till about 2 seconds. Then it stops abruptly for 3 seconds allowing the diaphragm to recoil.

b. **Ventral group of neurons**
   - Associated with expiration and inspiration
   - Present in the ventrolateral part of medulla—occupying the nucleus ambiguus and nucleus retroambiguus
   - They do not take part in the normal quiet respiration. Thus, inspiration is triggered by dorsal group of neurons and expiration is a passive process due to elastic recoil of lungs and diaphragm.
   - During exertion, when there is a requirement of more oxygen, these centers are triggered by an overflow of impulses from the dorsal group of neurons.
   - Some neurons in the ventral group are associated with inspiration and others with expiration.

c. **Pneumotaxic centre**
   - Present in the nucleus parabrachialis in the dorsal part of upper part of pons
   - It acts as a switch off point to control inspiration
   - Its action is to control the rate of respiration by causing the inspiration to stop and thereby expiration to begin.

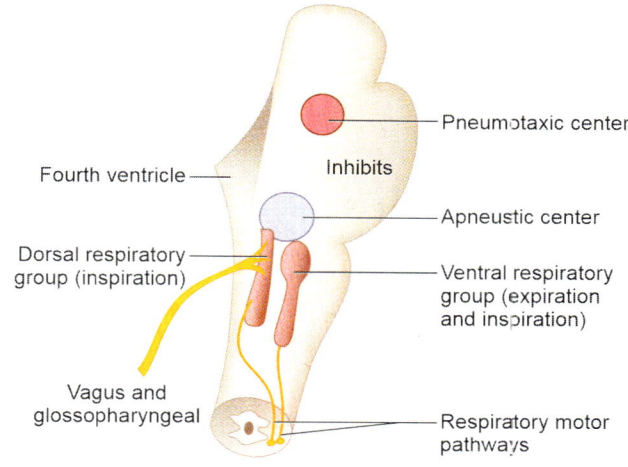

Fig. 6.5

   - A strong pneumotaxic signal has the ability to increase the rate of breathing up to 30 to 40 breaths per minute, whereas a weak pneumotaxic signal decreases the respiratory rate to only 3 to 5 breaths per minute.
   - Apneustic centre
     o It is present in the lower part of the pons.
     o It increases the depth of inspiration by acting on the dorsal group of neurons.

Neural Regulation of Respiration

Afferents from the peripheral chemoreceptors and peripheral baroreceptors via IX and X nerves and stretch receptors in the lungs via the vagus reach the respiratory centers

Respiratory centres
The outcome depends on the signals from various receptors like cortical, J receptors, baroreceptors, chemoreceptors, thermal receptors, pain receptors.

Nerves from the respiratory centres descend in the lateral column of spinal cord

Terminate in the anterior horn cells of cervical and thoracic segments: Phrenic nerve and intercostal nerves

Fig. 6.6

Hering-Breuer Reflex

- It is a protective reflex
- Objective is to prevent over inflation of lungs
- Pathway

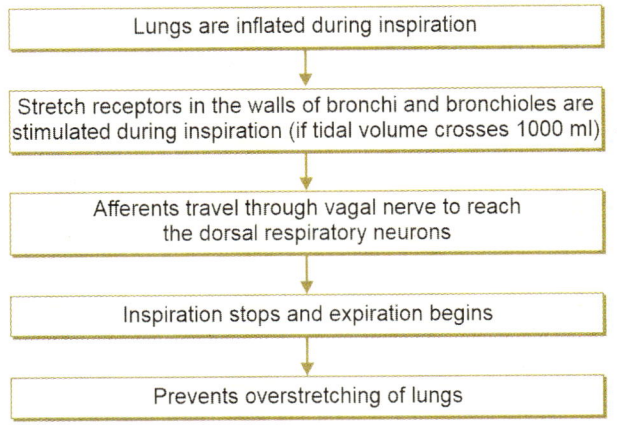

```
┌─────────────────────────────────────────┐
│   Lungs are inflated during inspiration  │
└─────────────────────────────────────────┘
                    ↓
┌─────────────────────────────────────────┐
│ Stretch receptors in the walls of bronchi│
│ and bronchioles are stimulated during    │
│ inspiration (if tidal volume crosses 1000 ml)│
└─────────────────────────────────────────┘
                    ↓
┌─────────────────────────────────────────┐
│  Afferents travel through vagal nerve to │
│  reach the dorsal respiratory neurons    │
└─────────────────────────────────────────┘
                    ↓
┌─────────────────────────────────────────┐
│ Inspiration stops and expiration begins  │
└─────────────────────────────────────────┘
                    ↓
┌─────────────────────────────────────────┐
│   Prevents overstretching of lungs       │
└─────────────────────────────────────────┘
```

Fig. 6.7

- The opposite happens during expiration and is called Hering-Breuer's deflation reflex.

Ondine's Curse

- It is known as congenital central hypoventilation syndrome
- It gets its name from a mythological character of a nymph who curses her unfaithful husband that he could breathe only if he was awake. So, the moment he fell asleep. He would stop breathing.
- It can be a congenital etiology or due to trauma to the lower medulla and there is a loss of neural control of breathing. It must be initiated voluntarily.
- These patients require mechanical ventilation through tracheostomy throughout their life.

4. A newborn child was admitted in NICU soon after childbirth. History revealed that it was a premature birth and the child was diagnosed to have respiratory distress syndrome. What is the role of surfactant in lungs? Where is it synthesized? What is its composition? What is lung compliance? What are the factors that affect it? Write a note on hyaline membrane disease.

Respiratory distress syndrome (RDS) of the newborn is a breathing disorder of premature babies. Also referred to as hyaline membrane diseases.

A. Role of Lung Surfactants

- Surfactant is a surface acting agent that decreases the surface tension of a fluid.
- Surfactant that lines the epithelium of the alveoli in lungs is known as pulmonary surfactant

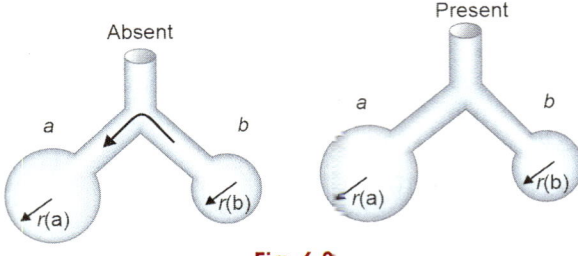

Fig. 6.8

- It decreases the surface tension of water film on the alveolar membrane and thus prevents collapse of the alveolus.
- The collapse of an alveoli is more when the radius is small and surfactant is less. So, the importance of surfactant is further exaggerated in smaller airways where collapse more plausible.

B. Source of Surfactant

1. Type II alveolar epithelial cells
- In the lungs, which are called type II pneumocytes.
- They have a granular cytoplasm
- They are roughly cuboidal with microvilli on their alveolar surface

2. Clara cells
- Which are situated in the bronchioles.
- These cells are also called bronchiolar exocrine cells.

C. Composition of Surfactant

Surfactant is a compound mixture consisting mainly of phospholipids.

1. Phospholipids
- Phospholipids form about 75% of the surfactant
- They have detergent-like action as they are bipolar. The lipid part is hydrophobic and the lipophobic part binds at the alveolar end.
- Major phospholipid present in the surfactant is dipalmitoyl phosphatidylcholine (DPPC)

2. Other lipids: Other lipid substances of surfactant are triglycerides and phosphatidylglycerol (PG)

3. Proteins
- Proteins of the surfactant are called specific surfactant proteins.
- There are four main surfactant proteins, called SPA, SPB, SPC and SPD.
- SPA and SPD are hydrophilic, while SPB and SPC are hydrophobic.
- They are vital to the activity of the surfactant.

4. **Ions:** Ions present in the surfactant are mostly calcium ions.

D. Lung Compliance

- Lung compliance refers to the ability of the lungs to expand
- Definition: It is defined as the change in volume per unit change in the pressure.
- Determination of compliance is useful as it is the measure of stiffness of lungs.

E. Factors Affecting Compliance

1. Elastic property of the lung

- Elasticity of the lung is determined by collagen and elastin fibers meshed inside the lung parenchyma.
- When the lung is outside the body system and in a deflated state, these fibers are fully contracted due to elasticity.
- When the lung expands, they elongate and exerts even more elastic force similar to a rubber band.
- Thus, the flexibility of these fibers determines the compliance of the lungs.

2. Surface tension elastic force

- The compliance of lung not only determined by the elastic forces of the tissue but also contributed to through surface tension exerted by the fluids lining the walls of the alveoli.
- When water forms a surface with air, the water molecules distribute strong attractive force for one another, causing contraction of the surface.
- Similarly, water lining the inner surface of the alveoli attempt to force air out of the alveoli and tries to collapse it.
- This force is termed the surface tension elastic force. Its minimum value is found to be 35–41 dyne/cm^2.
- A surfactant reduces the surface tension by partial dissolution.
- Due to its role in surface tension modification, it indirectly affects the compliance of the lung.

3. Lung volume

- Compliance is related to the lung volume, considering the formula relating volume and pressure.
- However, to eliminate this variable, specific compliance is measured using the formula:

Specific compliance = compliance/FRC (functional residual capacity).

4. Age

- This factor minimally influences compliance.
- Pulmonary compliance increases with age is owing to the structural changes in the lung elastin fiber.

F. Hyaline Membrane Diseases

- It is also called respiratory distress syndrome
- It is commonly seen in premature neonates due to their inability to secrete surfactant by the immature pneumocytes.
- As a result, the alveoli cannot open during inspiration.
- It affects about 1% of premature newborn infants and is the leading cause of death in such babies.

Pathogenesis

- The primary cause of RDS is inadequate pulmonary surfactant.
- Premature neonates, especially less than 28 weeks, have three features which make them susceptible to atelectasis of the alveoli and RDS.
  - The alveoli are small
  - There is inadequate surfactant production
  - They have a weak chest wall and hence lower compliance. The structurally immature and surfactant-deficient lung has compliance and a tendency to atelectasis (collapse)
- When the alveoli collapse, well perfused but poorly ventilated areas of lung lead to V/Q mismatch (with intra-pulmonary shunting) and alveolar hypoventilation results.
- As a result, there is hypoxemia and hypercarbia.
- Severe hypoxemia and systemic hypoperfusion result in anaerobic metabolism, and subsequent lactic acidosis.
- Hypoxemia and acidosis lead to pulmonary vasoconstriction causing pulmonary hypertension and resultant in right-to-left shunting at the levels of the foramen ovale and ductus arteriosus.
- Also, baro/volutrauma and high FiO_2, may initiate release of inflammatory cytokines and chemokines, causing more endothelial and epithelial cell injury.
- This further decreases surfactant synthesis and function as well as increased endothelial permeability leading to pulmonary edema. This goes into a vicious circle.

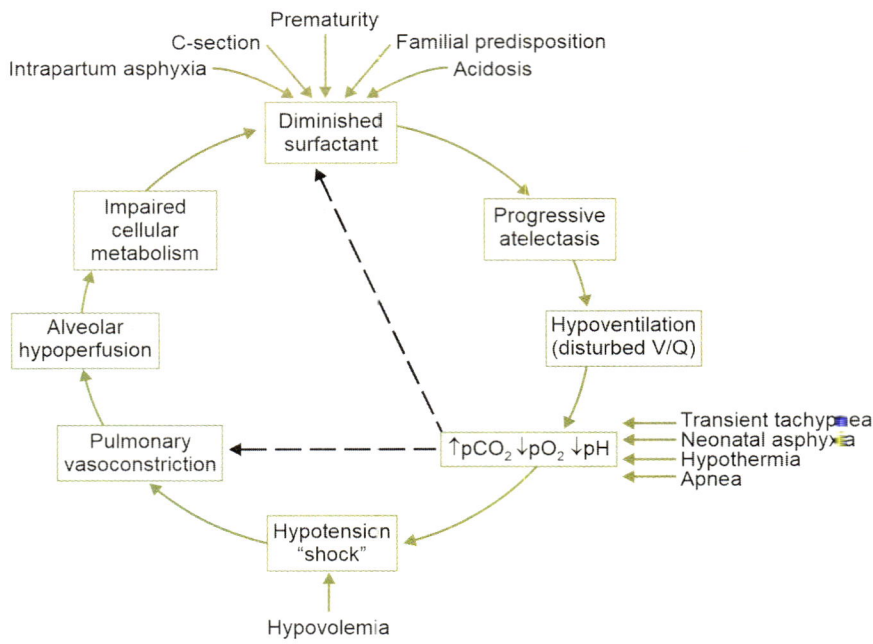

Fig. 6.9

- Leakage of proteins into the alveolar space further exacerbates surfactant deficiency by causing surfactant inactivation.
- An eosinophilic membrane composed of a fibrinous matrix of materials leaked from the blood constitute the hyaline membrane which lines the visible airspaces that usually constitute dilated terminal bronchioles and alveolar ducts.

Clinical Features

- Signs of RDS appear immediately after birth or within 4 h.
- The child may not cry at birth.
- There are signs of respiratory distress like tachypnoea, intercostal retractions, nasal flaring, grunting and cyanosis.
- Tachypnea is due to an attempt to increase minute ventilation to compensate for a decreased tidal volume and increased dead space.
- Retractions occur as the infant is an attempt to increase the negativity of the intrathoracic pressure so as to expand the poorly compliant lungs.
- Grunting results from the partial closure of the glottis during forced expiration in an effort to maintain FRC.

Treatment

Surfactant is added into the respiratory tract.

5. A 70-year-old male patient was admitted to medical ICU with symptoms of difficulty in breathing. He was diagnosed as pneumonia with COVID-19 positive. What is the pathophysiology in pneumonia? Explain VA/Q ratio, its normal and abnormal values, and conditions.

Pathophysiology of Pneumonia

- Pneumonia is an inflammatory response to either a microorganism or an irritant, following which there is edema, leucocytic response and blood in the alveoli.
- The affected part of the lung becomes consolidated and is unable to conduct air.
- Most common cause is bacterial infection. Others are viral, parasitic and toxin mediated. The abovementioned patient is diagnosed of a viral pneumonia which is presently a global pandemic.
- It is acquired through inhalation of the viruses through respiratory route.
- Coronavirus infection is a systemic infection. It causes interleukin mediated inflammatory

destruction of the alveoli and decreases the oxygen carrying capacity of the RBCs. Death is due to type 1 respiratory failure.

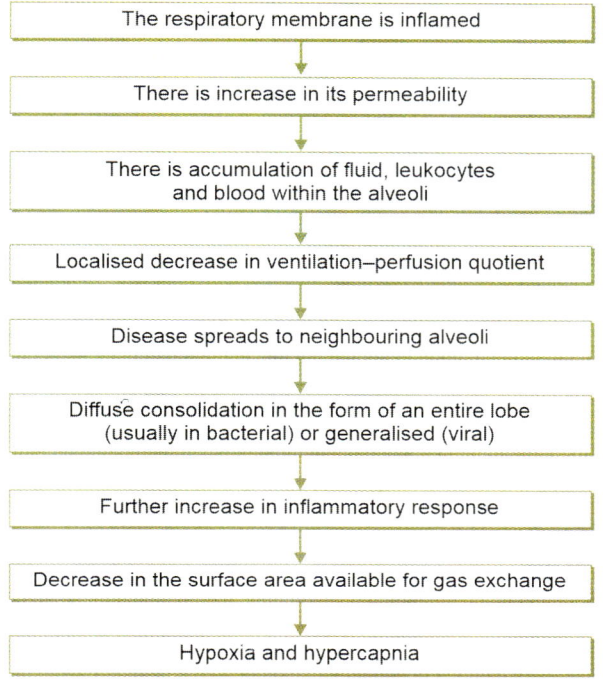

Fig. 6.10

Ventilation–Perfusion Ratio

- It is the ratio of alveolar ventilation to the amount of blood that perfuses the alveoli.
- It is written as VA/Q.

Normal Values

Normal value is about 0.84

1. **Apex of the lung or zone 1**
   - There is practically no blood flow in the capillaries, but only ventilation.
   - VA/Q is extremely high and approaches infinity
   - It is also called physiological dead space
2. **Midportion—zone 2**
   - Here the blood flow is intermittent, depends on the pulmonary artery pressure.
   - During systole, perfusion is less than the pulmonary artery pressure and during diastole, perfusion is more than the pulmonary artery pressure.
   - This zone is called area of intermittent blood flow.

3. **Lower portion—zone 3**
   - Here the blood flow is extremely high and is more than the alveolar pressure
   - VA/Q approaches zero.
   - This zone is called area of continuous flow.

Calculation

$$\text{Ventilation–perfusion ratio} = \frac{\text{Alveolar ventilation}}{\text{Pulmonary blood flow}}$$

Alveolar ventilation
= (Tidal volume – dead space) × respiratory rate
= (500 – 150) ml × 12/minute
= 4,200 ml/minute
Blood flow through alveoli
(Pulmonary blood flow) = 5,000 ml/minute
Therefore,

$$\text{Ventilation–perfusion ratio} = \frac{4,200}{5,000} = 0.84$$

Causes for Increased and Decreased VA/Q

Decreased ventilation perfusion quotient	Pneumonia, atelectasis
Increased ventilation–perfusion quotient	Emphysema, pulmonary embolism

6. Explain diffusion of gases across respiratory membrane. Describe the oxygen dissociation curve. What is P50? What happens to the curve in a 20-week foetus and why?

Diffusion Across Respiratory Membrane

Structure of Respiratory Membrane (Fig. 6.11)

- Also called alveolar membrane. It is very thin and has a thickness of 0.5 microns.
- It has six layers from inside outwards as described below:
  1. Monomicrolayer of surfactant
  2. It spreads on the inside of the alveolus
  3. Fluid layer that lines the alveoli
  4. Alveolar epithelium lying on a basement membrane
  5. Interstitial space
  6. Basement membrane of capillaries
  7. Capillary endothelial cells

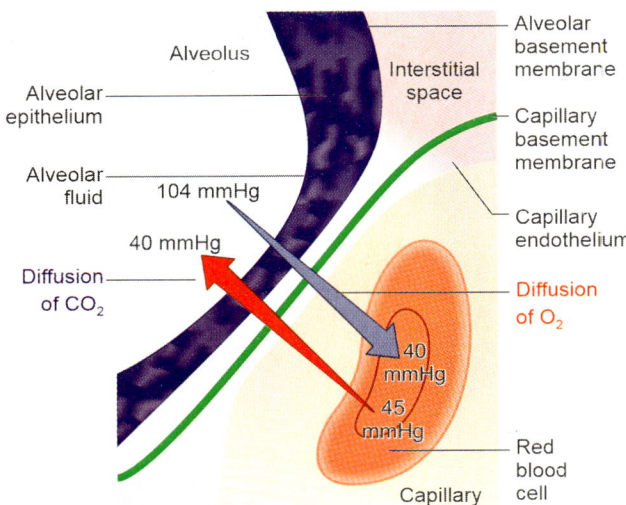

Fig. 6.11

Diffusion of Oxygen (Fig. 6.12)

- The partial pressure of oxygen in the atmosphere is 159 mmHg and in the alveoli is 104 mmHg
- There is gradient and as a result, oxygen easily flows from atmosphere into the alveoli.
- The factor that controls diffusion of oxygen through the alveolar membrane are its diffusion capacity. It is the volume of oxygen that diffuse across the alveolar membrane every minute along a pressure gradient of 1 mmHg. Diffusion capacity for oxygen is 21 ml/minute/mmHg.
- Diffusion capacity depends on the pressure gradient across the membrane, oxygen solubility

in the layers of the membrane and total surface area of the membrane. It is inversely proportional to the thickness of the membrane.

- When the oxygen in the pulmonary capillaries is exposed to oxygen in the alveoli, oxygen quickly and efficiently diffuses from alveoli into the pulmonary capillary. It has a partial pressure of 40 mmHg. Hence, oxygen diffuses from alveoli to the pulmonary capillary.

Diffusion of carbon dioxide		
Atmosphere	Alveolus	Blood vessels
CO_2 0.3 mmHg	40 mmHg	Pulmonary artery: 46 mmHg Pulmonary vein: 40 mmHg

- Carbon dioxide flows along the concentration gradient from blood vessels to alveoli and then atmosphere.

Oxygen Dissociation Curve (Fig. 6.13)

- It represents the relationship between partial pressure of oxygen in blood and the percentage saturation of hemoglobin with oxygen.
- It explains hemoglobin's affinity for oxygen.
- The curve has an initial staggering as binding of first molecule of oxygen to hemoglobin is difficult.
- Once this is established, there is positive cooperation which leads to increased affinity of hemoglobin to oxygen. Thereby the steep mid-portion results.

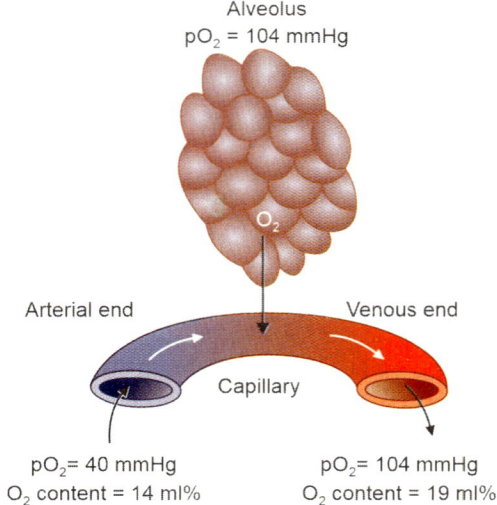

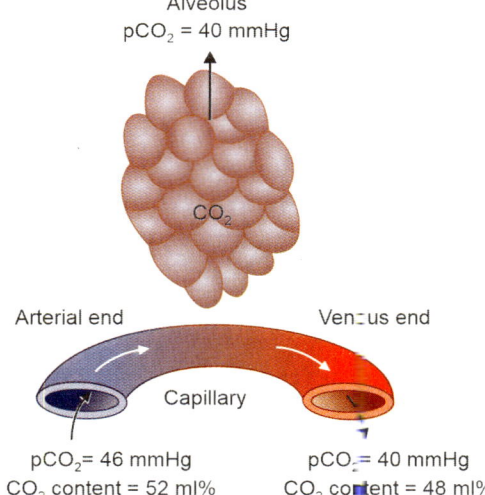

Fig. 6.12

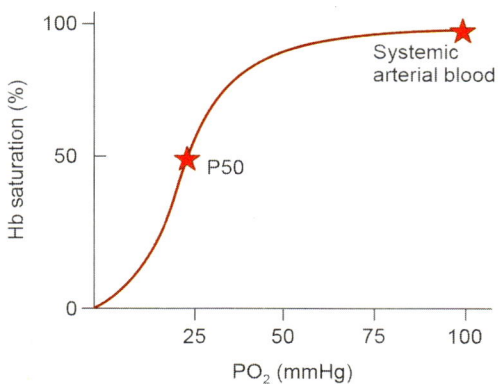

Fig. 6.13

- Once the partial pressure of oxygen nears 40 mmHg, the hemoglobin saturation is 75% and then there is slowing of binding process and finally the curve levels out as the hemoglobin is saturated with oxygen at around 60 mmHg.
- This is the reason for the sigmoid shape of the dissociation curve.
- Causes for shift of curve

Shift to left	Shift to right
It indicates increased affinity of hemoglobin to oxygen Examples are	It indicates decreased affinity of hemoglobin to oxygen (increase in dissociation)
1. Fetal hemoglobin	1. Decrease in partial pressure of oxygen
2. Decrease in H$^+$ ions in blood	2. Increase in partial pressure of CO_2
	3. Increase in H$^+$ ions in blood
	4. Raised body temperature
	5. Increase in 2,3 DPG in blood

P50

It is the partial pressure of oxygen at which the hemoglobin is 50% saturated. It is around 25–27 mmHg.

Fetal Hemoglobin

- In a 20-week fetus, hemoglobin is called hemoglobin F. it contains 2 alpha chains and 2 gamma chains.
- Hemoglobin F is fetal hemoglobin and has high affinity to oxygen.
- As a result, the oxygen hemoglobin dissociation curve is shifted to right as fetal hemoglobin has high affinity to oxygen. This is due to low partial pressure of oxygen in umbilical vein.
- At birth, 80% of Hb is HbF. During the first 6 months of life, it decreases to about 5% of total.
- HbF level may remain elevated in children with anemia and beta thalassemia, as a compensatory measure.

SHORT ESSAYS

1. Explain the mechanics of breathing under the following headings: (1 + 2 + 2 marks)
A. Muscles of respiration
B. Pressure changes during breathing
C. Explain static and dynamic compliance of lung

A. Muscles of Respiration

Are grouped as muscles of inspiration and muscles of expiration.

Muscles of inspiration	Muscles of expiration
1. Primary inspiratory muscles • Diaphragm • External intercostal muscles	1. Primary expiratory muscles • Internal intercostal muscles
2. Accessory inspiratory muscles • Sternocleidomastoid • Sternocleidomastoid • Scalene • Anterior serrati • Elevators of scapulae and pectorals	2. Accessory expiratory muscles • Abdominal muscles

B. Pressure Changes during Breathing (Fig. 6.14)

- There are two types of pressure exerted during respiration:
  1. **Intrapleural pressure or intrathoracic pressure**
     - It is the pressure existing in the intrapleural space (between the parietal and visceral layers of pleura).
     - It is a negative pressure. It is due to constant pumping out of fluid from the pleural cavity.
     - During inspiration: –6 mmHg, during expiration: –2 mmHg
     - At the end of forced inspiration: –30 mmHg
     - As a result of negative pressure, the alveoli are kept inflated. Also, the negative intrathoracic pressure pulls blood from the veins and thus increases venous return.

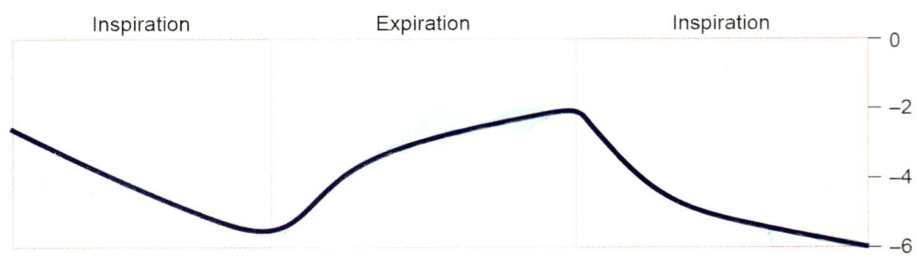

Inspiration	Expiration	Inspiration	0
			−2
			−4
			−6

Fig. 6.14

2. **Intra-alveolar pressure or intrapulmonary pressure**
   - It is the pressure existing in the alveoli in the lungs.
   - Normally, it is equal to the atmospheric pressure which is 760 mmHg.
   - During inspiration, it becomes 759 mmHg and during expiration, it becomes 761 mmHg.
   - During inspiration the negative pressure leads to entry of air into the alveoli and during expiration, it becomes positive and thus leads to exit of air from the alveoli.

C. Compliance of Lung
- It is defined as the capacity of the lungs and thorax to distend or expand.
- It is a measure of stiffness of lungs and is measured in change in volume per unit change in pressure (ml/cm of H_2O).
- It is of two types:

Static compliance	Dynamic compliance
• It is measured under static conditions, i.e. when breathing does not take place.	• It is measured during breathing.
• It is the pressure required to overcome the elastic recoil of the airway for a given volume of air	• It is decreased in pathological conditions

2. What is ventilation–perfusion ratio? Give its normal values at different levels of lung. How is V/P ratio affected?

Ventilation–Perfusion Ratio
- It is the ratio of alveolar ventilation to the amount of blood that perfuses the alveoli.
- It is written as VA/Q.

Normal Values
- Normal value is about 0.84

- Apex of the lung—zone 1
  - There is practically no blood flow in the capillaries, but only ventilation.
  - VA/Q is very high and approaches infinity
  - It is also called physiological dead space
- Midportion—zone 2
  - Here the blood flow is intermittent, depends on the pulmonary artery pressure.
  - During systole, perfusion is less than the pulmonary artery pressure and during diastole, perfusion is more than the pulmonary artery pressure.
  - This zone is called area of intermittent blood flow
- Lower portion—zone 3
  - Here the blood flow is very high and is more than the alveolar pressure
  - VA/Q approaches zero.
  - This zone is called area of continuous flow

Calculation

$$\text{Ventilation–perfusion ratio} = \frac{\text{Alveolar ventilation}}{\text{Pulmonary blood flow}}$$

Alveolar ventilation
= (Tidal volume – dead space) × respiratory rate
= (500 – 150) ml × 12/minute
= 4,200 ml/minute
Blood flow through alveoli
(pulmonary blood flow) = 5,000 ml/minute
Therefore,

$$\text{Ventilation–perfusion ratio} = \frac{4,200}{5,000} = 0.84$$

3. Draw a Spirogram. Explain the normal lung volumes and capacities.
Spirogram is a graphical record of different volumes and capacities of the lung measured using a spirometer (Fig. 6.15).

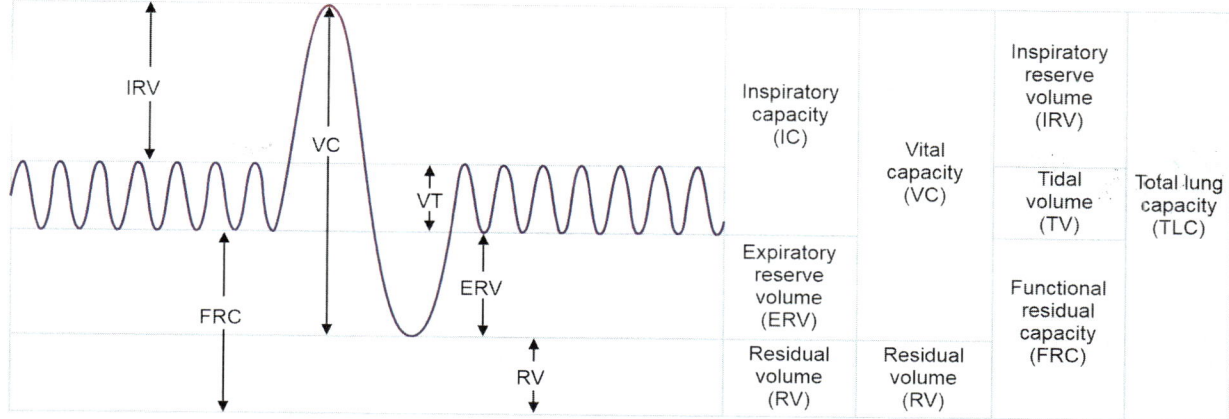

Fig. 6.15

Normal Lung Volumes

These are static measures of air breathed by an individual.

Tidal Volume

- Volume of air inhaled and exhaled out of lungs in a single normal quiet respiration
- Normal value: 500 ml

Inspiratory Reserve Volume

- It is the additional volume of air that can be inhaled forcefully after the end of a normal quiet inspiration
- Normal value: 3,300 ml

Expiratory Reserve Volume

- It is the additional volume of air that can be exhaled out forcefully after normal expiration
- Normal value: 1,000 ml

Residual Volume

- It is the volume of air remaining within the airways even after forced expiration (which cannot be emptied)
- Normal value: 1,200 ml

Lung Capacities (Fig. 6.16)

Lung capacities are a combination of two or more lung volumes

1. **Inspiratory capacity (IC)**
   - It is the maximum volume of air that can be inhaled after a normal expiration.
   - Inspiratory capacity = tidal volume + inspiratory reserve volume = 500 + 3,300 = 3,800 ml

2. **Functional residual capacity (FRC)**
   - It is the amount of air present in the lungs after normal expiration
   - Functional residual capacity = expiratory reserve volume + residual volume = 1000 + 1,200 = 2,200 ml

3. **Vital capacity (VC)**
   - It is the volume of air that can expelled out forcefully after a deep inspiration
   - Vital capacity = tidal volume + inspiratory reserve volume + expiratory reserve volume = 500 + 3,300 + 1000 = 4,800 ml

4. **Total lung capacity**
   - It is the total volume of air present in the lungs after a deep inspiration.
   - TLC= IRV + TV + ERV + RV = 6000 ml

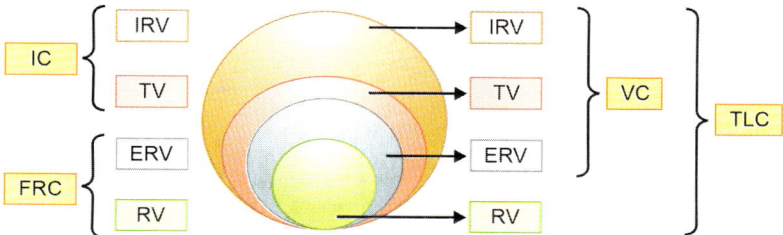

Fig. 6.16

4. Explain compliance of lungs. Name the clinical conditions which reduce the compliance of the lungs. In which condition is compliance of the lungs increased?

Compliance (Fig. 6.17)

- It is defined as the ability of the lungs and thorax to distend or expand. It is the extent to which the lungs will expand for each unit increase in pulmonary pressure.
- It is a measure of stiffness of lungs and is measured in change in volume per unit change in pressure (ml/cm of H_2O). The total compliance of both lungs in an average adult is 200 ml/cm of H_2O of transpulmonary pressure.
- The compliance diagram of the lungs is shown below. The transpleural pressure is increased step by step and the lungs can expand.
- It depends on the elasticity of the lung tissues and the elastic forces of the fluid that lines the inside of the alveoli. Greater part is played by the surfactant.
- It is of two types:

Static compliance	Dynamic compliance
It is measured under static conditions, i.e., when breathing does not take place. It is the pressure required to overcome the elastic recoil of the airway for a given volume of air.	It is measured during breathing. It is decreased in pathological conditions.

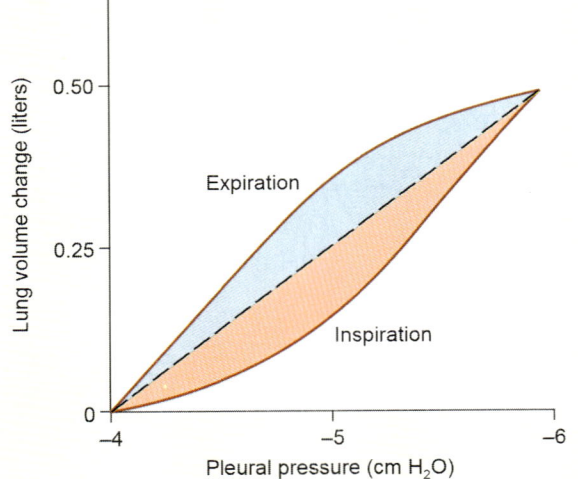

Fig. 6.17

Causes for Changes in Compliance

Decreased compliance	Increased compliance
Pulmonary fibrosis	Emphysema or chronic
Respiratory distress syndrome (absence of surfactant)	obstructive pulmonary disease
Pleural effusion and thickening	Bronchial asthma
Hydrothorax, pneumothorax	Old age
Respiratory paralysis	
Kyphosis, scoliosis	

5. Define and give its normal value:
A. Respiratory minute volume (RMV)
B. Maximum ventilatory volume (MVV)
C. Breathing reserve (BR)

Respiratory minute volume
- It is the volume of air that goes in and out of the lungs in one minute during a quiet respiration $500 \times 12 = 6000$ ml or 6 L
- It is calculated by multiplying tidal volume by respiratory rate

Maximum ventilatory volume
- It is the volume of air that can be forcefully breathed in and out of lungs within one minute   Males: 150–170 L/min Females: 80–100 L/min

Breathing reserve
- It is the difference between maximum breathing capacity and respiratory minute volume   145–165 L

6. What is FRC? Give its normal value. What is the physiological importance of FRC?

- Functional residual capacity (FRC) is the volume of air that remains in lungs after normal expiration (after normal tidal expiration).
- Functional residual capacity includes expiratory reserve volume and residual volume.
- It cannot be measured by spirometer. It can be measured by helium dilution method, nitrogen washout method and plethysmography.
- Functional residual capacity = Expiratory reserve volume + residual volume

$$2,200 \text{ ml} = 1,000 + 1,200$$

Physiological Importance of FRC
- FRC is the volume of air in the lungs that remains after a silent expiration.

- This air is responsible for keeping the alveoli from collapsing when the thoracic cage moves outward.
  - So it is equivalent to the elastic recoil.
  - Thus, it keeps the small airways open. If FRC drops below the equilibrium, the alveoli collapse.
- It helps in decreasing the work of breathing while initiating an inspiration.
  - It behaves as a gas reserve between breaths.
  - Because some residual gas remains in the lung, gas exchange can carry on during the entire respiratory cycle.
  - The implication of this is during induction of anaesthesia, the time between induction and intubation purely depends on the FRC as it acts as a reservoir of oxygen.
- The pulmonary vascular resistance is kept at a minimum
  - The resistance in alveolar and extra-alveolar vessels depend on lung volume changes.
  - When the small alveoli are collapsed, pulmonary vascular resistance is high because pulmonary arteries are narrowed.
  - As the lung inflates to FRC, arteries can increase in diameter and the resistance decreases.

Clinical Importance

- FRC is more in young adults, taller people and men. FRC is lesser in older people, pregnant ladies
- In restrictive lung diseases, there is reduced compliance of lung. As a result, there is increase in elasticity of the lung. As a result, less air enters the lung and TLC is decreased. As a result, FRC is decreased.
- In obstructive lung diseases, there is increased compliance of lung as expiration is obstructed. As a result, there is increase in TLC and therefore FRC.

7. Explain surfactant: Its composition, source of secretion and functions.

- Surfactant is a surface acting agent which lowers surface tension of a fluid.
- Water has high surface tension. As a result, the water molecules tend to concentrate leading to collapse of the alveolus.
- Surfactant that lines the epithelium of the alveoli in lungs is known as pulmonary surfactant.

Source of Surfactant (Fig. 6.18)

Pulmonary surfactant is secreted by two types of cells

1. **Type II alveolar epithelial cells**
   - In the lungs, which are called pneumocytes
   - These cells are cuboidal, have a granular cytoplasm and have microvilli on their surface.
2. **Clara cells**
   - These are present in the bronchioles.
   - These cells are also called bronchiolar exocrine cells.

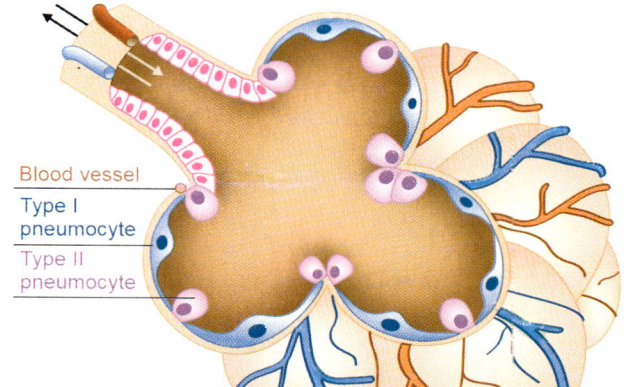

Blood vessel
Type I pneumocyte
Type II pneumocyte

Fig. 6.18

Composition of Surfactant

Surfactant is a complex mixture of phospholipids, proteins and ions.

1. **Phospholipids**
   - Surfactant mainly is formed by phospholipids
   - The most important is a phospholipid—dipalmitoyl phosphor—phosphatidyl choline.
2. **Other lipids:** Other lipid substances of surfactant are triglycerides and phosphatidylglycerol (PG)
3. **Proteins**
   - Proteins of the surfactant are called specific surfactant proteins.
   - There are four main surfactant proteins, called SPA, SPB, SPC and SPD.
   - These are vital for the action of surfactant.
4. **Ions:** Ions present in the surfactant are mostly calcium ions.

Functions (Fig. 6.19)

1. It reduces the surface tension of water by dissolving unevenly in water.

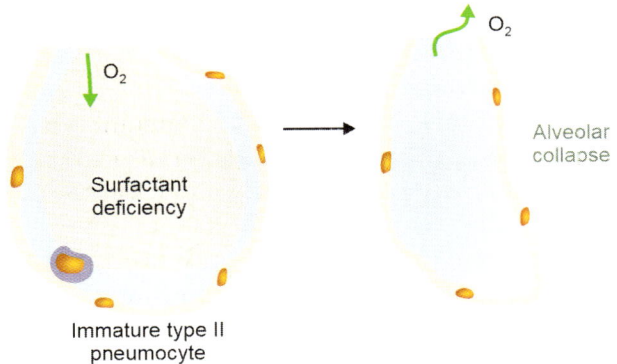

Fig. 6.19

2. Normal surface tension in the alveolus is 50 dynes/cm but is reduced to 5–10 dynes/cm due to the action of surfactant.

3. In the absence of air, the alveoli tend to shut as a result of negative intra-alveolar pressure and a positive surface tension. In the presence of surfactant, this collapse is prevented.

4. Its clinical implication is understood in respiratory distress syndrome of the newborn, especially premature, who are born without surfactant. They are therapeutically administered surfactant into the lungs.

SHORT ANSWERS

1. Describe Hering-Breuer's inflation reflex.

- It is a protective reflex
- Objective is to prevent over inflation of lungs
- The opposite happens during expiration and is called Hering-Breuer's deflation reflex
- Pathway:

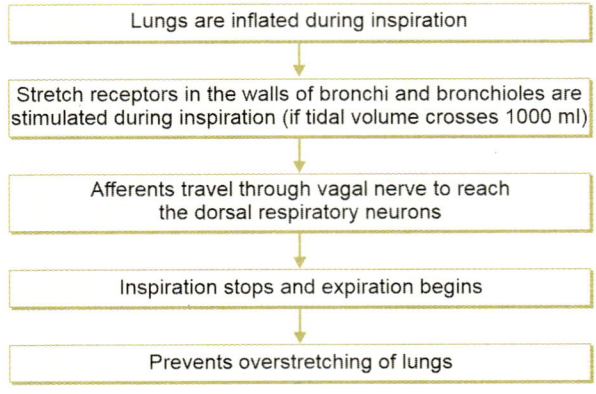

| Lungs are inflated during inspiration |
| Stretch receptors in the walls of bronchi and bronchioles are stimulated during inspiration (if tidal volume crosses 1000 ml) |
| Afferents travel through vagal nerve to reach the dorsal respiratory neurons |
| Inspiration stops and expiration begins |
| Prevents overstretching of lungs |

Fig. 6.20

2. Define dead space air. What are its types and give its physiological importance?

Definition

- Dead space is the region of the respiratory tract, which is not utilized for respiration, that is exchange of gases.
- Normal value is 150 ml.

Types

1. **Anatomical dead space:** It extends from nostrils to the terminal bronchiole.
2. **Physiological dead space**
   - It includes anatomical dead space plus air in the alveoli in which gas exchange is not happening due to dysfunction and air in the alveoli that are not receiving enough blood supply.
   - Normally, anatomical dead space = physiological dead space

Physiological Importance

- Tidal volume is 500 mL. of this, 150 ml is dead space. Hence, in a minute of 12 breaths, total amount of alveolar ventilation is 350 × 12 = 4200 ml/min. alveolar ventilation is the determinant for the amount of oxygen and CO_2 flowing in and out of the alveoli.
- Dead space increases in conditions which either destroy the alveolar membrane or when blood supply to alveoli is reduced. ARDS, emphysema, cigarette smoking and pneumonia increase dead space. As a result, the amount of oxygen reaching blood reduces.
- Short and shallow breaths increase dead space, whereas deep and slow breaths decrease dead space.
- The concept of dead space is important in mechanical ventilation. Capnography—measurement of alveolar CO_2 helps to know the actual dead space. Also, use of high-speed nasal cannula decreases dead space.

3. What are J receptors present in lungs? Give its physiological importance.

- 'J' receptors are juxta-capillary receptors
- They are present on the walls of the alveoli and are strongly associated with pulmonary capillaries. Some are present in the bronchi.
- They are sensory receptors of vagus nerve.

- The nerve fibers from these receptors are non-myelinated.

Functions

1. They are mainly involved in regulation of respiration.
2. They are stimulated mainly when the pulmonary capillaries are fully filled with blood.
3. Examples are pulmonary edema due to congestive heart failure, pneumonia, pulmonary embolism and chemicals like bradykinin, serotonin, halothane, and histamine.

Effect of Stimulation of J Receptors

1. Their stimulation gives rise to a feeling of dyspnea.
2. They cause hyperventilation, probably to remove the offending agent.
3. It is associated with bradycardia, hypotension, and weakness of skeletal muscles.

6.3 DESCRIBE AND DISCUSS THE TRANSPORT OF RESPIRATORY GASES: OXYGEN AND CARBON DIOXIDE

SHORT ESSAYS

1. Explain the different forms in which carbon dioxide is transported in the body. What is Hamburger's phenomenon.   (3 + 2 marks)

- Carbon dioxide is transported by blood from the tissue to alveoli and then from alveoli to the atmosphere air.
- Carbon dioxide diffuses from tissues into capillaries through the basement membrane by simple diffusion.

Step 1

In blood

CO_2 is transported in 4 ways.

1. Dissolved in plasma—about 3% is transported as a simple solution
2. As carbonic acid—minute amount of CO_2 combines with H_2O in plasma to form carbonic acid
3. As bicarbonate—about 63% is carried in this manner. This reaction takes place in a RBC in the presence of carbonic anhydrase H_2CO_3 is an unstable compound. It splits into H^+ and HCO_3^-.
4. As carbamino compounds—about 30% is transported in this manner. CO_2 combines with amino group in the Hb molecule and amino group if plasma proteins to form carbamino compounds. This bond is a weak bond, so that CO_2 diffuses easily from blood into alveoli.

Carbon dioxide dissociation curve (Fig. 6.21)

- CO_2 in blood depends on partial pressure of carbon dioxide

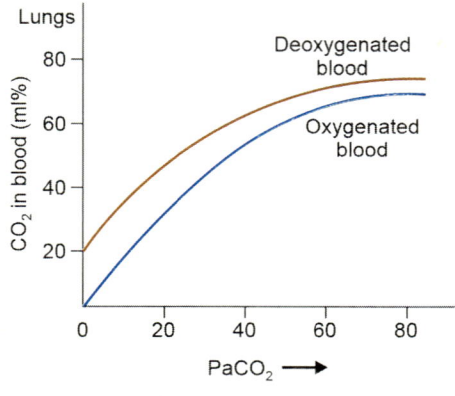

Fig. 6.21

- Increase in concentration of oxygenated hemoglobin causes CO_2 to diffuse out of the RBCs. This effect is essential for CO_2 to leave RBCs and enter alveoli of the lungs
- When $PaCO_2$ increases, the Hb becomes more attached to the CO_2 molecule
- When $PaCO_2$ increases, the hemoglobin shows more affinity to oxygen. The oxygen makes the RBS milieu more acidic which releases H^+ ions. These combine with. HCO_3^- for H_2O and CO_2.
- CO_2 diffuses out

Step 2

- Diffusion of CO_2 from blood into alveoli
- Pressure gradient in blood and alveoli (46 mmHg and 40 mmHg) causes simple diffusion of CO_2 into alveoli

Step 3

- Partial pressure of CO_2 in atmospheric air is 0.3% and in alveoli, it is 40 mmHg
- As a result, CO_2 escapes into atmosphere easily.

Hamburger's Effect (Fig. 6.22)

- Also called chloride shift
- It is a phenomenon of exchange of chloride ion for a bicarbonate ion
- Discovered in 1892.
- CO_2 diffuses into the RBC from plasma
- It combines with H_2O to form carbonic acid.
- Carbonic acid splits into H^+ and HCO_3^-
- Bicarbonate ion diffuses plasma in exchange of Cl^- ion in plasma through anion antiport channel.
- This phenomenon takes place in venous blood.

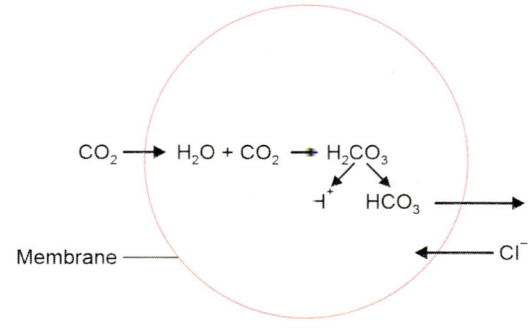

Fig. 6.22

- Importance
  - It maintains electro-neutrality as HCO_3^- easily diffuses out of the RBC
  - It increases CO_2 carrying capacity of the RBC
  - It increases unloading of oxygen, because of allosteric modification of hemoglobin tetramer by chloride.

2. What are the pressures at which gas exchange takes place at lung? Explain alveolar membrane. Mention the factors which alter the diffusing capacity of lungs.

A Gas Exchange Pressures

- The normal atmospheric pressure is 760 mmHg, of which 21% is contributed by oxygen. Thus, the partial pressure of oxygen in atmospheric air is 159 mmHg.
- The partial pressure of oxygen in the alveoli is decreased when compared to atmospheric proportion due to constant absorption into pulmonary capillaries, humidification, mixture of carbon dioxide and the fact that alveolar oxygen is constantly replaced by atmospheric air with each breath. Thus, it is 104 mmHg.

	Atmosphere	Alveolus	Blood vessels
Oxygen	159 mmHg	104 mmHg	Pulmonary artery: 40 mmHg, Pulmonary vein: 104 mmHg
CO_2	0.3 mmHg	40 mmHg	Pulmonary artery: 46 mmHg, Pulmonary vein: 40 mmHg

B. Alveolar Membrane (Fig. 6.22a)

- Also called respiratory membrane. It is very thin and has a thickness of 0.5 microns.
- It has six layers from inside outwards as described below:
  1. Monomicrolayer of surfactant
  2. It spreads on the inside of the alveolus
  3. Fluid layer that lines the alveoli
  4. Alveolar epithelium lying on a basement membrane
  5. Interstitial space
  6. Basement membrane of capillaries
  7. Capillary endothelial cells.

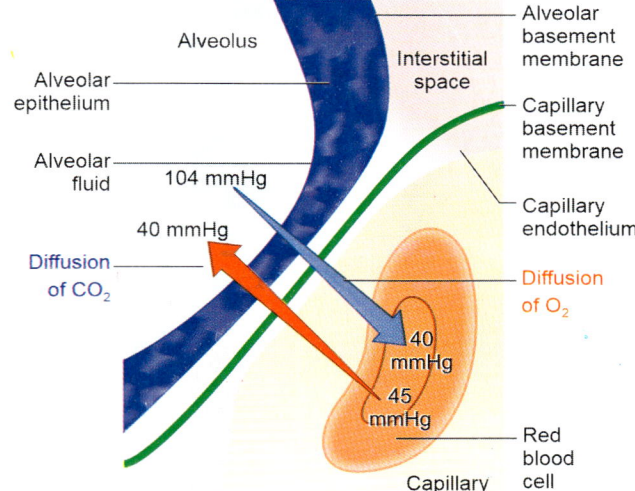

Fig. 6.22a

C. Factors Affecting Diffusing Capacity

Diffusing capacity is the volume of gas that diffuses across the respiratory or alveolar membrane in a given unit of time for a pressure gradient of 1 mmHg.
  1. Pressure gradient of a gas across the respiratory membrane
  2. Solubility of gas in fluid medium
  3. Surface area of the respiratory membrane
  4. Molecular weight of the gas
  5. Thickness of the respiratory membrane

3. Why is the oxygen dissociation curve sigmoid in shape? What are the factors which shift the curve?   (3 + 2 marks)

A. Oxygen Hemoglobin Dissociation Curve

- It represents the relationship between partial pressure of oxygen in blood and the percentage saturation of hemoglobin with oxygen (Fig. 6.23).
- It explains hemoglobin's affinity for oxygen.
- Normally, 1g of hemoglobin can carry 1.34 ml of oxygen. This is called oxygen carrying capacity of hemoglobin.
- Partial pressure of oxygen in mmHg is plotted in X axis and percentage of oxygenated hemoglobin saturation is plotted on the Y axis. Hemoglobin is saturated with oxygen when it is not able to further get oxygenated. The resultant sigmoid curve is called the oxygen hemoglobin dissociation curve.
- The steep portion of the curve represents the positive cooperation, i.e. increase in affinity of

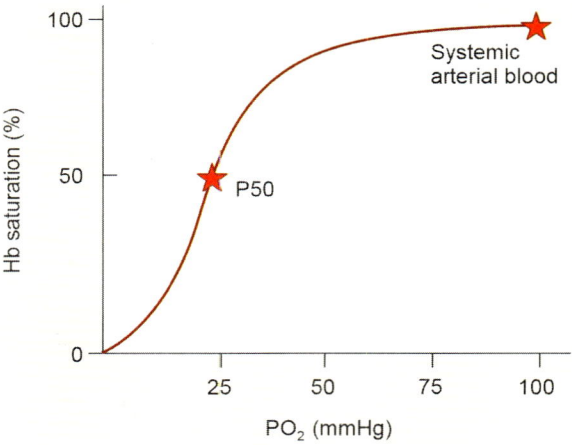

Fig. 6.23

hemoglobin to oxygen with increase in partial pressure of oxygen.

- P50 is the partial pressure of oxygen when the hemoglobin saturation is 50%. Its value is around 25–27 mmHg.
- When partial pressure of oxygen is 100 mmHg, hemoglobin saturation is 95%.

B. Causes for Shift of Curve

Shift to left	Shift to right
It indicates increased affinity of hemoglobin to oxygen Examples are 1. Fetal hemoglobin 2. Decrease in H⁺ ions in blood	It indicates decreased affinity of hemoglobin to oxygen (increase in dissociation) 1. Decrease in partial pressure of oxygen 2. Increase in partial pressure of CO_2 3. Increase in H⁺ ions in blood 4. Raised body temperature 5. Increase in 2,3 DPG in blood

SHORT ANSWERS

1. What is Bohr's effect? Give its physiological importance.

Bohr's Effect (Fig. 6.24)

- It is a concept by which oxygen hemoglobin dissociation curve shifts to right in presence of carbon dioxide.

- The mechanism under Bohr's effect is when CO_2 increases in blood, it diffuses into the red blood cell. Here CO_2 combines with H_2O to form carbonic acid. It dissociates into hydrogen ions which combine with oxyhaemoglobin to dissociate oxygen from the oxyhaemoglobin.

Physiological Significance

The advantage of shift of the hemoglobin dissociation curve is that in presence of carbon dioxide decreases haemoglobin's affinity to oxygen and thus it can carry CO_2 towards the alveoli.

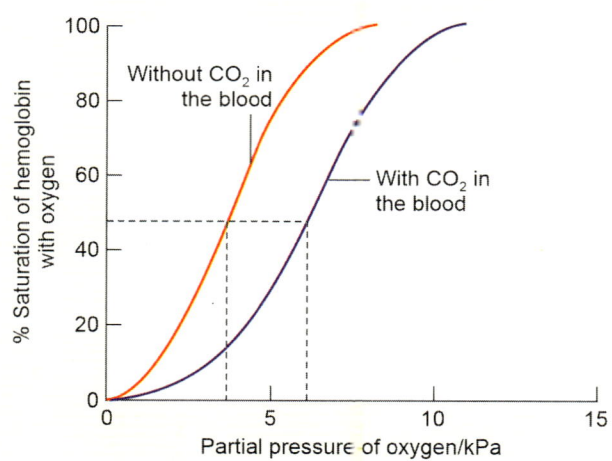

Fig. 6.24

2. Explain the differences between obstructive and restrictive lung diseases.

Parameter	Restrictive lung diseases	Obstructive lung diseases
Cause	Decreased compliance of the lung due to decreases expansibility of the lung parenchyma or the chest wall	Increased constriction of the airways causing decreased oxygenation of the lung parenchyma
Compliance and elasticity	Compliance is less, elasticity is more	Compliance is more, elasticity is less
	Examples	Kyphoscoliosis
	Interstitial lung disease (pneumoconiosis)	
	Idiopathic lung fibrosis	
	Flail chest	
	Diaphragmatic paralysis	
	Pleural effusion/hydrothorax	Bronchial asthma
		Chronic pulmonary obstructive disease
		Cystic fibrosis
		Laryngobronchitis
		Foreign body
Clinical signs	Rales, decreased chest expansion	Barrel-shaped chest
		Rhonchi, rales
Pulmonary function test	Mild decrease in FEV1/FVC	Marked decrease in FEV1/FVC
	FRC is decreased	FRC is increased
	TLC is decreased	TLC is increased

6.4 DESCRIBE AND DISCUSS THE PHYSIOLOGY OF HIGH ALTITUDE AND DEEP SEA DIVING

SHORT ESSAY

1. Explain Bends and Chokes disease. How do you prevent it?

- Decompression sickness is also called Bends and Chokes disease.
- It occurs when a person rapidly returns rapidly to normal surroundings from a region of elevated atmospheric pressure (deep sea).

Causes

1. Increased barometric pressure at the deep sea leads to compression of gases in the body.
2. Nitrogen is in the highest concentration which cannot be absorbed or utilized. Due to its fat solubility, it is in liquid state in high pressure.
3. Due to Boyle's law, volume of a gas is dependent on the pressure. Higher the pressure, lower is the volume.
4. Thus, when the person ascends suddenly to normal atmospheric pressure, the nitrogen increases in volume and forms bubbles and escapes the tissues
5. These bubbles can block vessels and ducts.

Symptoms

- Patients present with severe pain in tissues, joints
- Paranesthesia-numbness, tingling sensations and pricking pain
- There can be temporary paralysis—due to nitrogen bubbles in the myelin sheath
- Myocardial ischemia due to embolus in the coronary vessels, stroke due to emboli in the brain and spinal cord
- Finally fatigue, unconsciousness and death.

Treatment

- Prevention is the best way—there should be step-wise ascent
- Recompression chamber—patient is kept in a recompression chamber and then slowly the pressure is decreased.

6.5 DESCRIBE AND DISCUSS THE PRINCIPLES OF ARTIFICIAL RESPIRATION, OXYGEN THERAPY, ACCLIMATIZATION AND DECOMPRESSION SICKNESS

SHORT ANSWER

1. Explain hyperbaric O_2 therapy? Mention its indications. Give the significance of hyperbaric O_2 therapy.

Hyperbaric Oxygen Therapy

- In this method of treatment, pressure of oxygen used is 2–3 atmospheres.
- The patient is placed in a tank with high pressure oxygen delivered to the mouth and nose through a mask, whereas the rest of the body is surrounded by normal air compressed to the same amount of pressure.

Indications and Significance

1. In cases of carbon monoxide poisoning, central retinal artery occlusion, crush injury, compartment syndrome, severe blood loss and compromised grafts:
   - Under normal circumstances, the hemoglobin is saturated 97% under normal pressure. The dissolved oxygen is 1.5 ml/dl

- When pressure is raised to 3 atm, the dissolved oxygen content is 6 ml/dl. As a result, oxygen can reach places with compromised blood supply and thus salvages tissue from ischemic insult.

2. Air embolism:
   - With increase in pressure, volume of the gas bubble decreases (Boyle's law). Thus, it escapes and leads to reperfusion.

3. It also has effects on reducing lipid peroxidation and is thus used in crush injuries and compartment syndrome.

4. It synergises the effect of antibiotics and thus used in necrotizing infections like gas gangrene—caused by anaerobic bacilli *Clostridium perfringens*. The bacteria stop growing at a pressure of 70 mmHg. So, they are used to treat this potentially fatal condition.

5. Decompression sickness: It is formed when a person suddenly enters an area of less pressure from an area of severe high pressure (deep sea).

6. Others are osteomyelitis and myocardial infarction.

6.6 DESCRIBE AND DISCUSS THE PATHOPHYSIOLOGY OF DYSPNOEA, HYPOXIA, CYANOSIS ASPHYXIA; DROWNING, PERIODIC BREATHING

SHORT ESSAYS

1. Explain periodic breathing. Give one cause for each.

Periodic Breathing

- It is abnormal irregular respiratory rhythm.
- It is of two types: Cheyne-Stokes breathing and Biot's breathing.
  1. **Cheyne-Stokes breathing**
     - It is characterized by hyperpnea followed by periods of apnea
     - The breathing is shallow to begin with. Slowly the force of respiration increases and reaches a maximum (hyperpnea) followed by a period of minimum respiration (apnea)
     - There is over ventilation during hyperpnea which causes increased amounts of oxygen in blood. It takes several seconds to get reach the respiratory centres before it stimulates them.
     - Once the respiratory centres are damped due to over oxygenation, they lead to inhibition of respiration. As a result, the amount of oxygen in blood decreases.
     - Normally, this mechanism is damped by increased presence of oxygen and CO_2 in the cells of the respiratory centres.
     - In two conditions, these factors are impaired: Delay in transport of respiratory gases to the respiratory centres and increased negative feedback gain in the respiratory control areas. As the lungs cannot build up enough extra carbon dioxide or depress the oxygen

sufficiently in a few seconds, the next cycle of the periodic breathing begins.

Physiological causes	Pathological causes
Deep sleep	Raised intracranial pressure
High altitude	Advanced cardiac disease
After prolonged voluntary hyperventilation	Uremia
	Narcotics
After severe muscular exercise	Premature infants

  2. **Biot's breathing**
     - In this type of periodic breathing, there are periods of hyperpnoea and apnea without waxing and waning
     - During hyperventilation, carbon dioxide is washed out and the respiratory centres are not stimulated. As a result, apnea results. During apnea, increased CO_2 causes stimulation of respiratory centres leading to hyperventilation.
     - It occurs only in pathological conditions such as lesions in the brain

2. How are alveoli kept dry in the lungs? What is pulmonary edema?

Alveoli Kept Dry in the Lungs (Fig. 6.26)

- The alveoli are covered by sheets of capillaries.
- There are some features specific to pulmonary circulation that help to maintain the alveoli 'dry'.
- These differences between pulmonary capillaries and capillaries elsewhere help in keeping minimum water content in the alveoli.
  - The pulmonary capillary pressure is 7 mmHg, very low in comparison to that in peripheral tissues which is 17 mmHg.
  - The interstitial fluid pressure in the pulmonary interstitial fluid is more negative than in subcutaneous tissue present elsewhere.
  - The pulmonary capillaries are leaky to proteins than elsewhere. As a result, the oncotic pressure in the interstitium is around 14 mmHg, which is twice as much as that in peripheral tissues.
  - The surfactant which coats the inner layer off the alveolus, causes the surface tension to fall and thus does not attract more and more water molecules. This pressure is around –8 mmHg.

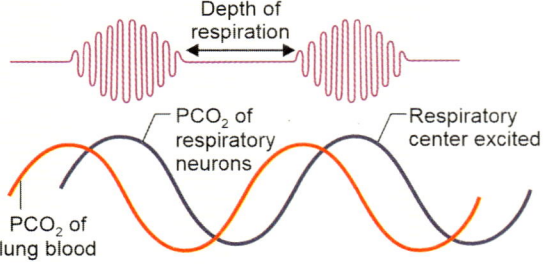

Depth of respiration

PCO$_2$ of respiratory neurons

Respiratory center excited

PCO$_2$ of lung blood

Fig. 6.25

- Also, there is evaporation of water from the alveolus.
- Thus, whatever fluid collects in the alveolus is immediately sucked into the interstitium and carried out by the lymphatics of the lung.
- Thus, it is clear that the negative pressure in the interstitium is the main factor which keeps the alveoli dry.
- The reasons for maintenance of negative pressure in the interstitium are discussed below.
- The forces which cause movement of fluid from capillaries into the interstitium
  - Interstitial fluid oncotic pressure: 14 mmHg
  - Pulmonary capillary pressure: 7 mmHg
  - Negative interstitial fluid pressure: 8 mmHg
    Total = 29 mmHg
- The forces which cause movement of fluid from interstitium into the capillaries: Plasma colloid osmotic pressure: 28 mmHg. As a result, the net filtration pressure is 1 mmHg.

Pulmonary Edema

It is the accumulation of fluid in the alveoli and pulmonary interstitium.

Causes (Fig. 6.27)

1. The alveolar membrane is made of a very thin layer of epithelium which increases its propensity to break off easily following a pressure rise in the interstitium compared to the alveolar pressure.
2. It is caused due to increased pressure by decreased pumping of left ventricle. As a result, there is back pressure on the pulmonary vessels and the

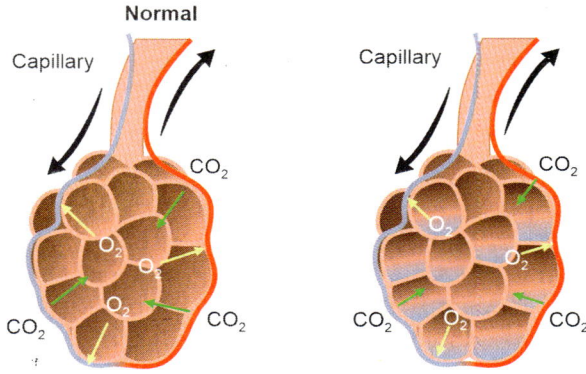

Fig. 6.27

capillaries which rupture leading to accumulation of blood in the alveoli and the pulmonary interstitium.
3. Also caused in inhalation of toxic gases like sulphur dioxide and chlorine.
4. Pneumonia also causes pulmonary edema.

Clinical Features

- Due to decreased ventilation, patients present with dyspnoea which increases on recumbent position.
- Pulmonary edema is associated with blood stained frothy sputum.
- On X-ray, it is seen as ground glass opacity of the lungs.
- Treatment is treatment of the underlying condition and loop diuretics to remove excess water from the lungs.

SHORT ANSWERS

1. Define hypoxia. Mention its types.

Definition

- Hypoxia is defined as reduced oxygen delivery to the tissues.
- Perfusion of a tissue requires 4 components to function well.
  1. Well-oxygenated blood
  2. An efficient oxygen carrying capacity of blood
  3. Adequate blood flow
  4. Ability of the cells to utilize the oxygen

Types

Based on pathologies involving each type, hypoxia can be grouped as:

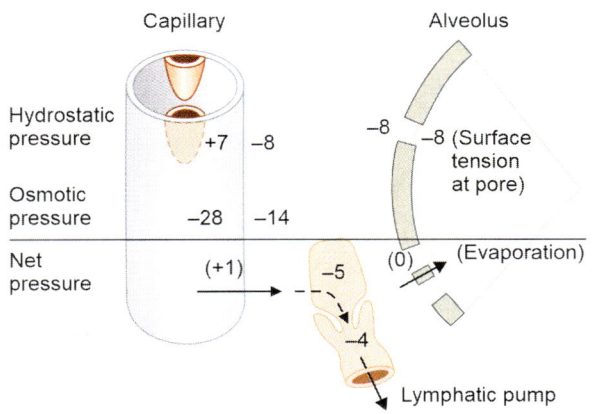

Fig. 6.26

1. **Hypoxic hypoxia**
   - Due to reduced partial pressure of oxygen in blood.
   - Causes are low oxygen tension in the inspired air, respiratory disorders causing decreased ventilation and cardiac disorders
2. **Anemic hypoxia**
   - Decreased ability of the RBCs to carry oxygen
   - It can be due to decrease in number of RBCs, decreased hemoglobin content in blood, altered hemoglobin which does not bind well to oxygen, and combination of hemoglobin with other gases like carbon monoxide.
3. **Stagnant hypoxia**
   - It results because of sluggish blood flow either due to decreased arterial blood or stasis of venous blood.
   - Causes are congestive cardiac failure, hemorrhage, circulatory collapse, thromboembolism
4. **Histotoxic hypoxia**
   - Here, the tissues are incapable of utilizing oxygen
   - Exposure to poisons and toxins (like cyanide) lead to inability of the tissues to utilize oxygen due to destruction of cellular enzymatic processes.

2. Define hypoxia, hypercapnea and hyperventilation.

A. Hypoxia

- Definition: Reduced availability of oxygen to the tissues.
- Hypoxia is encountered in pathophysiological conditions, such as atherosclerosis, obstructive sleep apnea, mountain sickness, ischemic diseases (stroke) and cancer
- Factors which lead to hypoxia are:
  - Oxygen tension in arterial blood
  - Oxygen carrying capacity of blood
  - Velocity of blood flow
  - Utilization of oxygen by the cells.
- Types of hypoxia
  1. Hypoxic hypoxia
  2. Anemic hypoxia
  3. Stagnant hypoxia
  4. Histotoxic hypoxia

B. Hypercapnea

- Definition: Hypercapnea is the increased carbon dioxide content in blood.

- Causes
- Asphyxia: blockage of respiratory pathway.
- It also occurs while breathing the air containing excess carbon dioxide content.
- Effects of hypercapnea.

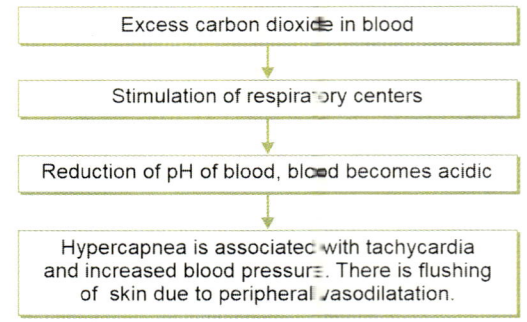

Excess carbon dioxide in blood

↓

Stimulation of respiratory centers

↓

Reduction of pH of blood, blood becomes acidic

↓

Hypercapnea is associated with tachycardia and increased blood pressure. There is flushing of skin due to peripheral vasodilatation.

Fig. 6.28

C. Hyperventilation

- *Definition:* Hyperventilation is defined as increased pulmonary ventilation or increased volume of air entering and leaving the respiratory tract.
- It is also called overventilation.
- In hyperventilation, both rate and force of breathing are increased.
- So, pulmonary ventilation also increased
- Hyperventilation mostly occurs in conditions
  - Exercise when partial pressure of carbon dioxide (pCO_2) is increased.
  - Excess of carbon dioxide stimulates the respiratory centres.
  - Voluntarily also, hyperventilation can be produced.
  - Hyper-excited states like emotional stress
- Effects of hyperventilation
  - Excessive carbon dioxide gets washed out leading to fall in partial pressure of carbon dioxide.
  - It causes suppression of respiratory centers, resulting in apnea.

3. What is hyperventilation? How does exercise-induce hyperventilation?

Definition

- Hyperventilation is defined as increased pulmonary ventilation. In hyperventilation, both rate and force of breathing are increased, and a large amount of air moves in and out of lungs. Thus, pulmonary ventilation is increased.

- It is also called overventilation.

Effects of Hyperventilation

- Excessive carbon dioxide gets washed out leading to fall in partial pressure of carbon dioxide.
- It causes suppression of respiratory centers, resulting in apnea.
- It causes suppression of respiratory centers, resulting in apnea. Apnea is followed by Cheyne-Stokes type of periodic breathing. After a period of Cheyne-Stokes breathing, normal respiration is restored.

Exercise-induced Hyperventilation

- During exercise, the skeletal muscles require more oxygen due to over work.
- As a result, more CO_2 is produced. Also, there is increase in lactic acid production in the muscles which flows into the circulation.
- Increased H^+ ions and CO_2 in blood lead to stimulation of the respiratory centres—especially the anterior group.
- It increases the rate of respiration and induces accessory muscles to work.
- As a result, depth of respiration also increases.
- Thus, it causes hyperventilation.

6.7 DESCRIBE AND DISCUSS LUNG FUNCTION TESTS AND THEIR CLINICAL SIGNIFICANCE

SHORT ANSWER

1. **What is $VO_{2\,max}$? Explain its physiological importance.**

$VO_{2\,max}$

- It is the amount of oxygen consumed under maximum aerobic respiration.
- It is calculated as a product of maximal cardiac output and maximum amount of oxygen consumed by the muscle.
- Normal values: Men: 30–35 ml/kg body wt/min, women: 30–35 ml/kg body wt/min

Physiological Importance

- It represents the amount of oxygen that is utilized by the body during maximum aerobic exercise.
- A high VO_{max} represents the endurance capacity of an athlete. It represents athletic fitness of the body.

6.8 DEMONSTRATE THE CORRECT TECHNIQUE TO PERFORM AND INTERPRET SPIROMETRY

SHORT ANSWERS

1. Explain and give the importance of forced expiratory volume 1 (FEV-1).

Forced Expiratory Volume 1

- It is the volume of air that can be expired forcefully in each unit of time: 1 second.
- It is also called timed vital capacity.
- It is a dynamic lung volume.

Importance

- Its value is 83% of total vital capacity
- It is decreased in obstructive lung diseases (like emphysema and asthma).
- It is slightly decreased in restrictive diseases like fibrosis.

2. Explain the indications and uses of spirometry.

Spirometry is a lung function test that measures lung volumes and capacities. It is used to measure the volume of air that moves in and out of the lungs.

Indications

1. The main indication is in assessment of patients who present with respiratory complaints of breathlessness, long standing cough, wheezing, etc. they help in differentiating obstructive from restrictive pulmonary disease.
2. Spirometry can be used to follow-up of cases with treatment.
3. It also helps to monitor disease progression
4. Preoperative risk assessment in a patient with underlying pulmonary pathology is done by spirometry
5. Many occupations are associated with lung damage. It can be assessed with pulmonary function test using spirometry.

Uses

1. It measures tidal volume, inspiratory reserve volume and expiratory reserve volume.
2. It measures vital capacity and inspiratory capacity.
3. It cannot measure residual volume, functional residual capacity and total lung capacity.
4. However, in clinical practice, FEV1 and FVC are commonly measured for assessing and follow up of respiratory illnesses.

6.9 DEMONSTRATE THE CORRECT CLINICAL EXAMINATION OF RESPIRATORY SYSTEM ON A NORMAL VOLUNTEER OR SIMULATED ENVIRONMENT

SHORT ESSAY

1. Perform the clinical examination of respiratory system in the given subject.

For examination purpose, the chest is divided into 9 regions on each side for the ease of examination and clarity of findings.

1. Supraclavicular area
2. Infraclavicular area
3. Mammary region
4. Inframammary area
5. Axillary region
6. Infra-axillary area
7. Suprascapular area
8. Interscapular area
9. Infrascapular area

Relevant Anatomy

- The ribs are counted from the sternal angle which forms the 2nd intercostal cartilage.
- It represents the bifurcation of trachea.
- A line drawn from the second thoracic spine to the sixth rib corresponds to the upper border of the lower lobe.
- On the right side, a horizontal line drawn from the fourth costal cartilage till the interlobar fissure marks the upper border of right middle lobe.

Respiratory System Examination

It includes:

1. Inspection of the chest
2. Palpation
3. Percussion
4. Auscultation

1. Inspection of the chest

Form of the chest
- Inspect the form of the chest. Normally, it is bilaterally symmetrical, elliptical in shape.
- Hutchison's index: The ratio of transverse to anteroposterior diameter is 7:5.
- There are usually no hollows or bulges
- In thin individuals, sternal angle may be prominent

Respiratory movements
- Look for the symmetry of movements of respiration.
- Accessory muscles of respiration like sterno-cleidomastoid may be prominent.

- Look for indrawing of intercostal muscles—a sign of respiratory distress
- The normal rate of respiration is 12–16/minute
- Type of respiration
  - Women usually have thoracic respiration
  - Men usually have abdominal respiration
  - Children have abdominal respiration
  - Some have a combination of both—thoracoabdominal and abdominothoracic.
- Also look for irregular respiration.

Apex beat
- It is the lowermost and outermost definitive cardiac impulse
- Look for the apex beat in the fifth intercostal space just medial to midclavicular line
- It is clearly seen in thin individuals but may be difficult to observe in females due to breasts and well-nourished individuals.

Position of trachea
- The position of trachea is determined by the prominence of the sternal heads of the sternomastoid muscle.
- If trachea is deviated to one side, then the sternal head on that side is prominent. This is called Trail's sign.

2. Palpation

- In this, the inspection findings are confirmed.
- Respiratory movements
  - The symmetry is checked by placing both hands on the chest at the level of the nipple such that both thumbs are approximated. When the patient takes a deep breath, both thumbs should move equally away from each other.
  - Also, chest expansion is measured with a tape. Normal expansion is around 2–4 cm.

Position of trachea
- The position of the trachea is confirmed by keeping the index finger and ring finger on the medial heads of either clavicle. The middle finger is run over the trachea.

Apex beat
- Normal position of apex beat is in the fifth intercostal space just medial to the left

midclavicular line. It is felt with the ulnar aspect of the palm.

- The apex beat can be shift based on underlying pathologies.
- Left or right ventricular hypertrophy causes left shift of the apex beat was found displaced to right suggestive of mediastinal shift.

Chest expansion
- Chest expansion is measured by keeping fingertips on either side of the midline such that the tips of thumbs meet at the midline.
- If one side moves more than the other, the movements on the other side is decreased as in this case.
- The total amount of chest expansion is measure with a measuring tape.

Vocal fremitus
- The ulnar border of the right hand is placed on various areas of the chest and the patient is asked to say 'ninety-nine' every time the hand is placed in a different area.
- It is decreased when there is pleural effusion/hydrothorax/pleural thickening. It is increased in consolidation.

3. Percussion
- The left middle finger (pleximeter finger) is placed flat on the intercostal spaces on each side and the index finger is used to percuss or strike at the distal interphalangeal joint.
- It is performed at the seemingly normal side and then the other side.
- It is best done in a methodical manner to not miss any part of the chest.
- The possible results are resonance, dullness, and tenderness.

Condition	Trachea/mediastinum
Consolidation	Central
Collapse	Pulled towards the affected side
Pleural effusion/hydrothorax	Pushed to the other side

- Apical percussion: is performed in the supraclavicular fossa
- Basal percussion: at the base of the lung to find the lung borders. Usually, liver dullness is in the sixth intercostal space on the right
- The lower border of the right lung is in the 6th intercostal space in the midclavicular line, 8th intercostal space in the midaxillary line and 10th intercostal space in the midscapular line.

4. Auscultation
- The diaphragm of the stethoscope is used to listen to breath sounds as they relatively high pitched.
- In adults, the quality of breath sounds is called vesicular. There is no pause between inspiration and expiration. The inspiratory sound lasts longer than the expiration.
- Normal vesicular sounds are heard when the lung is normally inflated.
- Vocal resonance is also performed in the same manner as tactile fremitus. The diaphragm of the stethoscope is placed in various areas and compared.
- Points to be borne in mind while auscultating
- Vesicular/bronchial breaths sounds
- Vocal fremitus/vocal resonance
- Aegophony, whispering pectoriloquy
- Added sounds like rhonchi, pleural rub, crackles

Characteristics of breath sounds				
	Duration of sounds	*Intensity of expiratory sound*	*Pitch of expiratory sound*	*Locations where heard normally*
Vesicular	Inspiratory sounds last longer than expiratory sounds	Soft	Relatively low	Over most of both lungs
Broncho-vesicular	Inspiratory and expiratory sounds are about equal	Intermediate	Intermediate	Often in the 1st and 2nd interspaces anteriorly and between the scapulae
Bronchial	Expiratory sounds last longer than inspiratory ones	Loud	Relatively high	Over the manubrium, (larger proximal airways)
Tracheal	Inspiratory and expiratory sounds are about equal	Very loud	Relatively high	Over the trachea in the neck

6.10 DEMONSTRATE THE CORRECT TECHNIQUE TO PERFORM MEASUREMENT OF PEAK EXPIRATORY FLOW RATE (PEFR) IN A NORMAL VOLUNTEER OR SIMULATED ENVIRONMENT

SHORT ESSAY

1. What is PEFR. Explain the method of measuring and interpretation of PEFR.

- PEFR is the maximum velocity of expiration (volume of air in liters per minute) that can be expelled with maximum force after a deep inspiration.
- Normal range is 350–600 liters per minute.

Method of Measurement

- The device is a small plastic cylinder with a mobile indicator within a slot that moves along a scale of numbers.

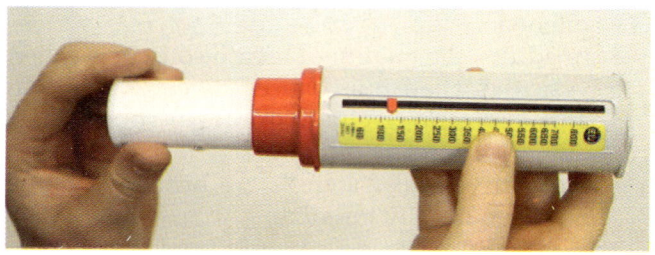

Fig. 6.29

- The opposite end has vents to let outflow of air.
- The patient is instructed to hold the mouthpiece in between the lips and seal the opening with mouth.
- He must take a deep breath and let go with a short sharp blast.
- The position of the indicator is noted, and this procedure is repeated 6 times at an interval of 1 minute.
- Best of the 6 is taken.

Interpretation

- It is decreased in obstructive lung diseases and restrictive disorders.
- The decrease is more in obstructive lung diseases— it is around 100 L/minute.
- In restrictive diseases, it is around 200 L/minute.
- It also helps to differentiate reversible from irreversible obstructive lung diseases. 20% improvement of PEFR is seen in bronchial asthma following inhalation of a short-term beta agonist. While in emphysema, there is no improvement.

Renal Physiology

7.1 DESCRIBE STRUCTURE AND FUNCTION OF KIDNEY

SHORT ESSAYS

1. Explain juxtaglomerular apparatus with a neat diagram.

Juxtaglomerular Apparatus

- It is a specialized structure found near the glomerulus.
- It is formed by three different structures: Macula densa, extraglomerular mesangial cells and juxtaglomerular cells.

  1. **Macula densa**
     - It is the thickened portion of the distal part of the thick ascending segment of the nephron.
     - It is near the afferent arteriole.
     - It consists of tightly packed cuboidal cells.

  2. **Extraglomerular mesangial cells**
     - These cells are present in the triangular space between the afferent arteriole, thick ascending limb and the efferent arteriole.
     - These are also called Lacis cells.
     - Mesangial cells within the glomerulus, surrounding the capillaries are involved in contraction of capillaries and regulating blood flow, not in juxtaglomerular system

  3. **Juxtaglomerular cells**
     - Specialized smooth muscle cells present in the wall of the afferent arteriole.
     - They are present at the junction of entrance into the glomerulus. The smooth muscles are present in the tunica media and adventitia.

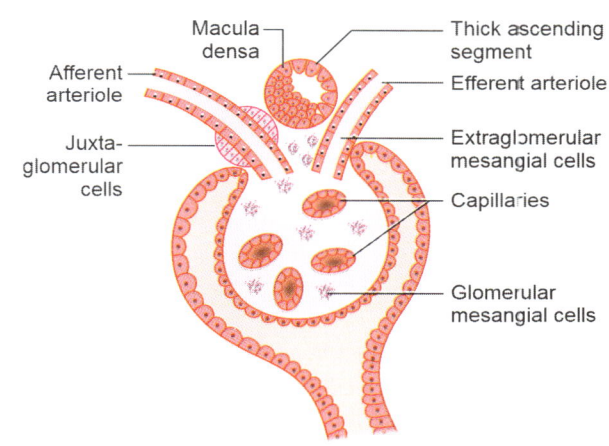

Fig. 7.1

Functions of the Juxtaglomerular Apparatus

1. Regulation of glomerular filtration
2. Secretion of renin and hormonal regulation of blood pressure.

Tubuloglomerular Feedback

- It is a local feedback mechanism for regulation of renal blood flow.
- The main component is the juxtaglomerular apparatus.

Afferent Limb

- Macula densa, a specialized part of the thick ascending limb of loop of Henle.

- It recognizes the amount of sodium concentration in the tubular fluid.
- It detects sodium concentration via the Na-K ATPase.
- The macula densa cells have Golgi apparatus directed towards the afferent arterioles.

Efferent Limb

- Juxtaglomerular cells around the afferent arteriole and the efferent arteriole.
- Mechanism
- Decreased GFR → decreased Na$^+$ ions in the macula densa

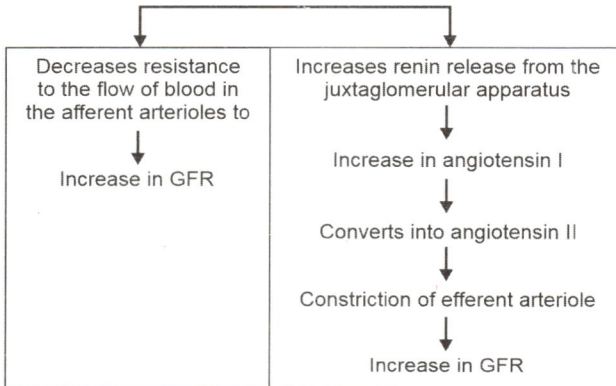

Fig. 7.2

2. Explain the peculiarities of renal circulation. What is the effect of sympathetic stimulation on renal blood flow?

Peculiarities of Renal Circulation

- As the renal arteries arise directly from the abdominal aorta, the pressure in the renal arteries is very high. As a result, it helps to filter the blood with increased filtration rate and overcoming other forces.
- The kidneys receive about 1,300 ml of blood per minute. Kidneys are the second to brain to receive maximum blood from the heart.
- Kidneys have dual circulation. The blood flows from arteries into a capillary network called glomerulus. Then, the efferent arteriole from the glomerulus divide to form peritubular capillaries. The blood reaching the peritubular capillaries is completely filtered through the glomerulus.
- As a result of high-pressure bed maintained in the glomerular capillaries, filtration results. This is the

highest pressure in capillaries in anywhere in the body.
- The peritubular capillaries form a low-pressure bed. As a result, the reabsorption form interstitium is easier.
- The vessels have a phenomenon called auto-regulation.
- It is done by two methods:
  1. **Myogenic response:** When there is increase in blood flowing in the afferent arterioles, the vessel wall is stretched. Calcium ions enter the muscle fibres. This leads to contraction of muscle fibers and causes decreased blood flow.
  2. **Tubuloglomerular feedback:** When there is increased sodium content in the distal tubule, the mesangial cells cause contraction of the afferent arteriole and reduces glomerular blood flow. This in turn reduces urine formation and also blood flow to the kidney.

Effect of Sympathetic Stimulation on Renal Blood Flow

- Increase in blood catecholamines (epinephrine and norepinephrine) causes vasoconstriction of the renal arteries and decreases the blood flow to the kidneys.

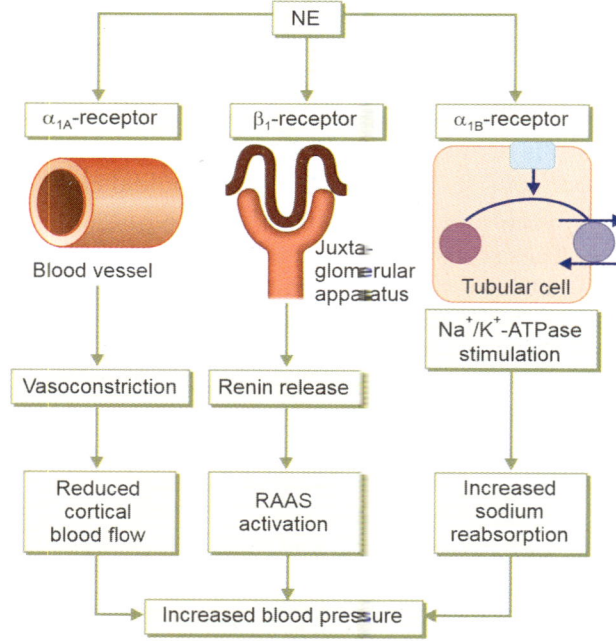

Effect of norepinephrine (NE) on renal blood flow

Fig. 7.3

- As a result, blood flowing through the afferent arteriole and thus, glomerulus decreases.
- This causes a reduction in urine formation.
- This reflex is especially helpful in cases of shock, where fluid is retained by kidneys by decreasing the urine output. Thus, decreased urine output is an important sign of circulatory shock or hypovolemic shock. Also, it helps to redirect blood to other important organs.
- The kidneys are innervated by sympathetic nerve through celiac plexus and splanchnic plexus. In times of decreased blood pressure, sympathetic nerves stimulate release of renin from kidneys.
- Renin converts angiotensinogen to angiotensin I which is converted to angiotensin II by angiotensin converting enzyme. Angiotensin II causes release of aldosterone which retains Na^+ ions from the tubules and thus retains water.

SHORT ANSWER

1. Mention the non-excretory functions of kidneys.

1. **Hematopoiesis:** Kidney secrete erythropoietin which is required for RBC production.
2. **Hormone production:** Erythropoietin, thrombopoietin, renin, calcitriol and prostaglandins.
3. **Regulation of blood pressure:** Kidneys regulate blood pressure through renin angiotensin system.
4. **Blood calcium:** Kidneys convert 1,25-dihydrocholecalciferol into calcitriol. Calcitriol helps in calcium absorption.

7.2 DESCRIBE THE STRUCTURE AND FUNCTIONS OF JUXTAGLOMERULAR APPARATUS AND ROLE OF RENIN-ANGIOTENSIN SYSTEM

LONG ESSAYS

1. A 45-year-old female patient comes for dialysis. She is suffering from end-stage renal disease with GFR <30 ml/min/1.73 m².
   - A. What is GFR? What is its normal value? **(2 marks)**
   - B. What are the factors that affect GFR? **(2 marks)**
   - C. How is GFR measured? **(2 marks)**
   - D. What is the role of dialysis in a renal disease? What are the different types and its adverse reactions? **(4 marks)**

A. Glomerular Filtration Rate

- The volume of filtrate that is formed through all the glomeruli from both kidneys in a unit of time is called glomerular filtration rate.
- Normal value is 125 ml/min.

B. Factors Affecting Glomerular Filtration Rate

- The GFR is determined by three factors: Hydrostatic pressure, colloidal osmotic pressure and Bowman's capsule pressure.
- From the above diagram, it is evident that glomerular hydrostatic pressure is positive towards formation of filtrate and the other two are opposing.
- The net filtration pressure is 10 mmHg.
- The factors that affect GFR are:
  1. Renal blood flow
  2. Tubuloglomerular feedback (autoregulation)

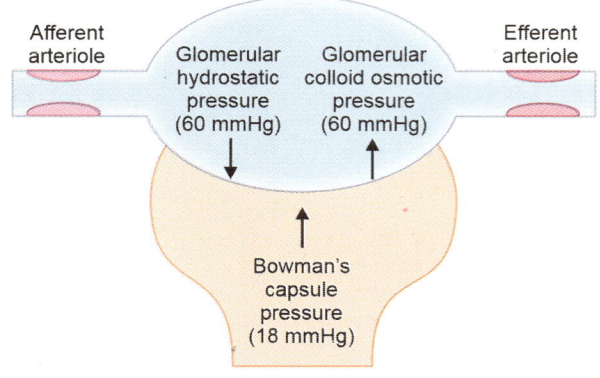

Fig. 7.4

3. Glomerular capillary pressure
4. Colloidal osmotic pressure
5. Hydrostatic pressure in the Bowman capsule
6. Pressure gradient between the afferent and the efferent arteriole
7. Systolic blood pressure
8. Sympathetic stimulation
9. Surface area of capillary basement membrane
10. Hormones like ANP, BNP, dopamine, PGE increase GFR. Hormones like angiotensin II, endothelins, noradrenaline decrease GFR.

C. Methods of GFR Measurement

1. **Inulin clearance**
   - Inulin is a substance that is neither absorbed nor digested but just excreted.
   - Thus, it is the ideal molecule that can be used to measure glomerular filtration.
   - A known quantity of inulin is injected into blood and its plasma (P) and urine (U) concentration are measured. The volume of urine (V) output is measured.
   - Glomerular filtration is calculated by the formula = UV/P

2. **Creatinine clearance**
   - It is easier than using inulin, as it is present in the blood.
   - Its concentration is calculated in urine and volume of urine is measured.
   - GFR is calculated in the same manner as inulin clearance.

D. Dialysis or Artificial Kidney

- Dialysis is a process by which solutes from an area of higher concentration to an area of lower concentration across a semipermeable membrane.
- In dialysis, patient's arterial blood passes through a dialyzer which contains minute channels placed between cellophane membranes which are porous.
- The outer surface of these membranes is surrounded by a dialysate.
- By dialysis, molecules like urea, creatinine, phosphate and others are removed from the blood.

- Dialysis is done in patients with end-stage renal disease (ESRD) which can result due to an acute or chronic insult to the renal parenchyma.

Types of Dialysis

1. **Peritoneal dialysis**
   - It is offered as first preference.
   - In this type, peritoneum of the patient acts as a dialyzing membrane.
   - The dialyzing fluid is placed in the intra-peritoneal space through a pre-placed catheter.
   - Solutes pass from the peritoneal vessels into the dialysate.
   - It is then removed after a certain amount of time.
2. **Hemodialysis**
   - A fistula is created between the radial artery and vein.
   - Blood is made to flow from the fistula into the dialyzing machine
   - The solutes from the blood pass through dialyzing membrane into the dialyzing fluid.

Complications

Peritoneal dialysis	Hemodialysis
Catheter related	Hypotension
• It inhibits movement of bowel leading to constipation	Cardiac arrhythmias—due to potassium derangement
• Intra-abdominal adhesions	and acid–base imbalance
• Catheter migration into the diaphragm	Sepsis
• Catheter kinking	Hemorrhage due to use of anticoagulants
Sclerosing peritonitis	Dialyzer hypersensitivity
Peritoneal membrane failure	

2. Explain the role of GFR, renin-angiotensin system, aldosterone and ANF in regulation of Na⁺ balance in the body.

GFR

Tubuloglomerular Feedback

- It is a local feedback mechanism for regulation of renal blood flow.
- The main component is the juxtaglomerular apparatus.
- Afferent limb
- Macula densa, a specialized part of the thick ascending limb of loop of Henle.

- It recognizes the amount of sodium concentration in the tubular fluid.
- It detects sodium concentration via the Na-K-ATPase.
- The macula densa cells have Golgi apparatus directed towards the afferent arterioles.
- Efferent limb
- Juxtaglomerular cells around the afferent arteriole and the efferent arteriole.
- Mechanism
- Decreased GFR → decreased Na⁺ ions in the macula densa.

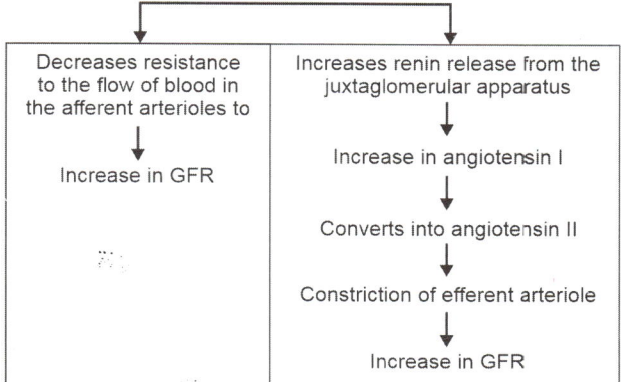

Fig. 7.4a

Renin–Angiotensin–Aldosterone System (RAAS)

- Renin is a hormone secreted by juxtaglomerular cells.
- Stimulants for renin secretion.
- It is secreted when there is a decrease in blood pressure or decreased Na⁺ concentration in the thick ascending limb.
- Sympathetic stimulation also causes renin release.
- Reduction in ECF volume.

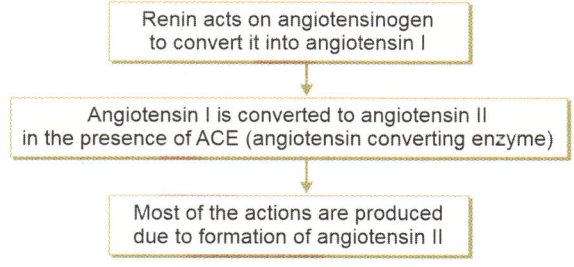

Fig. 7.5

Actions of Angiotensin II

Action on Adrenal Cortex

- It stimulates the zona glomerulosa to stimulate secretion of aldosterone, a mineralocorticoid.
- Aldosterone increases absorption of sodium from the distal convoluted tubule
- However, water is also reabsorbed. As a result, there is no hypernatremia.

Action on Kidney

- It constricts the efferent arteriole thus decreasing the glomerular filtration after an initial increase
- It decreases the surface area of the glomeruli by constriction of the mesangial cells.
- It increases sodium absorption from the proximal tubule.

Action on Brain

- It inhibits the baroreceptor area, thereby increases blood pressure.
- It stimulates the thirst centre and increases water intake.
- It also increases ADH secretion, increases water reabsorption.
- It increases CRH secretion and thus increases ACTH to release more cortisol.

Aldosterone

- It is secreted from the adrenal cortex.
- It acts primarily on the distal convoluted tubules to increase reabsorption of sodium.
- As a result, there is simultaneous water absorption.
- Thus, it increases sodium retention and increase in ECF volume and thus increases blood pressure.

ANP

- Atrial natriuretic peptide is secreted by atrial musculature of the heart.
- It is secreted in response to over stretching of atria due to increased venous return.
- Its action is mainly decreasing glomerular filtration rate by relaxation of mesangial cells and dilating afferent arterioles.

- It also causes decreased sodium reabsorption from distal tubule and collecting duct and natriuresis.

SHORT ESSAY

1. Explain tubuloglomerular feedback and glomerulotubular balance. How does it affect GFR?

Tubuloglomerular Feedback

- It is a local feedback mechanism for regulation of renal blood flow.
- The main component is the juxtaglomerular apparatus.

Afferent Limb

- Macula densa, a specialized part of the thick ascending limb of loop of Henle.
- It recognizes the amount of sodium concentration in the tubular fluid.
- It detects sodium concentration via the Na-K-ATPase.
- The macula densa cells have Golgi apparatus directed towards the afferent arterioles.

Efferent Limb

- Juxtaglomerular cells around the afferent arteriole and the efferent arteriole
- Mechanism
- Decreased GFR → decreased Na$^+$ ions in the macula densa

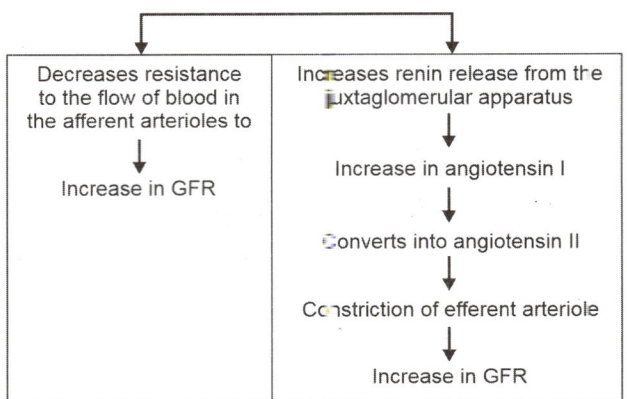

Fig. 7.5a

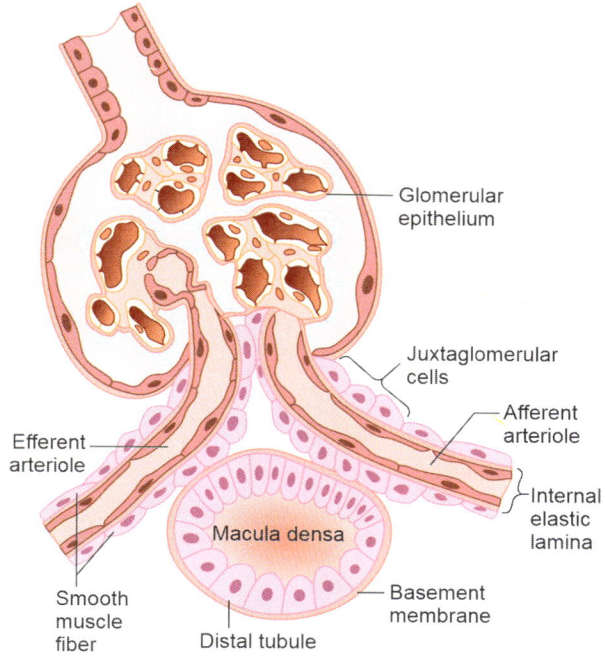

Fig. 7.6

Glomerulotubular Balance

- Normally, the GFR is 180 L/day and the tubular absorption is 178.5 L/day. As a result, only 1.5 litres of urine is formed and voided.
- If the glomerular filtration increases to 225 L/d in response to change in blood pressure of around 25 mm Hg, the urine output should magnanimously increase to 225–178.5 = 46.5 L/day which is deleterious to life.
- This does not happen, and this is due to glomerulotubular balance, due to which there is an intrinsic ability of the tubules to increase reabsorption rate in response to increased glomerular filtration.
- The amount of reabsorption in the proximal tubule is maintained at 65% of the filtrate. Some changes also take place in the loop of Henle.
- The exact mechanisms underlying these changes are not fully understood and not hormone dependent.
- Thus, glomerulotubular feedback and glomerulo tubular balance help in maintain the required osmolarity of the urine and the volume.

SHORT ANSWERS

1. Explain Starling's force. What is the net force with which water is filtered across the glomerular capillaries?

- Starling's law describes net filtration across a capillary membrane.
- Accordingly, the net filtration through capillary membrane is proportional to the hydrostatic pressure difference across the membrane minus the oncotic pressure difference.
- These pressures that determine net filtration are called Starling forces.
- There are 4 forces which determine whether the fluid flows out of blood into the interstitium or backwards.
- They are
  1. **The capillary pressure P_c:** It tends to force the fluid out of the capillary membrane.
  2. **The interstitial fluid pressure P_{if}:** If positive, it drives fluid into the capillary, and if negative, it drives fluid out of capillary.
  3. **The capillary plasma colloid osmotic pressure Π_p:** It tends to pull fluid into the capillary.
  4. **The interstitial fluid colloid osmotic pressure Π_{if}:** It tends to pull fluid into the interstitium and out of the capillary.
- If the sum of these forces is negative, there is net absorption of fluid into the capillaries from the tubular interstitium.
- If the sum of these forces is positive, there is net absorption of fluid into the interstitium from the capillaries.

$$NDP = P_c - P_{if} - \Pi_p + \Pi_{if}$$

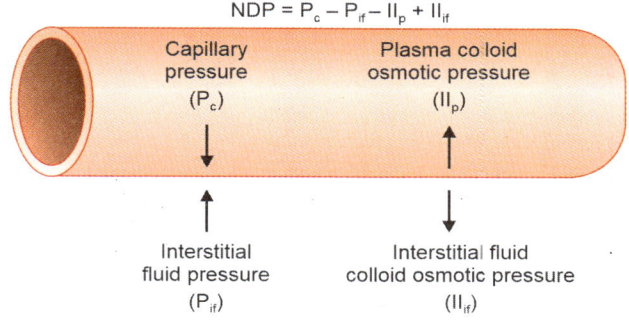

Fig. 7.7

Starling's Forces in Glomerular Filtration

- The GFR is determined by three factors: Hydrostatic pressure, colloidal osmotic pressure and Bowman's capsule pressure.
- From the above diagram, it is evident that glomerular hydrostatic pressure is positive towards formation of filtrate and the other two are opposing.
- The net filtration pressure is 10 mmHg.

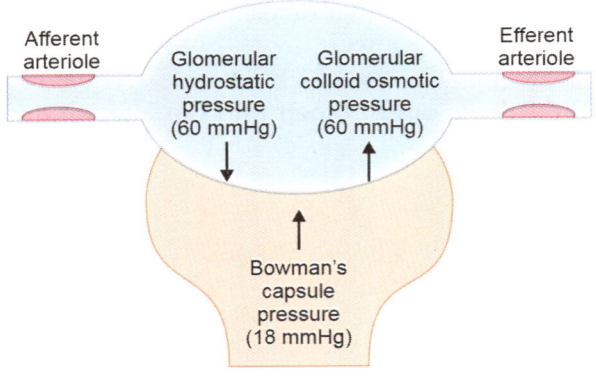

Fig. 7.7a

- As it is a positive pressure, there is a net filtration of fluid from capillaries into the interstitium.

2. What are GFR, filtration fraction and filtration coefficient?

A. Glomerular Filtration Rate

- It is the rate at which filtrate is formed from glomeruli of all nephrons of both the kidneys in each unit of time.
- Normal value is 125 ml/min or 180 L/day.

B. Filtration Fraction

- It is the fraction or part of the plasma that becomes a filtrate from the kidneys
- It is calculated as a ratio of GFR to renal plasma flow.
- Normal filtration fraction is around 15–20%.

C. Filtration Coefficient

- It is the coefficient of GFR in terms of the net filtration pressure.
- Net filtration pressure is around 20 mmHg.
- So, filtration coefficient is 125/20 = 6.25 ml/mm Hg

7.3 DESCRIBE THE MECHANISM OF URINE FORMATION INVOLVING PROCESSES OF FILTRATION, TUBULAR REABSORPTION AND SECRETION; CONCENTRATION AND DILUTING MECHANISM

LONG ESSAY

1. **Explain how renal medullary interstitium becomes hyperosmotic? What is the role of countercurrent multiplier and exchanger?**

Renal Medullary Interstitium

- The renal medullary interstitium is the surrounding tissue around the loop of Henle in the medulla.

- It is responsible for renal water reabsorption by the virtue of its high hypertonicity. As a result, water is drawn out of the thin descending limb of the loop of Henle and the collecting duct system.

- The osmolarity of the deep medullary interstitium is 1200 mOsm/L. The osmolarity gradually increases from cortex towards the medulla. This is called medullary gradient. Maintenance of osmolarity of the medullary interstitium is done by countercurrent mechanism (Fig. 7.8).

Factors Causing Hyperosmolarity of Medullary Interstitium
Countercurrent Mechanism

Countercurrent multiplier	Countercurrent exchanger
- Takes place in the loop of Henle as it extends deep into the medulla	- Takes place in the vasa recta which run parallel to the loop of Henle. Its descending limb is along the ascending limb of loop of Henle and ascending limb is along the descending limb of loop of Henle.
- This is caused by active reabsorption of Na$^+$ ions from the ascending limb into the medullary interstitium.	- Solutes which enter the medullary interstitium from ascending loop of Henle enter the descending limb of vasa recta in exchange for water molecules. So when blood reaches the ascending limb of vasa recta, it has high concentration of Na$^+$ ions. As a result, Na$^+$ ions diffuse into the medullary interstitium and water molecules enter the vasa recta. This cycle is repeated and thus the osmolarity of the medullary interstitium increases.
- As a result of increase in osmolarity of the medullary interstitium, sodium and chloride ions enter the descending limb. Thus, Na ions are circulated.	
- Urea absorption is an important step in formation of hypertonic interstitium. This is possible as most of the urea which is filtered remains in the tubule till the medullary part of the collecting ductule where it is actively absorbed. Due to its movement into the interstitium, the osmolarity increases.	- When blood passes through the ascending limb of vasa recta, sodium chloride diffuses out of blood and enters the interstitial fluid of medulla and water diffuses into the blood.
	- Recycling of urea also occurs similar to sodium chloride. When blood passes through the descending limb of vasa recta, urea diffuses into the medullary interstitium along with sodium chloride. When blood passes through ascending limb of vasa recta, urea diffuses back into the medullary interstitium along with sodium chloride. Thus, sodium chloride and urea are exchanged for water between the ascending and descending limbs of vasa recta hence this system is called countercurrent exchanger.

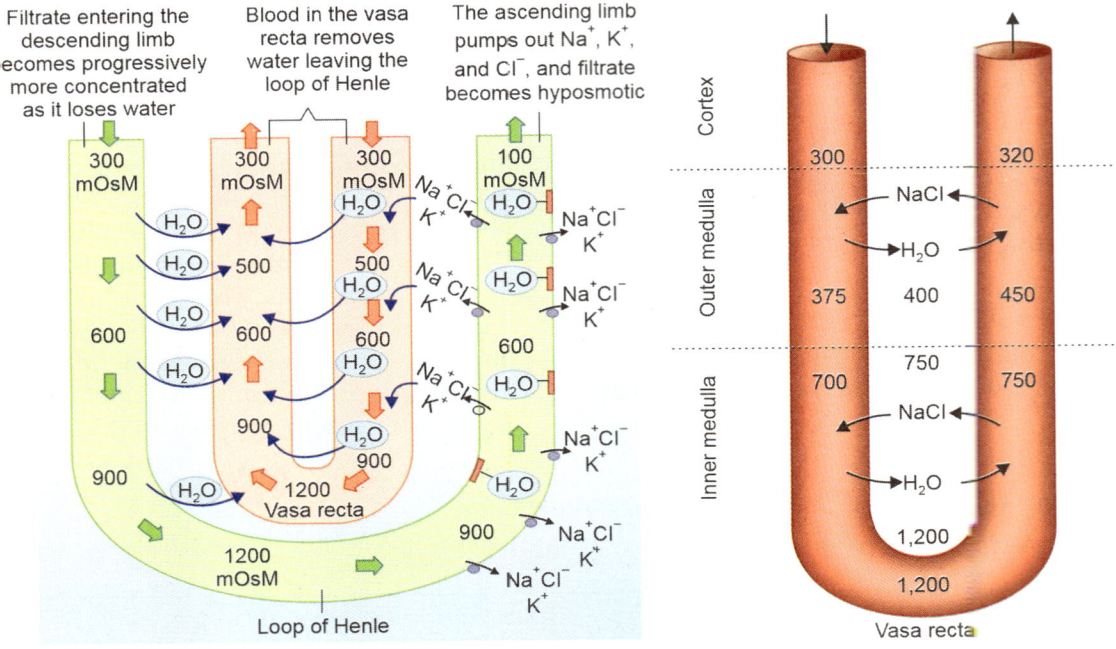

Fig. 7.8

SHORT ESSAYS

1. Explain renal handling of glucose. What is splay? Explain it with a graph.   (3 + 2 marks)

A. Renal Handling of Glucose (Fig. 7.9)

- Glucose gets filtered through the glomerulus.
- When it reaches the proximal convoluted tubule, it is completely reabsorbed along with Na ions by secondary active transport.
- Glucose and Na^+ ions bind to a carrier protein in the luminal membrane of tubular epithelium and get internalized into the cell.

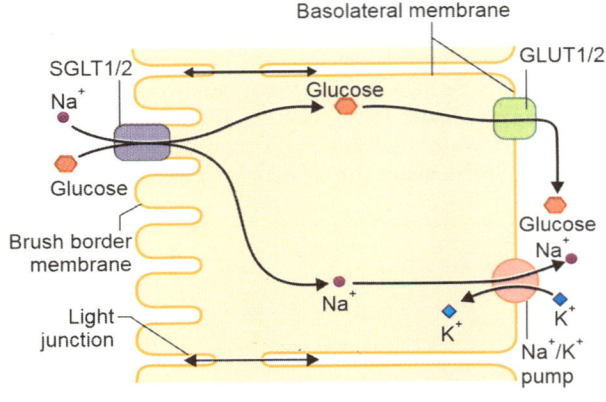

Fig. 7.9

- This carrier protein is called sodium-dependent glucose cotransporter 2 (SGLT2).
- Then glucose enters the medullary interstitium by another carrier protein called glucose transporter 2 (GLUT2).
- Renal threshold for glucose is 180 mg/dl. When blood glucose exceeds this level, it is not absorbed and appears in urine—this forms the basis for testing urine glucose in hyperglycemia/diabetes.

B. Splay (Fig. 7.10)

- Normal glomerular filtration is 125 ml/min. That means 125 mg of glucose is getting filtered every minute.
- Tubular maximum (T_m) for any compound is the maximum amount that can be absorbed by the renal tubule.
- Tubular maximum for glucose (T_{mG})
  – *Adult male:* 375 mg/minute
  – *Adult females:* 300 mg/minute.
- Thus normally, if glucose exceeds 375/125 = 300 mg/ml in blood, then it should appear in urine. But it is only 180 mg/dl.
- The main reason for this splay is that some nephrons excrete glucose in a lower than T_{mG}, and

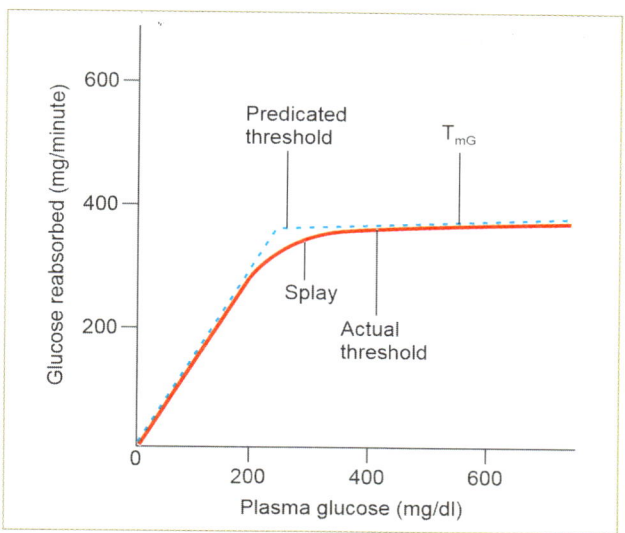

Fig. 7.10

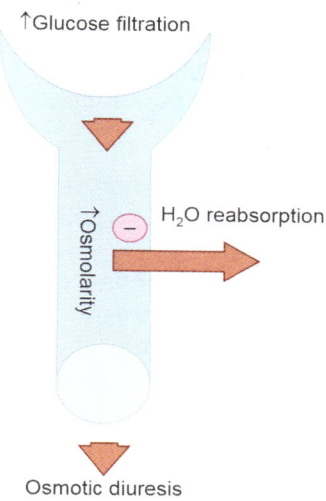

Fig. 7.11

the transport maximum for the kidneys is reached when all the nephrons reach their maximal capacity to reabsorb glucose.

- The red line represents glucose reabsorption rate with respect to blood glucose levels. It is observed that reabsorption starts well before T_m is reached.
- As a result, the curve in practicality deviates from the predicted or ideal curve.

2. What is osmotic diuresis? Explain the cause of osmotic diuresis in diabetes insipidus and diabetes mellitus.

Osmotic Diuresis

- It is the phenomenon by which there is increased urine formation due to increased osmolarity of blood due to introduction of a hyperosmolar substance in blood. These substances are freely filtered in the glomerulus but not reabsorbed.
- When the osmolarity of blood is high, the resultant filtrate in the proximal tubules is also high. As a result, the reabsorption of water is greatly reduced.
- As a result, large quantities of urine are formed.
- Substances that can cause osmotic diuresis are glucose (when more than 250 mg/dl in blood), mannitol, glycerol, etc.

Osmotic Diuresis in Diabetes Mellitus

- As stated above, plasma glucose more than 250 mg/dl causes the glomerular filtrate with high osmolarity.

- As a result, water reabsorption is decreased, and more water is lost in urine.

Diuresis in Diabetes Insipidus

- It is a condition with inadequate secretion of anti-diuretic hormone secreted from the posterior hypothalamus.
- As a result, water reabsorption is severely affected and diuresis results.

3. A 40-year-old male patient comes to medical OPD with symptoms of polyuria and polydipsia (excessive drinking of water). His blood sugars were normal, but his urine showed sugars present. He was diagnosed as renal diabetes.
A. What is renal threshold for a substance?
B. What is tubular maximum for glucose?
C. What is splay?
D. What are non-threshold substances? Give one example.

A. Renal Threshold for a Substance

- It is the concentration of a substance in plasma at which it appears in urine.
- It is specific for each substance. When it reaches the threshold in plasma, it is not reabsorbed and is excreted in urine.
- It is denoted by T_m.

B. Tubular Maximum for Glucose

- Tubular maximum (T_m) for any compound is the maximum amount that can be absorbed by the renal tubule.

- Tubular maximum for glucose (T_{mG})
  - *Adult male:* 375 mg/minute
  - *Adult females:* 300 mg/minute.

C. Splay (Fig. 7.12)

- Normal glomerular filtration is 125 ml/min. that means 125 mg of glucose is getting filtered every minute.
- Thus normally, if glucose exceeds 375/125 = 300 mg/ml in blood, then it should appear in urine. But it is only 180 mg/dl.
- Thus normally, if glucose exceeds 375/125 = 300 mg/ml in blood, then it should appear in urine. But it is only 180 mg/dl.
- The main reason for this splay is that some nephrons excrete glucose in a lower than T_{mG}, and the transport maximum for the kidneys is reached when all the nephrons reach their maximal capacity to reabsorb glucose.
- The red line represents glucose reabsorption rate with respect to blood glucose levels. It is observed that reabsorption starts well before T_m is reached.
- As a result, the curve in reality deviates from the predicted or ideal curve.

D. Non-threshold Substances

- These are substances which are not secreted or reabsorbed but simply excreted irrespective of their level in plasma.
- *Examples:* creatinine.

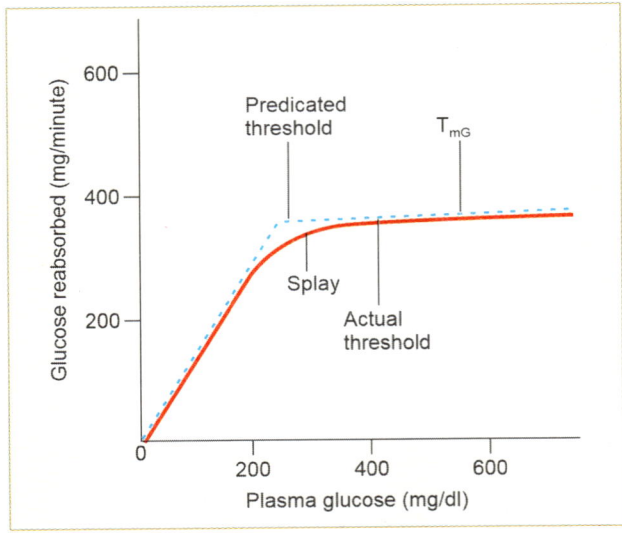

Fig. 7.12

4. Explain renal handling of sodium by kidneys. What is the role of aldosterone?

Renal Handling of Sodium

Sodium reabsorption occurs in various segments of the nephron.

1. **Proximal convoluted tubule (Fig. 7.13)**
   - Most of the sodium is reabsorbed in the proximal convoluted tubule.
   - Along with sodium, water molecules are also absorbed in high percentage.
   - Sodium is taken up within the luminal cells by active transport. It is sensitive to renin.
   - In the first part of the tubule, it is transported by sodium glucose symporter and sodium hydrogen antiport channels. It is also reabsorbed in conjunction with amino acids, phosphates.
   - In the distal part of the proximal tubule, there is high concentration of chloride ions in the lumen. Thus, chloride ions diffuse into the cells.

2. **Loop of Henle (Fig. 7.14)**
   - It contains a thin descending segment, thin ascending segment and a thick ascending segment.
   - The thick ascending segment of loop of Henle is involved in active reabsorption of sodium and water.
   - Na-K-ATPase on the basolateral surface of the luminal cells create a negative potential within the cell. The sodium-potassium-2 chloride channel on the luminal side of the cell helps in absorption of these ions within the cell.

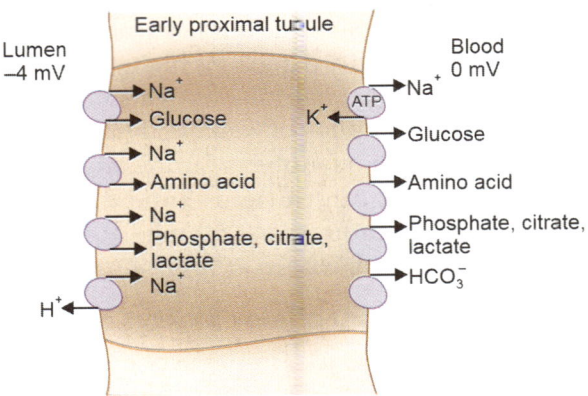

Fig. 7.13

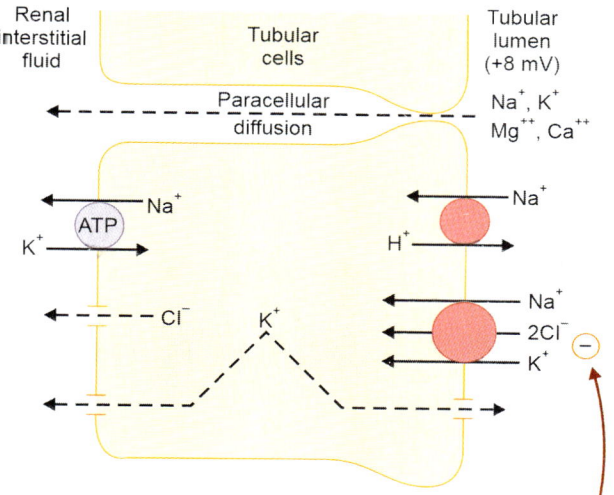

Fig. 7.14

- Sodium is also transported into the cell by Na-H antiport channel.
- There is also paracellular diffusion of Na⁺ ions.

3. **Distal tubule (Fig. 7.15)**
   - The early part of the distal tubule is a part of the juxtaglomerular apparatus. It is called diluting segment as it absorbs most of the solutes.
   - It reabsorbs sodium by sodium-chloride symporter. The sodium-potassium-ATPase transports sodium from cell into the renal inter-stitium. Thiazide diuretic acts at this symporter.
   - Late distal tubule consists of principal cells and intercalated cells. The principal cells are

involved in absorption of sodium and intercalated cells are responsible for absorption of potassium. It is sensitive to aldosterone and antinatriuretic factor. Thus, aldosterone antagonists which are used as diuretics act at this segment.

4. **Collecting duct**
   - It absorbs about 10% of sodium and water.
   - Na⁺ is absorbed through Na-H antiport.

Role of Aldosterone

- It has three main functions: Reabsorption of sodium from distal convoluted tubule and collecting ducts, excretion of potassium through renal tubules and secretion of hydrogen into renal tubules.
- In the absence of aldosterone, there is increased excretion of sodium ions into urine.
- When sodium is absorbed, proportionally water molecules are also absorbed leading to an increase in ECF volume. Thus, it leads to increase in blood pressure.

SHORT ANSWERS

1. What is the role of furosemide diuretic in reducing the blood pressure?

Role of Furosemide in Reducing Blood Pressure
- A diuretic is a substance that increases formation of urine.
- Most diuretics act by decreasing Na⁺ reabsorption and causing natriuresis (escape of sodium in urine) and thus leading to diuresis (Fig. 7.16).
- Loop diuretics like furosemide block active Na⁺ absorption from the thick ascending loop of Henle

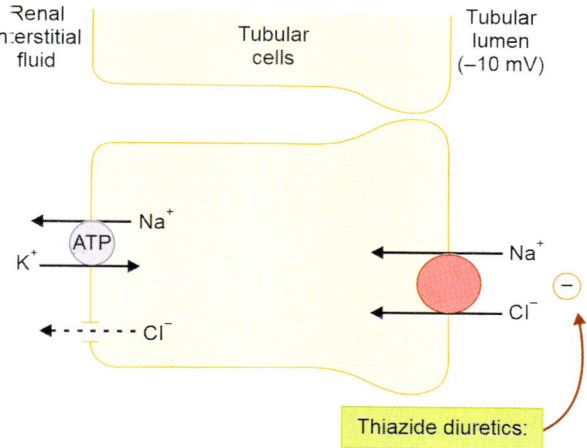

Fig. 7.15

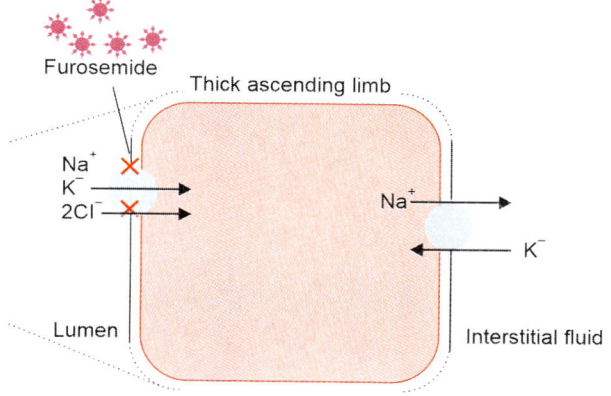

Fig. 7.16

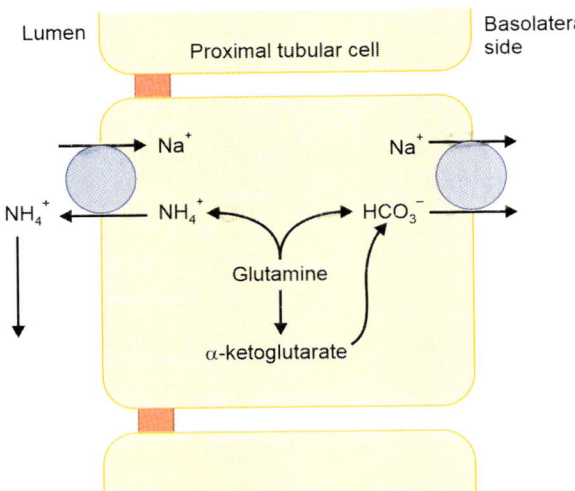

Fig. 7.17

by blocking the 1-Na$^+$, 2-Cl$^-$, 1-K$^+$ cotransporter on the luminal side of the tubular epithelium.

- As a result, the tubular fluid is rich in Na$^+$ ions and hence more sodium reaches the distal part of the nephron. As a result, more water is retained within the tubules.
- Also, they disrupt the countercurrent multiplier system by decreasing the absorption of ions from the loop of Henle into the medullary interstitium.
- As a result, a huge volume of extracellular fluid is lost.
- Thus, it decreases the blood pressure in a rapid fashion.

2. Explain obligatory loss of water. What is the minimum volume of urine required to be produced per day?

Obligatory Loss of Water

- It is the minimum amount of water that can be lost from the body.
- It is required to maintain balance of water in the body.
- Obligatory urine loss occurs to remove solutes from the body. Its value is 500 ml/day.

Components of Daily Obligatory Water Loss

Insensible loss	
• The amount of fluid lost from respiratory tract and skin	800 ml
• Occurs continuously and involuntarily	
• Cornified layer of epidermis is protective against water loss	
Minimum sweat loss	
• Highly variable, depending on temperature and physical activity	100 ml
Fecal loss	200 ml
Minimum urine to excrete solute waste	500 ml
Total:	1600 ml

3. Give the importance of ammonia secretion from renal tubules.

Ammonia Secretion (Fig. 7.17)

- Ammonia secretion in the tubules of the nephrons is an important step in acidification of urine.
- This is the most important step in acidification of urine.
- It takes place in the proximal tubule.
- Ammonia is generated within the tubular epithelium from glutamine.
- It is transported to the tubular lumen in exchange for Na$^+$ ions.
- The hydrogen that is normally excreted from the tubular epithelium combines with ammonia and forms ammonium.
- Thus, for each molecule of ammonia secreted, one H$^+$ is excreted and HCO$_3^-$ is retained.

7.4 DESCRIBE AND DISCUSS THE SIGNIFICANCE AND IMPLICATION OF RENAL CLEARANCE

SHORT ANSWER

1. What is the importance of urea clearance and creatinine clearance tests? Give its normal values.

Urea Clearance Test

- It is a clinical test done to calculate renal function of clearing urea from plasma.
- It is a metabolite of protein catabolism and blood urea is a very commonly performed renal function test.

Procedure

- It is normally occurring in the body and is secreted by the renal tubules.
- Plasma sample is tested for concentration of urea.
- Two samples of urine an hour apart is collected.
- It is calculated in the following way:

$$\text{Clearance} = \frac{UV}{P}$$

U: Concentration of urea in urine
V: Volume of urine excreted per minute
P: Concentration of urea in plasma

Normal Values

70 ml/minute

Creatinine Clearance Test

- Serum creatinine is a measure of renal function creatinine is a normally excreted end product of protein metabolism in urine.
- It is neither absorbed and secreted by the tubules of the nephron, and hence forms an ideal candidate for performing a clearance test.
- It is used to calculate the glomerular filtration rate.
- Glomerular filtration rate is calculated by the formula UV/P, where U is the concentration of creatinine in urine, V is the volume of urine per minute and P is concentration of creatinine in plasma.
- Normally glomerular filtration rate is 125 ml/min, thus 125 ml/min is the normal creatinine clearance.

7.5 DESCRIBE THE RENAL REGULATION OF FLUID AND ELECTROLYTES AND ACID-BASE BALANCE

SHORT ESSAYS

1. Explain the mechanism by which acid–base balance is maintained by the kidneys.

or

Explain the mechanism of secretion and excretion of H⁺ ions from the kidney.

- Kidney plays an important role in maintenance of acid–base balance in the plasma by excreting excess hydrogen ions (acidic) and retaining bicarbonate (basic) ions.
- Normal pH of urine 4.5

H⁺ Secretion (Fig. 7.18)

In Physiological Conditions

- Na^+–H^+ antiport: Ex-hydrogen ions are actively transported into the tubular lunar by Na^+–H^+ antiport system in exchange for Na^+ ions. This reaction is seen in proximal tubules.
- The Na^+–K^+ ATPase on the interstitial side of the tubular cells cause Na^+ ions to enter the cell.
- The H^+ ions are generated by the action of carbonic anhydrase on H_2CO_3.
- Thus, for each H^+ secreted into the lumen, one Na^+ and HCO_3^- enter the interstitium.

In Metabolic Acidosis

- Kidneys play an important role in preventing metabolic acidosis, by excreting excess H^+ ions.
- It is done by 3 methods.
  1. **Bicarbonate mechanism**
     - Excess bicarbonate and H^+ in urine combine to form H_2CO_3 (unstable). It dissociates to form H_2O and CO_2 which enter the tubular cell.
     - In presence of carbonic anhydrase, they form H_2CO_3 which is catalyzed into H^+ and HCO_3^-
     - Bicarbonate ions enter the interstitium
     - The H^+ ions are exchanged for Na^+ at the luminal end.
  2. **Phosphate mechanism**
     - In the tubular lumen, Na_2HPO_4 splits into Na^+ and $NaHPO_4^-$
     - In the tubular cell, $H_2O + CO_2 \rightarrow H_2CO_3$. It splits immediately into H^+ and HCO_3^-

- The H^+ is exchanged for Na^+
- The H^+ combines with $NaHPO_4^-$ to sodium dihydrogen phosphate

3. **Ammonia mechanism**
   - Ammonia is generated with the tubular cell from glutamine.
   - It is transported to the tubular lumen in exchange for Na^+
   - The hydrogen that is normally excreted combines with ammonia to form ammonium
   - Thus, for each molecule of ammonia formed one H^+ is excreted and NCO_3^- is retained.

Summary

1. Na^+–H^+ pump: Distal convoluted tubule
2. ATP driven proton pump: Distal convoluted tubule collecting duct
3. Bicarbonate mechanism—PCT, Henle's loop, DCT
4. Phosphate mechanism—DCT, collecting duct
5. Ammonia mechanism—PCT

2. Explain the renal reabsorption of water. What is the role of ADH and aldosterone hormone on reabsorption of water?   (3 + 2 marks)

A. Renal Reabsorption of Water (Fig. 7.19)

- Without water reabsorption, 180 ml of urine will be formed per day with an osmolality of 300 mosm/L.
- But the final osmolality of urine is 1200 mOsm/L

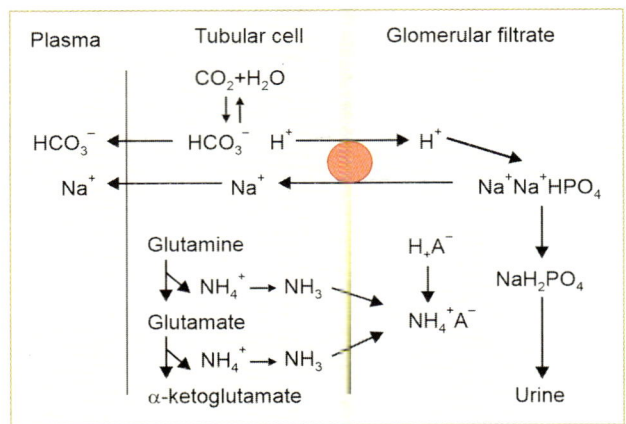

Fig. 7.18

- Tubular reabsorption is a process by which water is removed from the glomerular filtrate to return it back to circulation and cause a concentrated urine
- Osmolality of urine depends on the amount of water in the body and the role of ADH.
- The reason for concentration is the hyperosmolarity of the deep medullary interstitium which is 1200 mOsm/L. The osmolarity gradually increases from cortex towards the medulla. This is called medullary gradient. Maintenance of osmolarity of the medullary interstitium is done by countercurrent mechanism.

Countercurrent Mechanism

Countercurrent multiplier	Countercurrent exchanger
• Takes place in the loop of Henle as it extends deep into the medulla	• Takes place in the vasa recta which run parallel to the loop of Henle. Its descending limb is along the ascending limb of loop of Henle and ascending limb is along the descending limb of loop of Henle.
• This is caused by active reabsorption of Na$^+$ ions from the ascending limb into the medullary interstitium.	• Solutes which enter the medullary interstitium from ascending loop of Henle enter the descending limb of vasa recta in exchange for water molecules. So when blood reaches the ascending limb of vasa recta, it has high concentration of Na$^+$ ions. As a result, Na$^+$ ions diffuse into the medullary interstitium and water molecules enter the vasa recta. This cycle is repeated and thus the osmolarity of the medullary interstitium increases.
• As a result of increase in osmolarity of the medullary interstitium, sodium and chloride ions enter the descending limb. Thus, Na ions are circulated.	

Reabsorption of Water is Done in Five Stages

1. Bowman's capsule: The glomerular fluid is isotonic with plasma (300 mOsm/L). there is no concentration of urine in this segment.
2. Proximal convoluted tubule: In the PCT, there is active reabsorption of the sodium and chloride ions. Water molecules are driven in to maintain the osmolarity. As a result, water is absorbed but the osmolarity of the urine remains same.

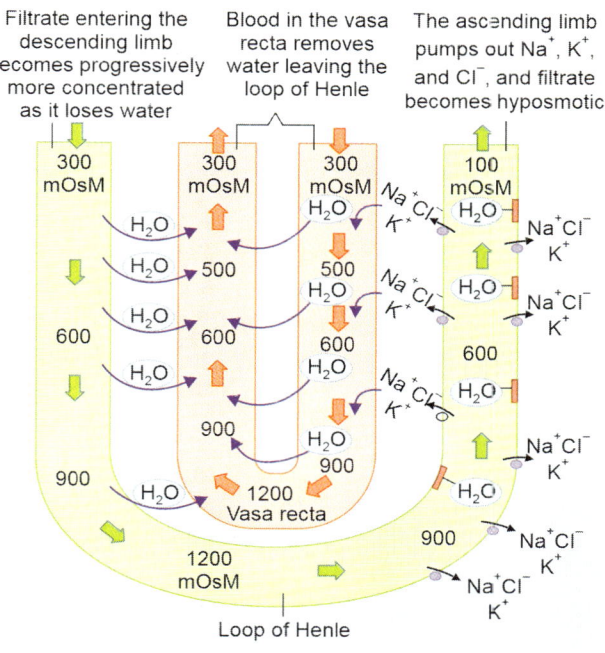

Fig. 7.19

3. Thick descending segment: This tube is slowly descending into the medullary interstitium. As a result, the water molecules are absorbed, and urine concentration becomes 450–600 mOsm/L.
4. Loop of Henle: During its descent in the loop of Henle, the concentration of urine increases to 1200 mOsm/L as it reaches the hair pin bend to match the osmolarity of the surrounding medullary interstitium. During its ascent, the concentration decreases again as the osmolarity of the surrounding interstitium also decreases.
5. Thick ascending segment: This segment is impermeable to water. But it allows exit of Na$^+$ and Cl$^-$ ions. Here fluid becomes hypotonic to plasma.

B. Role of ADH and Aldosterone in Water Reabsorption

ADH

- Final concentration of urine is achieved by the action of ADH anti-diuretic hormone
- When fluid enters the distal convoluted segment and the collecting duct, presence of ADH makes it permeable to water and water gets reabsorbed.
- Water is absorbed through aquaporin channels
- The fluid that reaches the DCT is hypotonic. In presence of ADH, the osmolarity of the urine becomes as high as the medullary interstitium.

- As large amounts of fluid enter the cortical interstitium, water is swept away by the peritubular capillaries. Also, it helps maintain the high osmolarity of the medullary interstitium.
- As the fluid enters the medullary part of the collecting ducts, there is further absorption of water into the interstitium.
- In the absence of ADH, the tubule is impermeable to water and thus dilute urine is formed. This condition is called diabetes insipidus (insipid = dilute)

Aldosterone

- It has three main functions: Reabsorption of sodium from distal convoluted tubule and collecting ducts, excretion of potassium through renal tubules and secretion of hydrogen into renal tubules.
- In the absence of aldosterone, there is hyper-excretion of sodium ions into urine.
- When sodium is absorbed, proportionally water molecules are also absorbed leading to an increase in ECF volume. Thus, it leads to increase in blood pressure.

7.6 DESCRIBE THE INNERVATIONS OF URINARY BLADDER, PHYSIOLOGY OF MICTURITION AND ITS ABNORMALITIES

SHORT ESSAYS

1. Describe micturition reflex. Write a note on atonic bladder.

Micturition Reflex

It is a reflex by which voiding of urine takes place.

Pathway

Afferent

- Stretch receptors are stimulated by the stretching of bladder when the volume of urine collected is around 300–400 ml.
- These relay in the S2, S3 and S4 segments of the spinal cord via the pelvic nerve (sensory fibers).

Efferent

- From the sacral segments of the spinal cord, the motor fibers travel through the pelvic nerve and innervate the detrusor muscle and the internal urethral sphincter.
- The detrusor contracts and as a result, the urine from bladder enters the urethra.
- Stretch receptors of the urethra get stimulated when urethra is distended with urine.
- They send impulses via the pelvic to the sacral segments.
- The efferent inhibits the pudendal nerve which relaxes the external urethral meatus and leads to voiding of urine.

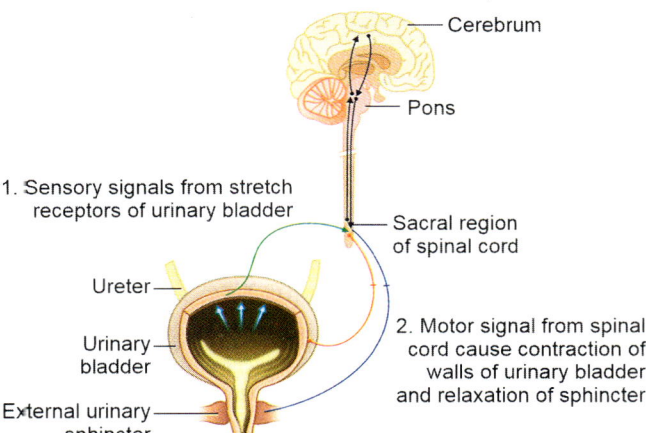

1. Sensory signals from stretch receptors of urinary bladder

Cerebrum

Pons

Ureter

Urinary bladder

External urinary sphincter

Sacral region of spinal cord

2. Motor signal from spinal cord cause contraction of walls of urinary bladder and relaxation of sphincter

Fig. 7.20

- Micturition reflex is self-regenerative, and the cycle continues till the bladder is completely empty.

Higher Centres for Micturition

Centres in midbrain ad cortex inhibit micturition by suppressing spinal micturition centres.

Atonic Bladder

- Usually seen in injury to spinal cord at the level of sacral segments. It is also seen in neurosyphilis.
- It is also called flaccid neurogenic bladder or hypoactive neurogenic bladder.

Characteristics

- The sensory supply is lost
- As a result, the bladder fills, and the patient does not have any sensation of filled bladder.
- When the volume of urine collected surpasses the bladder's capacity, the urine overflows.
- This is called overflow incontinence.

2. Explain micturition reflex. Write a note on spastic neurogenic bladder.

Micturition Reflex

It is a reflex by which voiding of urine takes place.

Pathway (Fig. 7.20a)

Afferent

- Stretch receptors are stimulated by the stretching of bladder when the volume of urine collected is around 300–400 ml.
- These relay in the S2, S3, S4 segments of the spinal cord via the sensory fibers of the pelvic nerve.

Efferent

- From S2, S3, S4 segments of the spinal cord, the motor fibers travel through the pelvic nerve and innervate the detrusor muscle and the internal urethral sphincter.
- The detrusor contracts and as a result, the urine from bladder enters the urethra.
- The stretch receptors of the urethra are stimulated when urethra gets distended by the filling of urine
- They send impulses via the pelvic to the sacral segments.

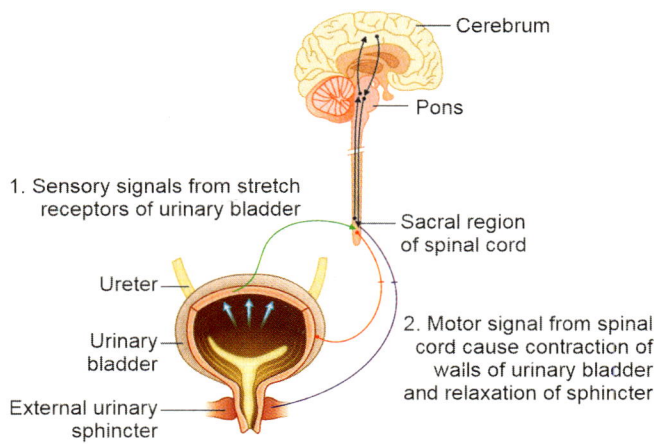

Fig. 7.20a

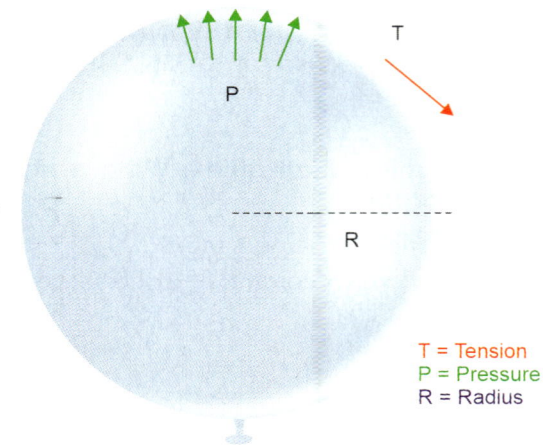

T = Tension
P = Pressure
R = Radius

Fig. 7.21

- The efferent inhibits the pudendal nerve which relaxes the external urethral meatus and leads to voiding of urine.
- Micturition reflex is self-regenerative, and the cycle continues till the bladder is completely empty.

Higher Centres for Micturition

Centres in midbrain and cortex inhibit micturition by suppressing spinal micturition centres.

Spastic Neurogenic Bladder

- It is due damage to the nerve above spinal level causing uninhibited signals from the brain
- It is caused by lesions in the midbrain
- In normal conditions, gradual filling of bladder causes excitation of the stretch receptors. Excitation of the pudendal nerve causes relaxation of the external and internal urethral sphincter. The parasympathetic nerves contract the detrusor muscles.
- In this condition, even small quantities of urine stimulate contraction of the detrusor and frequent voiding of urine. It becomes over reactive.

SHORT ANSWERS

1. Explain Laplace low. How does it explain micturition reflex?

Laplace's Law

- According to Laplace's law, the pressure within a sphere is inversely proportional to its radius, if the tone is kept constant (Fig. 7.21).
- That is, when radius increases, the pressure falls and vice versa provided the tone remains constant.

$P = T/R$ (P is pressure, T is tension and R is the radius)

Micturition Reflex and Implication of Laplace's Law

- Filling of the bladder studies using a cystometrogram.
- It has three phases: Phase 1—a steep slope, phase 2—a plateau and phase 3—a second sharp slope
- The phase 2 of this cystometrogram is explained by Laplace's law.
- In the phase 2, the volume of the bladder increases due to relaxation of the detrusor and thus it does not cause increase in pressure.
- The pressure in the bladder is around 10 cm of H_2O with a volume of 100 ml.
- It remains same even with increase in volume up to 400 ml as the detrusor relaxation.
- Thus, in the equation $P = T/R$, as the tension within the bladder wall increases with filling of urine, and radius also increases due to distension. P remains constant.
- After around 400 ml of urine collection, the pressure in the bladder rises sharply and Laplace's law does not hold good. The stretch receptors are stimulated leading to a micturition reflex.

2. What is automatic bladder? Mention one cause.

- Automatic bladder refers to a condition where urinary bladder is hyperactive and has lost voluntary control

- As a result, there is increase in frequency of urine.
- Whenever the bladder gets filled there is a desire to void urine, but there is no voluntary control
- It is also called detrusor sphincter asynergia as bladder and sphincter cannot coordinate.

Causes

1. It occurs in the second phase of recovery from complete transection of spinal cord above S2.
2. Following this type of injury, the urinary bladder loses the tone and becomes flaccid resulting in overflow incontinence.
3. During recovery, there is micturition reflex but no voluntary control. Voluntary control of the bladder is lacking because of inhibition micturition by higher centres.
4. There is hypertrophy of detrusor muscles so that the capacity of bladder reduces.

3. What type of bladder abnormality occurs in spinal shock?

- Spinal shock results due to acute spinal cord injury and causes an atonic bladder.
- Autonomic innervation of the bladder by the parasympathetic nerves is affected.
- When the sensory fibers of the pelvic nerve are destroyed, the bladder is filled but cannot conduct any sensory stretch signals to spinal cord.
- As a result, the bladder is completely filled with urine without any desire to micturition.
- Detrusor muscle loses its tone and becomes flaccid.
- Urine dribbles as and when it enters the bladder. It is called overflow incontinence or overflow dribbling.
- Conscious awareness of bladder filling is lost.
- Post spinal shock, involuntary and uncoordinated bladder contraction occurs.

7.7 DESCRIBE ARTIFICIAL KIDNEY, DIALYSIS AND RENAL TRANSPLANTATION

SHORT ANSWERS

1. What is artificial kidney? Mention the indications of dialysis.

Artificial Kidney (Fig. 7.22)

- It is the machine used for conducting dialysis.
- Dialysis is a process by which solutes from an area of higher concentration to an area of lower concentration across a semipermeable membrane.
- In the artificial kidney, patient's arterial blood passes through a dialyzer which contains minute channels placed between cellophane membranes which are porous.
- The outer surface of these membranes is surrounded by a dialysate.
- By dialysis, molecules like urea, creatinine, phosphate and others are removed from the blood.
- The rate at which blood gets dialysed is 200–300 ml/min. The total process takes 4–6 hours.

Indications for Dialysis

1. Uremia is the most important indication for dialysis. It can be due to chronic kidney disease or acute kidney injury.
2. Metabolic acidosis due to renal failure
3. Removal of certain toxins which are water-soluble like lithium, methanol, ethylene glycol, salicylates, valproate, etc.

4. Severe hyperthermia
5. Refractory hypercalcemia

2. Write a note on renal transplantation.

Renal Transplantation

- Transplantation is a process by which organ from a living donor is transplanted into a host.
- Organs that can be transplanted from live persons are liver, kidney (Fig. 7.23).

Indications

1. End-stage renal disease due to various reasons (infections, diabetic nephropathy, autoimmune conditions) not helped by dialysis
2. Malignancy of the kidney
3. Developmental anomalous kidneys (polycystic kidney)
4. Inborn errors of metabolism.

Contraindications

1. Cardiac and pulmonary insufficiency
2. Infections like HIV, hepatitis C

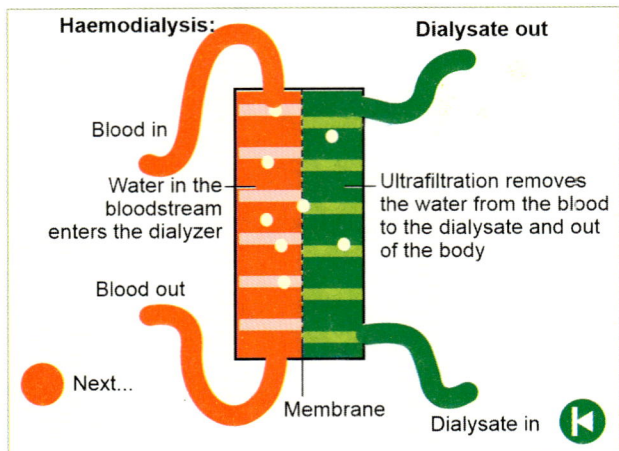

Fig. 7.22

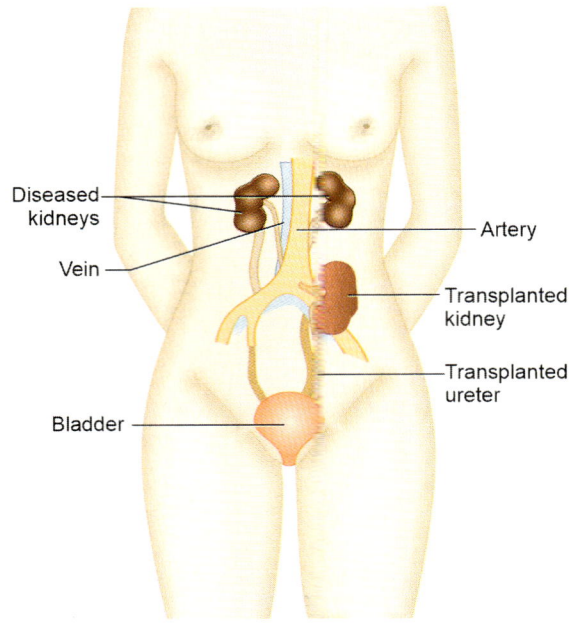

Fig. 7.23

Source of Donor Kidney

- Can be harvested from brain dead donor
- Living relative, HLA matched
- Living, HLA matched donor

Physiology of Organ Donation

- When a foreign substance is introduced into the body, the cells mount an immune reaction and damage it.
- As a result, the graft/transplant fails, and the purpose is defeated.
- The host is immunocompromised using various drugs.

- The donor blood and cells are taken, and HLA matching is done. There should be ABO and HLA compatibility.

Procedure

- The renal artery of the new kidney is attached to the external iliac artery of the host.
- The renal vein of the donor kidney relates to the external iliac vein of the host.
- Then the donor ureter is attached to the urinary bladder.

7.8 DESCRIBE AND DISCUSS RENAL FUNCTION TESTS

SHORT ESSAY

1. Explain 4 renal function tests.

- Renal function tests are tests performed to assess the functions of kidney.
- They are of three types
  1. **Urine analysis:** Macroscopic and microscopic analysis, biochemistry analysis for sugars, proteins, ketones, etc.
  2. **Serum analysis:** For urea and creatinine, blood urea nitrogen.
  3. **Clearance tests:** Tests both blood and urine

Urine Analysis

Physical Examination

- Urine is examined for color, specific gravity, pH and osmolarity.
- Increase in urine volume is associated with kidney disorders such as chronic renal failure, diabetes insipidus and glycosuria.
- Abnormal colour of urine is seen in disorders such as jaundice, hematuria, hemoglobinuria, medications, excessive urobilinogen.
- Specific gravity is low in diabetes insipidus and high in diabetes mellitus, acute renal failure and excess medications.
- Osmolarity of urine is decreased in diabetes insipidus.
- The pH decreases in renal diseases.

Microscopic Examination

- Presence of red blood cells in urine is suggestive of glomerular disease such as glomerulonephritis.
- White blood cells increase in urinary tract infection and acute glomerulonephritis.
- Presence of numerous epithelial cells indicates tubular necrosis and nephrotic syndrome
- Bacteria are commonly detected in urine specimens because of normal microbial flora of urinary tract, urethra. Due to their ability to multiply rapidly in urine.

Chemical Analysis

- Presence of glucose in urine is indicator for diabetes mellitus

- Presence of excess protein such as albumin (proteinuria) in urine indicates renal diseases.
- Ketonuria (presence of ketone bodies in urine) occurs in diabetes mellitus, prolonged starvation and glycogen storage diseases.
- Bilirubin appears in urine (bilirubinuria) in hepatic jaundice.
- Excess of urobilinogen in urine indicates hemolytic jaundice.
- Presence of bile salts in urine indicates jaundice.
- Presence of blood in urine (haematuria) indicates glomerulonephritis, renal stones
- Hemoglobin appears in urine (haemoglobinuria) during excess hemolysis.

Serum Analysis

Blood Urea

- It is a very commonly ordered simple renal function test
- Urea is formed when proteins are broken down in the liver
- Its normal value is 7–20 mg/dl or 2.5–7.1 mmol/L

Blood Urea Nitrogen

- Blood urea nitrogen, on the other hand, is a measure of the amount of nitrogen in the body.
- Each mol of urea contains 28 g of nitrogen. Thus, a serum concentration of 28 mg/dl of BUN is equivalent to 60 mg/dl of urea.
- BUN/creatinine gives the non-protein nitrogen value which is helpful in differentiating pre-renal and renal causes for acute kidney failure.

Clearance Tests

Urea Clearance Test

- It is a clinical test done to calculate renal function of clearing urea from plasma.
- It is a metabolite of protein catabolism and blood urea is a very commonly performed renal function test.

Procedure

- It is normally occurring in the body and is secreted by the renal tubules.
- Plasma sample is tested for concentration of urea.
- Two samples of urine an hour apart is collected.

- It is calculated by using the formula
  Clearance = UV/P
  U: Concentration of urea in urine
  V: Volume of urine excreted per minute
  P: Concentration of urea in plasma

Normal Values

70 ml/minute.

Creatinine Clearance Test

- Creatinine is a normally excreted product of protein metabolism in urine.

- Serum creatinine is a measure of renal function.
- It is neither absorbed and secreted by the tubules of the nephron, and hence forms an ideal candidate for performing a clearance test.
- It is used to calculate the glomerular filtration rate. Glomerular filtration rate is calculated by the formula UV/P, where U is the concentration of creatinine in urine, V is the volume of urine per minute and P is plasma concentration of creatinine.
- Normally glomerular filtration rate is 125 ml/min, thus 125 ml/min is the normal creatinine clearance.

7.9 DESCRIBE CYSTOMETRY AND DISCUSS THE NORMAL CYSTOMETROGRAM

SHORT ESSAY

1. Describe cystometrogram with graphical representation.

- Cystometry (cyst = bladder, metry = measurement) is a method used to study the relation between pressure within the urinary bladder and volume of urine in the bladder.
- Cystometrogram represents the changes in pressure with respect to differential change in volume of urine collected in the bladder.

Procedure of Recording Cystometrogram

- The urinary bladder is catheterized by a double lumen catheter.
- Through one of the lumens, fluid is infused into the bladder and the other port is used to insert a pressure sensor to record changes by connecting it to an amplifier.
- First, the bladder is emptied completely.
- Then, a known quantity of fluid is infused at regular intervals and the intravesical pressure is recorded continuously.
- A graph is plotted with intravesical pressure along the Y axis and volume inside the bladder along the X axis.

Description of Cystometrogram

A cystometrogram typically has three segments.

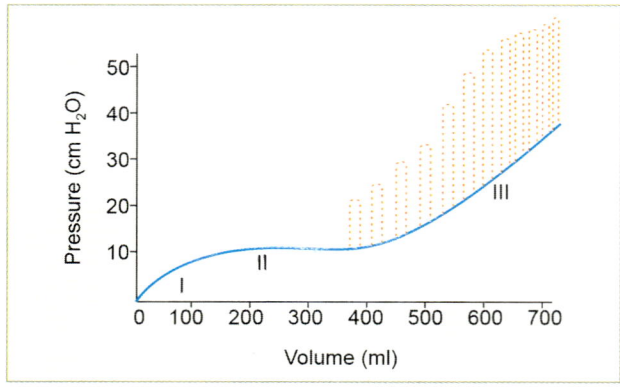

Fig. 7.24

Segment I

- Initially the pressure is zero when there is no urine inside.
- After 100 ml of infusion, the pressure rises sharply to about 10 cm H_2O.

Segment II

- Segment II is a plateau, i.e there is no change in pressure with a volume increasing even up to 300–400 Ml
- This is explained by Laplace's law and the tone in the wall of the bladder is constant.
- It is due to relaxation of the detrusor and thus accommodates more volume.
- When the intravesical volume rises beyond 400 ml, there is a steep increase in pressure.

  #### Laplace's law
  - In an isotonic spherical hollow organ, the pressure within it varies inversely to its radius.
  - If radius is more, the pressure is less and if radius is less the pressure is more, provided the tone remains constant.

  $$P = \frac{T}{R}$$

  - Where, P = Pressure T = Tension R = Radius
  - Accordingly, in the bladder, the pressure increases as the urine is filled provided tone is constant.

Segment III

- In this segment, there is a steep progressive increase in the intravesical pressure with collection of 300 to 400 ml of fluid, the tone of the detrusor muscle becomes more and more intense in a crescendo fashion, increasing the sensation and the urge to urinate.
- However, an individual can tolerate up to volume of 600 to 700 ml by voluntary control after which the intravesical pressure rises above 40 cm H_2O, the detrusor muscle contracts intensely and is beyond voluntary control of urination or micturition.
- At this stage, pain sensation develops and micturition results.

Chapter

8

Endocrine Physiology

LONG ESSAYS

1. Describe the hormonal regulation of calcium homeostasis. What is hypocalcemic tetany?
(7 + 3 marks)

Hormonal Metabolism of Calcium

- Calcium is involved in numerous biological processes throughout the body.
- Calcium homeostasis depends on the intricate yet meticulous interplay among its absorption, exchange between plasma and bone and finally its excretion.
- These three processes are governed by the action of parathormone and 1,25-dihydroxycholecalciferol.

Decrease in Serum Calcium

- It may be due to decreased uptake or due to increase in excretion or increased uptake by the bones.
- This causes release of parathormone from the parathyroid glands and release of 1,25-dihydroxycholecalciferol from the kidneys.
- Parathormone brings about resorption of calcium from the bones and increases serum calcium levels. Similar action is brought about by calcitriol.
- 1,25-dihydroxycholecalciferol increases absorption of calcium from the intestine.

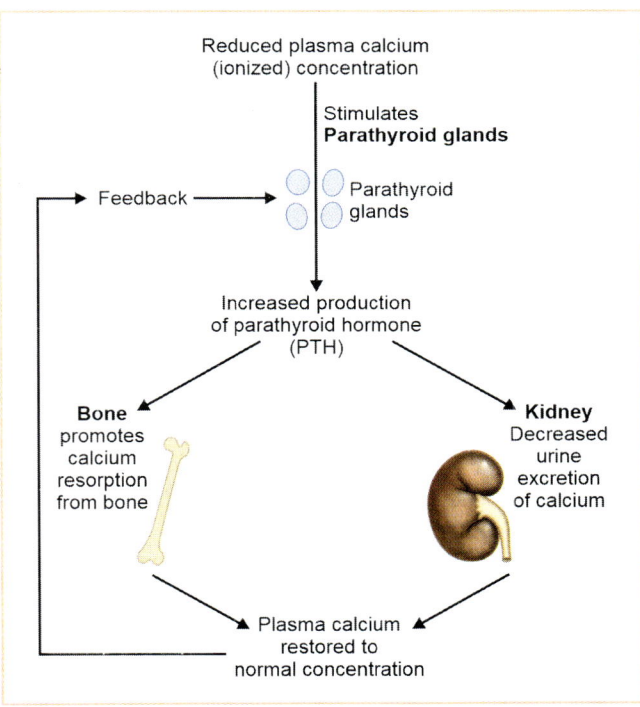

Fig. 8.1

Increase in Serum Calcium (Fig. 8.2)

Tetany

- It is abnormal painful spasm of muscles, especially of the extremities.

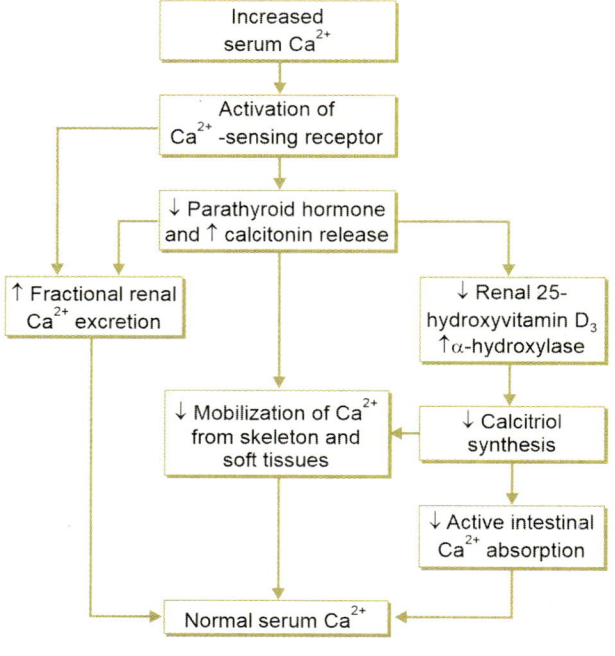

Fig. 8.2

- It occurs due to hyperexcitability of nerves and muscles due to hypocalcemia.

Causes

1. Hypocalcemia

- Normal range is 9–11 mg/dl in blood
- Tetany occurs when calcium levels fall below 6 mg/dl.
- Following massive blood transfusions—hypocalcemia occurs due to citrate overload.
- Hypoparathyroidism—primary or secondary
- Use of bisphosphonates for no metastasis
- Hyperventilation (either voluntary or involuntary) causes carbon dioxide wash out and causes respiratory alkalosis. Alkalosis precipitates calcium in blood. Vitamin D deficiency in infants can cause severe hypocalcemia and tetany.
- Severe vitamin D deficiency can cause hypocalcemia and tetany.

2. Hypomagnesemia

3. Alkalosis: It precipitates calcium ions and thus causes hypocalcemia

4. Oxalosis: Increased oxalates in blood precipitate calcium and cause hypocalcemia.

Clinical Features

- Hyperreflexia occurs due to hyperexcitability of nerves, which could later become convulsive.
- Carpopedal spasm
- It is pathognomonic for hypocalcemic tetany
- It is characterised by spasm of small muscles of hand in the form of a peculiar fashion, also known as main d'accoucheur (obstetrician's hand)
- It is characterised by:
  - Flexion at the wrist
  - Adduction of the thumb
  - Flexion at the carpometacarpal joints and hyperextension at the interphalangeal joints.
- Positive trousseau sign
- It is elicitation of carpopedal spasm by applying pressure over the brachial artery with a BP cuff and inflating it more than the systolic blood pressure for around 3 minutes.
- It may be accompanied by other signs of hypocalcemia like laryngeal stridor, positive Chvostek's sign and ECG changes.

SHORT ESSAY

1. State the normal serum calcium levels and give the important functions of calcium.　(5 marks)

Normal Serum Calcium Levels

9–11 mg/dl or 2.5 mmol/L

Diffusible: 6 mg/dl	Non-diffusible: 4 mg/dl	
Ionized: 5 mg/dl	Complexed: 1 mg/dl	Bound to albumin: 4 mg/dl (almost 40%)

Functions of Calcium

1. Calcium is an important component of bone and teeth and thus helps in their development. Calcium is also stored in the bones.
2. It is an important component for conduction at synapses. Inflow of calcium causes release of neurotransmitters. Also, calcium influx is associated with muscular contraction. It activates ATPase, which increases the interaction between actin and myosin.
3. Calcium forms an important part of blood coagulation. It is also called factor IV.
4. Calcium influences entry of many other solutes and water into the cell and thus helps in maintaining the integrity of the cell and its membrane.

5. Mediation of intracellular action of a hormone by acting as a second messenger in hormones like epinephrine.

6. It is necessary for activation of certain enzymes like pancreatic lipase, succinate dehydrogenase and ATPase. It also associates with calmodulin (calcium binding protein) and activates certain of the enzymes like adenyl cyclase.

7. It regulates cellular activities like endocytosis and exocytosis. Cell motility is also governed by calcium through its action on microtubules.

8. It prolongs systole of the heart by acting on the muscles.

8.2 DESCRIBE THE SYNTHESIS, SECRETION, TRANSPORT, PHYSIOLOGICAL ACTIONS, REGULATION AND EFFECT OF ALTERED (HYPO AND HYPER) SECRETION OF PITUITARY GLAND, THYROID GLAND, PARATHYROID GLAND, ADRENAL GLAND, PANCREAS AND HYPOTHALAMUS

LONG ESSAYS

1. Define signal transduction. Explain the events occurring inside a cell that is stimulated by norepinephrine.   (2 + 8 marks)

Signal Transduction

- Signal transduction is a process by which molecular signals from the exterior of the cell are transmitted to the inside.
- This is initiated by binding of the desired molecule to its respective receptor on the cell surface.
- Each cell has thousands of receptors, but they are highly specific to respective hormones or molecules.
- There are three general classes of methods for signal transduction by hormones:
  1. **Receptors that penetrate the membrane and alter permeability:** Example is neurotransmitter in a synapse increase the permeability of the post-synaptic membrane to sodium ions.
  2. **G protein coupled receptors activate intra-cellular enzyme:** *Example*—protein hormones and catecholamines.
  3. **Nuclear receptors:** Intracellular receptors which are linked to gene transcription.

Signal Transduction Following Norepinephrine

- When a catecholamine (primary messenger) like norepinephrine binds to its specific G protein coupled receptor, a complex is formed between hormone and the receptor.
- G proteins are GTP (guanosine triphosphate) linked proteins. It has a set of 7 transmembrane proteins which transverse in and out of the cell (secondary messengers). The intracellular parts of the membrane are associated with three subunits— α, β and γ. Some cells have IP3 as secondary messengers for alpha receptors.
- Binding of norepinephrine to its receptor causes a conformational change in the subunits and activates G protein.

- In inactivated state, G protein has GDP- guanosine diphosphate. After attachment with norepine-phrine, α subunit gets associated with the cytoplasmic portion of the receptor and gets phosphorylated to GTP.
- As a result, there is activation of ion channels and activation of an enzyme called adenyl cyclase.
- It converts ATP to cyclic AMP. This activates protein kinase A (PKA).
- Pyruvate kinase is associated with activation of required enzymes necessary for the action of nor-epinephrine.
- Phosphorylation of ion channels leads to the opening and entry of calcium ions → smooth muscle contraction → vasoconstriction
- Phosphorylation of ion channels → K⁺ influx → detrusor relaxation → no voiding of urine (through IP3).

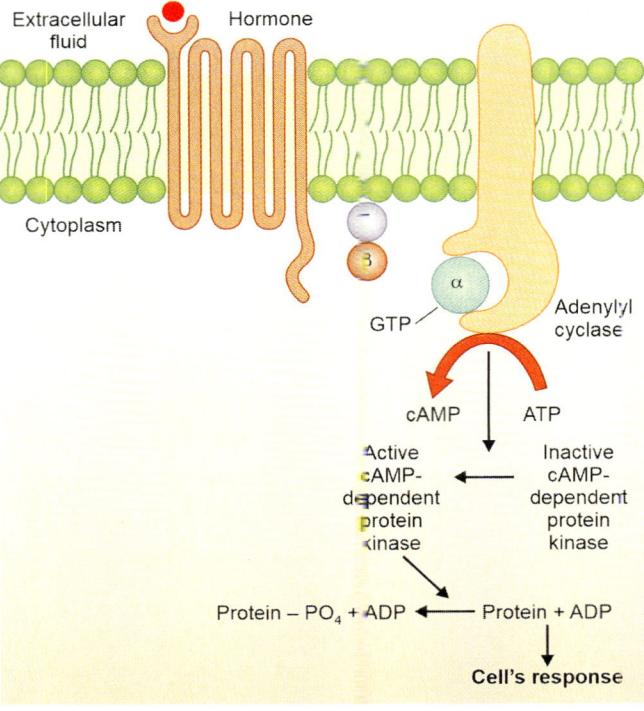

Fig. 8.3

Receptor	Mode of action	Response
Alpha-1 receptor	Activates IP3 through phospholipase C	Mediates more of noradrenaline actions than adrenaline actions
Alpha-2 receptor	Inhibits adenyl cyclase and cAMP	
Beta-1 receptor	Activates adenyl cyclase and cAMP	Mediates actions of adrenaline and noradrenaline equally
Beta-2 receptor	Activates adenyl cyclase and cAMP	Mediates more of adrenaline actions than noradrenaline actions

2. Describe the mechanism of action, functions, and regulation of growth hormone. Add a note on gigantism. (7 + 3 marks)

Growth Hormone

Mechanism of Action

- It is also called somatotropin and is responsible for postnatal growth.
- Growth hormone acts on the liver to form somatomedins or insulin like growth factor-1 and through insulin like growth factor-2.
- IGF-1 is the main component in post-natal life, whereas IGF-2 is responsible for intrauterine development.
- Growth hormone combines with its receptor-growth hormone secretagogue receptor (GHS-R).
- It is a transmembrane receptor. They are mainly present in the liver cells.
- Hormone receptor complex induces JAK-STAT pathway and transcription of genes responsible for production of proteins required for growth.

Functions

1. Promotion of growth

- It promotes linear growth by acting on bones and cartilages along with their connective tissue
- Growth hormone stimulates growth of chondrocytes and thus helps in growth of cartilage
- It increases osteoblastic activity and converts cartilage to bone. This helps in fusing the epiphyseal end of the bone during adolescence.

2. Metabolic effects

Proteins	Anabolic effect on protein metabolism	• Increases amino acid uptake by cells
	Positive nitrogen balance	• Increases protein synthesis in ribosomes
		• Stimulates transcription from DNA to RNA
Fats	Catabolic effect on fats	• Increases lipolysis in adipose tissue
		• Increases fat utilization
Carbohydrate	Positive glucose balance	• Increases gluconeogenesis by the liver
		• Decreases glucose uptake by cells and increases plasma glucose
		• Inhibits glycolysis and increases glycogen reserves in the body
Minerals	Positive calcium balance	• Promotes bone mineralization
		• Increases renal absorption of calcium, phosphate, and magnesium

3. Effects on lactation
- It has a prolactin like effect, thus causes milk production.

Regulation

Normally, growth hormone secretion is controlled by the hypothalamus through growth hormone releasing hormone and growth hormone inhibiting hormone.

Stimulants for GHRH Secretion

Hypoglycaemia, physical stress, emotions, slow wave phase of sleep, growth hormone releasing peptide or ghrelin.

Stimulants for GHIH Secretion (Inhibition of Growth Hormone)

- Hyperglycaemia and increased free fatty acids in plasma
- The insulin like growth factor or somatomedins inhibit secretion of growth hormone releasing hormone from hypothalamus and inhibits growth hormone release from pituitary.
- Growth hormone itself inhibits its release by inhibiting GHRH and stimulating somatostatin
- GHRH itself inhibits its secretion from hypothalamus.

Other Factors Involved in Growth Hormone Regulation

Thyroxine, cortisol	Stimulate production of growth hormone
Insulin	Suppresses growth hormone gene expression
Obesity	Decreases GH responses
Estrogen	Increases GH secretion

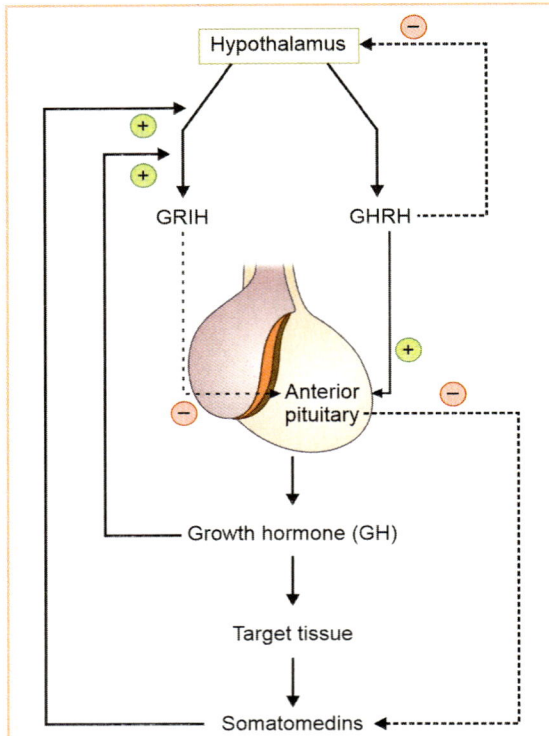

Fig. 8.4

Gigantism

- It is a clinical condition characterized by increased secretion of growth hormone prior to the epiphyseal closure.
- It is usually due to a pituitary tumour secreting excess growth hormone.

Clinical Features

1. Abnormal height: The affected individual is very tall—around 7–8 feet with long bones
2. Large hands and feet
3. Gynaecomastia due to prolactin like effect

4. Coarse facial features—thick lips, broad nose, macroglossia
5. Hyperglycaemia due to excess growth hormone secretion
6. Additionally, there may be features due to mass effect of the pituitary tumor which is the cause for gigantism. These may include headache, vomiting, diplopia, visual field defects.

3. Explain the synthesis of thyroid hormones. Describe its mechanism of action and physiological functions. How is pituitary dwarf different from hypothyroid dwarf?

(3 + 4 + 3 marks)

Thyroid Hormone Synthesis

T3 (triiodothyronine) and T4 (thyroxine) are the major thyroid hormone and they are synthesized from tyrosine, an amino acid and iodine, a trace element with the help of an enzyme complex: Peroxidase.

1. **Iodine trapping**
   - It is the first step in thyroid hormone synthesis.
   - It involves uptake of iodide that is circulating in blood
   - It is taken up by the cell by an active Na^+/I^- symporter on the apical membrane. The energy for this symporter is derived from Na^+-K^+-ATPase pump.
   - This step is influenced by the action of TSH.

2. **Thyroglobulin synthesis**
   - It is a continuous process that takes place in the endoplasmic reticulum and Golgi apparatus of the follicular cell of the thyroid gland.
   - It is a protein molecular with high molecular weight and serves as a reserve for hormone synthesis.
   - It is synthesized from tyrosine.
   - After production, it moves to the apex and gets secreted into the lumen of the follicle.

3. **Oxidation of iodide and organification of thyroglobulin**
   - Once taken up by the gland, iodide quickly moves to the apex from where it is transported into the lumen.
   - The apical membrane contains peroxidase enzymes which oxidize iodide to iodine.
   - This step is also influenced by TSH.

- Then, there is attachment of iodine to tyrosine residues of the thyroglobulin molecule.
- Tyrosine gets iodinated at the 3' position to form mono-iodothyronine and at the 5' position to form di-iodothyronine.
- This reaction also requires the help of thyroid peroxidase.

4. **Coupling reactions (Fig. 8.5)**
   - Two molecules of diiodothyronine form thyroxine (T4)
   - One molecule of monoiodothyronine and one molecule of di-iodothyronine forms tri-iodothyronine (T3)
   - The enzyme thyroid peroxidase is required again in this step
   - Once coupled, the hormones are stored in the colloid and can meet body requirements for 2–3 months.

5. **Release of hormones:** Hormones are released into the blood (Fig. 8.6).

Mechanism of Action

- They affect cellular activity of almost all cells in the body.
- Being lipophilic, thyroid hormones internalized easily within the cell.
- It has an intracellular receptor and it forms a complex with the receptor.
- This activated receptor enters the nucleus of the cell and binds to a respective part of the DNA called the hormone responsive element. This brings about gene transcription and then translation occurs.
- The necessary enzymes and proteins are synthesized.

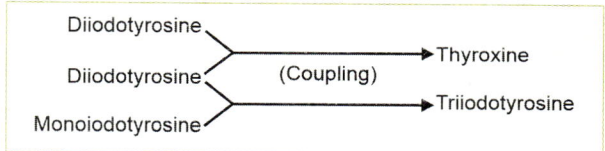

Fig. 8.5

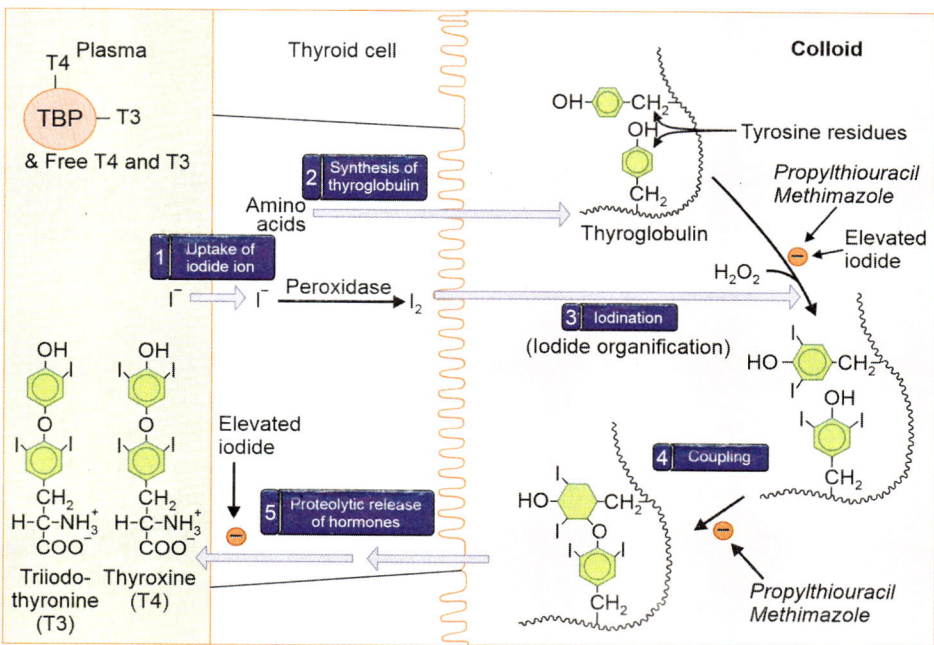

Fig. 8.6

Physiological Functions

Growth and development	• Increase in protein synthesis • Indirectly increase the effect of growth hormone • Skeletal development • Tissue differentiation • Development of neurons and dendritic development
Effect on metabolic rate	• Increases the basal metabolic rate and oxygen consumption in almost all cells except retina, brain, gonads, spleen and lungs

Effect on metabolism	1. *Carbohydrate metabolism*
	  – Accelerates all aspects of glucose metabolism
	  – Increased glucose uptake by cells, increased insulin secretion, increased gluconeogenesis
	2. Fat metabolism
	  – Increase in level of fatty acids in blood
	  – Mobilizes fat from adipose tissues
	  – Decrease in plasma cholesterol levels
	3. Protein metabolism
	  – Leads to positive protein balance due to increase in formation of proteins from amino acids. However, in hyperthyroid state, there is increased catabolism of proteins.
	4. Vitamin metabolism
	  – Due to increased demand due to high metabolic rate, there occurs a state of relative vitamin deficiency.

Effects on respiration	• Increases resting respiratory rate, minute ventilation and oxygen carrying capacity of blood.
Effects on CVS	• Increased heart rate and contractility by permissive action of adrenaline • Increased systolic blood pressure due to increased cardiac output • Decreased diastolic blood pressure due to peripheral vasodilatation (caused by increased generation of CO_2 and heat in the periphery)
Effects on CNS	• Critical for development of central nervous system • Increases awareness, wakefulness, responsiveness • Increases speed of reflexes • Potentiates catecholamine associated effects
Effects on GIT	• Increases appetite and food intake • Increases secretion of juices • Increases motility of the gut
Effects on reproductive system	• Responsible for proper functioning of reproductive system • In men, necessary for libido • In females, it is needed for regularity of menstrual cycle
Effects on kidney	• Increases GFR and T_{max}

Differences Between Pituitary Dwarf and Hypothyroid Dwarf/Cretinism

Aspect	Pituitary dwarf	Hypothyroid dwarf/cretinism
Cause or hormone effected	Decreased growth hormone secretion	Congenital absence of thyroid gland or iodine deficiency in infancy
Proportion	Body parts are proportionately small	There is disproportionate disturbance in growth abnormal
Neuronal growth	Normal	There is mental retardation as a rule Reflexes are sluggish
Facial features	Immature facies	Protruded tongue
Reproductive function	Normal	Abnormal

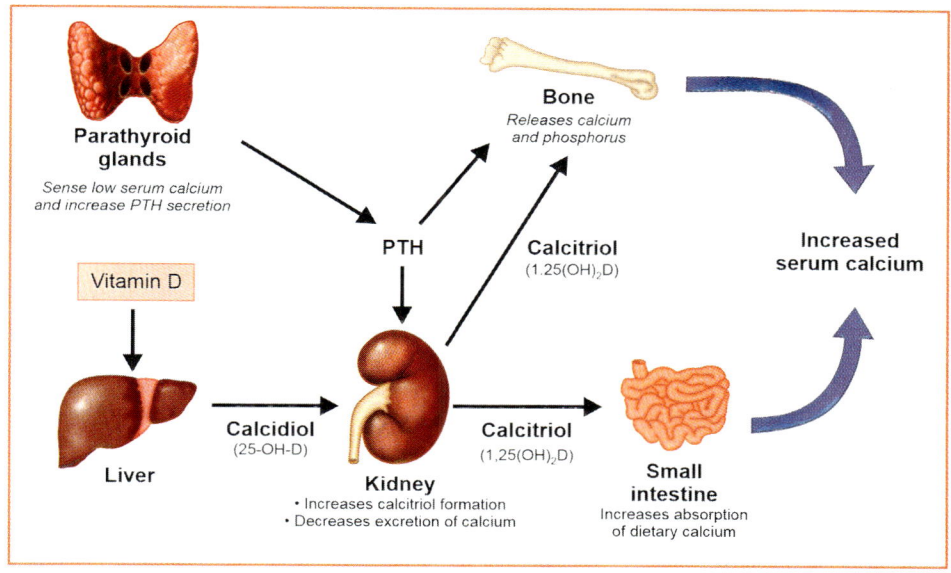

Fig. 8.7

4. Describe the role of parathyroid, calcitonin, and vitamin D in calcium homeostasis. Describe pathophysiology of rickets and its prevention. (6 + 4 marks)

Hormonal Metabolism of Calcium

- Calcium is involved in numerous biological processes throughout the body.
- Calcium homeostasis depends on the intricate yet meticulous interplay among its absorption, exchange between plasma and bone and finally its excretion.
- These three processes are governed by the action of parathormone and 1,25-dihydroxycholecalciferol.

Decrease in Serum Calcium (Fig. 8.7)

- It may be due to decreased uptake or due to increase in excretion or increased uptake by the bones.
- This causes release of Parathormone from the parathyroid glands and release of 1,25-dihydroxycholecalciferol from the kidneys.
- Parathormone brings about resorption of calcium from the bones and increases serum calcium levels. Similar action is brought about by calcitriol.
- 1,25-dihydroxycholecalciferol increases absorption of calcium from the intestine.

Increase in Serum Calcium

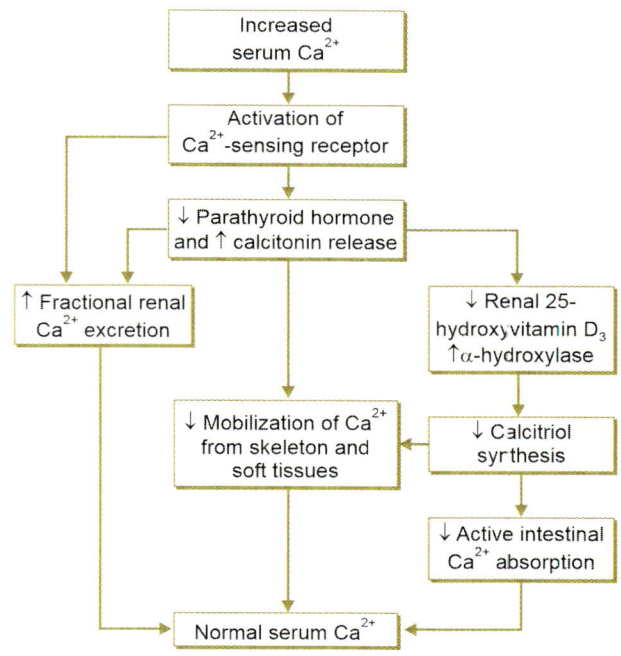

Fig. 8.8

Pathophysiology of Rickets

It is a metabolic bone disease characterized by defective bone mineralization of bone in growing children.

Vitamin D deficiency   **Dietary calcium deficiency**

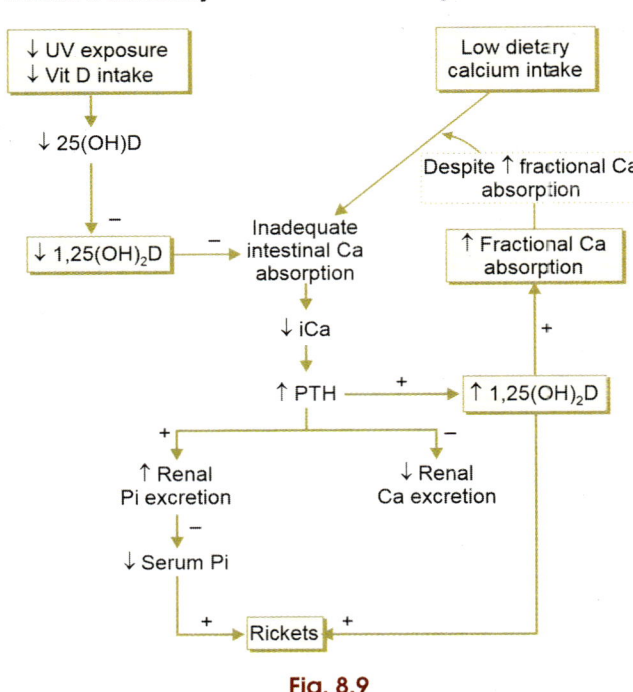

Fig. 8.9

Prevention

- Education about adequate breast feeding and improving nutritional conditions.
- Introduction of dietary sources of vitamin D—egg and fish oil.
- Adequate sun exposure: Traditional oil massage and sun exposure has been found to increase vitamin D formation in skin.
- Vitamin D_3 supplementation: 400 IU/day.

5. Name the catecholamines secreted by adrenal medulla. Mention the types of its receptors. Explain its role in fight and flight reaction. What is pheochromocytoma?

(2 + 2 + 4 + 2 marks)

Catecholamines

The adrenal medulla secretes
1. Adrenaline or epinephrine
2. Norepinephrine or noradrenaline
3. Dopamine

Receptors of Catecholamines

Catecholamine	Receptors
Adrenaline/ Epinephrine Norepinephrine/ Noradrenaline	1. Alpha 1 receptors • Present on the vascular smooth muscles, gastrointestinal and bladder sphincters, radial muscles of iris 2. Alpha 2 receptors • Present on the presynaptic nerve terminals 3. Beta 1 receptors • Present in the sinoatrial node, AV node and ventricular muscles of the heart. 4. Beta 2 receptors • Located in the vascular smooth muscles, bronchioles, bladder and walls of the GIT 5. Beta 3 receptors • Present in adipose tissues
Dopamine	1. D1 family • Present in basal ganglia, heart, kidney 2. D2 family • Striatum, substantia nigra, mesolimbic pathway

Fight and Flight Reaction

- It refers to simultaneous diffuse activation and discharge from all portions of the sympathetic system in case of heightened stress.
- It is also known as alarm response or mass reflex.
- It begins in the hypothalamus of the brain. It stimulates the adrenals to produce cortisol.
- Through reticular formation, the impulses reach the sympathetic plexus along the spinal cord and bring about sympathetic events.
- The effects are due to increased circulation of catecholamines and cortisol.
  - Increased blood pressure
  - Increased blood flow to skeletal muscles and relative decrease of blood supply from GIT and kidneys.
  - Increased metabolic rate throughout the body
  - Increased glucose production by glycolysis from liver and muscles

– Increased rate of blood coagulation
– Increased strength in muscles
– Increased mentation

Pheochromocytoma

- It is a tumor of chromophil cells of the adrenal medulla.
- When it arises from sympathetic ganglia, it is called extra-adrenal pheochromocytoma.
- As a result, there is increased secretion of catecholamines in blood and their effects.

Clinical Features

- Blood pressure is high (around 200/120 mmHg)
- Episodes of uncontrolled anxiety, rage
- Fear
- Headache
- Hyperpyrexia
- Palpitation
- Polyuria and glycosuria

6. A 32-year-old female no resumption of menses 6 months after lactating her baby. She then developed facial hair, a swollen upper back and acne. She subsequently developed back pain and was found to have a compression fracture of the lumbar spine. She saw a local physician who diagnosed her with Cushing's syndrome. What is the pathophysiology in Cushing's syndrome? Explain probable investigations to confirm the diagnosis.

(5 + 5 marks)

Cushing Syndrome

Cushing syndrome is a collective term used to describe the effects of increased cortisol and other glucocorticoids either from pituitary or from the adrenal cortex.

Pathophysiology

- CRH is secreted by the hypothalamus which stimulates production of ACTH by the anterior pituitary
- ACTH in turn stimulates the adrenal cortex to produce glucocorticoids which have effects on various tissues in the body
- Normal cortisol levels are maintained by negative inhibition to release of CRH and ACTH by serum cortisol levels.

- However, this negative feedback mechanism fails in certain ACTH secreting adenomas and resultant increase in serum cortisol results.

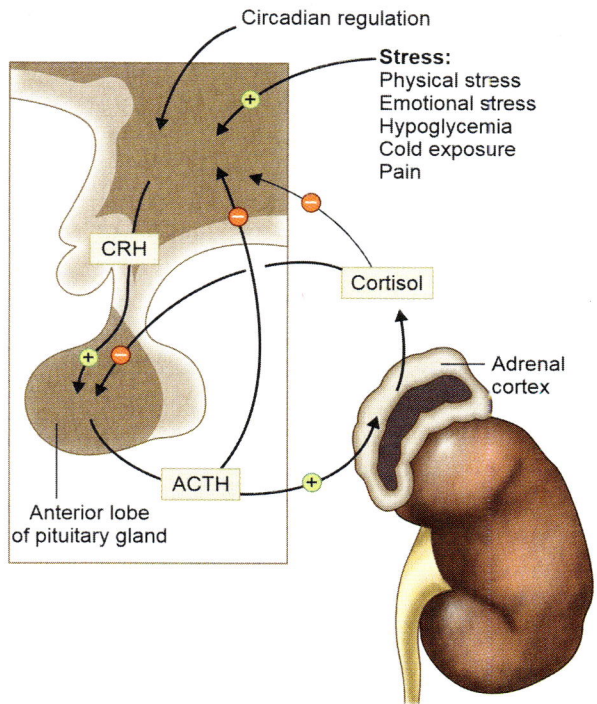

Fig. 8.10

Pituitary origin	Adrenal origin
• They are also called ACTH dependent Cushing's syndrome	• They are called ACTH independent Cushing's syndrome
• Tumours of pituitary that secrete excess ACTH	• Tumor of the adrenal cortex
• Neuroendocrine malignancy of lungs or other organs that secrete ACTH	• Exposure to high synthetic corticosteroids in treatment of conditions like nephrotic syndrome, rheumatoid arthritis, autoimmune conditions
• Secretion of increased corticotropin releasing hormone by hypothalamus.	• Prolonged treatment with ACTH

Diagnostic Workup (Fig. 8.11)

1. **Serum cortisol levels:** Cushing syndrome is a clinical syndrome and is confirmed by blood cortisol levels (normal is 10–20 microgram per decilitre)

2. **Low dose dexamethasone test**
   - It is done to diagnose cushing's syndrome. 1mg dexamethasone is given at 2300 hours a night and the serum cortisol are check at 0900 hours the following day. If the cortisol levels are low, there is no Cushing's syndrome. If the cortisol levels are still high, there is Cushing's syndrome.
   - However, to find the exact cause for elevated cortisol levels, a workup is required.
   - Serum ACTH can differentiate between ACTH dependent and ACTH independent Cushing's syndrome.
   - It is because large dose of steroid in the blood suppresses ACTH secretion from the adrenals, however, fails to do so in ectopic tumors.

3. **High dose dexamethasone suppression test**
   8 mg dexamethasone is used to suppress the ACTH. Possible results:
   - If the abnormal cortisol is arising from the adrenals, then ACTH is undetectable. These patients should undergo an imaging of the adrenals
   - If the abnormal cortisol is arising from an ectopic neuroendocrine tumor, then high levels of dexamethasone fails to suppress the ACTH. The same is the case with pituitary ACT secreting tumors. These patients require an imaging of the brain (MRI) and chest (CT).

4. **CRH stimulation test**
   - It is used to differentiate whether the source of abnormal ACTH is from pituitary or ectopic tumor.

- Ectopic tumors secreting ACTH will not be affected by CRH.
- Another invasive method is petrosal venous sampling to differentiate the two.

7. Explain glucose homeostasis. Discuss physiological basis of cardinal features of diabetes mellitus. (6 + 4 marks)

Glucose Homeostasis (Fig. 8.12)

It is the intricate balance between insulin and glucagon to maintain blood glucose levels.

Physiological Basis of Cardinal Features of Diabetes Mellitus

- Diabetes mellitus is characterized by hyperglycemia.
- Hyperglycemia results due to poor uptake of glucose by cells and increased output of glucose from liver.
- The three classical features of diabetes are:
  1. **Polyuria**
     - There is increased filtration of glucose in urine. When the plasma glucose surpasses the T_{max} (180 mg/dl), there is appearance of glucose in urine. This is called glycosuria.
     - Due to increased osmotic pressure of urine, there is increase in water losses in urine. This is called osmotic diuresis.
     - This causes polyuria.
  2. **Polydipsia**
     - Due to osmotic diuresis, there is also loss of electrolytes in urine.

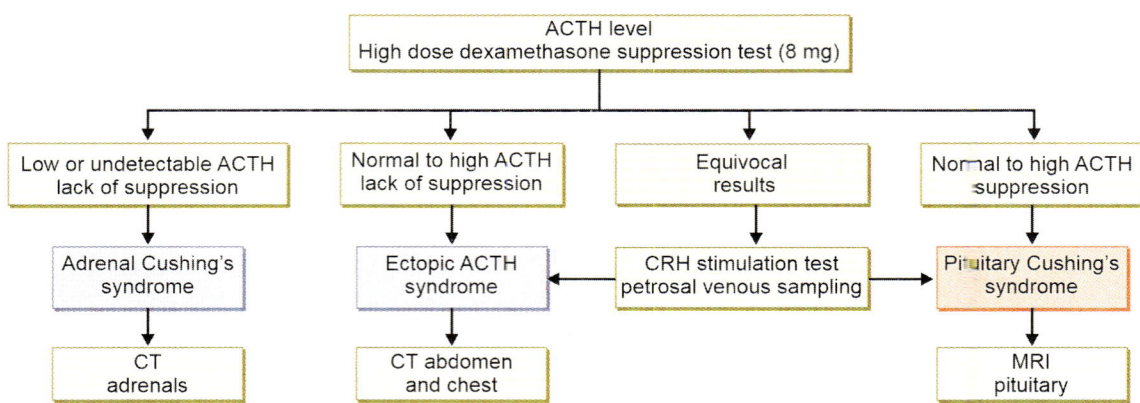

Fig. 8.11

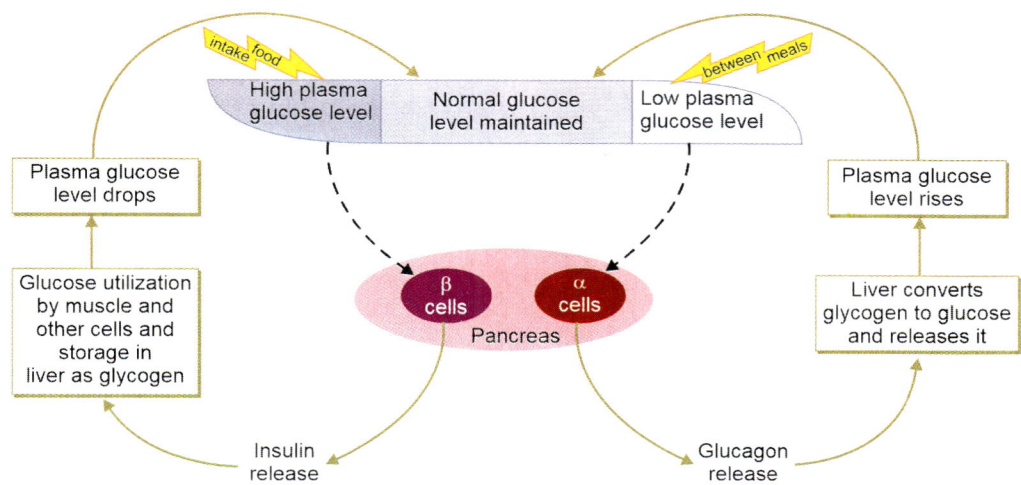

Fig. 8.12

- As a result, there is cellular dehydration.
- Osmoreceptors in the hypothalamus are stimulated and they increase thirst.
- This causes polydipsia.

3. **Polyphagia**
   - Due to loss of glucose in urine and poor cellular uptake, there is calorie loss
   - There is stimulation of the feeding centre in the hypothalamus and this causes an urge to eat more and thus there is polyphagia.

SHORT ESSAYS

1. Explain JAK-STAT pathway with example.

(5 marks)

JAK-STAT Pathway

It stands for Janus Tyrosine Kinase- signal transducer and activator of transcription pathway.

Mechanism (Fig. 8.13)

- When a hormone binds to its receptor, there is conformational change in the intracytoplasmic tail of the receptor.

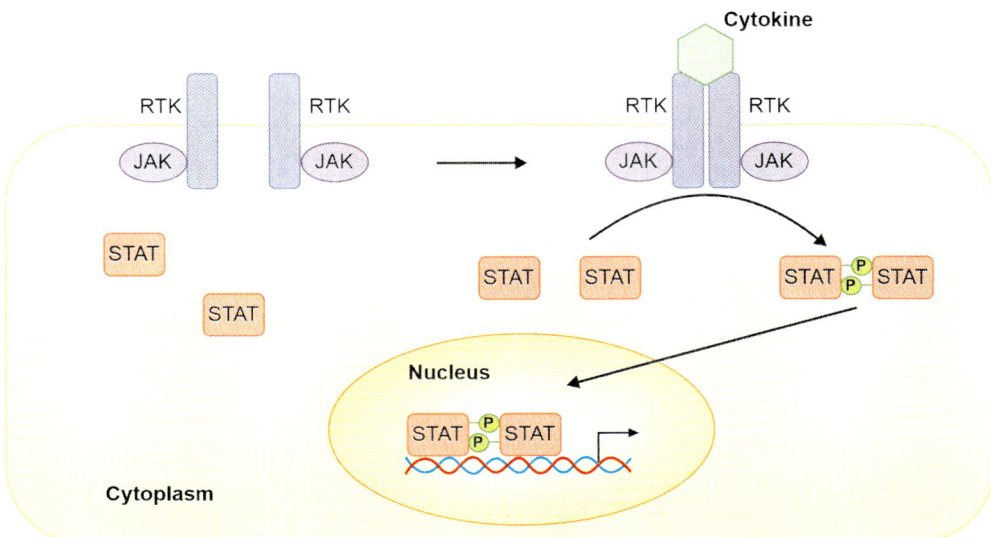

Fig. 8.13

- As a result, the cytoplasmic part of the receptor attracts the JAK molecules and dock them.
- This causes attraction of the STAT kinases to get attracted and their phosphorylation.
- This causes phosphorylation of transcription factor proteins which brings about gene expression of the desired effect.
- Examples: Growth hormone, cytokines, prolactin releasing hormones.

2. Describe the mechanism of action, functions and regulation of prolactin.

Prolactin

- It is a peptide hormone secreted by the acidophilic cells of the pituitary.
- It is secreted in pulses and is highest during sleep. Its production starts during pregnancy and peaks at term.
- It is secreted by the placenta and the amniotic membranes during pregnancy along with maternal pituitary.

Mechanism of Action

- It acts at the alveolar cells of the mammary glands to produce milk.
- It also acts on the epithelial cells of the mammary glands and increases their growth and proliferation.

Functions

- Potentiates breast growth during pregnancy and preps the breasts for lactation. The alveoli undergo distension and growth, there is increase in vascularity to the tissues and new vessels are formed.
- Increases production of milk—lactogenesis and maintenance of milk production—galactopoiesis.
- Inhibits ovulation by inhibiting FSH and LH.

Regulation

- The secretion from anterior pituitary is regulated by the hypothalamus. This is through prolactin inhibitory factor or dopamine.
- It is transported to the anterior pituitary through the hypothalamo-hypophyseal portal system.
- This hormone checks the production and release of prolactin.

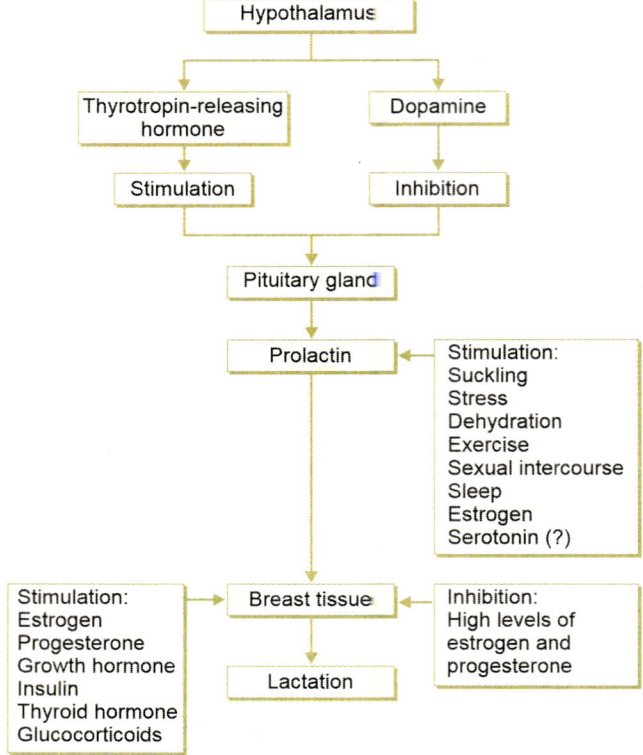

Fig. 8.14

3. A 40-year-old female presented with increased frequency of micturition, up to 18 L/day. Her sugar levels were normal with no other co-morbidity. She responded well to synthetic analogue of vasopressin. What could be the pathophysiology of this condition?

- This lady has a condition called diabetes insipidus—a disorder due to hyposecretion of antidiuretic hormone.
- Insipid = dilute
- The ability of the nephrons to concentrate urine is lost.

Action of Anti-diuretic Hormone or Vasopressin

- ADH is a neurohypophyseal hormone secreted when the osmolarity of blood is detected to be high. It acts on V2 receptors in the kidney.
- When fluid enters the distal convoluted segment and the collecting duct, presence of ADH makes it permeable to water and water gets reabsorbed. Water is absorbed through aquaporin channels.

- The fluid that reaches the DCT is hypotonic. In presence of ADH, the osmolarity of the urine becomes as high as the medullary interstitium (1200 mEq/L).
- As the fluid enters the medullary part of the collecting ducts, there is further absorption of water into the interstitium.

Pathophysiology of Diabetes Insipidus

Neurogenic or central diabetes insipidus	Nephrogenic diabetes insipidus
- Congenital hypoplasia of the pituitary - Malignancy of the pituitary or hypothalamus - Surgical resection of the pituitary or hypothalamus - Vascular lesions	- Mutation of gene responsible for production of expression of V2 receptors

- In the absence of ADH, the tubule is practically impermeable to water and thus dilute urine is formed. This condition is called diabetes insipidus (insipid = dilute)
- As a result, large amounts of hypotonic urine is lost and there is increased thirst. These patients have an increased risk of dehydration.

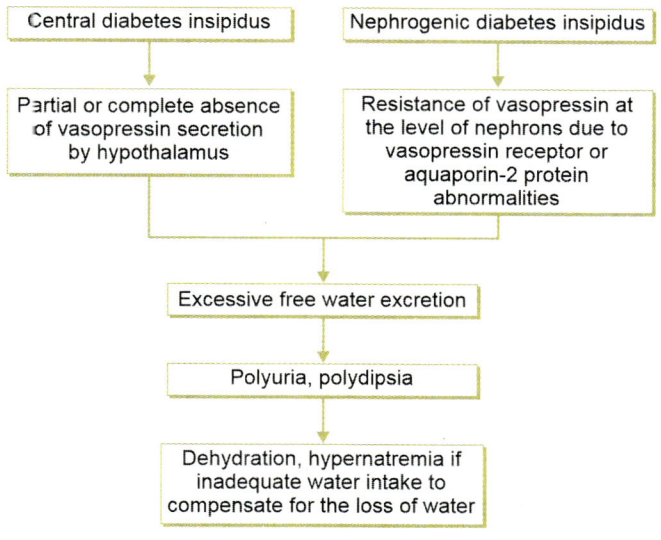

Fig. 8.15

4. Explain milk ejection reflex.

Milk Ejection Reflex or Milk Let Down Reflex

It is a neuroendocrine reflex.

Baby suckling at the nipple stimulates receptors at the nipple. Also, the thought, smell or sight of baby send signals to the hypothalamus.
↓
Somatic afferent nerve fibers to paraventricular and supraoptic nuclei of hypothalamus
↓
Hypothalamus send signals to posterior pituitary through hypothalamo-hypophyseal tract
↓
Release of oxytocin in blood
↓
Reaches the mammary gland to cause contraction of myoepithelial cells
↓
Ejection of milk from mammary glands

Fig. 8.16

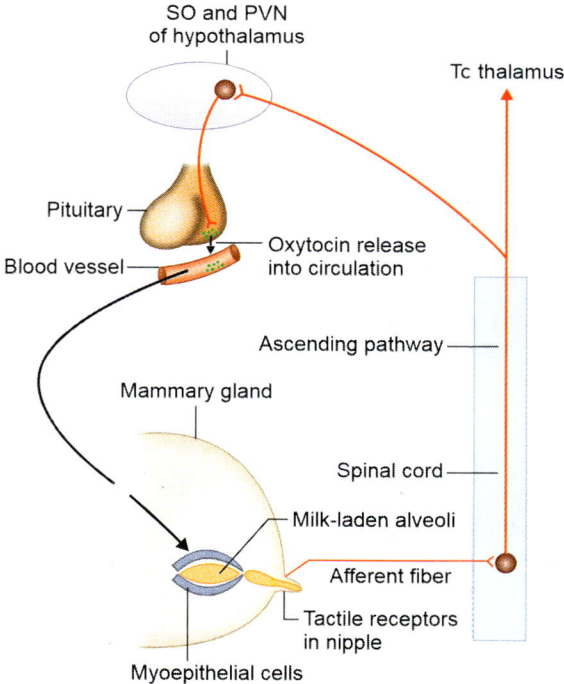

Fig. 8.17

5. A 20-year-old male presented with failure to gain height from the age of 8 years, poor secondary sexual characteristics and mental retardation. On investigations he was diagnosed to have cretinism. Describe cretinism and its aetiology.

Cretinism

- It is term used to describe features of congenital hypothyroidism and hypothyroidism occurring within the first year of life.
- It is characterized by extreme failure to grow physically and intellectually.

Etiology

Decreased thyroid hormones in blood in infancy has deleterious effects on the physical and mental growth.

- *Congenital cretinism*
    - *Maternal hypothyroidism*
        - o During the first three months, the foetus is entirely dependent on the maternal thyroid hormones for development.
        - o It may be due to iodine deficiency, radioactive iodine ablation of thyroid of mother or inflammatory thyroiditis in pregnancy.
        - o Use of antenatal use of antithyroid drugs also can cause cretinism.
        - o If the blood thyroxine levels are not corrected soon after birth, there may be permanent damage.
    - *Congenital absence of thyroid gland*
        - o It is due to unavailability of thyroid hormone because of agenesis of the thyroid gland which is rare
        - o Congenital inability of the gland to produce thyroxine due to genetic defects in thyroxine preparation.
- *Endemic cretinism*
    - Low iodine in diet.
    - It is more common in hilly areas as the iodine content of water in hilly areas is less.

Features of Cretinism

- Usually normal at birth due to maternal thyroid hormones.

- After a few weeks, the movements become sluggish and the child exhibits a hoarse cry.
- Thyroid hormone is required for normal development at this point, otherwise it results in permanent handicap.
- Skeletal growth is more inhibited than soft tissue growth, the child's height is less than 50th centile. As a result, the child has short, stocky appearance.
- These children have a thick tongue which may even impair them from swallowing or breathing
- Other features are flat nose, pot belly, dry skin and sparse hair.
- They have severe mental handicap.

6. Describe the synthesis and actions of vitamin D₃.

Vitamin D

- It is also called 'sunshine vitamin' as most of it is formed in sunlight.
- 7-dehydroxycholesterol or ergosterol is present in the Malpighian layer of the epidermis.
- When sunlight falls on skin, it is converted into vitamin D₃ or cholecalciferol.
- Vitamin D₂ is also received in the form of dietary sources like egg and milk.

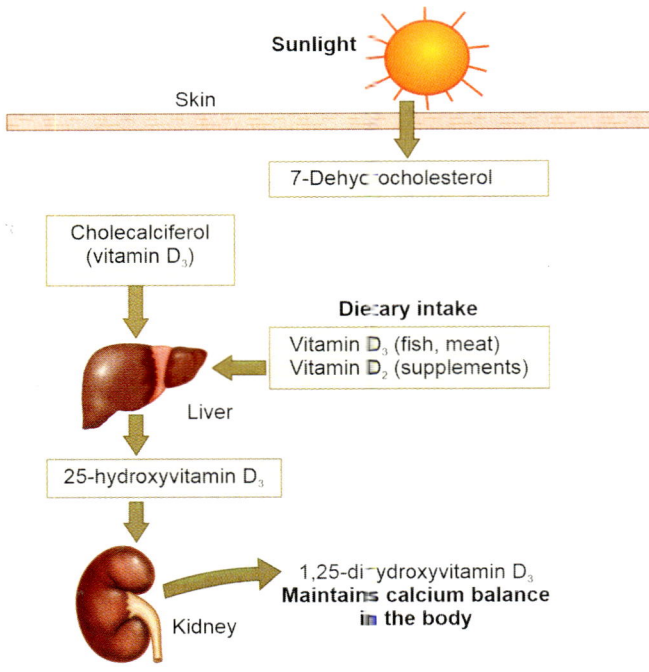

Fig. 8.15

- Cholecalciferol is hydroxylated in the liver at 25' position to form 25-hydroxycholecalciferol.
- It is then transported to the kidneys and converted to 1,25-dihydroxycholecalciferol. This is the active form of vitamin D and is also called calcitriol.

Actions of vitamin D₃

Action on Calcium and Phosphate Homeostasis

1. It increases absorption of calcium from the mucosa of the intestine by increasing permeability of the mucosa to calcium and through increased production of calmodulin.
2. It increases bone mineralization during osteogenesis. As a result, the calcium is taken into bones.
3. Under the influence of parathormone, it causes resorption of bone leading to osteoclastic osteolysis and increase in serum calcium levels.
4. It increases calcium and phosphate reabsorption by the tubules of the kidney.

Other Actions

1. It increases calcium uptake by skeletal muscles
2. It stimulates differentiation of keratinocytes
3. It stimulates differentiation of immune cells.

7. Explain the mechanism of action and functions of insulin.

Mechanism of Action of Insulin (Fig. 8.19)

- Insulin is a hormone secreted by the beta cells of the islet of Langerhans in the pancreas. It brings about its action through the insulin receptor present on the liver cells, muscles and fat.
- The insulin receptor has two parts: One extracellular and one cytoplasmic.
- The receptor for insulin is a tetramer, formed by two alpha and two beta subunits. They are bound together by disulphide bonds.
- The intracellular portions have protein kinase activity.
- Binding of insulin to its receptor causes autophosphorylation of two pathways
    1. *MAP kinase signalling pathway:* It is involved in cell growth and proliferation and gene expression
    2. *PI-3K signalling pathway:* It is involved in synthesis of lipids, proteins, glycogen. It also produces GLUT-4 receptors.
- Also, it causes production of GLUT-4 receptors by transcription and translocation to the plasma membrane and thus entry of glucose into the cell.

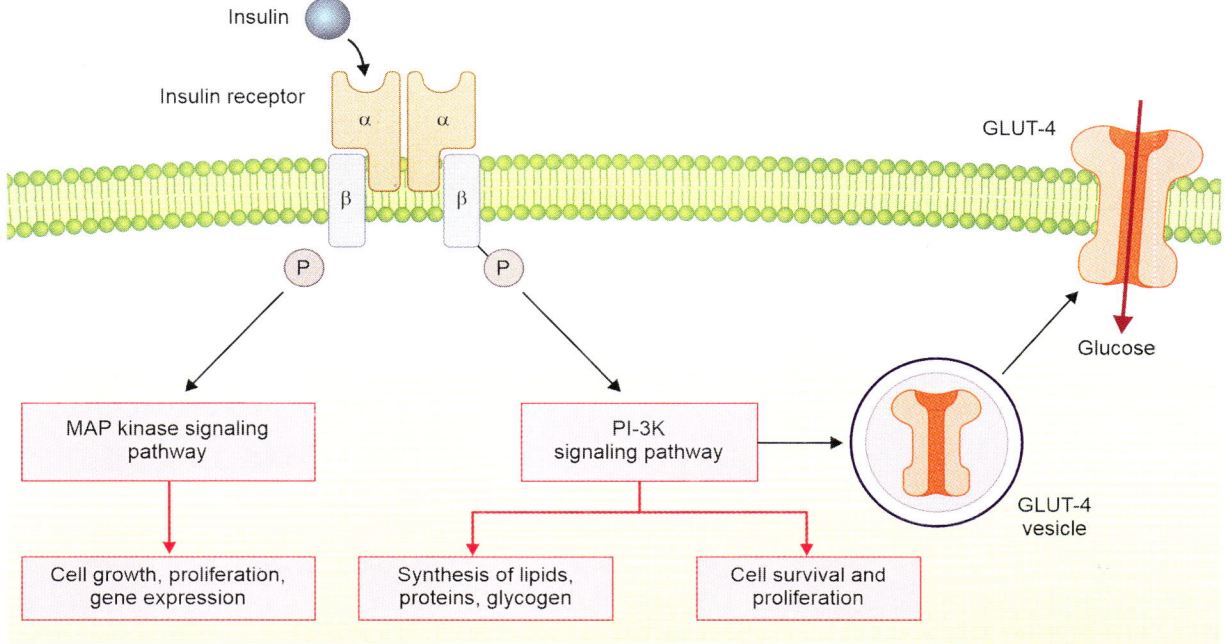

Fig. 8.19

Functions of Insulin

Cell	Increases permeability to glucose. Increase influx of potassium and phosphate ions and amino acids increases cell growth
Blood	Decrease in blood glucose by increasing glucose uptake by cells. But this mechanism does not apply to neurons
Liver	Promotes glycogenesis by activating glycogen synthase Inhibits liver phosphorylase that prevents glycogenolysis Increases the activity of glucokinase and increases glucose uptake.
Muscle	Increases glycogen formation and storage
Fat	Increases conversion of excess glucose into fatty acids and their subsequent conversion into triglycerides.

8. Name hormones that affect plasma glucose concentration and describe the functions of glucagon.

Hormones Affecting Glucose Homeostasis

Hyperglycemia inducing hormones	Hypoglycemia inducing hormone
Glucagon Cortisol Thyroxine Epinephrine	Insulin

Functions of Glucagon

- Glucagon is secreted by the alpha cells of the islet of pancreas.
- When glucose levels fall below 80 mg/dl, its secretion is triggered.
- Its main function is to increase plasma blood glucose by several ways.
  1. **Action on carbohydrate metabolism**
     - Its main action is on the hepatocytes.
     - It exerts glycolytic effect and activates enzymes responsible for glycogenolysis and gluconeogenesis.
     - Glucose is formed from fatty acids and amino acids.
  2. **Action on lipid metabolism**
     - It is a powerful lipolytic agent
     - It stimulates lipase and causes break down of triglycerides into free fatty acids.
     - Free fatty acids are utilized for generation of heat, as a result, ketones are produced.

3. **Effect on protein metabolism:** It lowers plasma amino acid levels and causes their uptake into liver. Thus, promotes gluconeogenesis.
4. **Effect on energy metabolism:** It has a calorigenic effect through glucocorticoids and thyroxine.

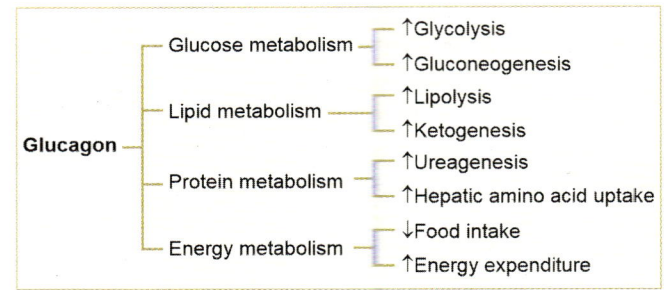

Fig. 8.20

SHORT ANSWERS

1. Describe the synthesis and release of insulin from pancreatic islet of Langerhans. (3 marks)

Synthesis and Release of Insulin

- It is a protein hormone synthesized in the rough endoplasmic reticulum of the beta cells of the islets of pancreas.
- It is synthesized as pre-pro insulin. (109 aminoacids)
- It is quickly converted into proinsulin in the RER by removal of 23 amino acid residues.
- The proinsulin is transported to the Golgi apparatus and then cleaved by protease to form insulin and C peptide.
- The insulin is packed in granules.

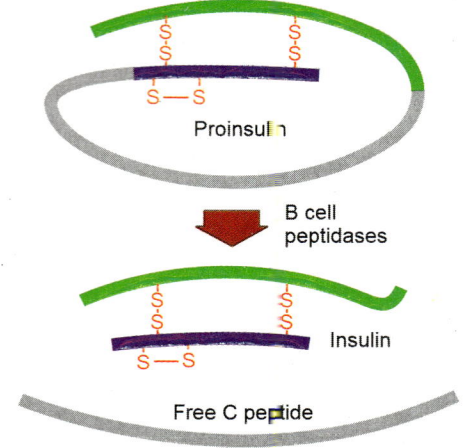

Fig. 8.21

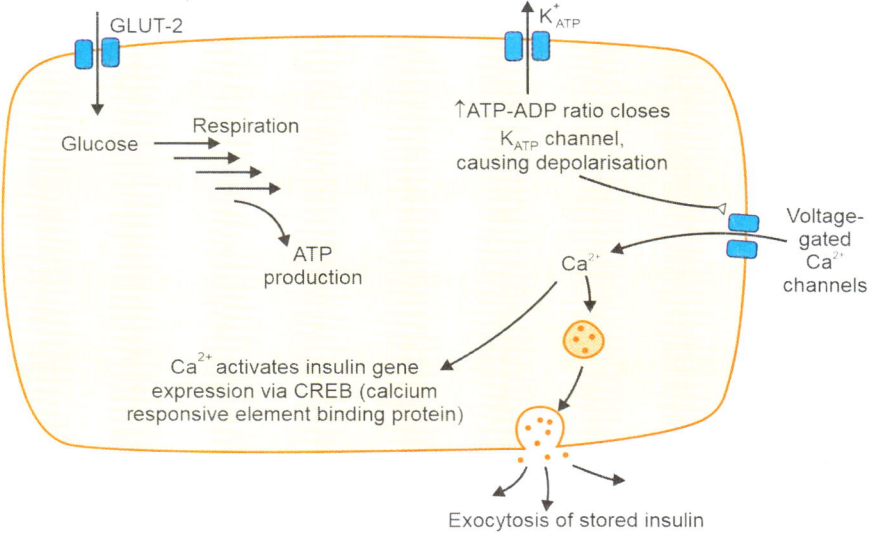

Fig. 8.22

Secretion or Release of Insulin (Fig. 8.22)

- When there is increase in blood glucose, the GLUT-2 receptors on the beta cells allow entry of glucose molecules, which produces ATP with the help of glucokinase enzyme.
- This causes closure of ATP sensitive potassium channels.
- The resultant depolarization causes opening of calcium channels
- Calcium influx causes fusion of the secretory vesicles and exocytosis.

2. What is permissive action of hormones. Give 2 examples. (3 marks)

Permissive Action of Hormones

- It refers to execution of action of other hormones only in the presence of the hormone.
- The hormone in question does not cause the required change but its presence in small quantities potentiates the action of the other.

Examples

1. **Permissive effect of thyroxine on adrenaline**
   - Presence of thyroxine increases the number of receptors on target cell for catecholamines.
   - This is evidenced by the clinical manifestation of hyperthyroidism causing features of increased sympathetic activity—like increased heart rate, blood pressure and decreased adipose tissue synthesis.

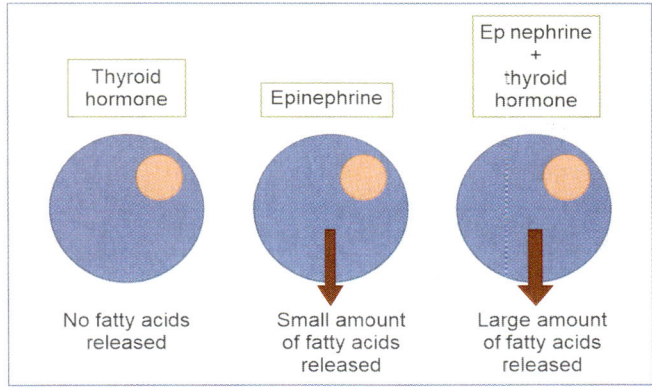

Fig. 8.23

2. **Permissive effect of glucocorticoids on glucagon and catecholamines**
   - Calorigenic effects of glucagon and catecholamines are increased by the action of glucocorticoids.
   - Bronchodilatation by beta adrenergic receptors by the action of catecholamines is enhanced by the presence of glucocorticoids.

3. What is congenital adrenal hyperplasia? Mention its causes. (3 marks)

It is a congenital disorder characterized by increase the size of the adrenal cortex.

Causes

- It is a genetically inherited condition
- Mutation of genes responsible for

- 21-hydroxylase
- 11β-hydroxylase
- 17α-hydroxylase
- 3β-hydroxysteroid dehydrogenase

• The normal pathway of formation of glucocorticoids, mineralocorticoids and sex steroids involves enzymes like

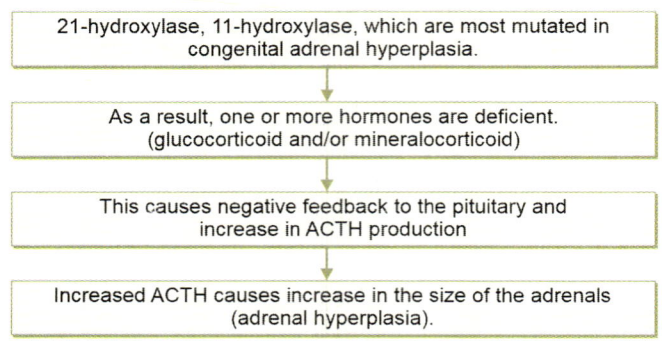

21-hydroxylase, 11-hydroxylase, which are most mutated in congenital adrenal hyperplasia.

↓

As a result, one or more hormones are deficient. (glucocorticoid and/or mineralocorticoid)

↓

This causes negative feedback to the pituitary and increase in ACTH production

↓

Increased ACTH causes increase in the size of the adrenals (adrenal hyperplasia).

Fig. 8.24

4. Name 3 hormones secreted by endocrine pancreas and list their functions. (3 marks)

Hormones secreted by endocrine pancreas—islet of Langerhans

Source of secretion	Hormones	Functions
A cells or alpha cells	Glucagon	1. It increases blood glucose levels 2. Promotes gluconeogenesis and glycogenolysis in liver 3. Increases uptake of amino acids into hepatocytes 4. It has lipolytic and ketogenic actions
B cells or beta cells	Insulin	1. Anti-diabetic hormone 2. Reduces blood sugar, increases glucose uptake by cells, promotes glycogenesis, stimulates production of fatty acids, promotes synthesis of proteins
D cells or delta cells	Somatostatin	1. It inhibits secretion of insulin and glucagon (paracrine function) 2. It decreases motility of stomach, duodenum 3. It decreases secretion of gastrin, CCK, GIP and VIP

5. Discuss the pathophysiological basis of:

A. Cretinism	(3 marks)
B. Myxedema	(3 marks)
C. Hyperthyroidism	(3 marks)

A. Cretinism

• It is the term used to describe features of congenital hypothyroidism and hypothyroidism occurring within the first year of life.
• It is characterized by extreme failure to grow physically and intellectually.

Etiology

1. **Congenital Cretinism**
   • *Maternal hypothyroidism*
     – It may be due to iodine deficiency, use of goitrogens, radioactive iodine ablation of thyroid of mother or inflammatory thyroiditis in pregnancy. Use of antenatal use of antithyroid drugs also can cause cretinism.
     – If the blood thyroxine levels are not corrected soon after birth, there may be permanent damage.
   • *Congenital absence of thyroid gland*
     – It is due to unavailability of thyroid hormone because of agenesis of the thyroid gland which is rare.
     – Congenital inability of the gland to produce thyroxine due to genetic defects in thyroxine preparation.

2. **Endemic cretinism**
   • Low iodine in diet in infancy.
   • It is more common in hilly areas as the iodine content of water in hilly areas is less.

Pathophysiology

• Decreased thyroid hormones in blood in infancy has deleterious effects on the physical and mental growth
• Due to low circulating thyroid hormones, there is defective growth of the skeletal system, although the connective tissue continues to grow. Hence there is disproportionate growth retardation. Bone age is lesser than normal.
• Because of thyroid of nervous growth, there is intellectual growth and delayed tendon reflexes. The child has short stature.

- The muscles are flabby due to hypotonia and may be associated with a pot belly.
- The child has coarse facial features and a thick protruding tongue.

B. Myxedema

- It is hypothyroidism occurring in adults.
- It is named so because, there is characteristic infiltration of skin with myxedematous tissue.

Causes for Hypothyroidism

1. Chronic autoimmune thyroiditis characterized by lymphocytic destruction of thyroid follicles
2. Iodine deficiency causes decreased by production of thyroxine
3. Use of goitrogens leads to decreased production of thyroxine
4. Radioactive iodine ablation causes damage to follicle
5. Central hypothyroidism (pituitary causes)
6. Following removal of thyroid gland

Pathophysiology

- Due to the abovementioned causes which lead to decreased or absent thyroid levels, hypothyroidism results.
- It causes varied manifestations.
- Pretibial myxedema is characteristic for hypothyroidism. There is deposition of glycosaminoglycans in the dermis which leads to thickening. Also, there is water retention due to imbalance of water homeostasis.

C. Hyperthyroidism

It is a state caused by increased thyroid hormones in the body.

Causes

1 **Graves' disease**
- It is an autoimmune condition which causes production of antibodies against thyroid follicles.
- These antibodies bind on the receptors for TSH on the thyroid follicles leading to stimulation of thyroid hormone production.
- As a result, there is hyperthyroidism.
2. **Thyroid adenoma:** This is a solitary tumor which autonomously produces thyroid hormone leading to hyperthyroidism.

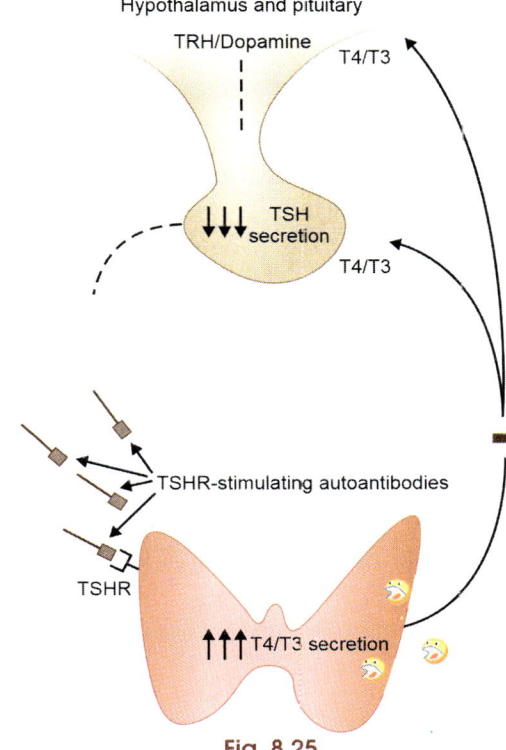

Hypothalamus and pituitary
TRH/Dopamine   T4/T3
↓↓↓ TSH secretion
T4/T3
TSHR-stimulating autoantibodies
TSHR
↑↑↑ T4/T3 secretion

Fig. 8.25

6. Define hormones and classify the hormones.

Hormones

Hormones are chemicals secreted from ductless endocrine glands, which when released in catalytic concentration into blood and transported to specific target cells (or organs) bring about physiological, morphological, and biochemical responses.

Classification of Hormones

- Based on their site of production

Endocrine hormones	• Secreted by a typical endocrine cell → transported through blood vessels → acts on a distal cell
Neurocrine hormones	• Secreted by a neurosecretory cell → transported through blood vessels → acts on a distal cell • Example: Oxytocin
Paracrine hormones	• Secreted by an endocrine cell → transported over a short distance through interstitial fluid → acts on target cell • Example: Somatostatin secreted by delta cells act on beta cells of pancreas
Autocrine hormones	• Secreted by cells → act on neighboring cells of similar type • Example: Prostaglandins

- Based on chemical nature

Proteins and Polypeptides	Amines (derivatives of tyrosine)	Steroids
1. Anterior and posterior pituitary hormones	1. Hormones of adrenal medulla	1. Adrenal cortex
2. Pancreatic hormones	2. Thyroid hormones	2. Ovaries
3. Parathyroid hormone		3. Testis
		4. Placenta

7. Explain second messenger system.

Second Messenger System

- When a hormone binds to its receptor, it activates another chemical within the cytoplasm. This is called second messenger, the hormone being the first messenger.
- This is mediated by G-proteins.
- Usually the hormone is water soluble and it binds to its receptor on the plasma membrane.
- This leads to activation of the G protein within the plasma membrane by the use of GTP.
- This activated G protein interacts with one or more effector proteins. These effector proteins may be enzymes (adenyl cyclase) or ion channels (calcium or potassium channels)
- This leads to activation or inhibition of these effector molecules.

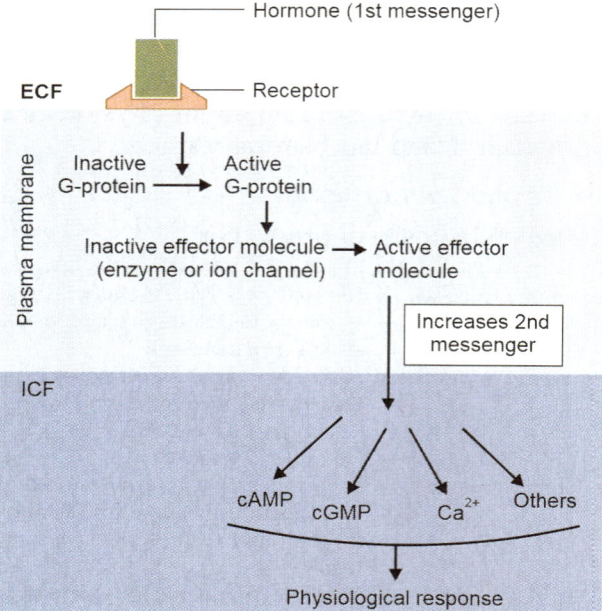

Fig. 8.26

- The changes effector molecules in-turn generate second messengers which bring about the desired effect of the hormone.
- The hormones involved in generating action through second messenger are called group II hormones.

Adenyl cyclase—activation or inhibition	• Production or decrease in cAMP
	• Example: ACTH, ADH, Angiotensin II
Guanylate cyclase—activation or inhibition	• Production or decrease in cGMP
	• Example: ANF and nitric oxide
Membrane phospholipase	• Activates protein kinase C and releases calcium ions
	• Example: PDGF
Calcium calmodulin system	• Activation of G protein causes entry of calcium ions
	• Example: Acetylcholine, catecholamines

8. List the anterior pituitary hormones.

Hormone	Functions
Growth hormone	• Stimulates physical growth
Adrenocorticoid stimulating hormone	• Stimulates secretin of adrenocorti-coids, mineralocorticoids and glucocorticoids
Thyroid stimulating hormone	• Stimulates production of thyroxine
Follicle stimulating hormone	• Females: Stimulates growth of Graafian follicles in ovaries, converts androgens to estrogens and stimulates theca cells to produce estrogen
	• Males: Stimulates spermatogenesis
Luteinizing hormone	• Females: Stimulates ovulation, induces synthesis of androgens from theca cell, improves formation of corpus luteum and secretion
Prolactin	• Acts on the epithelial cells of mammary glands to produce milk
Beta lipotropin	• Promotes lipolysis and forms precursor for endorphins

9. Enlist any 6 clinical features of an acromegaly.

1. **Acromegalic face:** Broad jaw, think lips, long face, prominent brows, broad nose, thickened skin
2. **Prognathism:** Forward protruding lower jaw

3. **Acromegaly**
   - Large feet and hands with long fingers, broad thick fingers
   - Height may be normal but built is stocky
4. **Kyphosis:** May result attributable to abnormal vertebral growth
5. **Overgrowth of internal organs:** Cardiomegaly, hepatomegaly, splenomegaly
6. **Increased sympathetic activity**

10. Explain the mechanism of action of aldosterone in sodium reabsorption.

Mechanism of Action of Aldosterone

- Aldosterone is a mineralocorticoid secreted from the zona glomerulosa of the adrenal cortex.
- 60% of the secreted aldosterone combines with plasma proteins and the rest in free form in the blood.
- After binding to its receptors on the tubular cell in the distal convoluted tubule, an aldosterone-induced protein is synthesized.

Effects on Distal Tubules

- Increases Na^+, hydrogen reabsorption

- Increases secretion of potassium, magnesium and ammonium.

Sodium Reabsorption (Fig. 8.27)

1. Aldosterone combines with its cytoplasmic receptors on target cells.
2. The hormone receptor complex initiates transcription of genes associated with new proteins.
3. Formation and synthesis of new ion channels and pumps.
4. Modulation of existing channels and pumps.
5. It increases sodium reabsorption by the following mechanisms
   - Increased permeability of the tubular cells to sodium along the electrical gradient (passive transport).
   - In the apical membrane, thiazide-sensitive NaCl cotransporters increase in number.
   - Increase in the number of Na^+-K^+-ATPase pumps on the basolateral surface of the tubular epithelium helps in absorption of sodium from the tubular cell into the interstitium.

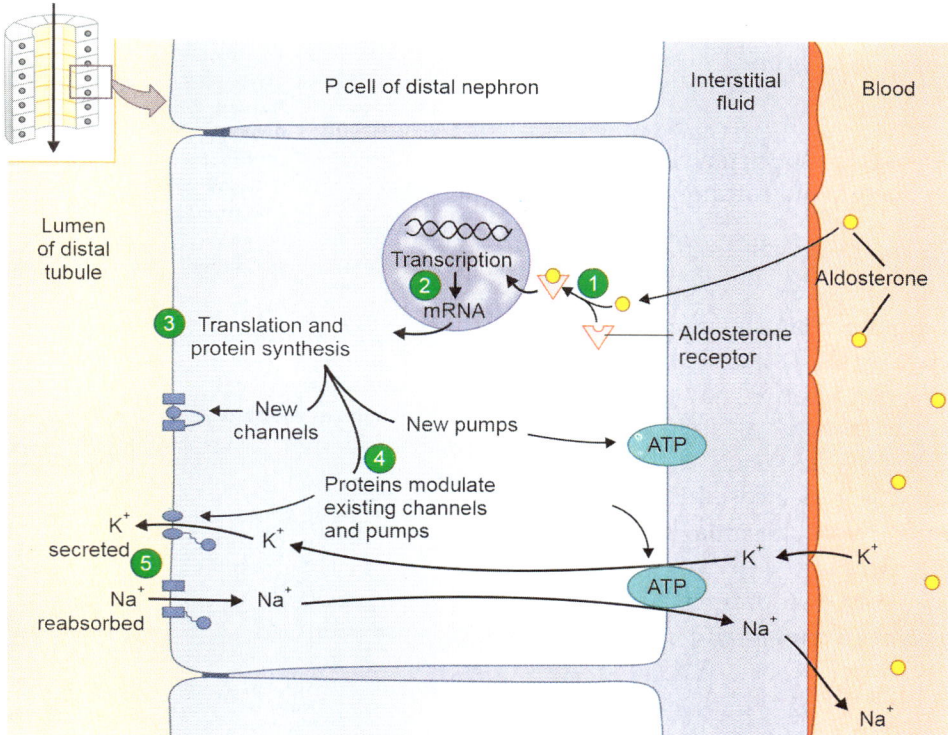

Fig. 8.27

Short-term Effects of Aldosterone

- Increase in aldosterone has transient effects of increasing serum sodium level and ECF volume for 1–2 days. There is also hypokalaemia.
- This is followed by pressure natriuresis and loss of sodium ions in urine and decrease in ECF volume.
- Also, there is secretion of ANP-atrial natriuretic factor due to increased venous return detected by right atrium. It causes increased loss of sodium in urine.
- This phenomenon is called aldosterone effect.

Long-term Effects of Aldosterone

- After the aldosterone escape, if a person continues to have excess aldosterone, there is no effect on sodium and water reabsorption.
- It solely depends on the intake of sodium and water. However, the blood pressure increases.

11. Discuss the clinical features with patho-physiological basis of:

A. Addison's disease, why hyperpigmentation occurs in it	**(3 marks)**
B. Cushing's syndrome	**(3 marks)**
C. Conn's syndrome	**(3 marks)**
D. Adrenogenital syndrome	**(3 marks)**

A. Addison's Disease

- Addison's disease is characterized by chronic deficiency adrenocorticoid hormone production.

Pathophysiology and Clinical Features

1. **Glucocorticoid deficiency**
   - The body cannot handle stress and can be fatal if encountered by mild stress (e.g. infection)
   - There is loss of appetite, nausea, vomiting, malaise, and diarrhoea.
2. **Mineralocorticoid deficiency**
   - Hypotension due to decreased ECF volume
   - Hyponatremia, hyperkalaemia, acidosis
3. **Sex hormone deficiency**
   - There is deficiency of androgens
   - Hypogonadism in males and sparse hair in females
4. **Pigmentation**
- It is characterized by melanin production and deposition of skin and mucous membranes. The deposition is uneven and may be in blotches and more under thin skin.

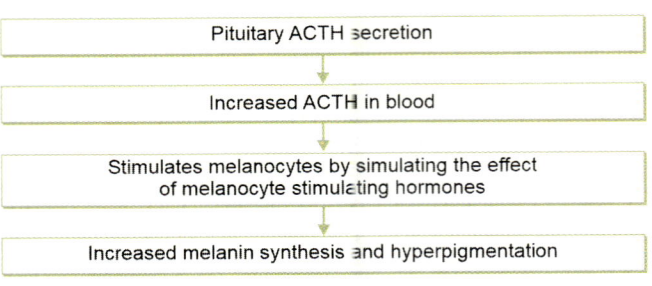

Fig. 8.28

B. Cushing Syndrome

It is a collection of signs and symptoms due to increased circulating cortisol due to any cause.

Pathophysiology

- The cortisol may be endogenous or exogenous in origin.
- It may also be secondary to hypersecretion of ACTH from the pituitary or an ectopic tumour.
- It is mainly divided as ACTH independent and ACTH dependent Cushing's syndrome

ACTH independent		ACTH dependent	
Hypersecretion of cortisol from the adrenal cortex due to an adrenal tumour	Treatment with exogenous steroids for pathological conditions (autoimmune conditions, nephrotic syndrome)	ACTH secreting pituitary tumor causing cortisol hypersecretion from adrenal	Ectopic neuroendocrine tumour secreting ACTH. ACTH stimulates adrenals to produce cortisol.

Clinical Features

Increased cortisol shifts the metabolism of carbohydrates and lipids towards a positive balance.	• Hyperglycaemia • Truncal obesity • Purple striae due to excessive stretching of skin by subcutaneous fat → rupture of subdermal tissues • Buffalo hump due to fat deposition
Cortisol has mild mineralocorticoid function	• Sodium and water retention • Increased blood pressure • Moon-like face or cushingoid facies: Due to increased fat deposition and water retention

Contd.

Contd.

Cortisol has catabolic effects on proteins	• There is proximal muscle weakness
Increased adrenal androgens	• Hirsutism and menstrual irregularity
Increased protein depletion and osteoclastic activity	• Increased chances of osteoporosis
Suppresses activity of the immune cells	• Susceptibility to infections, poor wound healing
Cortisol increases basal gastrin secretion	• Susceptibility to peptic ulceration
Hypersecretion of ACTH has melanocyte stimulating hormone like effect	• Pigmentation of skin
	• Acanthosis nigricans—darkened and thickened skin in axilla, groin (signifies insulin resistance)
Due to protein catabolism, thinning of skin and decreased clotting factors	• Easy bruisability

C. Conn's Syndrome

- It is hyperaldosteronism due to any cause.
- When primary, it is referred to as Conn's disease.
- Conn's disease is caused by a tumour of the zona glomerulosa secreting excess mineralocorticoids.
- Secondary Conn's syndrome is caused by hyper-activation of the RAAS leading to hyperaldosteronism and its effects.

Pathophysiology and Clinical Features

Primary Conn's disease	Pseudo-primary	Secondary
Tumour of the zona glomerulosa	Hypercortisolism Congenital adrenal hyperplasia (17α-hydroxylase deficiency) Activating mutation of mineralocorticoid receptor	Renal artery stenosis Toxaemia of pregnancy Aortic coarctation Cirrhosis of liver

Electrolyte Abnormalities

- Excess aldosterone causes sodium and water retention causing hypertension and pitting edema.

- There is no marked hypernatremia due to simultaneous water absorption.
- There is hypokalemia due to excretion of excess potassium.
- There is also alkalosis due to loss of hydrogen ions in urine. This leads to metabolic alkalosis and precipitate hypocalcemic tetany.

D. Adrenogenital Syndrome

- It is a constellation of signs due to abnormal amount of sex steroids secreted by the tumour of zona reticularis of the adrenal cortex.
- When there are excess androgens in the females, there is development of masculine features.

Pathophysiology

- There is a tumor of the zona reticularis of the adrenal cortex.
- The tumor can be adenoma (benign) or carcinoma (malignant)
- As a result, there is increased production of sex steroids.

Clinical Features

Features in females	Features in males
Adrenal virilism	Due to excess estrogen secretion
• Deepening of voice	• Feminization
• Masculinization, increased bulk of muscles	• Gynaecomastia
• Enlarged clitoris	• Testicular atrophy
• Male type of hair growth	• Decreased libido
• Amenorrhoea	

12. Describe the basis of classification of diabetes mellitus.

Classification of Diabetes Mellitus

- Diabetes mellitus is a disorder characterized by increased glucose in the blood and their manifestations in various tissues.
- It is primary or secondary.

Primary diabetes	Secondary diabetes
• Due to no underlying cause—unrelated to another disease It is further divided based on the dependency of insulin	• Due to an underlying disorder Example: Cushing's syndrome, hyperthyroidism, acromegaly, chronic pancreatitis and pancreatic damage due to hemochromatosis, cystic fibrosis, malignancy, pancreatectomy
Type 1 diabetes Type 2 diabetes	

Type 1 diabetes mellitus	Type 2 diabetes mellitus
• Previously known as insulin dependent diabetes mellitus	• Previously known as insulin resistant diabetes mellitus
• There is no family history	• It is an acquired condition with a strong family history
• It is due to autoimmune destruction of beta cells and manifests in childhood.	• Manifests in adulthood
• There is absolute insulin deficiency and hence progresses very fast and has early complications	• Insulin level may be low normal but the tissues have resistance to the action of insulin. Complications are lesser compared to type 1.

• Totally dependent on insulin
Other types
  1. Latent autoimmune diabetes in adults
  2. Maturity onset diabetes in young (hereditary)
	• Insulin dependence is partial
	Other types
	  1. Gestational diabetes
	  2. Impaired glucose tolerance

8.3 DESCRIBE THE PHYSIOLOGY OF THYMUS AND PINEAL GLAND

SHORT ANSWERS

1. What is the impact of melatonin on sleep wake cycle?

Melatonin (Fig. 8.29)

- The suprachiasmatic nucleus the master clock of the body and receives information from the pineal gland.
- The melanopsin containing retinal ganglion cells send information regarding presence or absence of light to the suprachiasmatic nucleus and pineal gland.
- Pineal gland produces melatonin and it controls various aspects of sleep like arousal, REM and NREM successions and consolidation of sleep.
- Melatonin is secreted in bursts in the night and their levels are maximum at around 3 am. This is regulated by the suprachiasmatic nucleus.
- Its effects are mediated through MT1 and MT2. They are densely situated in the suprachiasmatic nucleus.

Sleep Wake Cycle

- The daily sleep wake cycle is influenced by 2 factors: Process C and process S.
- Process C or circadian is an endogenous clock which helps in designing the timing for sleep and waking.
- Process S or sleep propensity determines the amount of sleep and wakefulness.
- Excitatory signals from the suprachiasmatic nucleus and melatonin suppression cause wakefulness, and inhibitory signals from suprachiasmatic nucleus and melatonin secretion cause sleep.

2. List functions of pineal gland.

- Pineal gland is a small conical structure present in the diencephalon and above the hypothalamus.
- It secretes the hormone melatonin from the epithelium.

Functions of Melatonin

1. **In circadian rhythm**

- The dark light cycle through the supraventricular nuclei of the hypothalamus are shown to exhibit a wide variation in circadian rhythm of melatonin secretion.
- It is secreted when there is dim light and plays an important role in sleep cycles.
- Many hormones and body functions have a circadian rhythm and melatonin helps in maintaining the body through it.
- Synthetic melatonin is being tried to help individuals with sleep problems.

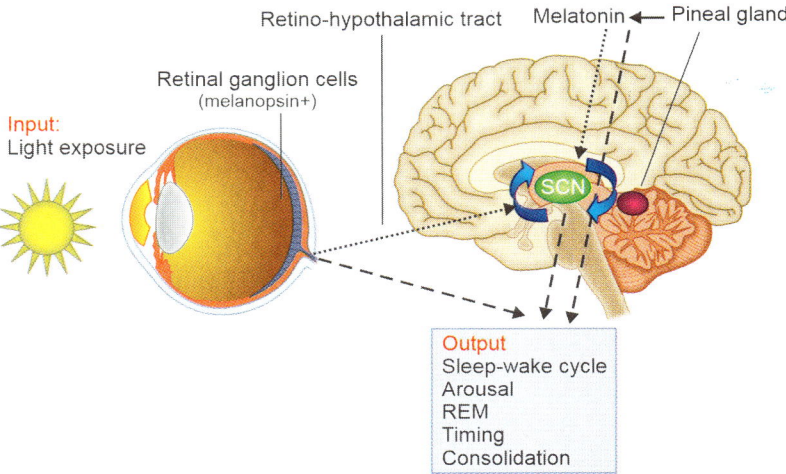

Retino-hypothalamic tract   Melatonin ← Pineal gland

Retinal ganglion cells
(melanopsin+)

Input:
Light exposure

SCN

Output
Sleep-wake cycle
Arousal
REM
Timing
Consolidation

Fig. 8.29

2. **On gonads**
   - In lower animals, melatonin is involved in increasing fertility during mating seasons.
   - In humans, they have stimulatory and inhibitory effects on the gonads.
   - It is also found to inhibit puberty.
3. **Melatonin exerts** an inhibitory effect on melanocyte stimulating hormone and adrenocorticotropic hormone.

3. What is the impact of thymectomy?

- Thymus is a small lymphoid tissue that is present just anterior to the trachea. Its main function is development of immunologically competent T cells.
- It also provides continuous source of T cells.

- Thymectomy is indicated in thymomas, which give rise to myasthenia gravis.

Effects of Thymectomy

Removal of Thymus in Newborn

- This causes depletion of T cells and immunodeficiency in neonates.
- This is shown by the fact that DiGeorge's syndrome (thymic aplasia) causes severe immunodeficiency.

Removal of Thymus in Adulthood

- It does not cause immediate effect on immunity
- However, it is therapeutic in myasthenia gravis and helps to avoid use of immunosuppressant drugs.

8.4 DESCRIBE FUNCTION TESTS: THYROID GLAND, ADRENAL CORTEX, ADRENAL MEDULLA AND PANCREAS

SHORT ANSWERS

1. Explain thyroid function tests.

Hormone Assays and Plasma TSH (Table 8.1)

- Most performed tests. They are usually performed together.
- It can be done by radioimmunoassay (RIA), enzyme-linked immunosorbent assay (ELISA), fluorescent immunoassay (FIA) or chemiluminescent immunoassay.

2. Discuss glucose tolerance test with its clinical significance.

Glucose Tolerance Test (Table 8.2)

- This test is used to understand the efficiency of glucose homeostatic mechanisms in the body.
- It is done by giving a fixed amount of glucose after an overnight fast and measuring the glucose levels.

Procedure

- After an overnight fast, blood is drawn for a fasting blood glucose sample.
- Later, the individual is given 75 g of anhydrous glucose with 250–300 ml of water. This dose is same for all individuals irrespective of age, sex and weight.
- Blood is drawn at one-hour post glucose and 2 hours post glucose and values are compared.

- This test is used to classify patients with impaired glucose tolerance and diabetes. It is also helpful in detecting gestational diabetes.

3. How do you diagnose pheochromocytoma with hormonal assay?

Pheochromocytoma

Urine Test

a. 24-hour urinary excretion of vanillylmandelic acid
   - VMA is a metabolic product of epinephrine.
   - Normal excretion in urine is 2–6 mg/day

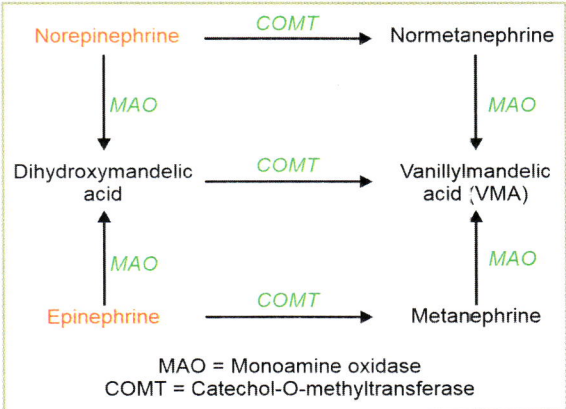

MAO = Monoamine oxidase
COMT = Catechol-O-methyltransferase

Fig. 8.30

Table 8.1			
Parameter	T3	T4	TSH
Normal levels	100–200 ng/dl	5.0–11.0 microgram/ml	0.4–.5 mIU/ml
Subclinical hypothyroidism		Normal	Elevated
Primary hypothyroidism	Decreased	Decreased	Elevated
Central hypothyroidism (following destruction of pituitary)	—	Decreased	Decreased
Primary hyperthyroidism	Elevated	Elevated	Decreased
Subclinical hyperthyroidism		Normal	Decreased
Central hyperthyroidism (pituitary tumor secreting TSH)	Elevated	Elevated	

Table 8.2			
Parameter	Normal persons	Criteria for diabetes	Criteria for diagnosing IGT
Fasting	<100 mg/dl	>126 mg/dl	110 to 126 mg/dl
1 hour (peak) after glucose	<160 mg/dl	Not prescribed	Not prescribed
1 hour after glucose	<140 mg/dl	>200 mg/dl	140 to 199 mg/dl

- It is increased in pheochromocytomas as there is increase in serum catecholamines (epinephrine)
- It is also increased in neuroblastomas. (due to increased norepinephrine)
- This test is performed after refraining the patient from intake of chocolates, vanilla flavoured food

b. Plasma epinephrine and norepinephrine levels are increased

c. Phentolamine suppression test
- Phentolamine is a short acting antagonist of epinephrine
- 2.5 mg injection of phentolamine is given intravenously and after 10 minutes, the concentration of serum epinephrine and norepinephrine is checked
- The levels are not affected as they are secreted from the tumor

8.5 DESCRIBE THE METABOLIC AND ENDOCRINE CONSEQUENCES OF OBESITY AND METABOLIC SYNDROME, STRESS RESPONSE. OUTLINE THE PSYCHIATRY COMPONENT PERTAINING TO METABOLIC SYNDROME

SHORT ANSWERS

1. Define obesity. List the criteria to diagnose metabolic syndrome.

Obesity

In terms of body mass index, obesity is defined as BMI >30 kg/m².

Diagnostic Criteria for Metabolic Syndrome

- The signs stem from increased weight gain and deposition of fat around the viscera
- This adipose tissue is resistant to the action of insulin.
- Features are
  - Obesity (especially abdominal fat accumulation) >40 inches in men and >35 inches in women
  - Insulin resistance
  - Fasting hyperglycemia (fasting blood glucose >100mg/dl)
  - Lipid abnormalities—hypertriglyceridemia (>150 mg/dl) and decreased HDL (<40 mg/dl)
  - Hypertension (BP >130/85 mm Hg)

2. Explain the effects of stress response.

Stress Response

- It refers to simultaneous diffuse activation and discharge from all portions of the sympathetic system in case of heightened stress.
- It is also known as alarm response or mass reflex.

Effects of Stress Response

The effects are due to increased circulation of catecholamines and cortisol.
1. Increased blood pressure
2. Increased blood flow to skeletal muscles and relative decrease of blood supply from GIT and kidneys.
3. Increased metabolic rate throughout the body
4. Increased glucose production by glycolysis from liver and muscles
5. Increased rate of blood coagulation
6. Increased strength in muscles
7. Increased mentation

3. Discuss the psychological/psychiatric components of bulimia nervosa.

Bulimia Nervosa (Fig. 8.31)

- It is a potentially life-threatening eating disorder characterized by episodes of binge eating followed by weeks of self-starving in order to avoid weight gain. Some individuals even resort to purging with the help of laxatives or induced vomiting.
- In this type of eating disorder, there is a body image disturbance and the affected individual is unable to perceive his body image accurately. There is intense fear of becoming obese.
- Also, there is heightened craving for food and the person is preoccupied with thoughts of food. This causes large amount of food to be ingested in a short span of time.
- This causes feelings of shame and self-hatred which leads the individual to diet restriction, purging by use of laxatives, induced vomiting and use of drugs which suppress appetite.

4. Enlist the adipose tissue hormones. Explain the mechanism of action of any one orexigenic hormone.

Adipose Tissue Hormones

1. Leptin   2. Adiponectin   3. Resistin

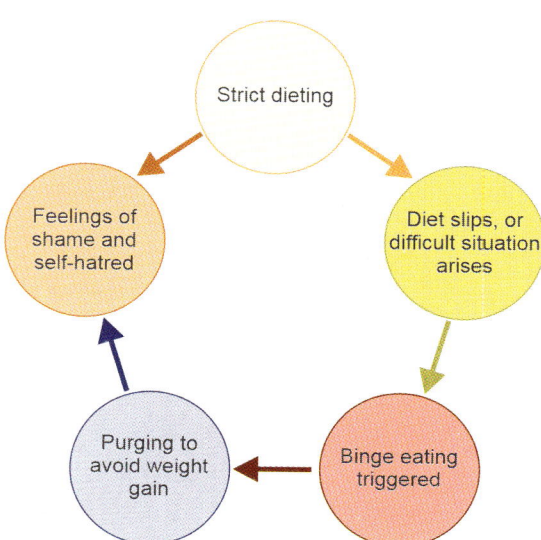

Fig. 8.31: The binge purge cycle

Orexigenic Hormone

That induce appetite—ghrelin

- An orexigenic, a substance which increases appetite and increases food intake.
- It plays a role in increasing hunger and adipose tissue volume.
- It is released by the oxyntic cells of the mucosa of the stomach and to a small extent by intestinal mucosa.
- Stimulants include fasting states.
- Ghrelin acts on the agouti-related peptide receptor and neuropeptide Y receptor on the arcuate nucleus.
- This causes stimulation of melanocyte stimulating hormone and cocaine-amphetamine relater transcripts to be produced proopiomelanocortin neurons.
- MSH activate melanocortin receptors 3 and 4 and cause increased appetite and thus increase weight gain.

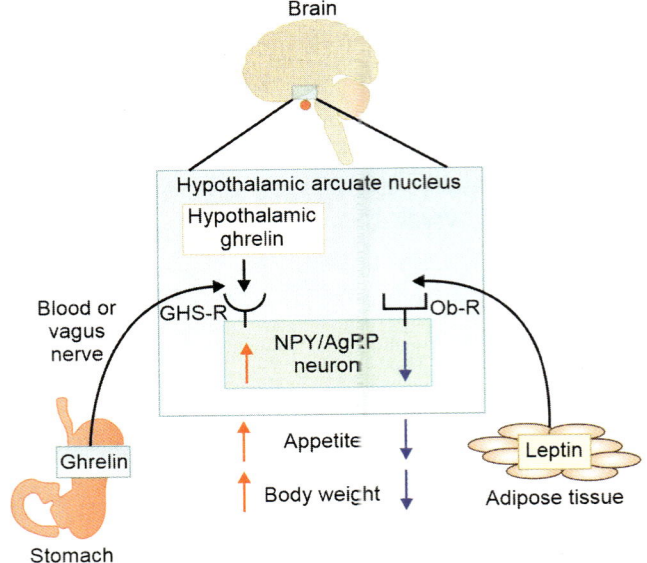

Fig. 8.32

8.6 DESCRIBE AND DIFFERENTIATE THE MECHANISM OF ACTION OF STEROID, PROTEIN AND AMINE HORMONES

SHORT ANSWERS

1. List the various types of hormone receptors with examples for each.

Hormone Receptors

Based on the location of receptors, they are divided as nuclear and cytoplasmic receptors.

A. Nuclear Receptors

- They are situated within the cytoplasm and bring about action through gene modification.
- Examples: Thyroid hormone receptor, steroid and retinoid receptor.

B. Cytoplasmic Receptors

- They are situated on the surface of the cell.
- Examples: Sex hormones, aldosterone.

2. Explain upregulation and downregulation of receptors.

- The number of receptors for a particular hormone varies according to the need.
- This is regulated tightly by upregulation and downregulation.

Upregulation

- It is increase in the number of active receptors on the cell surface.
- This causes an increase in sensitivity of a particular hormone, causes increased binding and therefore increase in its effect.
- This happens when the concentration of hormone in blood decreases. It also can happen when there is an increased need for the hormonal action.
- Example: Increase in oxytocin receptors on uterus during the end of pregnancy.

Downregulation

- It is the decrease in the number of receptors on the cell surface
- This decreases the hormone sensitivity and thus decreases the effects of the hormone
- It is seen when there is an excess of hormones in the circulating blood.

- It is also seen when there is chronic exposure to a particular drug or a toxin. This is called desensitization.
- Example: Decrease in insulin receptors in presence of excess insulin in blood.

3. Explain the mechanism of action of hormones action on intracellular receptors.

- Group I hormones bring about their effects through intracellular receptors.
- Examples: Thyroid hormone, steroid and retinoid hormones.

Steps

1. After being secreted, the hormone is transported to the target tissue with the help of a serum binding protein.

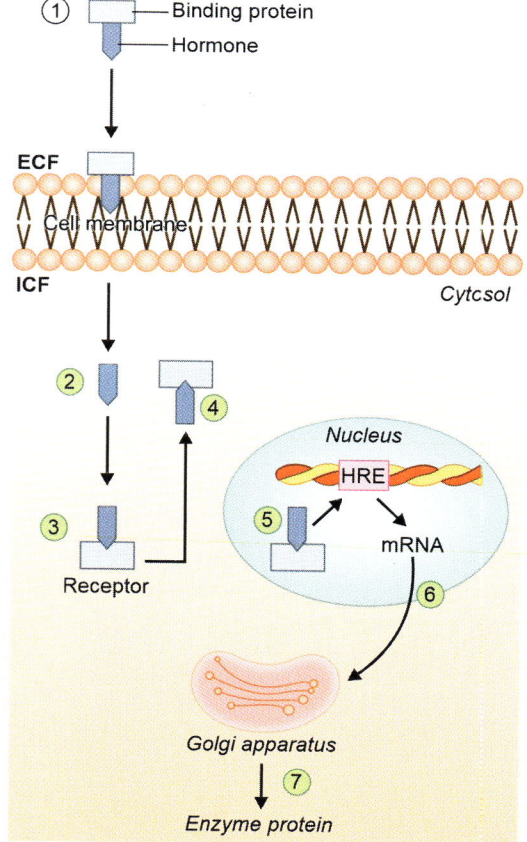

Fig. 8.33

2. Being lipophilic, the hormones internalized easily within the cell.

3. It binds to an intracellular receptor and it forms a complex with the receptor.

4. There is conformational change in the receptor and thus gets activated.

5. This activated receptor enters the nucleus of the cell and binds to a respective part of the DNA called the hormone responsive element.

6. This brings about gene transcription and then translation occurs.

7. The necessary enzymes and proteins are synthesized.

Reproductive Physiology

9.1 DESCRIBE AND DISCUSS SEX DETERMINATION; SEX DIFFERENTIATION AND THEIR ABNORMALITIES AND OUTLINE PSYCHIATRY AND PRACTICAL IMPLICATION OF SEX DETERMINATION

SHORT ANSWERS

1. What is karyotyping? What is its physiological importance?

Karyotyping

- Karyon = nucleus. Typing = studying
- It is the study of chromosomes.
- It is process by which the chromosomes of the nucleus are paired and arranged in sequential order.
- The cells in metaphase are arrested with the use of mitotic spindle inhibitors and stained. In metaphase, they take the form of two chromatids connected to a centromere.
- The karyotype is formed by arranging the autosomes according to length followed by sex chromosomes. They are numbered accordingly and there are 22 pairs of autosomal chromosomes and 1 pair of sex chromosomes: X and Y. Thus, normal genotype for female is 46 XX and for male it is 46 XY.

Physiological Importance

- Karyotyping is used to study the chromosomes. Euploidy is a state where the number of chromosomes is an exact multiple of 23.
- When the cell acquires the number of chromosomes which is not an exact multiple of 23, it is referred to as aneuploidy.

- Trisomy (n + 1) is a condition where there are three chromosomes for one haplotype. Monosomy (n – 1) is a condition where one chromosome represent one set.
- It is important in recognizing various structural and numerical abnormalities in an individual when in doubt. Various structural abnormalities like decrease or increase in length of the arms can be detected. Deletions, translocations can be detected. Thus, they help in detecting certain translocations which cause cancer.

2. Why is prenatal sex determination illegal in India?

Prenatal sex determination is knowing the sex of the fetus prior to its birth.

Implications

- In India, the tradition has been patriarchal and there is a tendency to want to have a male child for inheritance of property and performing of last rites and so on. There is also a notion of 'dynastical' continuation which is supposed to be brought about by the 'son'
- As a result, there has been a negative attitude towards female fetus.
- Due to all these inhumane reasons, there has been lot of female feticide in the past and now there is an imbalance with respect to sex ratio. Presently it is 924 females per 1000 males.

- This can have bad social repercussions in the form of increased sexual crimes against women and polyandry.
- These are the reasons why prenatal diagnosis of sex is a crime in India and the doctor who discloses sex of the baby is equally responsible.

3. Explain Klinefelter syndrome.

- Klinefelter syndrome is the most common sex chromosome disorder affecting 1:3000 individuals.
- It is a trisomy, characterized by an extra X chromosome in a phenotype male.
- It is produced due to fertilization of an egg containing two X chromosomes or by fusion of a sperm containing an extra X chromosome with a normal egg.
- As a result, there are two X chromosomes in a zygote.
- The extra X chromosome in a gamete is produced due to non-disjunction of X chromosomes during meiosis.

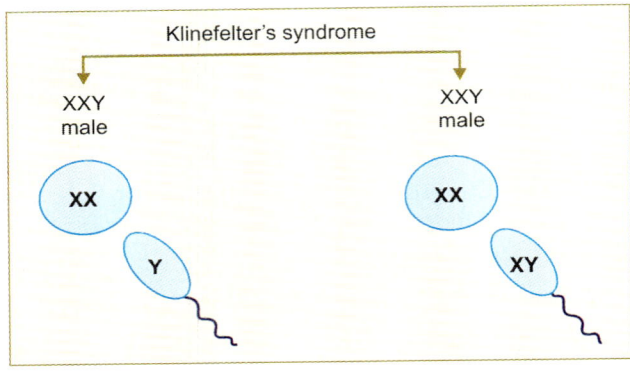

Fig. 9.1

Clinical Features

- The affected individual is tall, and lean built with gynecomastia (enlarged breasts)
- He has high pitched voice and poorly developed secondary sexual characters.
- Testis is poorly developed and there is hyalinization of seminiferous tubules, the individual is sterile.

Prenatal Diagnosis

In suspected individuals, it is done by karyotyping of amniocentesis and chorionic villus sampling.

4. Explain Turner's syndrome.

- It is a chromosomal abnormality (monosomy) caused by single X chromosome.
- This is due to during formation of an egg or a sperm, the gamete does not receive X chromosome.
- As a result, after zygote formation, the karyotype is 45, XO.

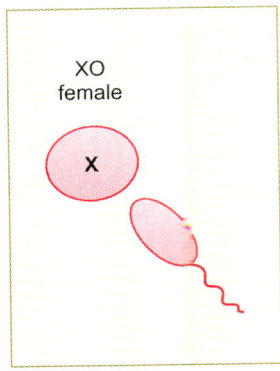

Fig. 9.2

Clinical Features

- These girl children are usually born with cystic hygromas in the neck.
- They are short and have webbed neck.
- They have characteristic facies: Ears are low set, small jaw and have low hairline.
- The elbow shows cubitus varus. Hands are small and chubby.
- They are predisposed to developing coarctation of aorta and mental retardation.
- Nipples are widely spaced and chest is broad.
- Ovaries are ill formed and are called streak ovaries. They have delayed puberty and infertility.

Prenatal Diagnosis

When suspected on an anomaly ultrasound scan, amniocentesis and chorionic villus sampling can be done.

5. What are hermaphrodites? Explain its types.

Hermaphrodite

- It is a condition characterized by sexual features of both the sexes.
- This is displayed in lower animals like frogs.
  1. **True hermaphroditism**
     - It is rare to have both sex organs in the same individual.

- They have testis on one side and ovary on the other. Sometimes, one gonad with both histological features of testis and ovary are present.
- It can present as bilateral ovotestes, or unilateral ovotestis and normal testis or ovary on the other side, one testis on side and ovary on the other.
- They display breast development and have menstruation.

2. **Pseudohermaphroditism:** It means having genotype of one sex and phenotype of the opposite sex. So, they have gonads of one sex and external genitalia and secondary sexual characteristics of the opposite sex.

Female Pseudohermaphroditism

- The individual has genotype XX
- They have ovaries and other internal genitalia
- At puberty, there is development of penis and male type of pubic hair growth.
- They have high plasma androgens
- It can be seen as a part of congenital adrenal hyperplasia where there is excess production of one type of sex steroids due to deficiency of enzyme necessary for glucocorticoid production.

Male Pseudohermaphroditism

- The individual has genotype of XY
- The testes may be undescended or small
- They develop feminine secondary sexual characters. It can occur in the following situations
- Testicular feminization syndrome: Here there is resistance to androgens. As a result, there are development of female secondary sexual characters and vagina which ends blindly. There is no uterus and thus no menstruation.

- It also seen in mullerian regression factor deficiency and 17α-hydroxylase deficiency.

6. Write a note on Barr body.

- During embryonic development, one X chromosome in the female zygote becomes inactive and the other is active.
- The exact underlying mechanism is not known.
- The inactive form of the X chromosome forms a condensed clump near the nucler membrane separate from rest of the chromosomes. This is called Barr body.

Importance

- Presence of Barr body in the somatic cells helps to readily know that the organism is female. The most suitable cells for this test are polymorphonuclear cells (neutrophils)
- In abnormal genotypes with multiple X chromosomes, only one X is active and the extra X chromosomes from Barr bodies. So, there may be two Barr bodies.

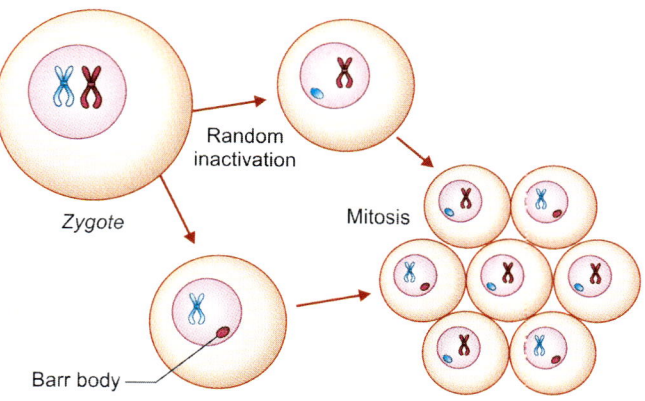

Fig. 9.3

9.2 DESCRIBE AND DISCUSS PUBERTY: ONSET, PROGRESSION, STAGES; EARLY AND DELAYED PUBERTY AND OUTLINE ADOLESCENT CLINICAL AND PSYCHOLOGICAL ASSOCIATION

SHORT ESSAYS

1. Explain the onset of puberty, changes that occur during puberty. Describe the factors that affect the onset of puberty.　(3 + 2 marks)

- Puberty is defined as the beginning of the ability to reproduce.
- It is marked by development and maturation of the gonads.

Onset of Puberty

- In prepubertal age, the hypothalamus keeps secreting GnRH and is under feedback control of estrogen and androgens secreted by the adrenal cortex and prepubertal testes.
- However, during puberty, the sensitivity to negative feedback decreases.
- The signals probably from the limbic system stimulate the hypothalamus according to preprogrammed (probably genetic and environmental influences) timetable.
- The hypothalamus directs the anterior pituitary to secrete gonadotropins (LH and FSH) which stimulate the gonads to secrete respective hormones.
- In females it is called menarche which marks the beginning of the first menstrual period. It is normally around 10–13 years of age.

- In males, one cannot demarcate the exact time of puberty, however, it is realized by a set of changes. It is around 12–15 years of age.

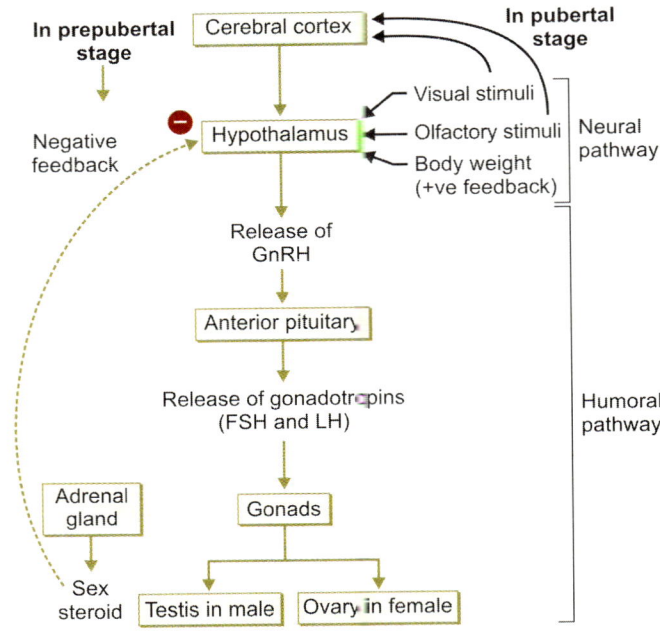

Fig. 9.4

Changes that Occur at Puberty

Stage of puberty	Age in years	In females	Age in years	In males
1	7 ½	Preadolescent age	7 ½	Preadolescent age
2	10 ½	Thelarche: Appearance of breast buds	12	Enlargement of testis
3	11 ½	Pubarche: Appearance of pubic hair Elevation of breast		
		Sudden increase in height	14	Pubarche: Appearance of pubic hair Enlargement of penis
4	13	Menarche: First menstrual period Elevation and projection of breasts	15	Sudden increase in height Enlargement of male external genitalia
5	14	Development of secondary sexual characteristics	16 ½	Development of secondary sexual characteristics

Factors that Affect Onset Puberty

Genetic predisposition is the most important factor.

Factors that hasten puberty	Factors that delay puberty
1. Increased BMI in females hastens menarche 2. CNS infections and tumors 3. Increased sex hormones in blood: Due to congenital enzyme deficiencies like congenital adrenal hyperplasia and tumors of the adrenal gland	1. Malnutrition 2. Malabsorption syndromes 3. Systemic illnesses like renal, cardiac and pulmonary disorders 4. Psychiatric syndromes like anorexia, bulimia, stress induced 5. Hormonal: Hypothyroidism, Cushing syndrome, diabetes mellitus 6. Recurrent infections and AIDS

2. A 17-year-old female is brought to the gynecology OPD by her mother with the complaint of primary amenorrhea. Define delayed onset of puberty. What are its causes?

Delayed Onset of Puberty

- Delayed puberty is defined when menarche fails to occur by the age of 17 years in a female or testicular development and maturation fails to occur in a male by the age of 20 years.

Causes

Nonspecific to gender	Specific to gender
General causes • Malnutrition • Total body irradiation prior to bone marrow transplantation *Systemic causes* • Cardiac illness • Renal disorders • Pulmonary diseases *Psychological causes* • Anorexia nervosa • Bulimia nervosa • Stress *Hormonal or metabolic* • Uncontrolled diabetes • Congenital hypopituitarism • Hypothyroidism • Cushing's disease *Infections like AIDS*	*Females* • Gonadal dysgenesis like Turner's syndrome • Polycystic ovaries *Males* • Klinefelter syndrome • Bilateral cryptorchidism

SHORT ANSWERS

1. Describe the secondary sexual characteristics in males and females.

Structural Characteristics

Parameter	Female	Male
Body structure	Lean, narrow shoulders, breasts, wider hips with converging thighs	Broad shoulder, narrow hips
Skin	Smooth and light	Thick, dark and oily
Subcutaneous fat	More around breasts and hips.	—
Hair	Fine and scanty body hair, no facial hair	Rough and dark body hair
		Moustache and beard
	Rounded frontal hairline	Frontal hairline indented on sides
	Triangular pubic hair with base up	Triangular with apex upwards—pubic hair
Muscles	Soft	Bulky and stronger
Accessory sex organs	Clitoris, labia majora and labia minora	Prostate, seminal vesicles and bulbourethral glands

Functional Characteristics

- Females: Soft and shrill voice, with a lower basal metabolic rate and lower RBC count and hemoglobin concentration.
- Males: Thickened and enlarged vocal cords giving rise to a deep voice. Higher basal metabolic rate and high RBC and hemoglobin concentration.

2. Explain precocious puberty. Mention its causes.

Precocious Puberty

- Precocious puberty refers to onset of puberty in a child of any sex prior to the age of 8 years.
- There is development of secondary sexual characters well before age and there is gametogenesis.
- There is a normal sequence of events but occurring early.
- There is hastened growth and the bone age is higher than normal. The bones ossify earlier than usual and thus they have short stature.
- Female children have menstruation, development of breasts and pubic hair well before their normal pubertal age.
- Male children have early development of external genitalia and pubic hair and development of facial hair.

Causes

1. True precocious puberty

- It is seen in irritative lesions of hypothalamus which cause increased secretion of GnRH causing excess secretion of sex hormones.
- Also called GnRH dependent precocious puberty.

2. Pseudo-precocious puberty

- It is seen when there is an exogenous source of sex hormones or due to excess production by the adrenals.
- It is seen in conditions like congenital adrenal hyperplasia, androgen secreting tumors in males and estrogen secreting tumors in females.

9.3 DESCRIBE MALE REPRODUCTIVE SYSTEM: FUNCTIONS OF TESTIS AND CONTROL OF SPERMATOGENESIS AND FACTORS MODIFYING IT AND OUTLINE ITS ASSOCIATION WITH PSYCHIATRIC ILLNESS

SHORT ESSAY

1. Describe spermatogenesis and the factors that control and affect spermatogenesis.

Spermatogenesis

- It is the process by which spermatozoa are produced from primitive primordial cells in the seminiferous tubules of the testes.
- It occurs in four stages
  1. **Stage of proliferation**
     - It begins with spermatogonium, a cell containing diploid number of chromosomes.
     - Spermatogonia divide by mitosis up to 5 times. So, from one spermatogonium, 32 spermatogonia are produced.
     - This process takes place in the base of seminiferous tubules.
     - They divide again by mitosis to form primary spermatocytes. During this stage, spermatogonia migrate towards the lumen of the seminiferous tubules along with Sertoli cells.
  2. **Stage of growth:** The primary spermatocyte grows in this stage.
  3. **Stage of maturation**
     - After reaching full size, these cells undergo meiosis.
     - During meiosis I, primary spermatocyte divides into two secondary spermatocyte having haploid number of chromosomes, i.e. 22 autosomal chromosomes and one X/Y chromosome.
     - This is followed by meiosis II, where two spermatids are formed, each having haploid number of chromosomes.
  4. **Stage of transformation**
     - In this stage, morphological changes take place in the spermatids to become a sperm or spermatozoan.
     - This process is called spermiogenesis. It is characterized by loss of cytoplasm, placement of nucleus at one end with an acrosomal cap, development of a flagellum from the centromeres.

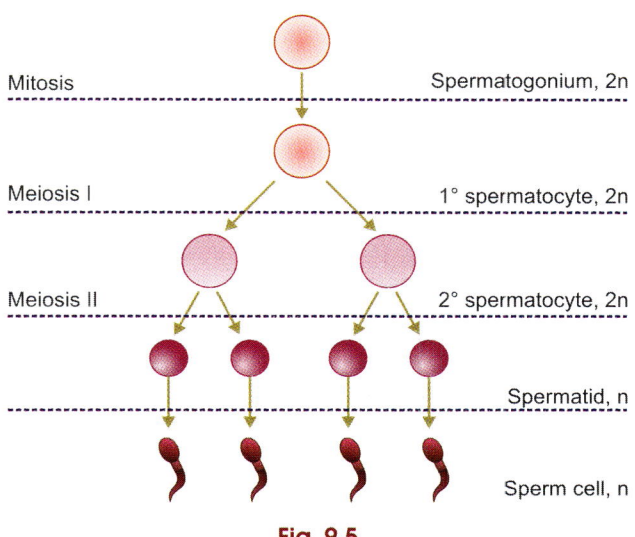

Fig. 9.5

Factors that Control and Affect Spermatogenesis

1. Hormones

Testosterone	Most important for spermatogenesis
Luteinizing hormone	Stimulates Leydig cells to stimulate testosterone
Estrogen	Decreases spermatogenesis

2. External factors

  i. Temperature
     - Cooler temperatures are preferred for spermatogenesis.
     - This is the reason why varicocele causes infertility. There is venous congestion around the testis raising the temperature.
  ii. Environmental toxins
  iii. Infections like mumps causes orchitis and degeneration of seminiferous tubules.
  iv. Seasonal variations—spermatogenesis is better in winter.

3. General factors

- Vitamins like B_{12}, C, E, A are required for spermatogenesis.
- General health affects spermatogenesis.
- Genetic predisposition may cause oligospermia.
- Chronic malnutrition and illnesses decrease spermatogenesis.

SHORT ANSWERS

1. Explain the functions of Sertoli cells.

- Sertoli cells are the supporting cells in the seminiferous tubules of testis.
- They are also called sustentacular cells.
- They are elongated and have cytoplasmic extension to which many germ cells are attached.

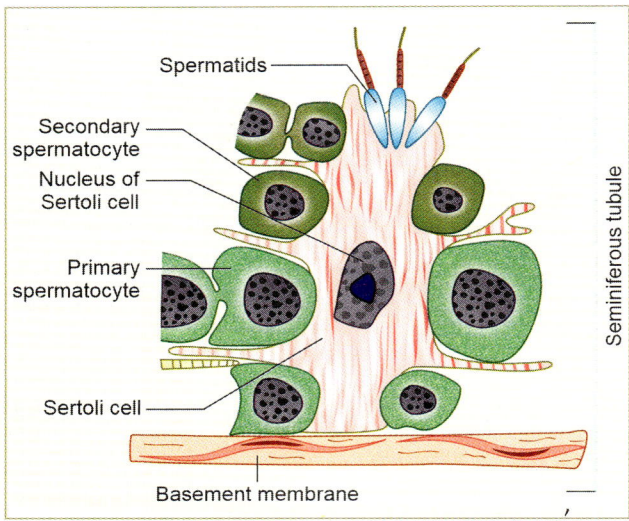

Fig. 9.6

Functions

1. Support and nourishment of spermatozoa through all stages of spermatogenesis.
2. They secrete androgen binding protein, which is required for transport of testosterone
3. Secretion of aromatase, which is necessary for conversion of androgens to estrogens.
4. Secretes activin and inhibin, which stimulates and inhibits the secretion of FSH respectively.
5. Secretes estrogen binding protein.
6. In the fetus, it is responsible for production of MIS or Mullerian Inhibiting substance under the influence of which there is regression of the structures of the Mullerian duct.

2. Describe the actions of testosterone.

- In testes, testosterone is secreted by interstitial cells of Leydig and zona reticularis of the adrenal cortex.
- Its actions are different in fetal and in adult life.

In Fetal Life

- Testosterone is secreted by genital ridge in the fetus beginning by about 7th week.
- It causes regression of Mullerian duct and development of male sex organs like epididymis, seminiferous tubules and vas deferens through Wolffian duct.
- It is also responsible for development of penis, scrotum, genital ducts and prostate.
- Initially, the testes are developed from the bipotential gonads in the abdomen. Under the influence of testosterone, they descend into the scrotum through the inguinal canal.

In Adult Life

Effects on Sex Organs

- It is required for growth of testes, penis and scrotum after puberty.
- It is also required for spermatogenesis.

Effects on Secondary Sexual Characters

- Testosterone increases muscle mass by about 50% in puberty due to anabolic effect on proteins.
- Increases thickness of bones, increases calcium deposition and early fusion of epiphysis of long bones.
- It makes the shoulders wide and pelvis narrow. The pelvis becomes funnel shaped
- It increases thickness of skin and sebum secretion from skin
- The body hair becomes coarse and dark, causes growth of facial hair in the form of moustache and beard
- There is hair growth in the pubic area, and it extends up to the umbilicus along the linea alba. There is also development of chest hair.
- Testosterone causes deepening of voice by increasing the thickness of the vocal cords, hypertrophy of laryngeal muscles, lengthening of larynx.
- Testosterone has an anabolic effect on proteins. It increases basal metabolic rate.
- It has a mineralocorticoid like action on salt and water absorption, thus causes sodium and water retention.
- It also has erythropoietic action as a result, it increases hemoglobin concentration and RBC count.

3. Describe the endocrine functions of testis.

- Testis contains three types of cells—seminiferous cells take part in spermatogenesis.
- Interstitial cells of Leydig secrete androgens
- Sertoli cells secrete estrogen, inhibin and activin.

Androgens

- Androgens are male sex hormones and include testosterone, androstenedione and dihydrotestosterone.
- They are secreted mainly in fetus and neonates and then at puberty. Androgen secretion starts decreasing by the age of 40 years and then becomes nil at around 80 years.
- They are secreted by the interstitial cells of Leydig.
- Normal secretion of testosterone is 4–9 mg/day, androstenedione is 2.5 mg/day and dihydrotestosterone are formed by reduction of testosterone by Sertoli cells and in periphery.
- They are responsible for development of sex organs and secondary sexual characters in male. Also, they are necessary for spermatogenesis.

Estradiol and Inhibin

They are secreted by the Sertoli cells and they inhibit LH secretion by the anterior pituitary.

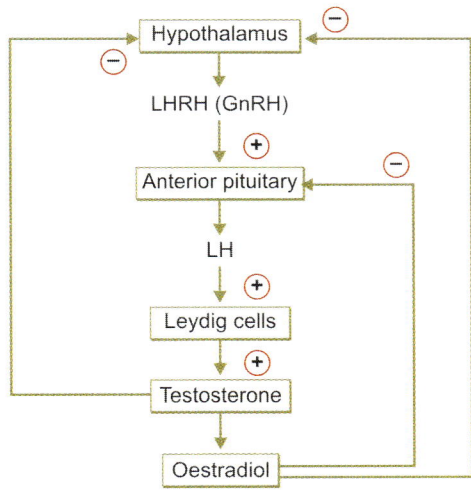

Fig. 9.7

Activin

It is secreted by the Sertoli cells and activates secretion of LH and GnRh by the pituitary and hypothalamus respectively.

4. A newborn child on examination found to have one testis undescended. What is this condition called? What would be the consequences if left untreated and why?

Condition Called

- This condition is called cryptorchidism (cryptus-hidden, orchid-testis)
- It is a congenital condition characterized by partial or complete failure of the testis to descend into the scrotum through the inguinal canal (Fig. 9.8).

Consequences of Undescended Testis

- The testes require cooler temperature to form adequate sperms. In the abdomen, they are unable to do so. As a result, sterility results. It should be corrected within 6–12 months.
- These undescended testes are highly prone for malignancies specially, germ cell tumors.
- They are also prone to testicular torsion and inguinal hernias.

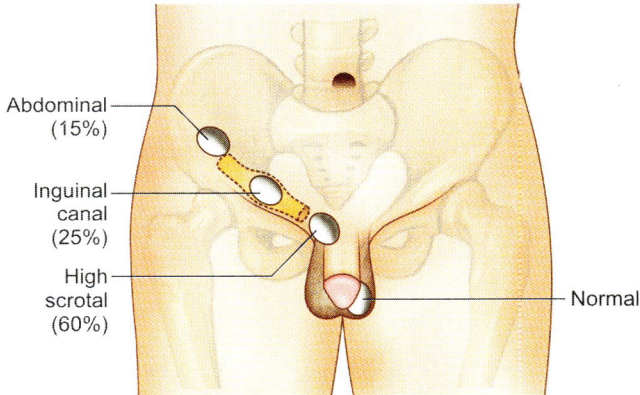

Fig. 9.8

9.4 DESCRIBE FEMALE REPRODUCTIVE SYSTEM: (A) FUNCTIONS OF OVARY AND ITS CONTROL; (B) MENSTRUAL CYCLE: HORMONAL, UTERINE AND OVARIAN CHANGES

LONG ESSAY

1. Explain the changes that occur during the menstrual cycle. Explain the role of hormones in menstrual cycle.   (5 + 5 marks)

Menstrual cycle is a constellation of changes occurring in the female reproductive organs in a rhythmic fashion in the reproductive age of a woman's life.

Changes Occurring during Menstrual Cycle

During menstrual cycle, simultaneous changes occur in the ovaries, endometrium of uterus, cervix and vagina.

A. Ovarian Cycle

The changes in the ovary occur in two phases

1. Follicular phase
- It extends from day 5 of the menstrual bleed to around day 14 when ovulation occurs.
- The main function of this phase is growth of the ovum.
- During this phase, 10–15 primordial follicles start maturing, but only one follicle matures, and the rest disappear by apoptosis. This follicle is called Graafian follicle.
- They undergo the following phases: Primordial follicles → primary follicles → vesicular follicle → Graafian follicle.
- Ovulation
- It is expulsion of the ovum by rupture of the Graafian follicle. It takes place by rupture of the follicle at stigma followed by oozing of fluid and freeing of the germ hillock form the wall. Ovum is expelled out and reaches the abdominal cavity, enters the fimbrial end of the fallopian tube and then enters the uterus.

2. Luteal phase
- It extends from day 15 to day 28 of the menstrual cycle.
- The Graafian follicle after expulsion of the ovum is converted into a corpus luteum.
- It remains in the ovary till the end of the cycle.
- The granulosa cells and theca interna cells are transformed into granulosa lutein cells and theca lutein cells.

B. Endometrial Cycle

It goes hand in hand with the ovarian cycle.

1. Menstrual phase
- It is the part of the menstrual cycle characterized by shedding of the endometrium.
- It lasts for 3–7 days.
- The process by which the decidual endometrium is shed is called menstruation.
- There is sudden vasoconstriction of endometrial vessels due to drop in levels of estrogen and progesterone followed by hypoxic necrosis of the endometrium.
- Necrosis causes rupture of blood vessels and there is bleeding which comes out of vagina as menstrual blood.
- The desquamated endometrium is expelled out by uterine contraction.

2. Proliferative phase
- It lasts from day 6 to day 14 of the cycle.
- It corresponds to follicular stage of the ovarian cycle.
- During this stage, there is proliferation of endometrial glands within the endometrial stroma.
- The endometrial thickness is 1 mm at the end of menstruation and becomes 3–4 mm at the end of proliferative phase.
- At the end of proliferative phase, there is ovulation.

3. Secretory phase
- It follows ovulation.
- The changes in the endometrium are due to the hormones secreted by the corpus luteum.
- The vessels in the endometrium become more tortuous as they increase in their length. New blood vessels appear.
- Thickness of the endometrium increases up to 6 mm.
- Cytoplasm of the endometrial stroma get accumulated with lot of glycogen vacuoles in order to prep the endometrium for the nourishment of embryo.

C. Changes in Vagina and Cervix

• In proliferative phase, the mucosa is thinner and more alkaline and favours entry of sperms.
• In secretory phase, the mucosa is thicker and adhesive.

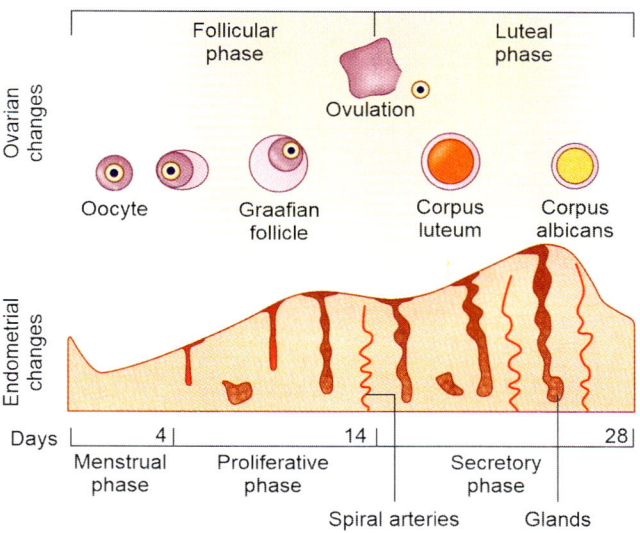

Fig. 9.9

Role of Hormones

Phase of menstruation	Hormone involved	Actions
Menstruation	—	—
Follicular stage	GnRH is secreted by the hypothalamus in pulsed manner (every 2 hours)	GnRH stimulates the anterior pituitary to secrete FSH and LH FSH stimulates development of the Graafian follicle, promotes aromatase activity which converts androgens to estrogens
	FSH is the predominant pituitary hormone, LH is also secreted	LH simulates theca cells to produce androgens
	Estrogen is secreted by the theca cells	Estrogen brings about changes in endometrium It also causes a negative feedback on hypothalamus and anterior pituitary It increases FSH and LH receptors on theca cells Facilitates faster growth of Graafian follicle
Ovulation	LH surge happens 36 hours prior to ovulation	Brings about rupture of Graafian follicle
Secretory stage	LH is secreted by the anterior pituitary	LH is necessary for maintenance of corpus luteum Stimulates corpus luteum to secrete progesterone
	Progesterone is secreted by corpus luteum under the influence of LH	Progesterone causes inhibit secretion of FSH and LH from the pituitary. Causes secretory changes in the endometrium and genesis of new vessels.
	FSH is secreted in low quantities	FSH stimulates the theca cells to secrete inhibin which inhibits the secretion of FSH and LH form pituitary. FSH maintains the secretory function of corpus luteum

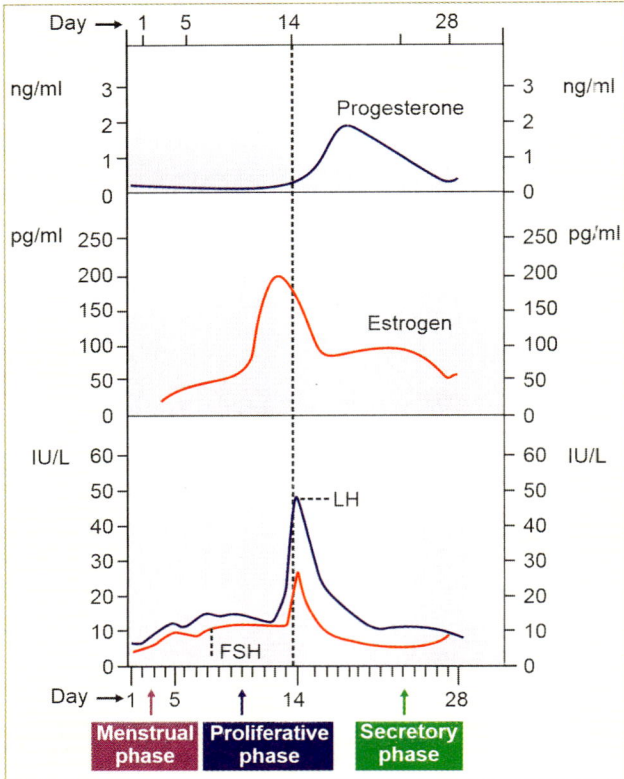

Fig. 9.10

SHORT ESSAY

1. List the ovarian hormones and describe the physiological actions of each.

Estrogen and progesterone are the ovarian hormones.

Estrogens

Related to Reproductive System

- Estrogens bring about growth and development of the reproductive organs.
- They take part in growth of the Graafian follicle and bring about proliferative changes in the endometrium. There is increase in the thickness of the endometrium.
- The fallopian tube becomes more functional.
- There is increase in size of the uterus and cervix.
- The vagina becomes longer in size and with the epithelial lining more cuboidal.
- There is increase in size of the clitoris and the labia majora and labia minora.
- Estrogens bring about secondary sexual characters like development of breasts and feminine appearance of a woman. There is deposition of subcutaneous fat more near the breasts and hips, smoothening of skin and female pattern of pubic hair.
- During pregnancy, it supports pregnancy.

Other Actions

- It increases bone density and ossification of the epiphysis.
- It enlarges the hip and widens the pelvic inlet.
- It has positive anabolic effect on the proteins and causes fat deposition under skin.
- It causes sodium and water retention.
- It has mild vasodilator effect.
- It increases libido in females.
- It makes skin thin and reduces the viscosity of sebum.

Progesterone

Reproductive Actions

- It is progestational: It supports pregnancy by all possible mechanisms. It helps in growth of the uterus, helps in maintain the endometrium, relaxes the smooth muscles of the uterus and decreases motility.
- It causes glycogen storage in the stroma of the endometrium in the secretory phase and prepares for nutrition of the embryo to be.
- The cervical discharge becomes thick and viscous.
- Vaginal epithelium becomes thickened and cornified.
- In the fallopian tube, progesterone increases the secretions enriched with nutritive material.
- In the breast, there is increase in the lobular and alveolar growth.

Other Actions

- Increases basal body temperature by about 0.5 degree
- It alters certain areas in the CNS and decreases appetite and increases somnolence.
- Progesterone has a pro-atherogenic effect by decreasing the HDL levels
- It also tends to cause hyperglycemia.
- There is smooth muscle relaxation in many tissues causing vasodilatation and lowering of blood pressure. Also, the lower esophageal sphincter is relaxed. Thus, pregnant women experience more belching and gastric reflux. Also, there is slowing of the bowel movements leading to constipation.

SHORT ANSWERS

1. What are the tests for ovulation?

- Ovulation is expulsion of the ovum from the Graafian follicle into the abdominal cavity.
- Tests for ovulation are important during fertility assessment and treatment procedures.
- It can be assessed by the following methods

Basal body temperature	Just prior to ovulation, there is a mild drop in the temperature. (0.3–0.5 degrees). However, it is non-specific
Determination of LH in serum	This test is commonly used. After 36 hours of LH surge, ovulation occurs.
Determination of hormonal excretion in urine	During ovulation, there is increased excretion of urinary estrogen and end products of progesterone metabolism which can be detected simple tests
Ultrasound scan	Transvaginal ultrasound shows absence of the Graafian follicle and collection of fluid in the cul-de-sac. It is difficult to obtain live ovulation as it cannot be predicted to that extent
Cervical pattern	When the cervical mucus spread on a slide is examined under microscope, it shows a fern pattern. This pattern is absent after ovulation

2. Explain the following terminologies:

- **A. Amenorrhea**
- **B. Menorrhagia**
- **C. Dysmenorrhea**

A. Amenorrhea

- It is absence of menstruation.
- Primary amenorrhea is absence of first menstrual period. It can occur in delayed puberty, Turner syndrome and pseudohermaphroditism.
- Secondary amenorrhea is absence of menstruation after a normal menstrual cycle is established. Pregnancy is the most common cause.

B. Menorrhagia

- It is increased bleeding during menstruation. It may be in relation to the number of days of bleeding or volume of blood lost.
- The cycles are regular.
- Common causes are anovulatory cycles, fibroid uterus and dysfunctional uterine bleeding.

C. Dysmenorrhea

- Pain associated with menstruation is called dysmenorrhea. It may be accompanied by nausea and vomiting depending on the severity.
- Mild cramp like pain is normal during menstruation.
- When the pain is too bad or starts prior to bleeding, it is pathological.

9.5 DESCRIBE AND DISCUSS THE PHYSIOLOGICAL EFFECTS OF SEX HORMONES

SHORT ESSAYS

1. Explain the synthesis, actions and regulation of ovarian hormones.

Estrogen and progesterone are ovarian hormones.

Estrogens

Synthesis

- It is synthesized mainly from theca interna and granulosa cells of the ovarian follicle
- A small quantity is secreted by the zona glomerulosa of the adrenal cortex.
- Estradiol, estriol and estrone are three forms of estrogens present in the body.

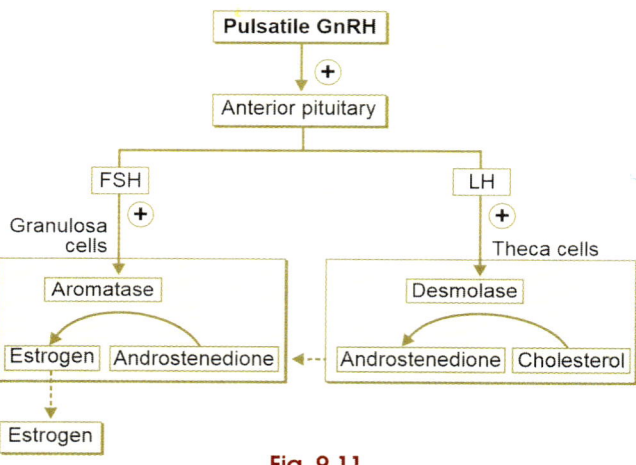

Fig. 9.11

Actions

Related to reproductive system

- Estrogens bring about growth and development of the reproductive organs.
- They take part in growth of the Graafian follicle and bring about proliferative changes in the endometrium. There is increase in the thickness of the endometrium.
- The fallopian tube becomes more functional.
- There is increase in size of the uterus and cervix.
- The vagina becomes longer in size and with the epithelial lining more cuboidal.
- There is increase in size of the clitoris and the labia majora and labia minora.
- Estrogens bring about secondary sexual characters like development of breasts and feminine appearance of a woman. There is deposition of subcutaneous fat more near the breasts and hips, smoothening of skin and female pattern of pubic hair.
- During pregnancy, it supports pregnancy.

Other actions

- It increases bone density and ossification of the epiphysis.
- It enlarges the hip and widens the pelvic inlet.
- It has positive anabolic effect on the proteins and causes fat deposition under skin.
- It causes sodium and water retention.
- It has mild vasodilator effect.
- It increases libido in females.
- It makes skin thin and reduces the viscosity of sebum.

Regulation

- Secretion of estrogen is under the influence of GnRH and FSH through the hypothalamo-pituitary ovarian axis and ACTH through the hypothalamo-pituitary-adrenal axis, the former being more predominant.

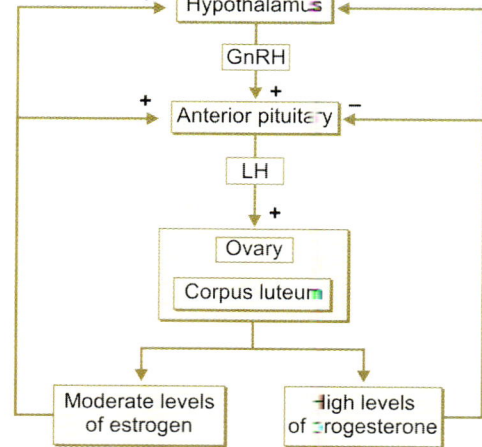

Fig. 9.12

Progesterone

Synthesis

- It is synthesized from cholesterol and forms an intermediary product during formation of all kinds of steroids in the body.

- In non-pregnant women, progesterone is secreted by the corpus luteum and in pregnant women, it is secreted by the placenta.

Actions

Reproductive actions

- It is pro-gestational: It supports pregnancy by all possible mechanisms. It helps in growth of the uterus, helps in maintain the endometrium, relaxes the smooth muscles of the uterus, and decreases motility.
- It causes glycogen storage in the stroma of the endometrium in the secretory phase and prepares for nutrition of the embryo to be.
- The cervical discharge becomes thick and viscous.
- Vaginal epithelium becomes thickened and cornified.
- In the fallopian tube, progesterone increases the secretions enriched with nutritive material.
- In the breast, there is increase in the lobular and alveolar growth.

Other actions

- Increases basal body temperature by about 0.5 degree
- It alters certain areas in the CNS and decreases appetite and increases somnolence.
- Progesterone has a pro-atherogenic effect by decreasing the HDL levels
- It also tends to cause hyperglycemia.
- There is smooth muscle relaxation in many tissues causing vasodilatation and lowering of blood pressure. Also, the lower esophageal sphincter is relaxed. Thus, pregnant women experience more belching and gastric reflux. Also, there is slowing of the bowel movements leading to constipation.

Regulation

- It is secreted in response to LH which is under the influence of GnRH.
- When progesterone level is high in blood, it causes negative feedback inhibition on GnRH and FSH and LH secretion from hypothalamus and pituitary.

SHORT ANSWER

1. Explain the physiological actions of hormone testosterone

- In testes, testosterone is secreted by interstitial cells of Leydig and zona reticularis of the adrenal cortex.
- Its actions are different in fetal and in adult life.

In Fetal Life

- Testosterone is secreted by genital ridge in the fetus beginning by about 7th week.
- It causes regression of Mullerian duct and development of male sex organs like epididymis, seminiferous tubules and vas deferens through Wolffian duct.
- It is also responsible for development of penis, scrotum, genital ducts and prostate.
- Initially, the testes are developed from the bipotential gonads in the abdomen. Under the influence of testosterone, they descend into the scrotum through the inguinal canal.

In adult life

Effects on Sex Organs

- It is required for growth of testes, penis and scrotum after puberty.
- It is also required for spermatogenesis

Effects on Secondary Sexual Characters

- Testosterone increases muscle mass by about 50% in puberty due to anabolic effect on proteins.
- Increases thickness of bones, increases calcium deposition and early fusion of epiphysis of long bones.
- It makes the shoulders wide and pelvis narrow. The pelvis becomes funnel shaped
- It increases thickness of skin and sebum secretion from skin
- The body hair becomes coarse and dark, causes growth of facial hair in the form of moustache and beard
- There is hair growth in the pubic area, and it extends up to the umbilicus along the linea alba. There is also development of chest hair.
- Testosterone causes deepening of voice by increasing the thickness of the vocal cords, hypertrophy of laryngeal muscles, lengthening of larynx.
- Testosterone has an anabolic effect on proteins. It increases basal metabolic rate.
- It has a mineralocorticoid like action on salt and water absorption, thus causes sodium and water retention.
- It also has erythropoietic action as a result, it increases hemoglobin concentration and RBC count.

9.6 ENUMERATE THE CONTRACEPTIVE METHODS FOR MALE AND FEMALE. DISCUSS THEIR ADVANTAGES AND DISADVANTAGES

SHORT ESSAYS

1. Mention the contraceptive methods in females. What is the mechanism of action of copper T?

Contraceptive Methods in Females

Based on the duration and mechanism of action, contraceptives in females are classified as:

A. Spacing Methods

- **Barrier:** Female condom, diaphragm
- **Chemical:** Use of spermicidal agents like nonoxynol-9
- **Hormonal:** Inhibition of ovulation with use of estrogen and/or progesterone
- **Intrauterine contraceptive devices:** Devices placed inside the uterine cavity

B. Terminal Methods

- Tubectomy—ligation of fallopian tube
- Laparoscopic occlusion of fallopian tube.
- Medical termination of pregnancy

Mechanism of Action of Copper-T

- Copper T is a "T"-shaped copper intrauterine device and is most used.
- It is inserted through the cervix and is suited for parous women.
- It prevents fertilization

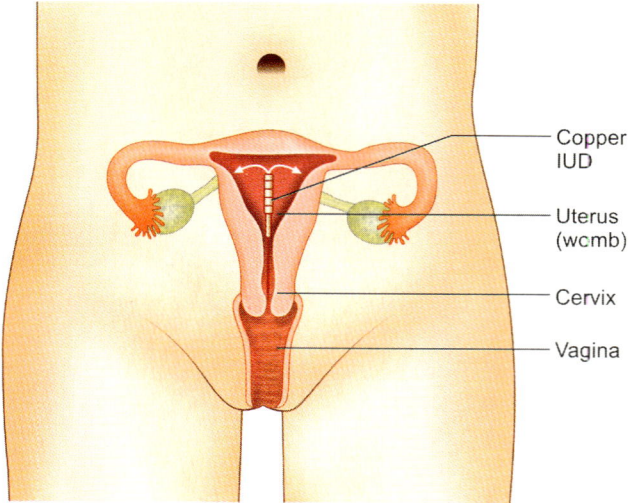
Copper IUD
Uterus (wcmb)
Cervix
Vagina

Fig. 9.13

- It causes aseptic inflammation of the endometrium and thus makes it unfavorable for implantation of the zygote
- It also has spermicidal action.

2. A young newly married couple came to OBG department for advice on contraceptive methods. What do you advice?

- A couple wanting to delay conception should be counselled together.
- A proper history taking about the lifestyle of the couple is important.
- Whether are more sedentary or workaholic, how often they consummate and other health problems, age at marriage and family history of frequent loss of fetus, infertility, breast cancer is important to elicit.
- Also, it is important to know how serious the couple is about contraception.
- After individualizing, proper regimen is selected.

Ovulation Inhibiting Hormones or Oral Contraceptive Pill

- In a young, healthy couple with no comorbidities, this is a safe option.
- It takes 2–3 months to be efficient, so barrier methods have to be used till then
- The regimen is easy—one pill per day for 21 days and then iron supplements.

Advantages	Disadvantages
1. Easily available	1. Tendency to put on weight
2. Efficacious, fertility is easily gained after withdrawal of drug	2. Not advisable in family history of breast and endometrial cancer
3. Few side effects with low dose pill	3. Tendency to form gall stones
4. Decreases bleeding and pain during menstruation by inhibiting ovulation	
5. Does not interfere with the act of coitus	

Contraceptive Injections and Implant

- Long-acting progesterone is given intramuscularly, and its effect lasts for 3 months.

- This changes the cervical mucus and makes it hostile for entry of sperm. Also, it inhibits ovulation.

Advantages	Disadvantages
1. Need not worry about it every day and does not interfere with the act	1. Painful injection

Combination of Barrier and other Methods

- In a couple with risk factors, these methods may be tried.
- Calendar method + barrier
- Male barrier + spermicidal agent
- Male barrier + female barrier + calendar
- Barrier + coitus interruptus

SHORT ANSWERS

1. What is barrier method of contraception in males? What are its advantages?

Barrier Method of Contraception in Males

- Barrier method is use of a condom, that is, worn on the erect penis prior to the act of coitus.
- It is usually made of fine latex.
- The end of the condom has a small bulb-shaped space for collection of semen after ejaculation.

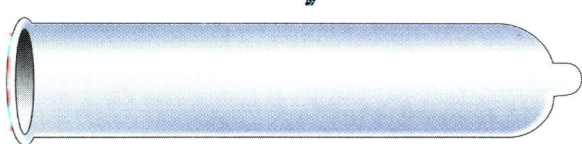

Fig. 9.14

Advantages

1. It can be easily worn prior to the act of coitus.
2. Condom is safe, inexpensive, and easily available.
3. It provides protection to both partners against sexually transmitted diseases.
4. It does not require any medical supervision.

2. What is safe period? What is calendar method of contraception?

Safe Period

- Safe period is that part of the menstrual cycle when ovulation does not occur, and chances of conceiving is very minute.

- In a regularly menstruating woman with a 28-day cycle, ovulation occurs on the 14th day.
- Safe period lasts during the first 7 days of the cycle and after 18th day of a regular 28–32-day cycle.
- Danger period lasts from 8th to 18th day.

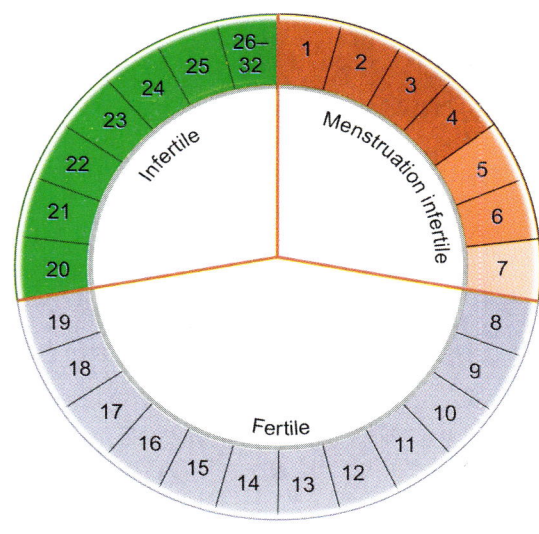

Fig. 9.15

Calendar Method

- Also known as Rhythm method.
- In this method the couple is advised to avoid intercourse during 8–18th day or the danger period.
- It is not a reliable method of contraception as ovulation may occur outside the fertile period. Also, a certain degree of will has to be practiced by the couple.
- It is a natural method. It is successful only if the menstrual cycles are normal and the woman keeps a record of basal body temperature and notes the timing of ovulation.

3. Describe the permanent methods of contraception in male and female.

In Males

1. **Vasectomy (Fig. 9.16)**
   - In this procedure, 1 cm of vas is removed by surgery and the ends are ligated.
   - As a result, the sperms that are formed are not able to reach the bulbar urethra.
2. **Vas occlusion with no scalpel:** In this technique, an elastomer is injected into the vas deferens which gets hardened and occludes the vas.

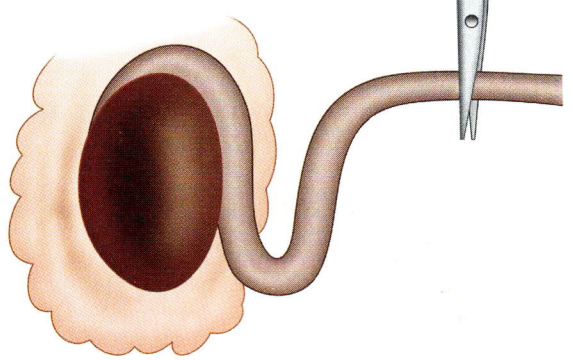

Fig. 9.16

In Females

1. **Tubectomy**
   - It is performed when the family of the couple is complete.
   - Here the fallopian tube is identified by making a small incision in the abdomen, and the tube is cut on both sides and ends are ligated.

2. **Laparoscopic occlusion**
   - It is done by inserting a laparoscopic instrument through minute incisions.
   - The fallopian tubes are occluded using silicone rubber bands.

9.7 DESCRIBE AND DISCUSS THE EFFECTS OF REMOVAL OF GONADS ON PHYSIOLOGICAL FUNCTIONS

SHORT ANSWERS

1. Explain the terms hypogonadism and eunuchoidism in males.

Hypogonadism

- Hypogonadism is a term used to denote small size of testes in adult males or decreased functional ability of testes.
- It is seen in many conditions like chromosomal abnormalities (Klinefelter's syndrome), decreased androgen in the body.

Eunuchoidism

- It is seen when extirpation of testes is done prior to puberty.
- As a result, the primary and secondary sexual characters do not develop.
- The individual has small-sized male external genitalia.
- There is no development of facial hair, affected individual is usually taller with thin long and slender bones. He has a childlike voice and abnormal fat deposition in hip and breasts in a feminine pattern.

2. Describe the effects of removal of ovaries.

- Removal of ovaries is called oophorectomy and it is indicated in suspicious tumors of ovary.
- If ovaries are removed, menopause-like situation is induced.
- There is sudden drop in blood levels of estrogen and progesterone.
- As a result, there is cessation of menstruation.
- If ovaries are removed prior to puberty (no clinical indication), secondary sexual characters do not develop.

Associated Functional Symptoms

- Mood swings
- There is high risk of cardiovascular diseases as estrogen is cardioprotective.
- Development of hot flushes or vasomotor changes is characteristic of menopause. These changes are produced due to low FSH and corresponding high GnRH pulses (which is in very close association with the thermoregulatory system) which occur every 2 hours causing hot flushes.
- Increased chances of osteoporosis.
- Increased chances of developing Alzheimer's disease.
- Atrophic changes in genitourinary tract
- Sexual dysfunction—loss of sexual drive.

9.8 DESCRIBE AND DISCUSS THE PHYSIOLOGY OF PREGNANCY, PARTURITION AND LACTATION AND OUTLINE THE PSYCHOLOGY AND PSYCHIATRY DISORDERS ASSOCIATED WITH IT

SHORT ESSAYS

1. Explain the fertilization of ovum and implantation of the zygote.

Fertilization of Ovum (Fig. 9.17)

- Fertilization is fusion of egg with sperm.
- It takes place in the middle of ampulla of the fallopian tube. It involves the following steps

  1. **Transport of gametes**
     - The ovum is expelled into the abdominal cavity but picked up by the fimbrial end of the fallopian tube. By the action of cilia, the ovum is transported towards the ostium of the tube.
     - The sperm after entering the uterine cavity, swims towards the ovum by flagellar movements.

  2. **Sperm capacitation**
     - It is the morphological change that occurs in the sperm after entering the uterine cavity.
     - The sperm becomes more permeable to calcium and there is decrease in the cholesterol content of the acrosomal cap.

  3. **Fusion of gametes**
     - There is chemoattraction of ovum and sperm due to chemicals produced by them.
     - Many proteolytic enzymes in the acrosome of the sperm cause lysis of the zona and permits entry of the sperm into the egg.
     - After entry of a sperm, there is activation of the ovum leading to depolarization. This causes some structural changes in the egg which prevent entry of more than one sperm.
     - This is done by spread of cortical granules along the perivitelline space.

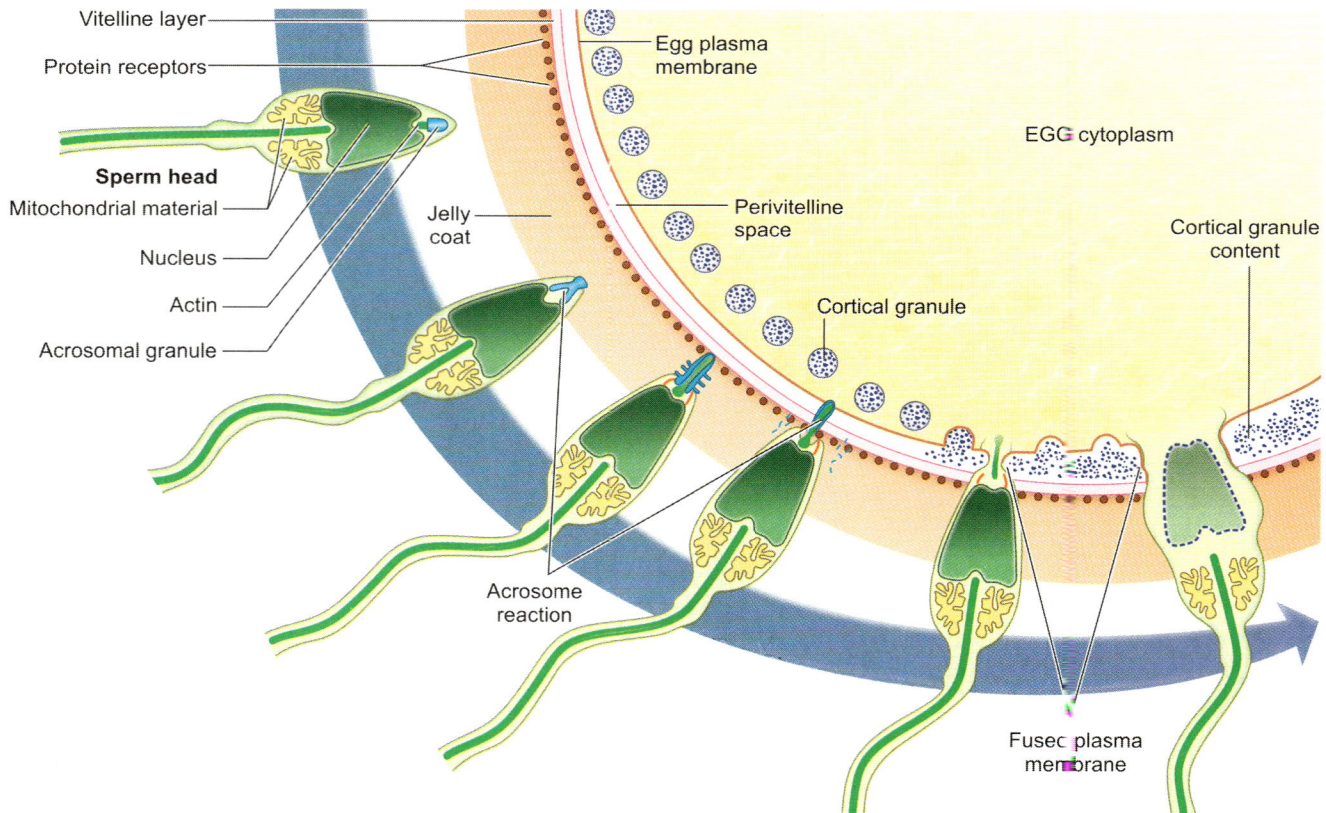

Fig. 9.17

Implantation of Zygote (Fig. 9.18)

- The fertilized ovum is called a zygote and starts dividing. A 16-cell stage is called morula.
- Following this, there is further division of cells leading to blastocyst formation. The blastocyst has an outer covering called trophoblast which later gives rise to placenta and its membranes.
- Implantation usually occurs on day 6–8 following fertilization.
- The embryo travels in the way as depicted in Fig. 9.18.
- The blastocyst corrodes the stroma of the endometrium and buries itself within it.
- The syncytiotrophoblast also causes proliferation into the blood vessels to acquire nutrition through uterine blood vessels.

2. List the placental hormones and describe their functions.

1. Beta human chorionic gonadotropin

- Its action is similar to LH.
- It maintains the corpus luteum till 7 days post-conception till the chorionic villi are formed.
- It stimulates the fetal testes to secrete testosterone which is responsible for development of male genitalia.

2. Human chorionic somatotropin

- Its secretion begins from the fifth week of pregnancy and continues till parturition.
- Its functions are similar to growth hormone and brings about growth of fetus.
- It causes deposition of protein in the tissues and brings about nitrogen, calcium and potassium retention.

3. Human chorionic thyrotropin: Functions like thyroid stimulating hormone.

4. Placental estrogen

- Growth and development of maternal reproductive organs
- Stimulates development of lactiferous ductules of the mammary glands
- Stimulates synthesis of thyroxine binding globulins and other plasma proteins

5. Placental progesterone

- It is initially produced by corpus luteum and later by the fetoplacental unit.
- It helps in growth of the uterus, relaxes smooth muscles of uterus
- It converts secretory endometrium to decidua of pregnancy
- It has immunosuppressive role in protecting fetus
- Acts as a precursor for generation of adrenal hormones in the fetus.
- Along with estrogen, it prepares the breast for lactation.

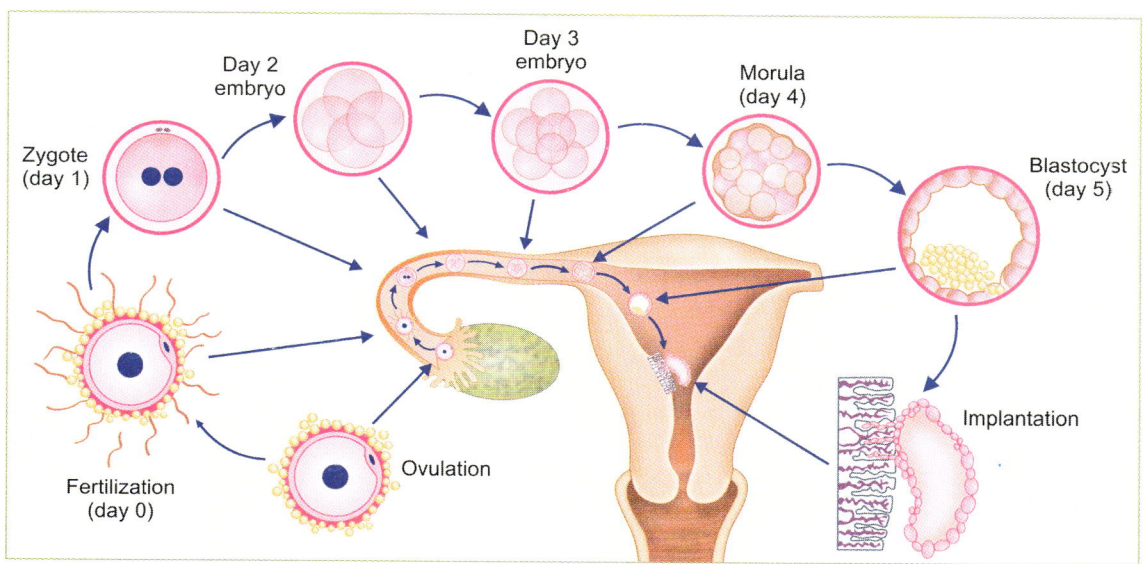

Fig. 9.18

6. **Relaxin**
   - It is of importance during onset of labor
   - There is relaxation of ligaments of the pelvis and cervix.
   - It increases oxytocin receptors on myometrium.

3. Briefly describe the physiological changes in the mother during pregnancy.

Various structural, functional and physiological changes take place in a woman's body during pregnancy.

1. **Changes in blood**
   - There is increase in plasma volume and this leads to increase in total blood volume.
   - There is hemodilution and resulting anemia.
   - There is hyperdynamic circulation.

2. **Changes in cardiovascular system**
   - During the first trimester, there is increase in the cardiac output. Then it gradually decreases and reaches normal during the later stages of pregnancy.
   - Physiologically, there is fall in blood pressure. However, increase in blood pressure is deleterious to the health of the fetus. This is called pregnancy-induced hypertension (PIH).

3. **Changes in respiratory system**
   - Tidal volume, respiratory minute volume, pulmonary ventilation increase.
   - This is to compensate for the increased physiological demand.

4. **Changes in excretory system**
   - Renal blood flow and GFR increases. There is increase in urine formation.
   - There is decrease in the specific gravity of urine
   - During first trimester, there is frequency micturition as the gravid uterus presses on the bladder.

5. **Changes in digestive system**
   - Progesterone increases the bowel transit time by decreasing the tone of the smooth muscles.
   - As a result, constipation occurs.
   - Also, due to relaxation of sphincters, there is gastroesophageal reflux causing heart burn.
   - There is an increased tendency to formation of gall stones.

6. **Changes in nervous system**
   - There is generalized excitation and the woman is susceptible to mood swings and anxiety.

- HCG triggers the CTZ causing nausea and vomiting in the first trimester. Later, it gets acclimatized.

7. **Changes in endocrine system**
   - There is increase in size of the pituitary gland.
   - FSH and LH secretion is reduced due to negative inhibition by the estrogens and progesterone.
   - There is increase in synthesis of cortisol, aldosterone and thyroxine.
   - Pregnancy is a hyperglycemia effect on the mother due to progesterone and human placental lactogen.

4. Describe the milk ejection reflex.

Milk Ejection Reflex or Milk Let Down Reflex (Fig. 9.19)

- It is the reflex by which there is milk being secreted by the mammary glands during a baby suckling at it and is a neuro-endocrine reflex.
- It is mediated through oxytocin.

Baby suckling at the nipple stimulates receptors at the nipple. Also, the thought, smell or sight of baby send signals to the hypothalamus
↓
Somatic afferent nerve fibers to paraventricular and supraoptic nuclei of hypothalamus
↓
Hypothalamus send signals to posterior pituitary through hypothalamo-hypophyseal tract
↓
Release of oxytocin in blood
↓
Reaches the mammary gland to cause contraction of myoepithelial cells
↓
Ejection of milk from mammary glands

SHORT ANSWERS

1. Explain fetoplacental unit.

- It is the interaction between the fetus and the placenta in the formation of steroid hormones.
- Some enzymes involved in steroid synthesis that are present in the fetus are absent in the placenta and viceversa (Fig. 9.20)
- Thus, the placenta and fetus complement and complete each other's requirement in production of progesterone during pregnancy.

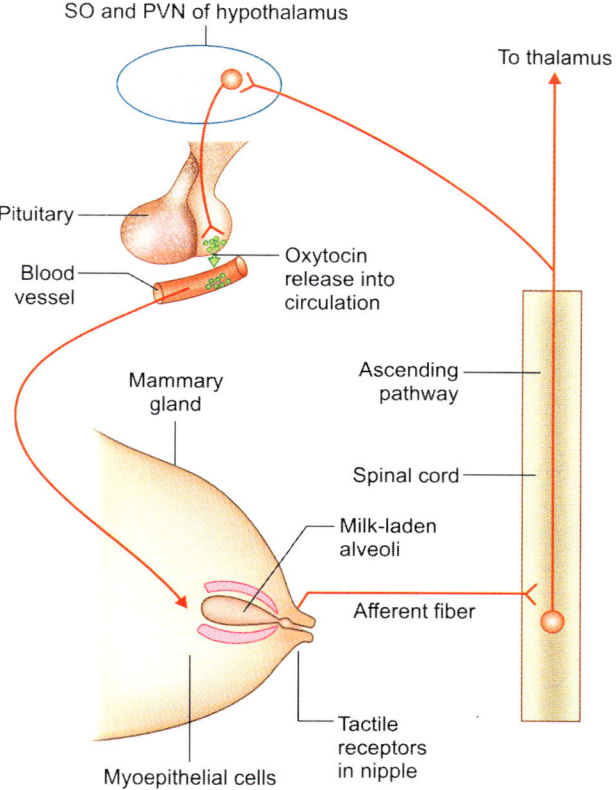

Fig. 9.19

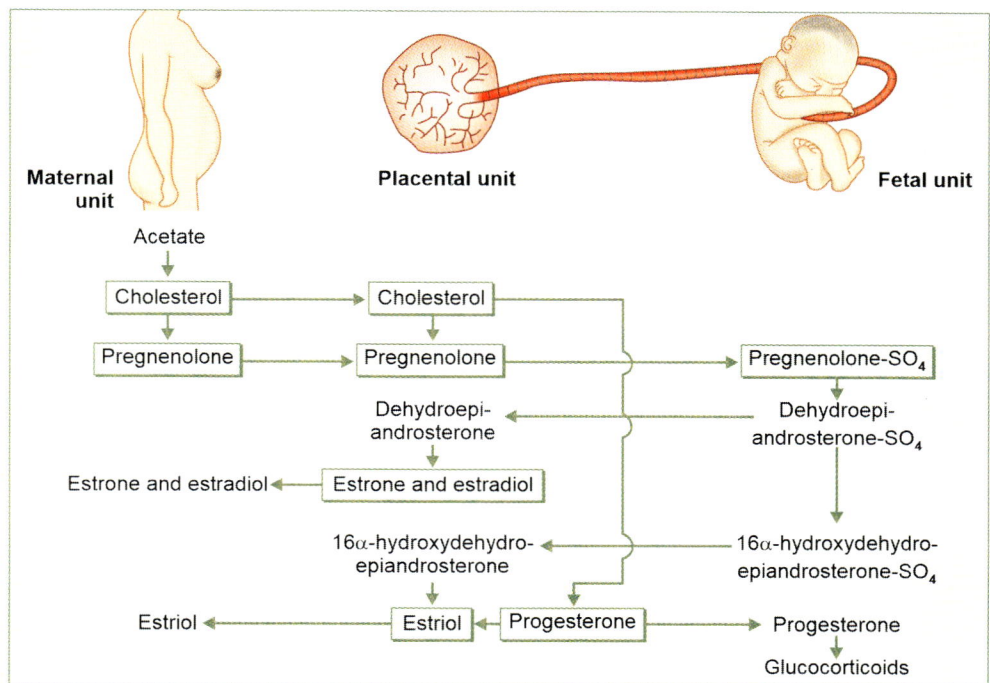

Fig. 9.20

2. What is Sheehan's syndrome? Briefly describe the emotional changes that a mother experiences during and after pregnancy.

Sheehan's Syndrome

- It is also known as pituitary apoplexy.
- It is a dreaded complication of postpartum hemorrhage. As a result of loss of blood, there is necrosis of the pituitary gland.
- During pregnancy there is increase in size of the pituitary. This makes it very susceptible to ischemic necrosis.
- As a result, there is cessation of secretion of pituitary hormones and causes hypopituitarism.

Emotional Changes during Pregnancy

- There is an exuberance of estrogens and progesterone during pregnancy.
- They have impact on the mood and psychology in pregnancy.
- Craving and aversion to food are two extremes. A pregnant lady can experience any type of emotion in this range.
- There is an increased incidence of anxiety, mood swings and irritability. Some experience increased sex drive and some women may experience the opposite.

Emotional Changes after Pregnancy

- After parturition, there is sudden withdrawal of estrogen and progesterone.
- This may cause a type of depression called post-partum depression. It is physiological. It may range from mild insecurity to severe forms of depression.
- Also, there is a tendency to protect the newborn.

9.9 INTERPRET A NORMAL SEMEN ANALYSIS REPORT INCLUDING (A) SPERM COUNT, (B) SPERM MORPHOLOGY AND (C) SPERM MOTILITY, AS PER WHO GUIDELINES AND DISCUSS THE RESULTS

SHORT ANSWERS

1. Describe the normal semen parameters in terms of (A) volume, (B) sperm count, (C) sperm morphology, and (D) sperm motility.

a. **Volume:** 2–6 ml per ejaculation
b. **Sperm count**
   - 100–150 million sperms/ml is normal
   - Less than 20 million causes sterility
c. **Sperm morphology:** Minimum of 30% of the total sperms must have normal morphology
d. **Sperm motility:** Minimum of 50% of sperms must be motile and in forward direction

2. Discuss the factors that can affect sperm count and quality.

The fertility worldwide is decreasing over the last century.

Factors affecting sperm count and quality are:

Generalized
- Old age
- Lifestyle—physical exercise improves quality of sperms
- Smoking and alcohol decrease sperm count and quality.
- Chronic diseases and infections
- Malnutrition
- Obesity

Local causes
- Increased temperature as in undescended testes, wearing tight clothes around the testes, occupational exposure, varicocele causes decrease in sperm count
- Trauma and previous infections (orchitis)
- Exposure to radiation and drugs

3. Define the following terms (A) oligospermia, (B) azoospermia.

Oligospermia

Total sperm count less than 20 million per ml is considered oligospermia causing infertility

Azoospermia

Complete lack of sperms in semen is called azoospermia.

9.10 DISCUSS THE PHYSIOLOGICAL BASIS OF VARIOUS PREGNANCY TESTS

SHORT ANSWER

1. Discuss the immunological test used to confirm pregnancy.

- Pregnancy is easily confirmed at 4–5 weeks of amenorrhea by simple immunological tests.
- After implantation, there is secretion of beta human chorionic gonadotropin by the chorionic villi.
- So, it is secreted in urine. Pregnancy can be confirmed by measuring plasma levels of beta hCG or in urine.

Principle

- Sheep RBCs or latex particles coated with hCG antisera are incorporated onto a plastic sterile disc.
- It can also be used to perform on a glass slide.
- When the urine of the pregnant lady (containing beta hCG is added, there is agglutination).

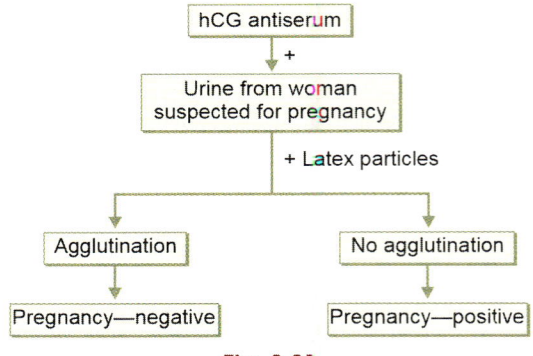

Fig. 9.21

Procedure

- On a clean glass slide, one drop of hCG antiserum is taken.
- One drop of urine (from a woman to be tested) is added to the antiserum.
- Latex particles are added and mixed.
- If hCG is present in urine, there is agglutination. Otherwise, there is no agglutination.

9.11 DISCUSS THE HORMONAL CHANGES AND THEIR EFFECTS DURING PERIMENOPAUSE AND MENOPAUSE

SHORT ESSAY

1. A 50-year-old female comes with the complaint of hot flushes after menopause. Discuss the indications, uses and side effects of hormone replacement therapy (HRT).

Menopause is a phase in the female reproductive life when the female sex hormones cease to be produced.

Indications

1. Hormone replacement therapy is providing exogenous estrogen with or without progesterone in women with post-menopausal symptoms.
2. Women at high risk of developing coronary artery disease, osteoporosis, stroke, colonic cancer
3. Premature menopause or post-surgical (oophorectomy)
4. Gonadal dysgenesis as a therapeutic intervention.

Uses

1. Drugs usually used are estrogen, progesterone, androgens
2. There is improvement of vasomotor symptoms
3. Increase in bone mineral density and reduced risks of fractures
4. Reduced risk of developing Alzheimer's disease.

Side Effects

Estrogen Associated

1. Breast tenderness, leg cramps, bloating, nausea
2. Increased risk of developing endometrial cancer
3. Increased chances of breast cancer, gall stones and liver diseases

Progesterone Associated

1. Premenstrual symptoms (depression, fluid retention)
2. Increased chances of cardiovascular diseases
3. Increased chances of hyperglycemia
4. Venous thromboembolism.

SHORT ANSWER

1. Define menopause. Discuss the hormonal changes that occur during menopause and functional changes that occur in different systems.

Menopause

Menopause is permanent cessation of the menstrual cycle in a female's lifetime.

Hormonal Changes

- A few years prior to menopause attainment, there is steady depletion of ovarian follicles and they even become resistant to gonadotropins.
- There is significant fall of estrogen from 50–300 pg/dl to 10–20 pg/dl.
- So, due to loss of negative feedback mechanism, there is increase in secretion of FSH. As a result, there is inadequate ovulation and estrogen excess.
- These result in disturbances in the length of the cycle and dysfunctional bleeding.
- As corpus luteum is not produced, there is deficient progesterone.

Functional Changes

- Mood swings
- There is high risk of cardiovascular diseases as estrogen is cardioprotective.
- Development of hot flushes or vasomotor changes is characteristic of menopause. These changes are produced due to low FSH and corresponding high GnRH pulses (which is in very close association with the thermoregulatory system) which occur every 2 hours causing hot flushes.
- Atrophic changes in genitourinary tract
- Sexual dysfunction—loss of sexual drive

9.12 DISCUSS THE COMMON CAUSES OF INFERTILITY IN A COUPLE AND ROLE OF IVF IN MANAGING A CASE OF INFERTILITY

SHORT ESSAY

1. A couple with the married life of 7 years comes for infertility treatment. List the new reproductive technologies that are available for an infertile couple. What do you suggest?

- Every case of infertility needs to be thoroughly investigated and the treatment is individualized.
- The options are based on the severity of infertility.

  1. **Ovulation assessment and follow-up**
     - If the sperm count is normal and the female has no detectable structural deformity or hormonal abnormality, the couple can be helped with ovulation study with the help of either urine strips or ultrasound assessment.
     - Transvaginal ultrasound is performed every day between 8th and the occurrence of ovulation. The couple is advised to try conceiving at the time of ovulation.

  2. **Ovulation induction and intrauterine insemination**
     - When ovulation is not regular and the sperm count is slightly on the lower side but there are no structural abnormalities in the uterus or fallopian tube, this method is advised.
     - The ovaries are stimulated with GnRH analogs and an increase in the number of eggs is brought about. This increases the chances of pregnancy.
     - The husband's sperm is injected into the cervical cavity after ovulation occurs. Ovulation also may be regulated with hCG.
     - This procedure overcomes local cervical sperm inhibiting factors.
     - In case the husband's count is very low, a donor's semen sample can be used.

  3. **Ovulation induction and IVF**
     - When the sperm count is very low or the female has structural abnormalities like cornual block or intrapelvic adhesions, IVF is the procedure of choice.
     - The egg is retrieved by cordocentesis after stimulation and ovulation.
     - Simultaneously, the husband's sperms are collected, and they are mixed to form zygote.
     - If either partner has no sperm or egg, a donor can be used. Surrogacy is another option if the female does not provide an appropriate environment for the embryo (autoimmune conditions)
     - Depending on the situation, there are three types
       i. **ICSI:** Intracytoplasmic sperm injection: If sperms are not able to enter the egg
       ii. **GIFT:** Gamete intrafallopian transfer
       iii. **ZIFT:** Zygote intrafallopian transfer.

SHORT ANSWERS

1. What are the common causes of infertility in the males?

Decreased Sperm Count

- Normal count is around 100–150 million/mm^3
- Infertility occurs when the count is less than 20 million/mm^3
- It can happen in orchitis, destruction of seminiferous tubules following orchitis, varicocele (varicosities of the veins around testis), undescended testis.
- It may be seen in antisperm antibodies also (post-traumatic orchitis).

Abnormal Sperms

Abnormal morphology of sperms like loss of head or tail or motility.

Obstruction to Reproductive Ducts

Obstruction of vas deferens due to infections like filariasis or sexually transmitted diseases.

Systemic Causes

- Diabetes
- Generalized debility
- Sedentary lifestyle
- Alcoholism
- Use of recreational drugs

2. What is IVF? Describe its role in managing a case of infertility.

IVF

- IVF is *in vitro* fertilization meaning, the egg from the female is procured and sperm from the male is taken.
- They are allowed to form a zygote in a laboratory under sterile conditions.
- Then the embryo is allowed to grow in an incubator.
- It is transferred into the uterus of the mother to be at 8 or 16 cell stage. The embryo attaches itself and grows as a fetus.

Role in Infertility

IVF is helpful in female infertility, male infertility and also in combined causes.

Female Infertility

- Diseases of the ovary like endometriosis or polycystic ovary diseases
- Diseases of the fallopian tube causing and cornual block
- Diseases of the uterus
- Repeated loss of conceptus due to luteal phase deficiency and autoimmune conditions.

Male Infertility

- Severely reduced sperm count or motility or unsuitable morphology of sperms
- In these cases, the conception becomes more controlled in terms of monitoring the ovulation, selection of good eggs and sperms and finally finding good embryos suitable for implantation.

Neurophysiology

10.1 DESCRIBE AND DISCUSS THE ORGANIZATION OF NERVOUS SYSTEM

SHORT ESSAYS

1. Explain the composition, circulation, absorption, and functions of CSF. Add a note on hydrocephalus. (1 + 1 + 1 + 2 marks)

Composition of CSF

- It occupies the space between the pia mater and the arachnoid.
- Normally CSF is a clear fluid is made up of the following.
- Water: >99% of CSF is made up of water.
- The remainder is made of solids

Organic solutes	Inorganic solutes
Proteins and amino acids	Sodium
Glucose	Potassium
Uric acid	Calcium
Urea	Magnesium
Creatinine	Chlorides
Lactic acid	Bicarbonates
Cholesterol	Sulfates

Circulation of CSF

- It is produced by the choroid plexus found in the ventricles.
- Choroid plexuses are a tuft of capillaries within the ventricles and are covered by piamater and ependymal cells.

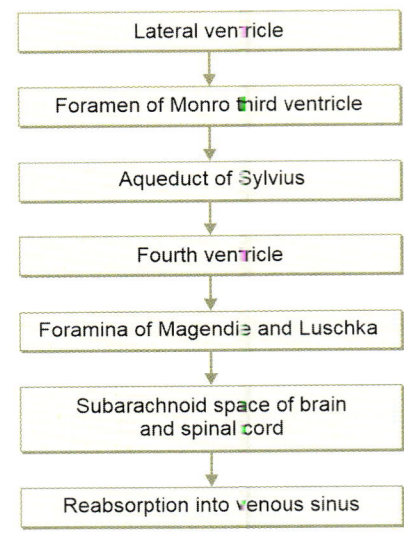

| Lateral ventricle |
| Foramen of Monro third ventricle |
| Aqueduct of Sylvius |
| Fourth ventricle |
| Foramina of Magendie and Luschka |
| Subarachnoid space of brain and spinal cord |
| Reabsorption into venous sinus |

Fig. 10.1

Functions of CSF

1. **Protective function**
   - It forms a shock absorber around the brain within the cranial cavity.
   - It prevents the movement of brain against the skull.
2. **Regulation of intracranial contents:** Whenever there is increase in volume of the cranial cavity, there is reflex increase in CSF absorption and thus volume is regulated.

3. **Medium of exchange**
   - It forms a medium for exchange of materials between brain and blood.
   - Also transports hormones.

Hydrocephalus

- It is a state characterized by increased CSF in the cranial cavity.
- It can be due to increased production or due to decreased absorption or due to an obstruction to outflow of CSF.
- Based on whether there is adequate drainage or not, hydrocephalus is classified as communicating or non-communicating hydrocephalus.

Communicating hydrocephalus	Non-communicating hydrocephalus
Meningitis—bacterial, viral Encephalocele	Arnold-Chiari malformation Dandy-Walker syndrome Tuberculous arachnoiditis

Clinical Features

- In young children, as the anterior fontanelle is open, elevation can be felt.
- They have headache and projectile vomiting
- After the fontanelles have fused, there is papilledema or edema of the optic disc.
- Also, there is sixth nerve palsy due to compression of the 6th nerve
- If uncorrected, there is optic nerve atrophy due to sustained pressure
- Death may result due to tentorial herniation.

Treatment

Medical

- Drugs to reduce CSF formation like carbonic anhydrase inhibitors.
- Drugs to increase excretion of water: Osmotic diuretics.

Surgical: Ventriculoperitoneal shunt.

SHORT ANSWERS

1. Write a neat labelled diagram of a neuron. Mention its types.

Types of Neurons

a. **Depending on the number of poles**
   1. Unipolar neurons

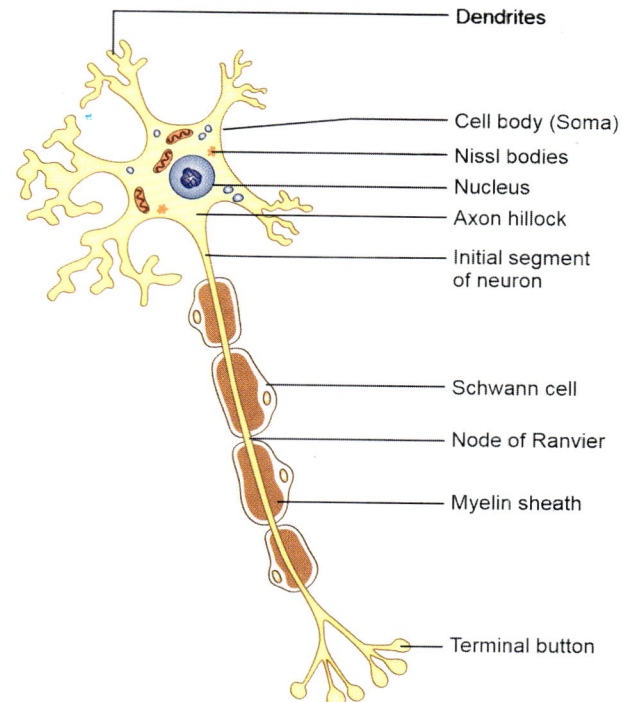

Fig. 10.2

   2. Bipolar neurons
   3. Multipolar neurons

b. **Depending on function**
   1. Motor neurons
   2. Sensory neurons

2. Explain the types of glial cells and functions.

Neuroglia

These are supporting cells present in the brain and the spinal cord.

Types of Neuroglia

Macroglia	Microglia
Large cells of ectodermal origin 1. Astrocytes 2. Oligodendrocytes	Smaller, mesodermal in origin

Astrocytes

Structure	Functions
• These are star-shaped cells • They have multiple processes that envelop the synapse. • They are of two types: Fibrous astrocytes and protoplasmic astrocytes	1. They help in forming the blood–brain barrier around the endothelial cells of the capillaries. 2. They help in providing nutrition to the neurons 3. They help in maintaining ion balance across the cell membrane 4. Help in repair processes following trauma

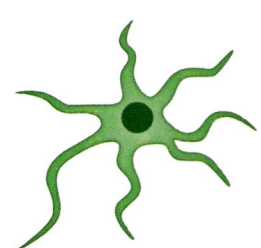

Oligodendrocytes

Structure	Functions
• They are large glial cells. • They have a few dendrons compared to other glia and neurons	1. They are responsible for production of myelin sheath 2. They also provide trophic support to the neurons

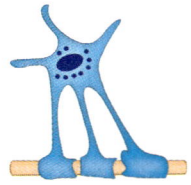

Ependymal Cell

Structure	Functions
• These are ciliated flat cells that line ventricles	1. They line ventricles and spinal canal 2. They secrete CSF (cerebrospinal fluid)

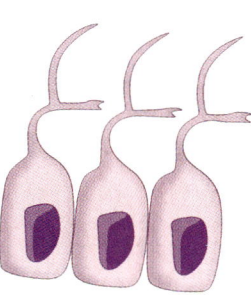

Schwann Cell

Structure	Functions
• The cell wraps around the neuron many layers and nucleus are pushed to one side	1. It helps if formation of myelin sheath 2. Myelin sheath is an important requirement of saltatory conduction

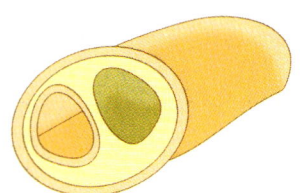

Microglia

Structure	Functions
• They are small cells with multiple dendritic projections	1. They have macrophage like function and thus protect the neurons from external agents. 2. They are constantly scavenging the brain for plaques, damages neurons and microbes. 3. They are also involved in antigen presentation

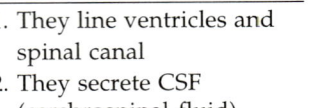

3. Explain blood–brain barrier.

- It is a neuroprotective layer of cells that controls entry of various chemicals and pathogens into the brain tissue from blood (Fig. 10.3).
- The endothelium present within the capillaries of the brain are attached tightly through tight junctions and thus entry of various molecules is restricted.
- Also, this barrier is reinforced by cytoplasmic foot processes of astrocytes. They envelop the blood vessels almost completely
- It functions as a gateway and allows only certain molecules to enter.

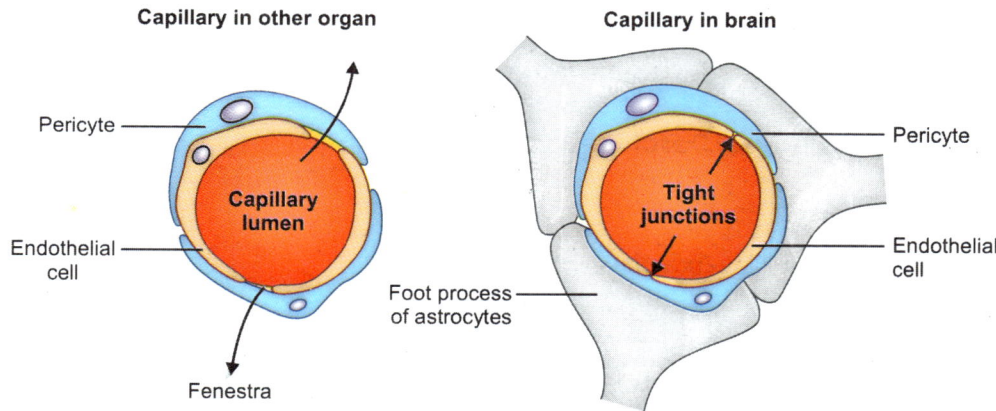

Fig. 10.3

Substances which can cross BBB	Substances which are restricted
• Oxygen	• Injurious chemicals
• Carbon dioxide	• Bacteria
• Water	• Catecholamines
• Glucose	• Bile pigments
• Amino acids	
• Electrolytes	
• Certain lipophilic drugs	

4. Discuss clinical applications of CSF analysis.

1. External appearance
- It is normally clear
- Turbid CSF is seen in bacterial meningitis and tubercular meningitis
- In tubercular meningitis, there is cobweb formation of standing

2. Opening pressure of CSF
- It is an indication of the intracranial pressure
- Normal is less than 200 cm of water
- Increased opening pressure is seen in hydrocephalus and intracranial space occupying lesions

3. Biochemistry panel
- Glucose and proteins are routinely measured in CSF

Causes for decreased glucose	Increased proteins
All types of infective meningitis Tubercular meningitis	Bacterial meningitis

- Certain other tests like ADA and LDH are also measured.

4. Microbiology
- Gram stain and culture is used to know the infection causing agent.
- Certain antibodies can help detect infections and autoimmune conditions.

5. Cytology
- Mainly done to rule out presence of cancer cells.
- Increased blood cells (RBCs) are seen in sub-arachnoid hemorrhage
- Leukocytosis is seen in bacterial infections, lymphocytosis is seen in viral and tubercular meningitis.

10.2 DESCRIBE AND DISCUSS THE FUNCTIONS AND PROPERTIES OF SYNAPSE, REFLEX, RECEPTORS

SHORT ESSAYS

1. Enlist the properties of synapse. Describe any 3 properties in detail.

Properties of Synapse

1. One-way conduction or Bell-Magendie law
2. Synaptic delay
3. Synaptic fatigue
4. Summation property of synapse
5. Convergence and divergence property
6. Occlusion phenomenon
7. Subliminal fringe effect
8. Facilitation
9. Synaptic plasticity and learning
10. Reverberation

1. One-way conduction

- It is also called Bell-Magendie law or law of dynamic polarity.
- Even though the axon can conduct impulses in both directions, a chemical synapse allows movement of impulse from the presynaptic neuron to post-synaptic neuron.
- It can never be in the opposite direction.

Causes

– The reason is that the presynaptic membrane contains the neurotransmitter and the post-synaptic membrane only has receptors for the neurotransmitter.
– When the impulse travels in opposite direction, it dies off due to absence of neurotransmitter in the cell body of the post-synaptic neuron.

2. Synaptic delay (Fig. 10.4)

- It refers to the time lapse between arrival of an impulse at the presynaptic nerve terminal and its passage into the post-synaptic membrane.
- Normally it is 0.5–1.0 millisecond

Causes

– Time taken for release of neurotransmitter and its diffusion through the presynaptic membrane
– Attachment of neurotransmitter to the specific receptor and opening of ion channels
– Diffusion of ions into or out of the post-synaptic membrane

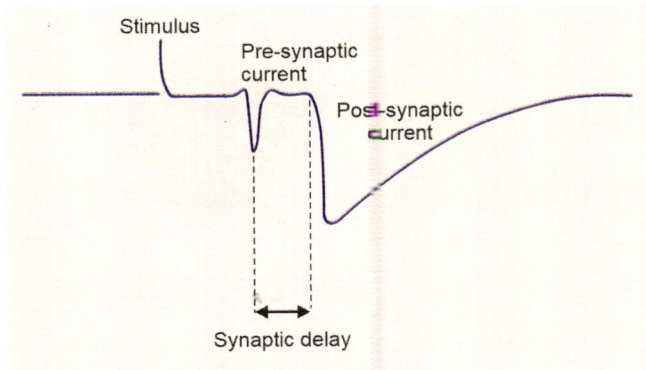

Fig. 10.4

3. Fatigue property of synapse

- When a presynaptic neuron is simulated repeatedly, the transmission is high in the beginning.
- With increase in rate of firing, the strength of post-synaptic response decreases step by step and finally dies off.
- It is also known as habituation
- After a particular recovery period, the neuro-transmission is possible again.

Causes

– This happens due to exhaustion of neuro-transmitter in the presynaptic neuron. The neurotransmitter needs to be produced/recycled continuously and when the emptying of the neurotransmitter exceeds its production, there is fatigue.
– Other causes are inactivation of calcium channels, accumulation of waste products and refractoriness of the post-synaptic membrane to the neurotransmitter.

2. Define receptors. Describe the mechanism of genesis of receptor potential in pacinian corpuscle.

Receptors

They are specialized sensory nerve ending which carry specific sensation from the periphery to a relay station.

Pacinian Corpuscle

It is a large receptor and is easily accessible. It detects pressure.

Structure

- It consists of large concentric lamellae of connective tissue around an unmyelinated portion of a nerve fibre.
- Myelination of nerve begins within the nerve such that the first node of Ranvier is within the corpuscle and the second lies outside.
- The potential is recorded placing electrodes—one on the unmyelinated nerve ending and the other on the second node of Ranvier.

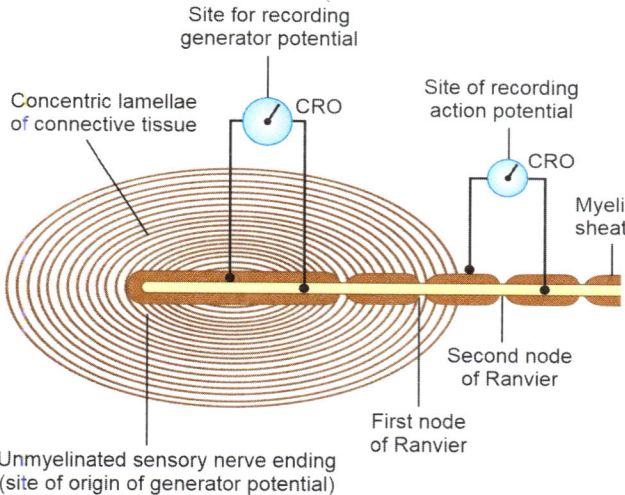

Fig. 10.5

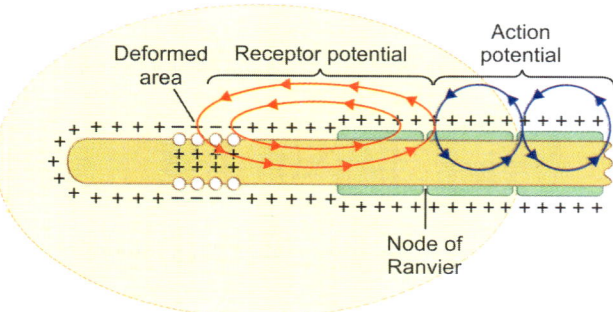

Fig. 10.6

Formation of Local Potential in Pacinian Corpuscle

- In the terminal part of the unmyelinated nerve ending, the sodium channels are opening causing a continuous influx of sodium ions from the surrounding.
- This creates positivity within the fibre. This is called 'receptor potential'. This is seen when mild pressure is applied. This causes a local circuit of flow of ions.
- When the pressure stimulus is progressively increased, the magnitude of the receptor potential increases. There is depolarization in the first node of Ranvier.
- When the receptor potential is great enough (>10 mV), it causes generation of action potential.

3. Classify sensory receptors. Describe local potential and its properties seen in pacinian corpuscle.   (2 + 3 marks)

Sensory receptors are designed to receive stimuli from external or internal environment and their transduction into neuronal impulses.

Classification of Sensory Receptors

A. Depending on the Source of Stimulus

Exteroceptors
- They gather information from the exterior of the body
- *Example:* Pain receptor, touch receptor

Enteroceptors
- They gather information within the body
- *Example:* Chemoreceptors, baroreceptors

Telereceptors
- They gather information present at a distance.
- *Example:* Rods and cones: vision, organ of Corti: auditory stimulus.

B. Depending on the Stimulus Energy

Mechanoreceptors
- Respond to mechanical stimulus
- Examples: Touch receptors, baroreceptors

Thermoreceptors
- Respond to changes in temperature
- *Examples:* Thermoreceptors in hypothalamus, Krause's organ

Photoreceptors
- Respond to changes in light
- *Examples:* Rods and cones

Chemoreceptors
- Responds to changes in the chemical composition
- *Examples:* Taste receptors, olfactory receptor, osmoreceptors in the hypothalamus.

Nociceptors: They are receptors which respond to extreme pressure in the form of pain.

Pacinian Corpuscle

It is a large receptor and is easily accessible. It detects pressure.

Formation of Local Potential in Pacinian Corpuscle

- In the terminal part of the unmyelinated nerve ending, the sodium channels are opening causing a continuous influx of sodium ions from the surrounding.
- This creates positivity within the fibre. This is called 'receptor potential'. This is seen when mild pressure is applied. This causes a local circuit of flow of ions.
- When the pressure stimulus is progressively increased, the magnitude of the receptor potential increases. There is depolarization in the first node of Ranvier.
- When the receptor potential is great enough (>10 mV), it causes generation of action potential.

Properties of Pacinian Corpuscle

1. **Wide range of detection**
   - When there is a threshold stimulus applied, there is generation of action potential which causes awareness of the stimulus.
   - When the strength of the stimulus is gradually increased, the response also increases incrementally.
   - When a very intense stimulus is provided, the increment is lesser and lesser.
   - Maximum firing limit is not reached until the stimulus is extremely high. This gives the receptors a large range of intensity of stimuli to pick up.

2. **Adaptability**
   - When a continuous stimulus is applied to a receptor, there is increased response in the form of generation of an action potential.
   - When this continues, the magnitude of the action potential gradually decreases and finally dies off.
   - Pacinian corpuscle has a very short duration of adaptability, within 1/100th of a second.

4. Explain the properties of receptors.

1. **Specificity of response**
   - Each receptor has a specificity for a single type of stimulus even at low threshold.
   - This is also called Muller's doctrine of specific nerve endings.
   - One type of sensory receptor can also get stimulated (by low threshold stimulus) by the particular sensation it has been designated for.
   - The rule against this law is that, if the intensity is increased, then the specificity is lost.

Examples

Receptor	Sensation	Receptor	Sensation
Meissner's corpuscle	Touch	Ruffini's end organ	Warmth
Pacinian corpuscle	Pressure	Free nerve endings	Pain
Krause end bulb	Cold	Rods and cones	Light

2. **Production of a receptor potential**
   - In the terminal part of the unmyelinated nerve ending, the sodium channels are opening causing a continuous influx of sodium ions from the surrounding.
   - This creates positivity within the fibre. This is called 'receptor potential'. This is seen when mild pressure is applied. This causes a local circuit of flow of ions.
   - When the pressure stimulus is progressively increased, the magnitude of the receptor potential increases. There is depolarization in the first node of Ranvier.
   - When the receptor potential is great enough (>10 mV), it causes generation of action potential.

3. Weber-Fechner law

- This law states that the intensity of response of a receptor varies directly as the logarithmic increase in the intensity with which it is stimulated.
- So, if the response from a receptor is to be doubled, then the strength of the stimulus must be increased 100 times.
- This allows receptor to pick up very subtle stimuli and at the same time, tolerate very gross stimulus. There is a huge range.

4. Law of projection

- There is extremely meticulous point to point representation of the body in the sensory homunculus.
- As a result, the stimulus is readily recognized.
- When a fibre is experimentally stimulated anywhere along its course, it is localized to its receptor.
- Following amputation, phantom limb is a known complication.
- There is irritation of the nociceptive and proprioceptive fibres at the stump of the amputated limb.
- Hence, a person may feel that his limb is still there and may experience pain along the same area.

5. Adaptability

- When a receptor is continuously stimulated with the same strength of stimulus, the receptors respond at a very high impulse rate at first, but the frequency of action potential in its sensory nerve goes on progressively decreasing, until finally some of the receptors do not respond.
- Based on this property, receptors can be of two types: Tonic (which do not adapt completely) and phasic receptors (which rapidly adapt)
- Examples of tonic receptors are baroreceptors, chemoreceptors, temperature-sensitive receptors and muscle spindles.
- Examples of phasic receptors are olfactory receptors, Meissner's corpuscles and pacinian corpuscle.

5. Explain reflex arc. Classify reflexes and discuss their properties.

Reflex Arc

- Reflex arc is anatomical neuromuscular pathway for completion of reflex action.

- It consists of 5 main components:
  1. **Receptor:** It is the end organ which following a stimulus creates an impulse.
  2. **Afferent nerve:** It is the pathway for transmission of impulse from the receptor to the centre.
  3. **Centre:** It receives impulse form the end organ through the afferent nerve and processes the impulse.
  4. **Efferent nerve:** It is a motor nerve which transmits the impulse to the effector organ.
  5. **Effector organ:** It is usually a muscle or a gland which produces the desired effect.

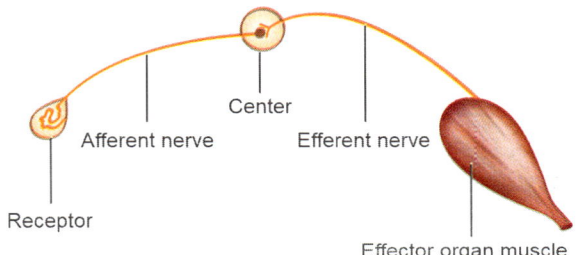

Fig. 10.7

Classification of Reflexes

Depending on period of acquisition	Inborn or unconditioned and acquired or conditioned
Depending on the anatomy	Cortical, cerebellar, midbrain, bulbar, and spinal
Depending on the purpose	Protective or flexor and anti-gravity or extensor
Depending on the number of synapses	Monosynaptic and polysynaptic
Depending on whether somatic or visceral	Somatic reflex and autonomous reflex
Depending on clinical basis	Superficial reflex, deep reflex, Visceral reflex and pathological reflex

Properties of Reflexes

1. One-way conduction or Bell-Magendie law

- The impulse always passes from the receptor to the effector organ
- The direction is always one way

2. Reaction time:
It is the time taken for the impulse to move through the reflex arc and is influenced by the length of the nerve fibers and the time taken at the centre of reflex.

3. **Summation**
   - When two afferent nerves of the same muscle are stimulated at the same time with subliminal stimulus, there is additive response (spatial summation).
   - When one nerve fiber is stimulated with two or more stimuli of subliminal strength, there is additive response (temporal summation)

4. **Occlusion:** When a muscle supplied by two motor nerves are stimulated, the effective contraction due to stimulation of both nerves is less than the sum of contraction when each nerve is stimulated individually.

5. **Subliminal fringe:** In some reflexes involving two motor nerves stimulating a muscle, the effective contraction of the muscle when both nerves are simultaneously stimulated is more than the sum of each nerve when each nerve is stimulated individually.

6. **Recruitment**
   - It is successive activation of more and more motor units when there is progressive increase in force of contraction
   - It is also called quantal summation.

7. **After discharge**
   - It is persistence of discharge of the effector end even after the stimulus has ceased to stimulate.
   - This is seen in conditions where there is continuous stimulation.

8. **Rebound phenomenon:** When the inhibition on a reflex is suddenly removed, there is increase in the effect of the stimulus.

9. **Fatigue:** When a reflex is elicited continuously for a long time, there is slowing down of reflex and after a time, the reflex dies off.

SHORT ANSWERS

1. Define synapse. Explain transmission across a synaptic junction.

Synapse

Synapse is a physiological continuity between two neurons (Fig. 10.8).

Steps in Synaptic Conduction

- Depending on whether the synaptic transmission causes excitation or inhibition of the post-synaptic neuron, the potential generated is classified as excitatory or inhibitory response.
- When the action potential arrives at the presynaptic membrane, calcium influx causes the vesicles containing neurotransmitters to rupture.
- In excitatory neurons, it is acetylcholine.
- The neurotransmitter binds to the receptor present on the post-synaptic membrane.
- This causes opening of sodium channels to cause influx of sodium ions leading to generation of positive potential.
- This causes production of excitatory local potential. When many such potentials sum up, it gives rise to action potential.
- In inhibitory neurons, the neurotransmitter is GABA. GABA binds with its receptor on the

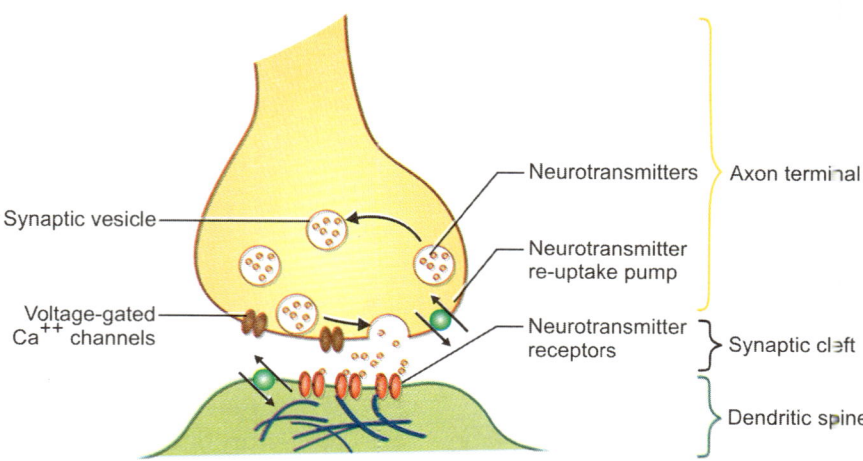

Fig. 10.8

post-synaptic membrane leading to efflux of potassium and influx of chloride ions. As a result, there is hyperpolarization and the action potential die.

2. Explain EPSP and IPSP.

EPSP: Excitatory Post-synaptic Potential

- When the action potential arrives at the presynaptic membrane, calcium influx causes the vesicles containing neurotransmitters to rupture.
- In excitatory neurons, it is acetylcholine.
- Acetylcholine binds to the receptor present on the post-synaptic membrane.
- This causes opening of sodium channels to cause influx of sodium ions leading to generation of a small positive potential.
- This is a non-propagative end plate potential, which does not obey all-or-none law. It is called excitatory post-synaptic potential.
- When many such potentials sum up, it gives rise to action potential.

IPSP: Inhibitory Post-synaptic Potential

- In inhibitory neurons, when action potential arrives at the presynaptic membrane, calcium influx from the ECF into the axon terminal causes rupture of vesicles containing GABA.
- GABA binds with its receptor on the post-synaptic membrane leading to efflux of potassium and influx of chloride ions.
- As a result, there is more negativity inside the neuron
- This results in hyperpolarization and an inhibitory post-synaptic potential
- The action potential dies and is not propagated.

3. What is inverse stretch reflex? Name the receptor involved.

Receptor Involved

- Golgi tendon organ is the receptor involved in this inverse stretch reflex.

- It is in the tendon of the muscle and is sensitive to extreme increase in tension of the muscle.
- They are placed in line with the tendon and muscle fibres and around 10–15 muscle fibres are associated with one Golgi tendon organ.

Inverse Stretch Reflex

- The Golgi tendon organ is supplied by the Ib sensory fibres.
- When a muscle contracts, there is increase in tension in the muscle and is picked up by the Golgi tendon organ.
- It sends impulses via the Ib sensory fibres to the dorsal root ganglion to the spinal cord.
- In the spinal cord, these Ib fibers stimulate the inhibitory interneurons.
- The interneurons release an inhibitory neuro-transmitter—glycine. Glycine inhibits the alpha-motor neurons and causes relaxation of the contracted muscle.

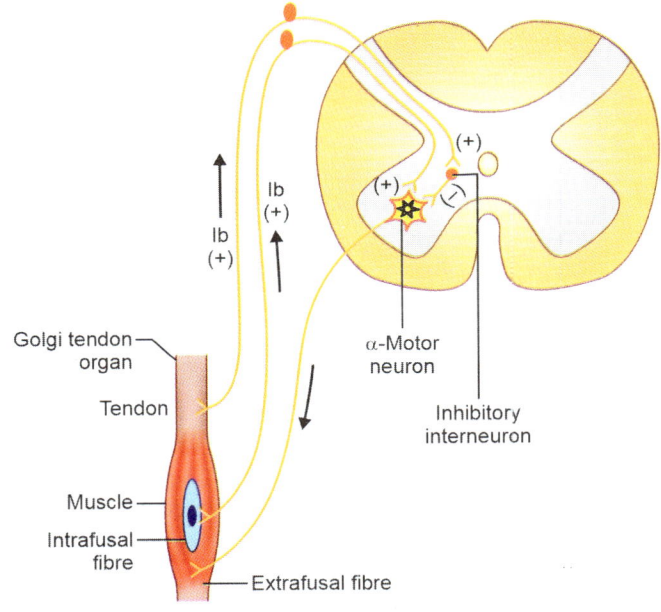

Fig. 10.9

10.3 DESCRIBE AND DISCUSS SOMATIC SENSATIONS AND SENSORY TRACTS

LONG ESSAY

1. **Draw a neat-labelled diagram of origin, course and termination of anterior spinothalamic tract and describe the sensations carried by it.**

Anterior Spinothalamic Tract (Fig. 10.10)

- Anterior spinothalamic tract is formed by fibres of second-order neurons and conducts impulses regarding crude touch.
- It is situated in the anterior white funiculus near the periphery.

Origin

- They receive sensory signals from cutaneous receptors which relay in the spinal ganglia. The processes from these ganglia terminate in the chief sensory neurons of posterior grey horn.
- The anterior spinothalamic tract originates in the chief sensory neurons of the posterior grey horn.
- They form the second-order neurons.

Course

- These fibres ascend on the same side along the spinal cord for 2–3 segments, after which most of the fibres cross to the contralateral side.
- Then these fibres pass through the medulla oblongata, pons, midbrain and terminate in the thalamus.
- Along with fibres of the lateral spinothalamic tract, these fibres form the spinal lemniscus in the brain stem.
- They terminate in the thalamus-ventral posterolateral nucleus of thalamus. The neurons of thalamus form the third order neurons and these fibres relay in the somatosensory area of the cerebral cortex.

Sensations Carried

- The anterior spinothalamic tract carries sensations regarding crude touch and pressure.
- The receptors for crude touch are free nerve endings and hair end organs.
- Crude touch is the ability to detect contact with skin and the exact localization is difficult.

SHORT ESSAYS

1. **Explain the anterolateral pathway and the sensations carried by it.**

Anterolateral Pathway (Fig. 10.10)

- Begins at the anterior white funiculus near the periphery and the lateral spinothalamic tract begins at the lateral funiculus near the medial side.
- The first-order neurons of this pathway are the spinal ganglia and receive information from cutaneous receptors.
- The second-order neurons are formed by the chief sensory neurons in the posterior grey horn of the spinal cord.
- The axons of these neurons form the spinothalamic tract.
- The anterior spinothalamic tract ascends on the same side of the spinal cord for 2–3 segments and then cross onto the opposite side.
- The fibres of the lateral spinothalamic tract cross to the opposite side in the same spinal segment and ascend along the lateral column of the spinal cord.

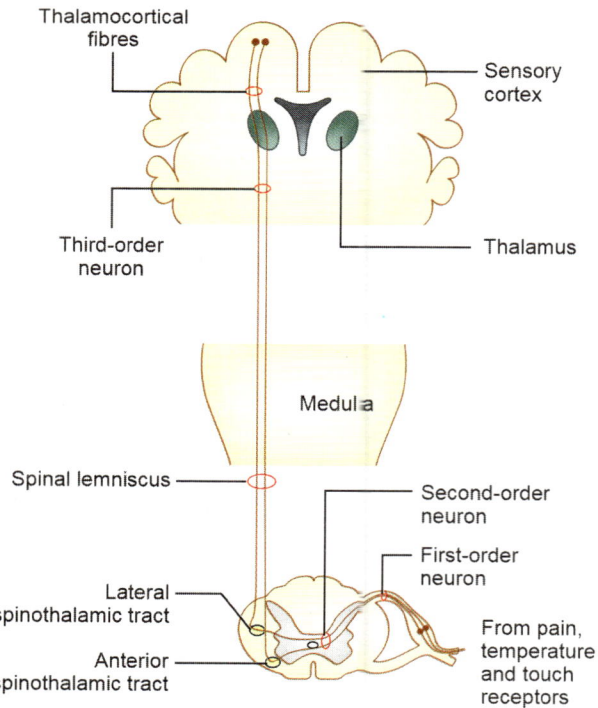

Fig. 10.10

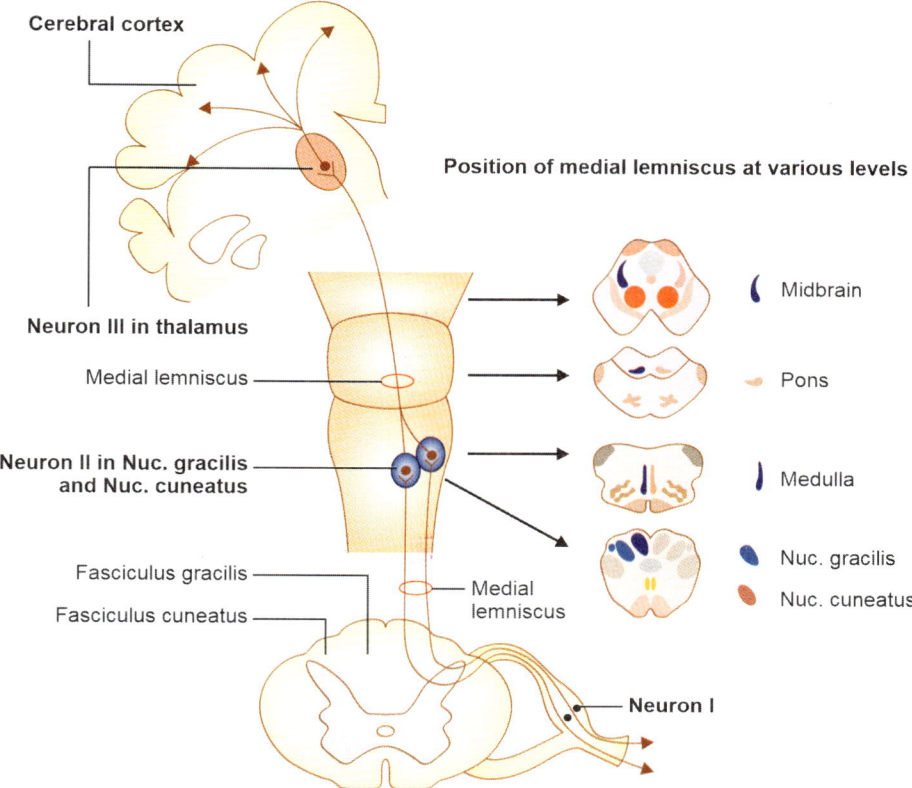

Position of medial lemniscus at various levels

Cerebral cortex

Neuron III in thalamus

Medial lemniscus

Neuron II in Nuc. gracilis and Nuc. cuneatus

Fasciculus gracilis

Fasciculus cuneatus

Medial lemniscus

Neuron I

Midbrain

Pons

Medulla

Nuc. gracilis

Nuc. cuneatus

Fig. 10.11

- These two tracts carry about 10% of fibers from the same side and ascend along the spinal lemniscus and run through the spinal cord, medulla, pons and midbrain and finally terminate in the thalamus.
- The neurons of the thalamus form the third-order neurons and relay in the somatosensory cortex.
- Sensations carried by lateral spinothalamic tract: Pain and temperature.

2. Describe the dorsal column pathway and list the sensations carried by it.

Origin (Fig. 10.11)

- The first order neurons are in the dorsal root ganglia.
- The axons from these forms a fasciculus (a group of axons)
- Fasciculus gracilis is formed by the distal most fibers—coccygeal, sacral, lumbar and lower thoracic ganglia. This occupies the medial part of the posterior column tracts.

- Fasciculus cuneatus is formed by the axons of the proximal fibers—upper thoracic and cervical ganglia.
- They occupy the posterior funiculus of the spinal cord.

Route

- They occupy the posterior column and pass uncrossed till the medulla.
- They synapse in the nucleus of gracilis and cuneatus in the medulla.
- They form the second order neurons.
- The fibers from here form the internal arcuate fibers and arch medially and anteriorly and cross the midline (sensory decussation).
- They form the medial lemniscus in the medulla and terminate in the ventral, posterolateral aspect of the thalamus.
- Axons of the third-order neurons pass through the internal capsule and corona radiata to reach the somatosensory areas of the cerebral cortex.

Functions

1. Sense of touch: Deep touch, fine touch, tactile localization, tactile discrimination, stereognosis
2. Sensations of proprioception: Received from various joints and muscles.
3. Sense of vibrations

3. What is classic defect below the level of lesion in Brown-Séquard syndrome?

Brown-Séquard Syndrome

It is a collection of symptoms and signs associated with hemisection of the spinal cord (Fig. 10.12).

Effects of Hemisection of Spinal Cord, below the Level of Injury

On the same side	On the opposite side
Sensations lost • Fine touch • Tactile localization • Tactile discrimination • Vibration sense • Stereognosis	Sensations lost • Crude touch • Pain • Temperature
Motor changes • Spastic paralysis • Rigidity • Babinski sign • Exaggerated tendon reflexes • Loss of superficial reflexes	Motor changes • Very mild weakness, if it occurs, it is UMN type
Autonomic • Fall in blood pressure due to loss of sympathetic tone	

4. Enumerate types of pain and trace the pain pathway.

Types of Pain

1. **Fast pain:** It is the first sensation whenever a pain stimulus is given. It is felt as a sharp, bright and localized pain sensation.
2. **Slow pain:** Dull, diffuse unpleasant pain.

Clinical Types of Pain

1. Somatic pain
2. Visceral pain
3. Referred pain
4. Radiating pain
5. Projected pain

Pain Pathway (Fig. 10.13)

1. **Fast pain**
   - Transmitted by A delta fibers
   - Nerve endings → spinal root ganglia → tract of Lissauer and terminate in the neurons of lamina 1. → fibers immediately cross to the opposite side → ascending in the spinal cord of the anterolateral column → neospinothalamic tract → few fibers terminate in the reticular formation → project in the VPL of the thalamus → primary sensory cortex.

2. **Slow pain**
   - Transmitted by C fibers
   - Through the dorsal root ganglion → terminate in the lamina II and III of spinal cord (substantia

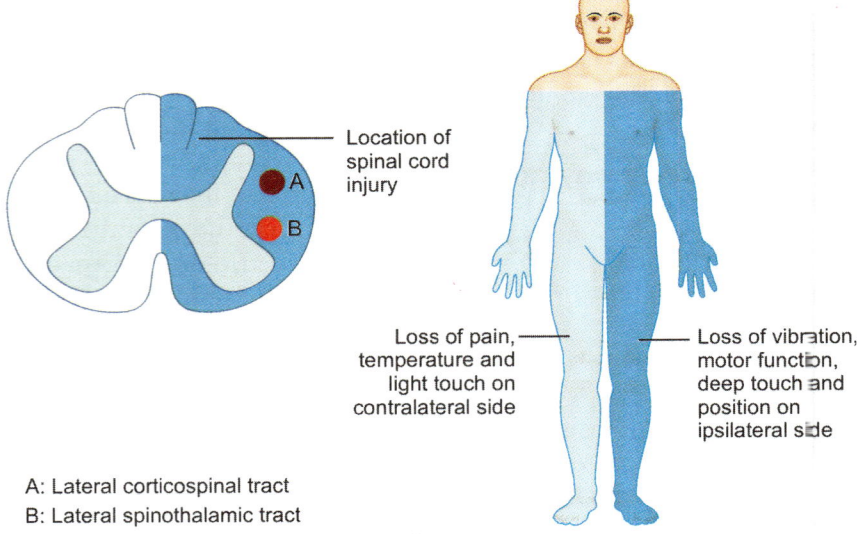

Location of spinal cord injury

Loss of pain, temperature and light touch on contralateral side

Loss of vibration, motor function, deep touch and position on ipsilateral side

A: Lateral corticospinal tract
B: Lateral spinothalamic tract

Fig. 10.12

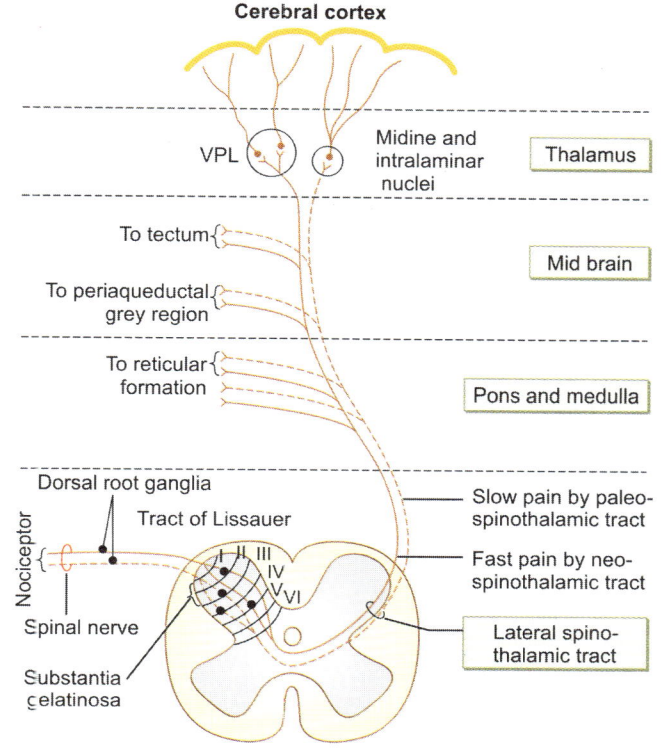

Fig. 10.13

gelatinosa) → lamina V of the dorsal grey horn → cross the midline → form the paleospinothalamic tract → relay widely in the reticular formation, superior colliculus and periaqueductal grey region → a few fibers relay in the posterior part of the thalamus → relay in all parts of the brain.

5. Define Weber-Fechner law and Muller's doctrine of specific nerve energies. Describe the phenomenon of phantom limb.

These are the properties of the sensory receptors.

Weber-Fechner Law

- This law states that the intensity of response of a receptor varies directly as the logarithmic increase in the intensity with which it is stimulated.
- So, if the response from a receptor is to be doubled, then the strength of the stimulus must be increased 100 times.

Muller's Doctrine of Specific Nerve Energies

- Muller's law: One type of sensory receptor can also get stimulated (by low threshold stimulus) by the particular sensation it has been designated for.

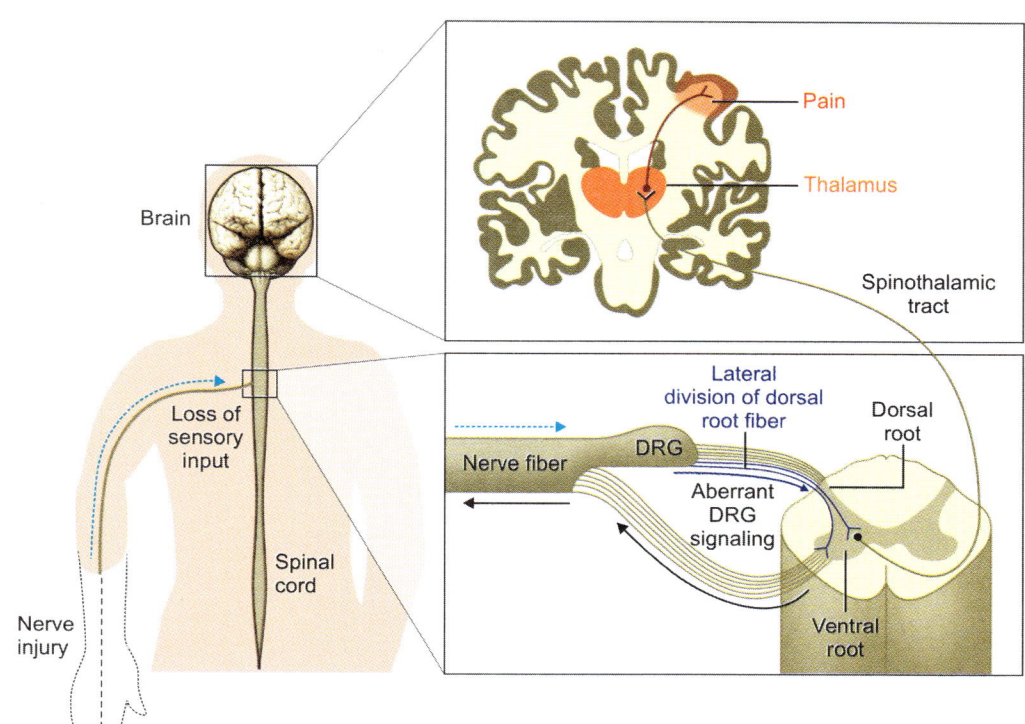

Fig. 10.14

- The rule against this law is that, if the intensity is increased, then the specificity is lost.

Examples

Receptor	Sensation	Receptor	Sensation
Meissner's corpuscle	Touch	Ruffini's end organ	Warmth
Pacinian corpuscle	Pressure	Free nerve endings	Pain
Krause end bulb	Cold	Rods and cones	Light

Phantom Limb (Fig. 10.14)

- It is a sensation of presence of a limb even after its amputation. Some patients may even experience pain.
- This is due to law of projection for a sensory nerve.

Law of Projection

- There is extremely meticulous point to point representation of the body in the sensory homunculus.

- As a result, the stimulus is readily recognized.
- When a fibre is experimentally stimulated anywhere along its course, it is localized to its receptor.
- Following amputation, phantom limb is a known complication.
- There is irritation of the nociceptive and proprioceptive fibers at the stump of the amputated limb.
- Hence, a person may feel that his limb is still there and may experience pain along the same area.

6. What is gate control theory of pain? Describe the descending pain suppressing pathways.

Gate Control Pathway (Fig. 10.15)

- According to this theory, pain impulses reaching the cortex are controlled by a "gate" mechanism at the posterior grey horn of the respective segment and also at the brain level.
- If the gate is open, pain is felt and if the gate is closed, the pain is not felt.

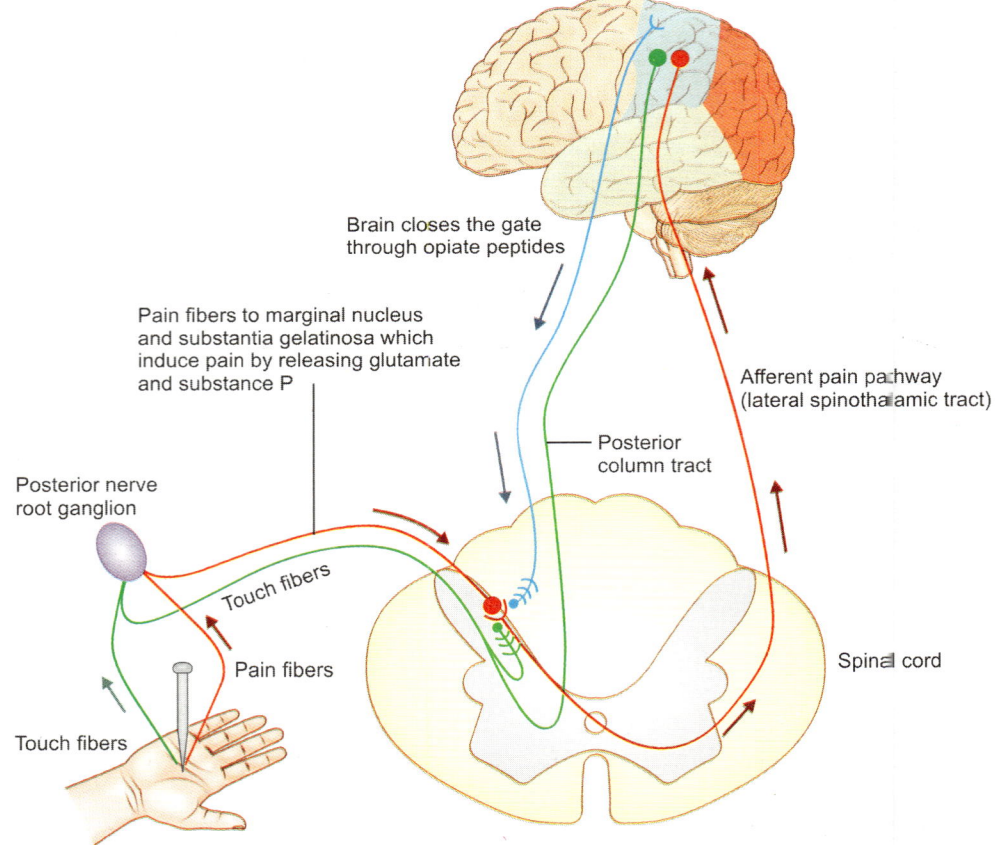

Brain closes the gate through opiate peptides

Pain fibers to marginal nucleus and substantia gelatinosa which induce pain by releasing glutamate and substance P

Posterior column tract

Afferent pain pathway (lateral spinothalamic tract)

Posterior nerve root ganglion

Touch fibers

Pain fibers

Spinal cord

Touch fibers

Fig. 10.15

Mechanism of Pain Control at Spinal Level

- When pain stimulus is applied to any point on the body, along with pain, touch receptors are also stimulated.
- Fibres of touch sensation pass through collateral through marginal cells and substantia gelatinosa. These fibres inhibit the release of glutamate and substance P.
- This causes pain sensation to be not transmitted.

Mechanism of Pain Control by Brain

- If the gate is not closed at spinal level, pain sensations reach the brain. These signals are processed in the thalamus and then sent to the somatosensory cortex.
- The cortex detects and assesses the amount of pain depending on the individual's capacity of tolerating pain.
- When intolerable, the brain releases opiates and thus closes the gate at spinal level.

SHORT ANSWERS

1. Define referred pain. Explain the theories of referred pain.

Referred Pain

- It is a pain that originates in a visceral organ but is referred to a somatic component.

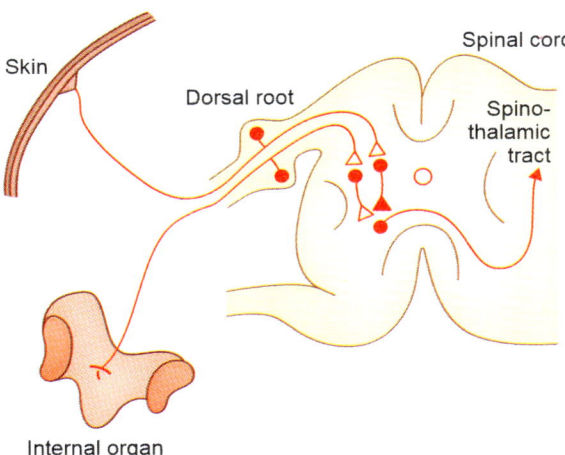

Fig. 10.16

- They are supplied by the same neural segment.
- *Examples:* Pain in cholecystitis is referred to tip of shoulder, pain in lower ureter is referred to inner side of thigh.

Theories of Referred Pain

1. **Convergence theory**
   - When the first order nerve supplying the skin and the visceral organ synapse on the same spinal segment, the brain is unable to identify the site of pain.
   - As a result, the pain is perceived to be in the corresponding somatic segment.

2. **Facilitation theory**
   - According to this, the visceral irritation is insufficient to produce a response and hence it is aided by the pain from the somatic component.
   - Thus, even minor irritation is picked by the somatic counterpart.

2. Name any 6 extrapyramidal tracts.

Rubrospinal tract	Red nucleus → interneurons of corticospinal tracts
Reticulospinal tract	
Medial	Medial pontine reticular formation → laminae VII and VIII of spinal cord
Lateral	Medullary reticular formation → VII, VIII and IX of the spinal cord
Olivospinal tract	Inferior olivary nucleus → laminae V and VII of spinal cord
Vestibulospinal tract	
Medial	Medial vestibular nucleus → laminae VII and VIII of spinal cord
Lateral	Lateral vestibular nucleus → laminae VII and VIII of spinal cord
Tectospinal tract	Superior colliculus → laminae V and VII of spinal cord
Medial longitudinal fasciculus	Different nuclei of brainstem → ventral horn cells of spinal cord

10.4 DESCRIBE AND DISCUSS MOTOR TRACTS, MECHANISM OF MAINTENANCE OF TONE, CONTROL OF BODY MOVEMENTS, POSTURE AND EQUILIBRIUM AND VESTIBULAR APPARATUS

LONG ESSAYS

1. Explain the corticobulbar and corticospinal tracts.

Corticobulbar Tracts (Fig. 10.17)

Also called corticonuclear tracts.

Origin

They begin in the cerebral cortex along with the corticospinal tracts.

Course

These fibres descend along with corticospinal tract fibres as part of corona radiata and then pass through the genu of the internal capsule.

Termination

In the brain stem, they cross to the opposite side at various levels and terminate onto cranial nerve nuclei, either direct or through interneurons.

Oculomotor nerve	Midbrain
Trochlear nerve	
Trigeminal nerve	Pontomedullary junction
Abducens and facial nerve	Upper medulla
Glossopharyngeal, vagus and hypoglossal nerve	Lower medulla
Accessory nerve	Upper cervical cord

Functions

They are motor to various skeletal muscles controlled by cranial nerves.

Pyramidal Tracts or Corticospinal Tracts (Fig. 10.18)

Origin

- The corticospinal tracts originate in the primary motor cortex (area 4), premotor cortex (area 8) and supplementary motor area and the somatic sensory areas.
- These form the fibers of the upper motor neuron.

Course

- They descend as a part of the corona radiata and posterior part of the internal capsule

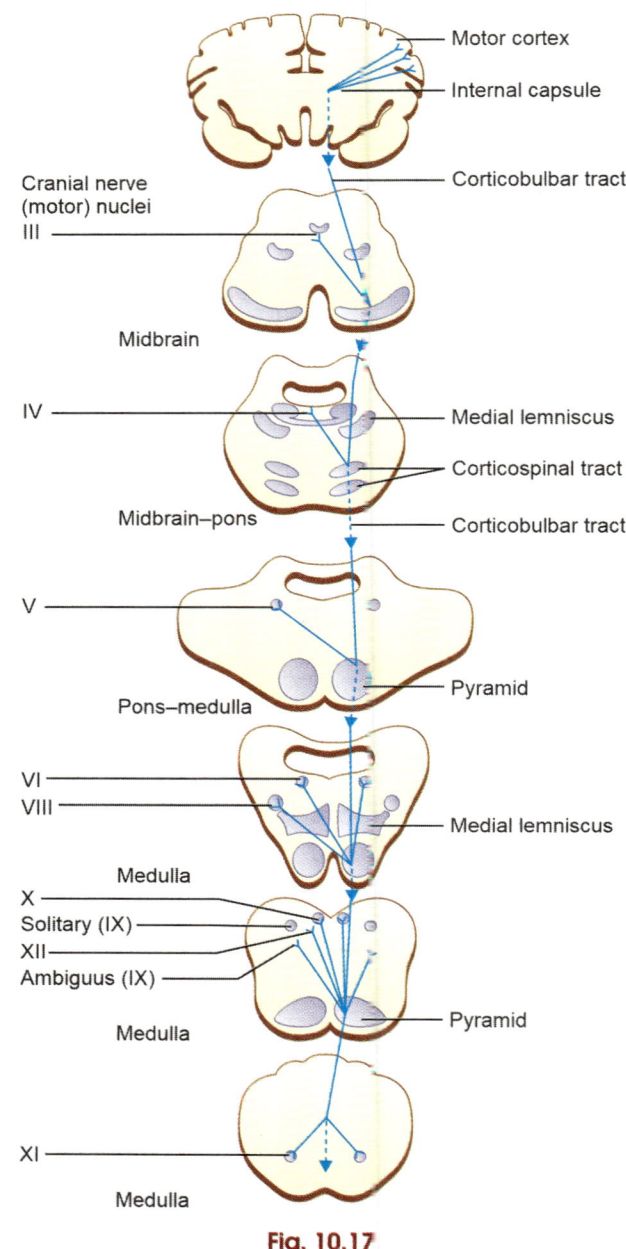

Fig. 10.17

- They descend through the medulla as pyramids and thus named as pyramidal tracts
- In the lower part of the medulla, 80% fibers decussate to the opposite side and form the lateral corticospinal tracts.

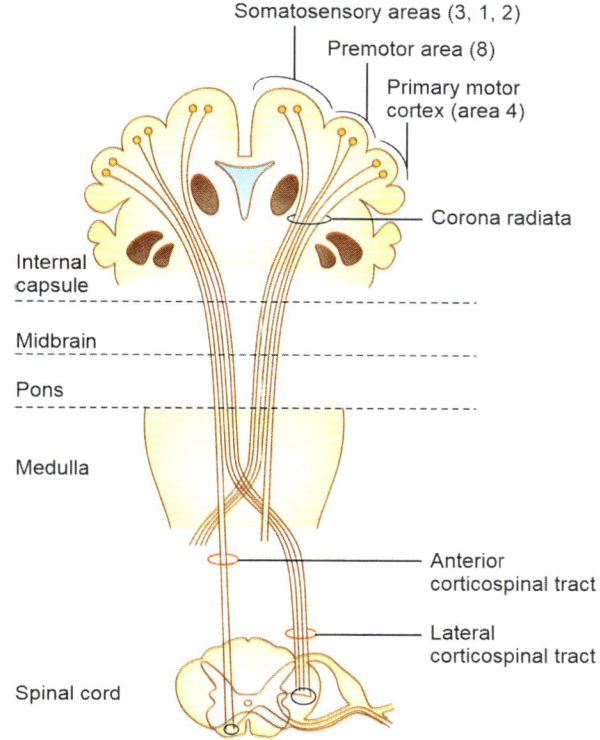

Fig. 10.18

Lateral corticospinal tract

- It descends through the entire length of the spinal cord along the posterior part of the lateral white funiculus.
- They terminate on the internuncial neurons of the spinal grey matter
- Some terminate directly on the alpha motor neurons
- The motor neurons supply respective skeletal muscles.

Anterior corticospinal tract

- It is formed by the remaining 20% uncrossed fibers
- They pass along the length of the spinal cord in the anterior white funiculus.
- On reaching an appropriate level in the spinal cord, they decussate to the opposite side and terminate similar to the lateral corticospinal tract.

Functions

1. These tracts are associated with voluntary motor activities
2. Fine skilled movements are done with the help of this tract

3. Some fibers from the pyramidal system relay in the nuclei of the cranial nerves in the brainstem.
4. These are termed corticonuclear fibers.
5. They are associated with cranial nerve functions.

2. Trace the extrapyramidal tracts and give their functions.

- The descending tracts of the spinal cord other than the pyramidal tract are called extrapyramidal tracts.
- They are:

1. Rubrospinal tract

Origin: This tract starts at the magnocellularis or red nucleus of the midbrain.

Course

- Immediately, they crossover to the opposite side in the lower part of the segmental of the midbrain (ventral segmental decussation)
- Then it descends in the pons and medulla contained in the lateral lemniscus.

Termination: They terminate in the internuncial neurons and the alpha motor neurons of upper three segments of the spinal cord.

Functions: It forms an alternate route through corticorubrospinal tract for pyramidal system to influence the lower motor neurons.

2. Vestibulospinal tracts

a. *Lateral vestibulospinal tract:* Origin, course and termination

- Lateral vestibular nucleus is the origin.
- The fibers supplying the cervical segments arise in the upper part of the nucleus, thoracic part arises from the middle part and lumbar from the lower part of the nucleus
- It remains uncrossed and lies in the anterior funiculus of the spinal cord
- They relay onto the laminae VII and VIII and influence the alpha and gamma neurons through internuntial neurons.

Functions

1. They are associated with postural muscle after receiving afferents form the utricle
2. Excites the extensors and inhibits the flexors.

b. *Medial vestibulospinal tract:* Origin, course and termination

- It originated in the medial vestibular nucleus

– They majorly remain uncrossed and descend through the anterior funiculus
– They terminate onto the anterior motor neurons directly or through internuncial neurons in the cervical segments of the spinal cord

Functions
1. They receive afferent from the semicircular canals
2. Provides a pathway for reflex movements of head, neck and eyes in response to auditory and visual stimuli.

3. **Reticulospinal tracts**
   a. *Medial or pontine reticulospinal tracts:* Medial reticular formation → descends uncrossed along the anterior funiculus → terminates in the laminae VII and VIII.
   b. *Lateral or medullary reticulospinal tracts:* Medullary reticular formation → descends in the lateral funiculus medial to the pyramidal tract → terminate in laminae VII, VIII and IX of spinal cord.

   Functions
   1. The reticular formation receives information from the motor cortex.
   2. Thus, they form an alternate pathway to the pyramidal system.
   3. They are concerned with maintenance of muscle tone.
   4. Convey autonomic information.

4. **Tectospinal tract**
   - Arises in the superior colliculus → cross midline in the lower part of segmental of midbrain → descends along the brainstem and enters the spinal cord
   - Terminates in the laminae V and VII of spinal cord

   Functions: They are concerned with movements of head, eyes and limbs in response to visual and auditory stimuli.

5. **Olivospinal tract**
   - Originates in the inferior olivary nucleus ' descends and terminates in the anterior grey horn of the spinal cord.

   Functions: Olive receives information from ipsilateral cortex and is involved in reflex movements following stimuli from proprioceptive stimuli.

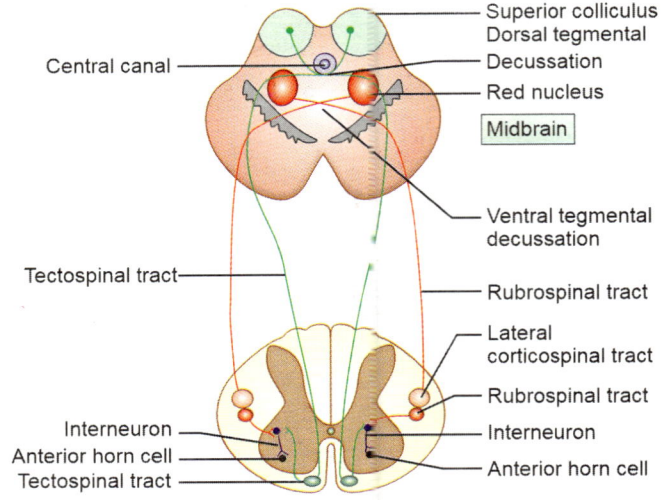

Fig. 10.19

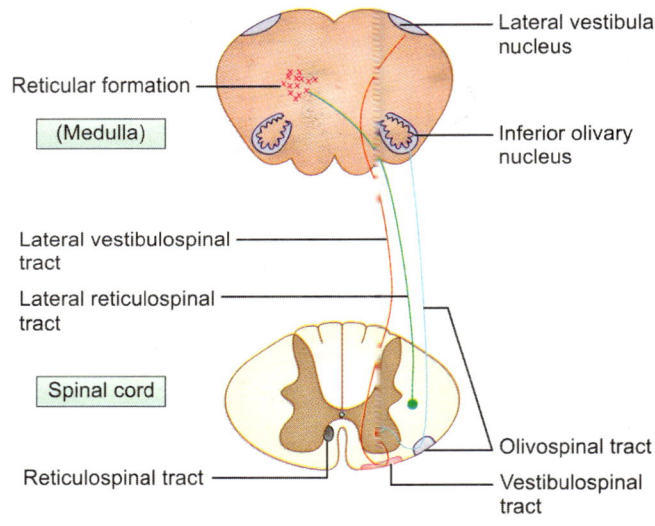

Fig. 10.20

6. **Medial longitudinal fasciculus**
   - It originates from the midbrain downwards.
   - The vestibular nucleus, reticular formation, superior colliculus, interstitial nucleus of Cajal and nucleus of the posterior commissure take part in origin of this tract.
   - It is closely related to the third, fourth and sixth nuclei. It is also closely associated with 7th nerve, 8th nerve and 12th nerve.
   - It becomes continuous with the intersegmental part of spinal cord.

- They terminate in the anterior grey horns of the spinal cord supplying the neck muscles.

  Functions: They are involved in horizontal eye movements. Also, in simultaneous movement of lips during speech.

SHORT ESSAYS

1. List the descending tracts. Add a note on Brown-Sequard syndrome.   (2 + 3 marks)

Descending Tracts

1. Pyramidal tracts—anterior and lateral corticospinal tracts
2. Corticonuclear tracts
3. Corticopontocerebellar pathway
4. Rubrospinal and vestibulospinal tract
5. Medial and lateral reticulospinal tract
6. Tectospinal tract

Brown-Sequard Syndrome

- It is a collection of symptoms and signs associated with hemisection of the spinal cord.

Effects of Hemisection of Spinal Cord—below the Level of Injury

On the same side	On the opposite side
Sensations lost	**Sensations lost**
• Fine touch	• Crude touch
• Tactile localization	• Pain
• Tactile discrimination	• Temperature
• Vibration sense	
• Stereognosis	
Motor changes	**Motor changes**
• Spastic paralysis	• Very mild weakness if it occurs it is UMN type
• Rigidity	
• Babinski sign	
• Exaggerated tendon reflexes	
• Loss of superficial reflexes	
Autonomic	
• Fall in blood pressure due to loss of sympathetic tone	

2. A 25-year-old male came to the emergency with history of fall from a height that injured his thoracic spinal cord. He was unable to move both the lower limbs. On examination, he presented with features of paraplegia. What type of lesion is this and describe the other features seen in this condition?

Paraplegia

This is a complete transection of the spinal cord—stage of spinal shock.

Features of Complete Transection of Spinal Cord

1. **Paralysis of both lower limbs**
   - As the lesion at the thoracic level, all motor functions of both flexor and extensor group of muscles are lost in both limbs.
   - There is flaccidity as the nerve from the anterior motor neuron cannot travel to the respective muscle.
   - All deep tendon reflexes are lost. In this case, knee jerk and ankle jerk would be lost.

2. **Loss of sensory functions:** All the sensations below the designated level are lost due to injury to the posterior nerve roots and sensory neurons in the spinal cord.

3. **Effect on bladder**
   - The bladder becomes atonic of flaccid.
   - As a result, the detrusor cannot detect filling of urine in the bladder. The urine goes on collecting till the maximum capacity is achieved.
   - Then there is overflow incontinence.

4. **Effect on bowel:** The bowel movements become sluggish and thus leads to constipation.

5. **Effect on the heart**
   - The venous return in resting condition significantly decreases as the tone in the muscles in lost.
   - As a result, preload decreases and thus cardiac output decreases.
   - The pulse is weak and blood pressure is low.
   - As the lesion is at the thoracic level, there is damage to some sympathetic fibres leading to failure of regulatory mechanisms of blood pressure.

6. **Effect on skin**
   - There is decreased blood supply and sensations leading to an increased risk of developing bedsores.
   - The skin is dry and scaly.

7. **Others:** Penis is flaccid and erection becomes impossible.

3. Compare and contrast upper and lower motor neuron lesion.

Parameter	Upper motor neuron lesion	Lower motor neuron lesion
Site of affection	Anywhere from the cerebral cortex to the synapse with the alpha motor neuron or internuncial neuron	Anywhere between the alpha motor neuron to the neuromuscular junction
Common causes	Poliomyelitis Transverse myelitis	Stroke Space occupying lesions
Single or multiple	Usually a group of muscles is affected	A single muscle is usually affected
Type of paralysis	Spastic paralysis	Flaccid paralysis
Deep tendon reflexes	Exaggerated	Lost
Plantar reflex • A gentle stroke over the outer edge of the sole of the foot causes plantar flexion and adduction of all toes Atrophy of muscle with long-standing paralysis	Babinski sign (extensor) Unlikely due to constant firing of the muscle with nerve impulse	Flexor Likely as there is no firing from the alpha motor neuron
Superficial reflexes	Lost	Lost
Clonus	Present	Absent
Clasp knife rigidity • It is resistance offered by a muscle to passive stretch. Initially there is resistance due to initiation of stretch reflex followed by a feeling of let-go due to inverse stretch reflex.	Present	Absent

4. Explain stretch reflex. Explain alpha-gamma coactivation.

Stretch Reflex (Fig. 10.21)

* It is a reflex characterized by reflex contraction of a stretched muscle.
* It is a monosynaptic reflex.
* Stimulation of muscle spindle → afferent through sensory nerve (group Ia and II) → reaches the dorsal horn of the spinal segment → stimulation of all anterior group of neurons associated with the muscle → efferent axon causing contraction of the muscle.

Role of Alpha-Gamma Coactivation (Fig. 10.22)

* During active movement, there is shortening of extrafusal fibres causing the tension in the muscle spindles to decrease.
* But during voluntary contraction of muscle, there is activation of both alpha and gamma neurons.

As a result, there is no unloading action of the muscle spindle.
* Thus, there is constant alpha motor discharge.

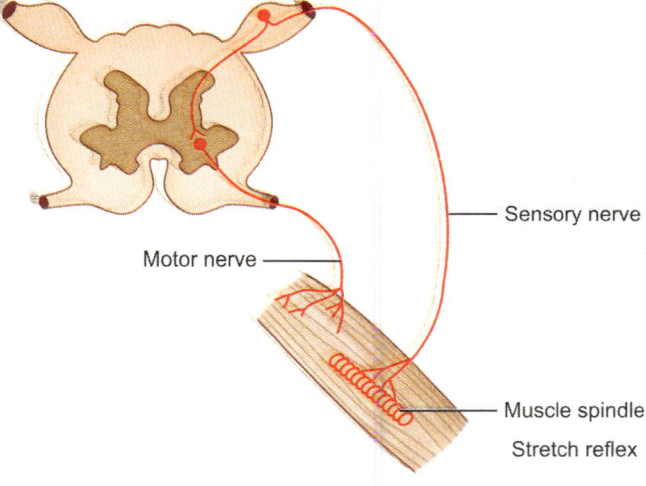

Sensory nerve

Motor nerve

Muscle spindle

Stretch reflex

Fig. 10.21

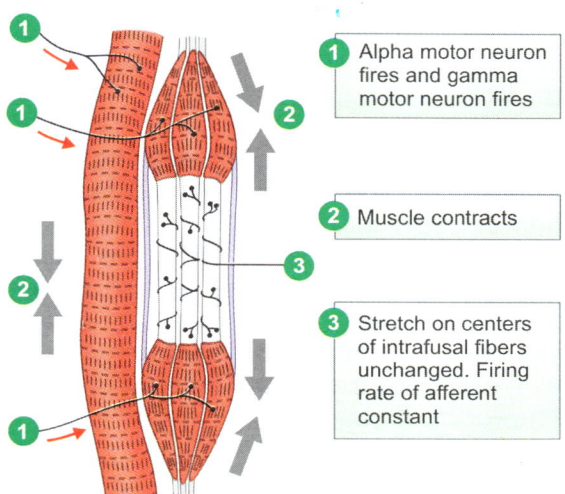

1. Alpha motor neuron fires and gamma motor neuron fires

2. Muscle contracts

3. Stretch on centers of intrafusal fibers unchanged. Firing rate of afferent constant

Fig. 10.22

5. Define muscle tone. What is the effect of UMN lesion on muscle tone?

Muscle Tone

- Muscle tone is a resistance offered to active or passive stretch.
- It is a sustained partial state of contraction of a muscle.
- It is due to low amplitude asynchronous firing of the gamma neuron.

Effect of UMN Lesion on Muscle Tone (Fig. 10.23)

- The tone of skeletal muscles is increased in UMN lesions (hypertonia).
- The type of hypertonia is called spasticity
- This happens due to continuous discharge from the alpha motor neuron as the inhibition is lost.

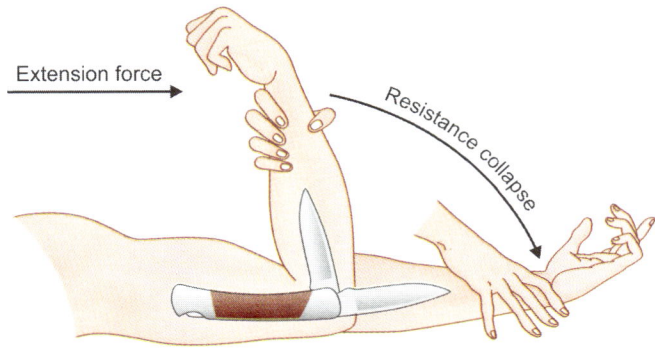

Extension force

Resistance collapse

Fig. 10.23

- There is resistance offered by a group of muscles—usually flexors.
- It is velocity dependent, that is, faster is the stretch, more is the resistance offered.
- Also, there is exaggerated deep tendon reflexes.
- There is clasp knife rigidity: It is resistance offered by a muscle to passive stretch. Initially there is resistance due to initiation of stretch reflex followed by a feeling of let-go due to inverse stretch reflex.

6. Knee jerk is a type of deep reflex. Describe the receptor structure and the reflex arc involved in elicitation of knee jerk reflex.

Deep Tendon Reflex

- Deep reflexes are basically stretch reflexes and can be elicited by stroking a tendon. So, they are also called deep tendon reflexes.
- The principle behind this stretch reflex: When a muscle spindle is suddenly stretched, it contracts.

Knee Jerk

- It is a commonly performed clinical test
- In sitting position with legs not in coming in contact with the ground, the patellar tendon just below the patella is struck gently with a knee hammer.
- This causes stretching of the quadriceps and reflex contraction causing mild transient extension of knee.

Receptor Involved (Fig. 10.24)

- Muscle spindle: Detects change in length of the muscle
- Each muscle spindle is made up of 3–10 intrafusal fibers and encapsulated in a thin capsule containing fluid.
- They are placed parallel to the extrafusal fibres.
- It consists of a central noncontractile element that lacks actin and myosin. Portion on either sides of this contain actin and myosin.
- The intrafusal fibers are of two types:
  1. **Nuclear bag fibers:** Each intrafusal fibre consists of 2–5 nuclear bag fibers and centre has a congregation of nuclei.
  2. **Nuclear chain fibers**
     - Nuclei are arranged in the form of a chain.
     - Around 6–10 nuclear chain fibres are present in one intrafusal fibre.

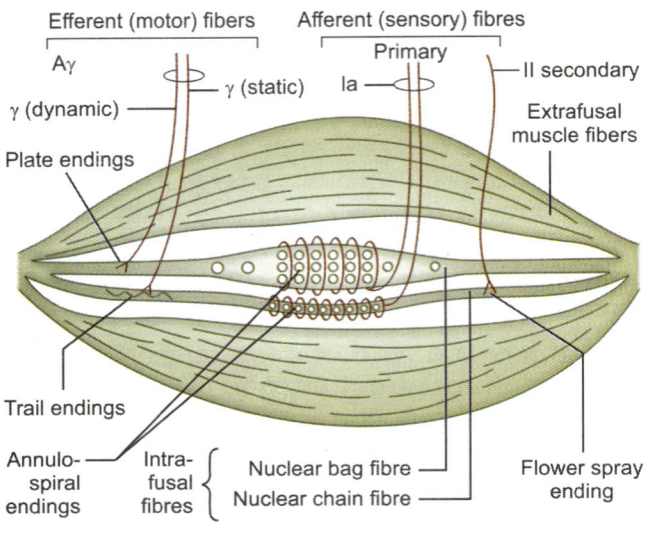

Fig. 10.24

Reflex Arc (Fig. 10.25)

- Knee jerk is a monosynaptic spinal reflex.
- The spinal segment involved is L3, L4
- Stimulation of muscle spindle → afferent through sensory nerve → reaches the dorsal horn of the

spinal segment → stimulation of the anterior group of neuron → efferent axon causing contraction of quadriceps.

7. A 40-year-old female dancer presented with inability to complete a pre-fixed motor task. She has been unable to dance due to sudden jerky movements of limbs which are not under her control. On examination, she had reduced tone in both lower limbs, pendular knee jerk and ataxia. Which region of the brain is involved? Describe any 4 functions of the same in motor control.

Region of the Brain is Involved

Based on the symptoms explained, this person has damage to the cerebellum.

Functions of Cerebellum

1. **Comparator function**
   - Cerebellum is responsible for integration and coordination of various movements of fingers, hands and feet.

Reflex reaction

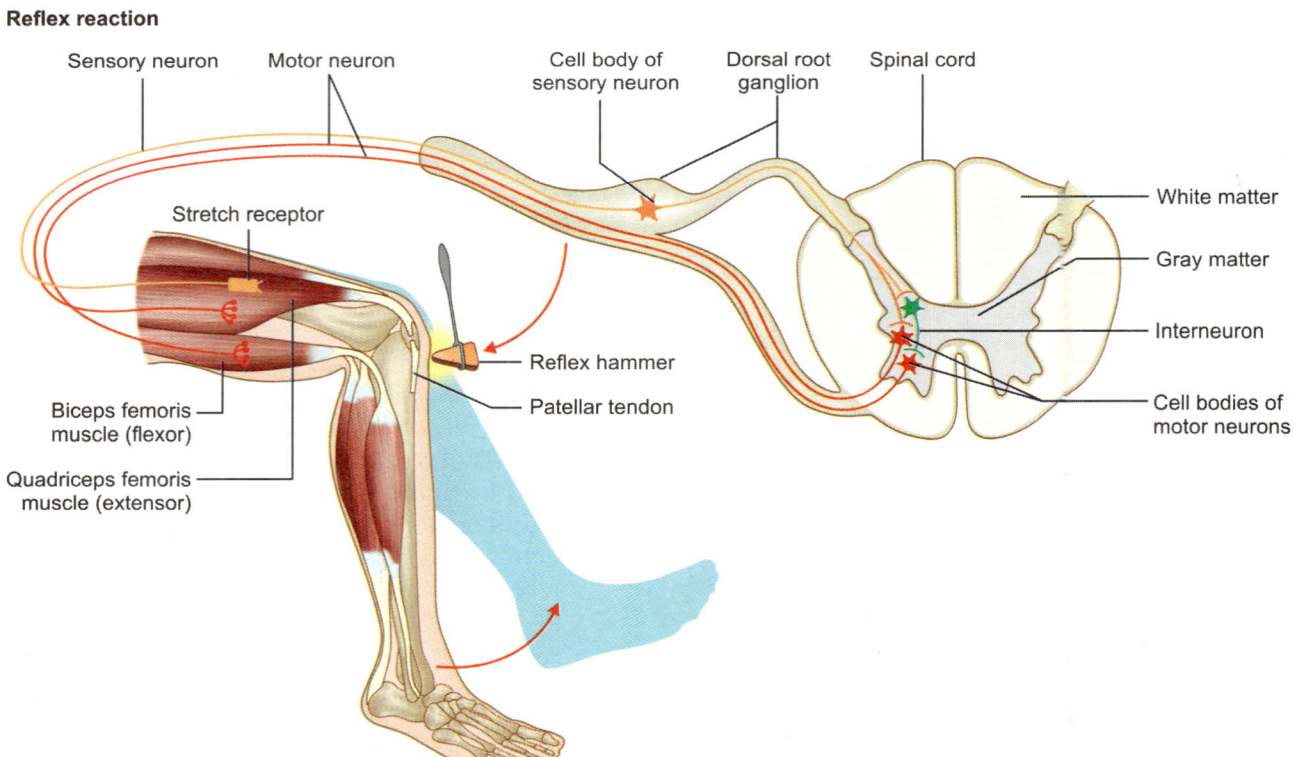

Fig. 10.25

- During a planned movement of a joint, the concerned motor cortex sends impulses to the respective muscle through corticospinal tract.
- En route, these fibres relay in the paravermal cerebellum. This part of cerebellum also gets a feedback from the distal parts of the body through proprioceptive receptors from the joints, muscles and tendons.
- The paravermal cerebellum compares the intended movement and the actual movement and sends corrective impulses to the cortex through thalamus and the red nucleus.
- This task gets completed with 20 ms.

2. **Damping action**
   - Even after comparator function is done by the cerebellum, the actions tend to be pendular and may overshoot.
   - The corticocerebellum then sends impulses to the motor cortex, so that if any exaggeration of muscular activity is reduced.
   - The movements are made smooth.

3. **Timing and programming of movements**
   - This is done by the lateral part of the cerebellum.
   - The cerebellum communicates with the premotor and sensory portions of the cerebellum and there is a two-way communication created. A plan is created and is stored in the cerebellum as memory this is the basis for skill development.
   - The timing is also decided by the cerebellum, as a result, one function follows the other without overlap.
   - Cerebellum also plays an important role in predicting the next outcome through visual and auditory feedback.

4. **Control of ballistic movements**
   - These are rapid alternative movements of the body.
   - These are also controlled by the cerebellum. This is done by the cerebellum by coordination of actions of the agonist muscles and antagonist muscles.

8. Describe the following reflexes:
   A. Inverse stretch reflex
   B. Withdrawal reflex
   C. Crossed extensor reflex

A. Inverse Stretch Reflex (Fig. 10.26)

- Golgi tendon organ is the receptor involved in this inverse stretch reflex.

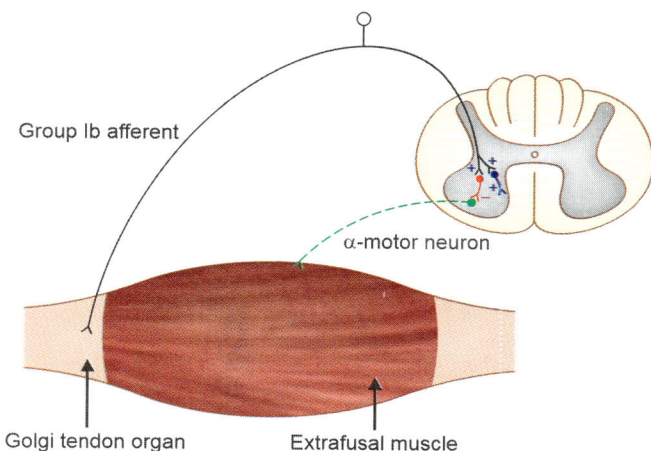

Group Ib afferent

α-motor neuron

Golgi tendon organ   Extrafusal muscle

Fig. 10.26

- It is in the tendon of the muscle and is sensitive to extreme increase in tension of the muscle.
- The Golgi tendon organ is supplied by the Ib sensory fibres.
- When a muscle contracts, there is increase in tension in the muscle and is picked up by the Golgi tendon organ.
- It sends impulses via the Ib sensory fibres to the dorsal root ganglion to the spinal cord.
- In the spinal cord, these Ib fibres stimulate the inhibitory interneurons.
- The interneurons release an inhibitory neuro-transmitter—glycine. Glycine inhibits the alpha motor neurons and causes relaxation of the contracted muscle.

B. Withdrawal Reflex (Fig. 10.27)

- It is a polysynaptic, superficial, flexor reflex.
- It occurs in response to nociceptive stimuli and is characterised by withdrawal of the body part from the area of painful stimulus.

Pathway for Withdrawal Reflex

- Receptors for pain are free nerve endings and these sensations are carried by A delta and C fibres.
- Fibers carrying pain sensations relay in various interneurons of the spinal cord.
- Some neurons relay on themselves forming reverberating circuits, some relay on the alpha motor neurons and some relay on inhibitory neurons.

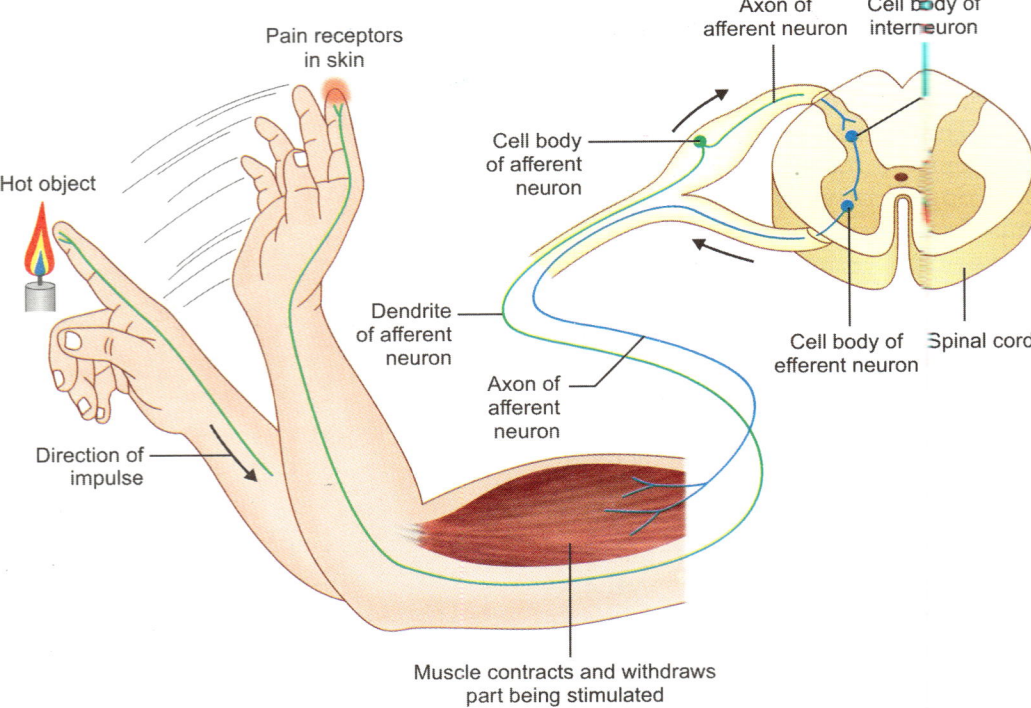

Fig. 10.27

- The effector organs—skeletal muscles are stimulated causing the withdrawing actin of the involved region.
- There is stimulation of flexors and inhibition of extensors.

C. Crossed Extensor Reflex (Fig. 10.28)

- When a strong stimulus is given to a particular limb, there is flexion of the affected limb along with extension of the other limb.

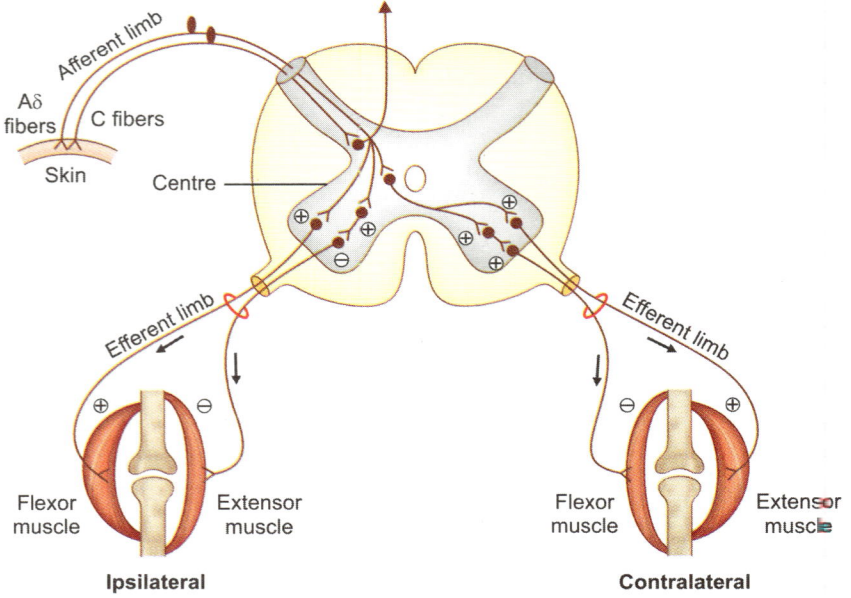

Fig. 10.28

- This is called crossed extensor reflex.
- It is produced by interneuron that crosses the midline and brings about extension of the other limb.
- The purpose of this reflex is, to support the body with the extending limb when the flexing limb is withdrawn from the stimulus.

SHORT ANSWERS

1. Compare and contrast decerebrate and decorticate rigidity.

	Decerebrate rigidity	Decorticate rigidity
Increase in tone	Extensors	Flexors
Cause	In man, occurs due to midbrain lesion	In man, it occurs in intracranial hemorrhage, brain abscess and brain tumor
Posture	Opisthotonus (hyperextension of back, extension of all limbs and tail)	Rigid extension of lower limbs, flexion of upper limbs, wrists and fingers flexed
Preparation	It is prepared by removing all connections from cerebral hemispheres	Removal of cerebral cortex, leaving basal ganglia intact

2. Describe the Golgi tendon organ and its functions.

- These are high threshold stretch receptors present in the muscle tendons.
- They are placed in series with the muscle fibres and tendons.
- Usually 10–15 fibers are associated with one Golgi tendon organ.
- It is basically a specialized receptor and thus has a group of neurons surrounded by a capsule of connective tissue.

Pathway of Reflex

- Afferent: Ib nerves
- When there is muscular contraction, the tension in the tendon increases.
- The afferents from here relay in the spinal cord. There is activation of inhibitory neurons.
- There is inhibition of alpha motor neurons and the muscle relaxation.

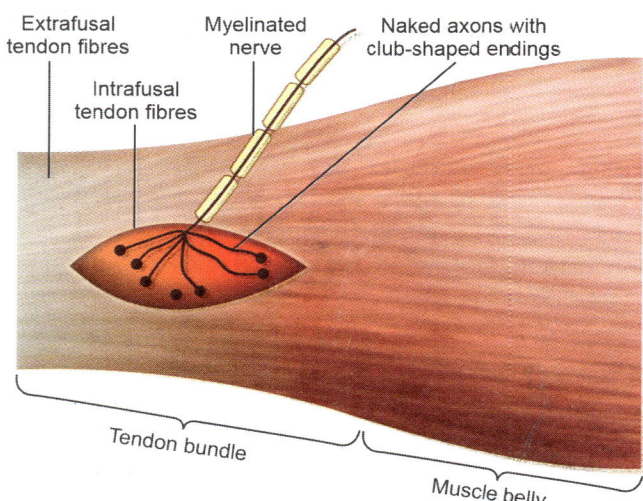

Fig. 10.29

Functions

1. It acts as a regulator of tension in the muscle. The increase in force of contraction is inhibitory to its muscle.
2. It is a protective reflex. This causes the muscle to lengthen in times of intense contraction.

3. What are the organs that help in maintaining balance in the body? Add a note on motion sickness.

Organs Concerned with Maintaining Balance

1. Inner ear or the labyrinth.
2. The utricle and saccule are concerned with linear motion
3. Semicircular canals are concerned with angular motion detection.

Motion Sickness

- It occurs due to excessive and repeated stimulation of vestibular apparatus.
- It is experienced during travel in automobile, ship, aircraft or spacecraft.
- There is also a psychological component that may increase the sickness.
- Some individuals may be stimulated by riding in fantasy rides in amusement parks.

Features

- It usually begins with sensation of unpleasantness with nausea, vomiting

- Some individuals may even develop sweating and pallor.

Treatment

- It is best avoided by premedication with anticholinergics and drugs like cinnarizine which decrease the sensitivity of the inner ear.
- Individuals should try not to move their head much during a travel.

4. What is Babinski's sign?

Babinski Sign

- A gentle stroke over the outer edge of the sole of the foot causes plantar flexion and adduction of all toes.
- Babinski sign is an abnormal plantar reflex where the response is dorsiflexion of the great toe and abduction or fanning of toes. It is accompanied by flexion of the knee and dorsiflexion of the ankle.
- It is also called extensor plantar.

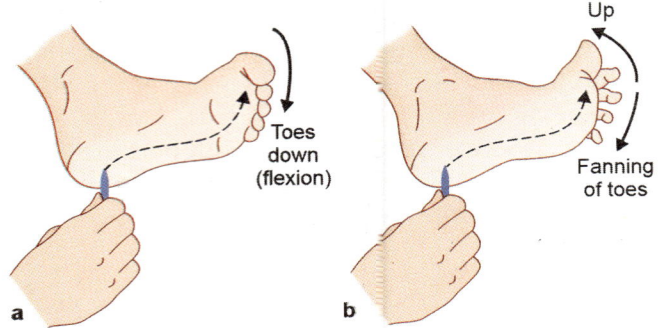

Fig. 10.30: (a) Normal planlar response, (b) Extensor plantar response (Babinski sign)

Significance

- It is an important clinical test in a neurological examination.
- Babinski sign is seen classically in upper motor neuron lesions.
- Physiologically, it is seen in infants and in deep sleep.

10.5 DESCRIBE AND DISCUSS STRUCTURE AND FUNCTIONS OF RETICULAR ACTIVATING SYSTEM, AUTONOMIC NERVOUS SYSTEM (ANS)

SHORT ESSAY

1. Explain the connections and functions of reticular activating system.

- It is an ill-defined mass of neurons and network situated in the brainstem.
- It is divided into a midbrain, pontine and medullary reticular system.

Connections of Reticular Activating System

Afferent Connections (Fig. 10.31)

- Reticular formation receives impulses from sensory pathways like optic, auditory, olfactory and taste pathways.
- Through the spinal cord, it gets connections for sensations of touch, temperature, kinesthetic sensation.
- Cerebral cortex, cerebellum, thalamus and corpus striatum.

Efferent Connections (Fig. 10.32)

- Reticular formation sends information to cerebral cortex, cerebellum
- Thalamus, hypothalamus, subthalamus
- Midbrain and basal ganglia
- Spinal cord.

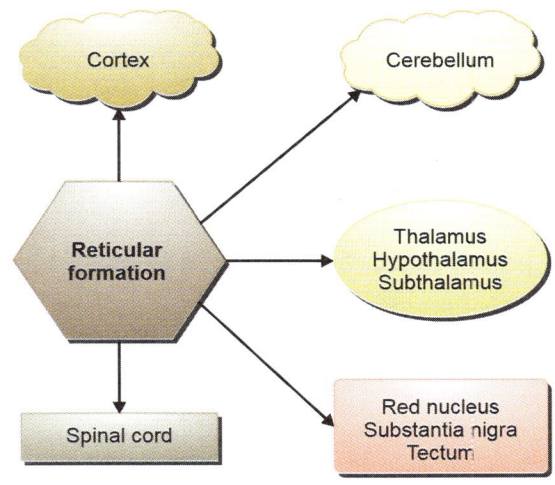

Fig. 10.32

- Based on these connections, RF forms several pathways
- Corticoreticulospinal pathways
- Corticoreticulocerebellar and corticoreticulo-basal ganglia pathway
- Visceral control pathway
- Reticular activating system

Functions of Reticular Activating System

1. **Sleep and wakefulness**
   - RAS sends strong excitatory drive to the central neurons and increases their excitability and responsiveness.
   - Stimulation of RAS causes alertness and arousal
2. **Attention and inattention**
   - RAS is necessary for selective attention and sensory inattention.
   - It takes part in processes like habituation and thus brings about inattention.
3. **RF plays an important role in learning and conditioning**
4. **RF plays an important role in autonomic function by exerting the effect of higher centres on autonomic ganglia**
5. **Control of muscle tone and postural reflexes**
   - RF is responsible for maintaining tone of antigravity muscles.

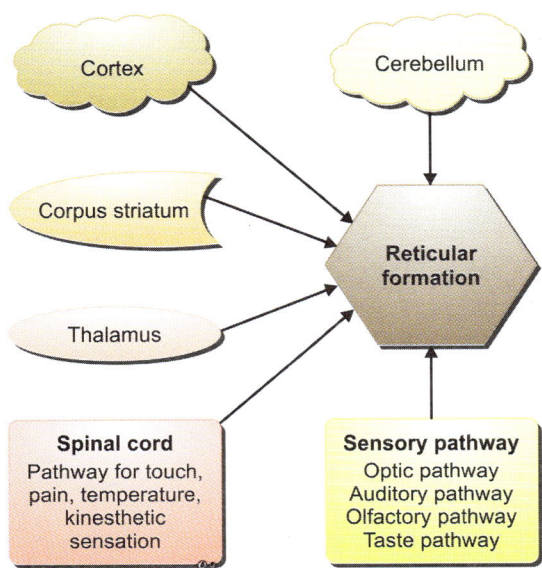

Fig. 10.31

- Pontine RF has excitatory function, whereas the medullary RF has inhibitory action on extensor muscle tone.

6. **Modulation of pain**
   - They form an endogenous pain relief system
   - Through the visceral regulating system

7. **RF is also involved in control of neuroendocrine system of the hypothalamus.**

SHORT ANSWERS

1. Explain 3 autonomic function tests.

1. **Valsalva maneuver test**
   - It is a measure of cardiovascular function
   - It is performed by making an individual blow through a pipe connected to a sphygmomanometer by keeping both his nostrils closed for 15 seconds.
   - The ECG during the process is recorded.
   - During strain, there is tachycardia and when released, there is bradycardia.
   - The RR interval is calculated during strain and during rest.
   - The ratio is normally >1.2.
   - If autonomic function is deranged, it is less than 1.2.

2. **Sudomotor function**
   - It is a test for sweating caused by heat exposure.
   - The individual is exposed to heat from an electrical heater and an area of skin is painted with iodine starch.

- When there is sweating, there is change in color of the dye.
- Sweating indicates an intact autonomous system.

3. **Pupillary testing**
- In Horner's syndrome the affected pupil has dilatation lag.
- When 4% cocaine is instilled in the affected eye, there is no dilatation, whereas the normal pupil dilates.
- Also, when 1% adrenaline or phenylephrine is added to the affected eye, the pupil dilates more than the normal eye due to denervation hypersensitivity.

2. List any 6 functions of sympathetic nervous system.

Functions of Sympathetic System

Heart	Positive inotropism, positive chronotropism
Blood vessels	Vasoconstriction, except those in heart and skeletal muscles
Eye	Pupillary dilatation and ciliary relaxation
Gastrointestinal tract	Inhibits motility, decreases secretion, constricts sphincters, relaxes smooth muscles
Urinary bladder	Relaxes detrusor, constricts sphincter
Bronchioles	Bring about dilatation

10.6 DESCRIBE AND DISCUSS SPINAL CORD, ITS FUNCTIONS, LESION AND SENSORY DISTURBANCES

LONG ESSAY

1. Explain the effects of complete transection of the spinal cord and the features of spinal shock.
(6 + 4 marks)

Complete Transection of the Spinal Cord

- Complete transection of spinal cord can occur in gun shot injuries, occlusion of blood vessels or dislocation of vertebrae.
- The effects are divided into three phases:

1. **Stage of spinal shock**
   - Cessation of all functions and activity below the level of transection.
   - Also called stage of flaccidity as there is loss of tonic discharge form the upper brainstem.
2. **Stage of reflex activity**
   - There is gradual gain of functions.
   - After about three weeks, there is patchy improvement of muscle functions.
3. **Stage of reflex failure**
   - There is deterioration of general health due to malnutrition, infections, toxaemia
   - Muscles undergo wasting.

Features of Spinal Shock

- Features depend on the level of injury.
- Any injury above C5 is fatal as connections are cutoff between the respiratory centres and muscles.
- In humans, the duration of spinal shock is long due to encephalization (greater dependence of spinal cord on higher centers)

1. **Paralysis of motor functions**
   - Below the level of lesion, there is loss of function of muscles
   - All motor functions of both flexor and extensor group of muscles are lost in both limbs.
   - There is flaccidity as the nerve from the anterior motor neuron cannot travel to the respective muscle.
   - All superficial and deep tendon reflexes are lost.
2. **Loss of sensory functions:** All the sensations below the designated level are lost due to injury to the posterior nerve roots and sensory neurons in the spinal cord.
3. **Effect on bladder**
   - The bladder becomes atonic of flaccid.
   - As a result, the detrusor cannot detect filling of urine in the bladder. The urine goes on collecting till the maximum capacity is achieved.
   - Then there is overflow incontinence.
4. **Effect on bowel:** The bowel movements become sluggish and thus leads to constipation.
5. **Effect on the heart**
   - The venous return in resting condition significantly decreases as the tone in the muscles in lost.
   - As a result, preload decreases and thus cardiac output decreases.
   - The pulse is weak and blood pressure is low.
   - As the lesion is at the thoracic level, there is damage to some sympathetic fibres leading to failure of regulatory mechanisms of blood pressure.
6. **Effect on skin**
   - There is decreased blood supply and sensations leading to an increased risk of developing bed-sores.
   - The skin is dry and scaly.
7. **Others:** Penis is flaccid and erection becomes impossible.

SHORT ANSWER

1. Explain Syringomyelia

- Syrinx = cavity, myelia = spinal cord
- It is a rare disorder of the spinal cord characterized by excessive growth of neuroglial tissue and cavity formation within the spinal cord.
- The grey matter surrounding the canal is affected first.

Causes

- A cavity forms near the spinal canal and expands horizontally to involve the white matter
- It also extends vertically involving more segments.
- Lower cervical and upper thoracic regions are affected first.

Clinical Features

Depends on the site of the cyst or cavity and the level of spinal cord at which it is present.

Around the spinal canal	• Loss of temperature, pain and crude touch sensations
Posterior grey horn	• All sensations are lost
	• As a result, the individuals are more prone to injuries
Anterior gray horn	• Flaccid paralysis of muscles
	• Later stages, pyramidal and extrapyramidal structures are involved.
	• As a result, spastic paralysis occurs.
	• Winging of scapula and scoliosis are seen in higher lesions

10.7 DESCRIBE AND DISCUSS FUNCTIONS OF CEREBRAL CORTEX, BASAL GANGLIA, THALAMUS, HYPOTHALAMUS, CEREBELLUM AND LIMBIC SYSTEM AND THEIR ABNORMALITIES

LONG ESSAYS

1. A 52-year-old male came with complaints of gait disturbances, and tremors in the hands. On examination, the patient had short shuffling gait, mask-like face and pill rolling movements in the hands along with. He was thus diagnosed to have Parkinson's disease. What is the pathophysiology in Parkinson's disease? Explain basis of probable treatment options for the same.

- It is also called paralysis agitans
- It is a degenerative condition of the basal ganglia.

Pathophysiology of Parkinson's Disease

- When the aetiology is ageing or idiopathic, it is called Parkinson's disease. If associated with other intracranial causes or secondary to drugs, it is known as Parkinson's syndrome or Parkinsonism nigra.
- Its pathophysiology revolves around the basal ganglia. The basal ganglia are connected to the cerebral cortex and are required for fine work. Almost all the fibres of the corticospinal tract pass through the basal ganglia.

Normal Putamen Circuit

- The principal pathways for basal ganglia begin the premotor and supplementary areas of cortex.
- From the cortex, there pass to the putamen → internal portion of the globus pallidus → substantia nigra → ventroanterior and ventrolateral nuclei of thalamus → back to cortex.
- Dopamine is an inhibitory neurotransmitter.
- Voluntary movements are initiated by the cortex and controlled through the basal ganglia.

What Happens in Parkinson's Disease (Fig. 10.33)

- A variety of causes lead to degeneration of the basal ganglia. Oxidative stress due to ageing, genetic factors lead to formation of abnormal proteins (Lewy bodies, alpha synuclein) which cause damage to the cells of the substantia nigra and thus there is decrease in production of dopamine from these cells.
- There is loss of inhibition due to deficient dopamine.

- Thus, there is increase in inhibitory output to the external globus pallidus → decreased inhibitory output from the subthalamic nucleus → increased excitatory output to the internal segment of globus pallidus → increased inhibitory output to thalamus → reduction in excitatory drive to the cerebral cortex.

Basis of Treatment in Parkinsonism

Dopamine agonists	Increase in the level of dopamine in the brain and are the first line of drugs used. They are very effective in controlling the symptoms.
MAO inhibitors	Dopamine is destroyed by monoamine oxidase. Enzyme inhibitors thus help to increase the quantity of dopamine available to the neurotransmitters
Fetal dopamine cells	These cells are transplanted into the caudate nuclei and they produce dopamine
Anticholinergics	Block the hyperexcitability caused by cholinergic neurotransmitters

2. Explain the nuclei, connections and functions of thalamus. Add a note on thalamic syndrome.

Nuclei of Thalamus (Fig. 10.34)
Anatomical Classification

Midline nuclei
- These are a group of small nuclei present in the midline near the medial surface

Intralaminar nuclei
- They are present in the medullary septum of thalamus

Media mass of nuclei
- They are situated medial to the septum.
- It consists of anterior and dorsomedial nucleus.

Lateral mass of nuclei
- They are situated lateral to the septum

Dorsal group	*Ventral group*
• Dorsolateral	• Ventral anterior nucleus
• Posterolateral	• Ventral lateral nucleus
• Ventral posterior nucleus.	

Posterior group of nuclei
- Continuation of lateral group
  1. Pulvinar
  2. Metathalamus which consists of two structures:
     a. Medial geniculate body, b. Lateral geniculate body.

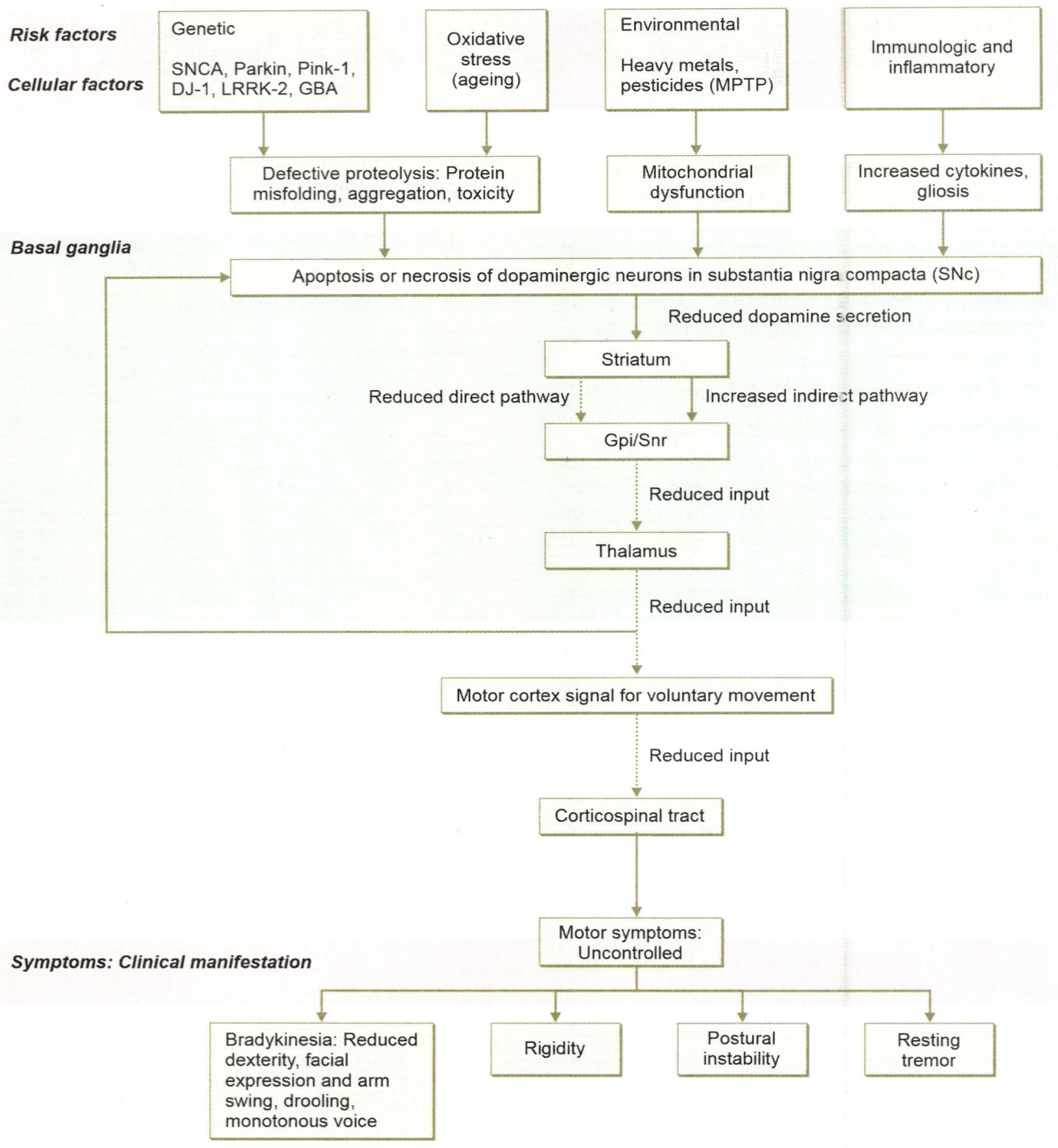

Fig. 10.33

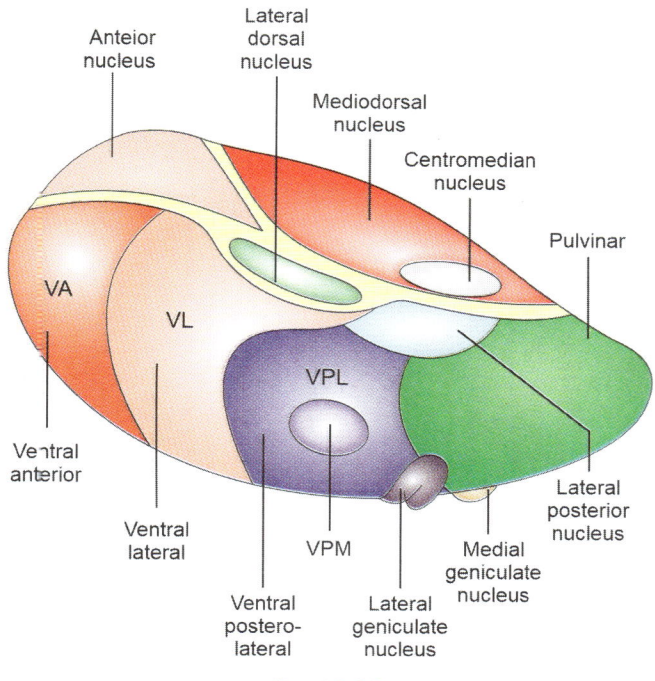

Fig. 10.34

Functional Classification

Non-specific projection nuclei	Specific projection nuclei

They receive impulses from the RAS for secondary responses
• Midline nuclei
• Centromedian nuclei
	They receive from specific sensations and project into specific portions of the cortex.
	1. Specific sensory relay nuclei
	  • Medial geniculate body
	  • Lateral geniculate body
	  • Posteroventral group of nuclei
	2. Motor control nuclei
	  • Ventrolateral group of nuclei
	  • Ventral anterior nucleus
	3. Visceral efferent control nuclei
	  • Anterior group of nuclei
	  • Dorsomedial nucleus
	4. Integrative and perceptual function control nuclei
	  • Pulvinar nucleus
	  • Lateral posterior nucleus
	  • Dorsal lateral nucleus.

Connections (Fig. 10.35)

1. Connections of nonspecific projection nuclei

Afferent	Efferent
RAS Basal ganglia Other thalamic nuclei	Stratum Neocortex

2. Connections of specific projection nuclei

Nuclei	Afferent	Efferent
Specific sensory relay nuclei		
Medial geniculate body	Auditory fibers from cochlear nerve	Auditory area (area 41, 42)
Lateral geniculate body	Projection from optic tracts	Striate cortex of occipital lobe (17,18,19)
Ventral posterior nucleus	From ascending tracts through spinal, medial and trigeminal lemnisci	Sensory cortex (3, 1,2,4)
Motor control nuclei		
Ventrolateral group of nuclei	Dentate nucleus of opposite side	Primary motor cortex
Ventral anterior nucleus	Globus pallidus, cerebellum, substantia nigra	Premotor cortex
Visceral efferent control nuclei		
Anterior group of nuclei	Hippocampus via the mammillothalamic tract	Cingulate gyrus (area 24)
Dorsomedial nucleus	Has reciprocal connections with prefrontal cortex and hypothalamus	
Integrative and perceptual function control nuclei		
Pulvinar nucleus	Superior and inferior colliculi	Parietal, occipital and superior temporal cortex
Lateral posterior nucleus	Superior colliculus	Superior parietal lobe
Dorsal lateral nucleus	Superior colliculi	Hippocampus

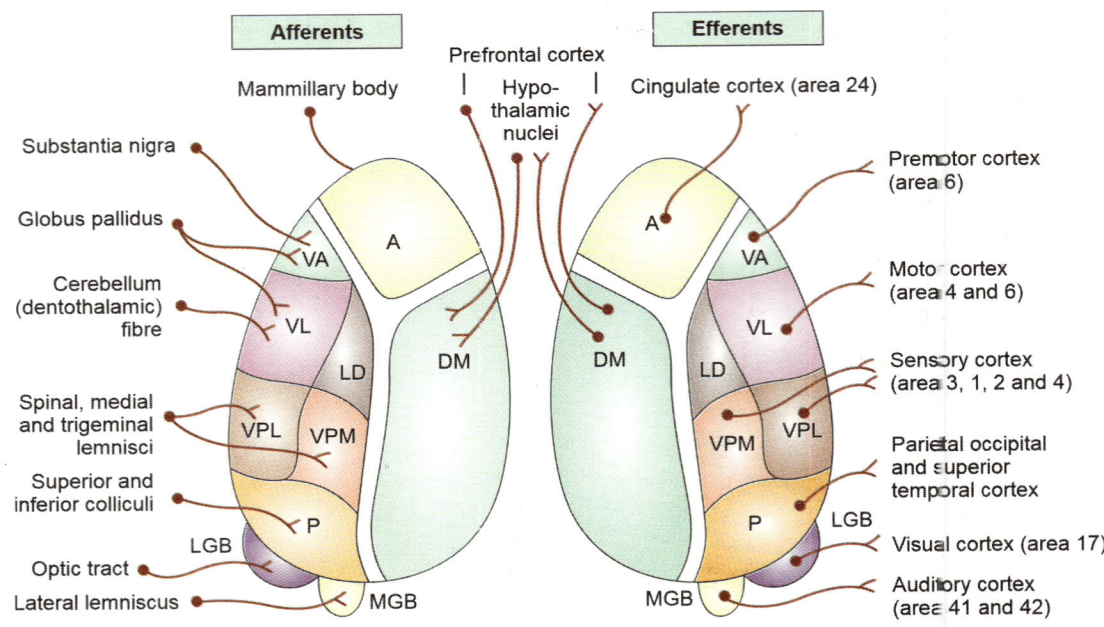

Fig. 10.35

Functions of Thalamus

1. **Thalamus forms a sensory relay centre**
   - Almost all sensory impulses relay in thalamus before being projected into the somatosensory cortex in the form of thalamic radiation.
   - An exception for this is olfactory sensation.

2. **Integration of sensory impulses**
   - There is not only relay of signals, but also modification and integration of peripheral sensation.
   - So, thalamus is called 'functional gateway' of cerebral cortex.

3. **Crude centre for perception of sensations**
   - Whether a sensation is painful or not is decided by the thalamus. It is called the affective nature.
   - However, differentiating the type of sensation is a task of the cortex.

4. **Integration of motor functions**
   - Thalamus receives signals from the basal ganglia and cerebellum before integration into the motor cortex.
   - Thus, it helps in integration of motor functions by unconscious regulation of muscle tone.

5. **Role in arousal and alertness reaction:** Due to the associations of the thalamus with reticular formation, it plays an important role in alertness and arousal.

6. **Role in emotional aspect of behaviour**
   - It is closely related to the frontal cortex and hypothalamus.
   - It plays an important role in subjective feeling of various emotions.
   - It is also associated with perception of sexual function.
   - It forms a part of the Papez circuit and so, it is associated with recent memories and emotions.

7. **Integration of somatic and visceral function:** It forms a relay centre for many autonomic impulses and somatic sensations, it helps in building an integration between the two.

Thalamic Syndrome

It is an emotional disturbance to sensory experience.

Cause

Ischemic damage to the posteroventral and posterolateral nuclei due to thrombosis of thalamogeniculate branch of posterior cerebral artery.

Clinical Features

Sensory	Motor
Astereognosis	Due to involvement of posterolateral nucleus
• Loss of tactile localization	Ataxia
Thalamic phantom limb	• Decreased muscle tone
• Inability to locate own limb with eyes closed due to loss of proprioception	• Muscular weakness
Thalamic over-reaction	Involuntary movements
• Decreased threshold for pain, temperature and touch	• Athetosis
• Exaggerated sensations	• Intentional tremors
	Thalamic hand
	• Abnormal posture of hand—moderate flexion of wrist and hyperextended fingers

3. Explain the nuclei, connections and functions of hypothalamus.

Nuclei of Hypothalamus (Fig. 10.36)

Anterior or preoptic nuclei	Middle or tuberal group	Posterior or mammillary group
1. Preoptic nucleus	1. Dorsomedial nucleus	1. Posterior nucleus
2. Paraventricular nucleus	2. Ventromedial nucleus	2. Mammillary body
3. Anterior nucleus	3. Lateral nucleus	
4. Supraoptic nucleus	4. Arcuate nucleus	
5. Suprachiasmatic nucleus		

Connections of Hypothalamus (Fig. 10.37)

Afferent connections	Efferent connections
• From rhinencephalon (limbic cortex) to preoptic nucleus, lateral nucleus and mammillary body	• From mammillary body to anterior thalamic nuclei
• From hippocampus to mammillary body	• From mammillary body to tegmental nuclei
• Stria terminalis: From amygdala to preoptic nucleus	• Posterior, supraoptic and tuberal nuclei to reach reticular formation, dorsomedial nucleus of thalamus and frontal lobe.
• From prefrontal area (8) and precentral area (6) of cerebral cortex to the supraoptic and paraventricular nuclei of hypothalamus	• From supraoptic and paraventricular nuclei to posterior pituitary.
• From globus pallidus to diffused areas of hypothalamus	
• From dorsomedial and midline nuclei of thalamus to diffused areas of hypothalamus	
• From reticular formation of brainstem to diffused areas	
• Fibers from retina to supraoptic, suprachiasmatic and ventromedial nuclei of hypothalamus	

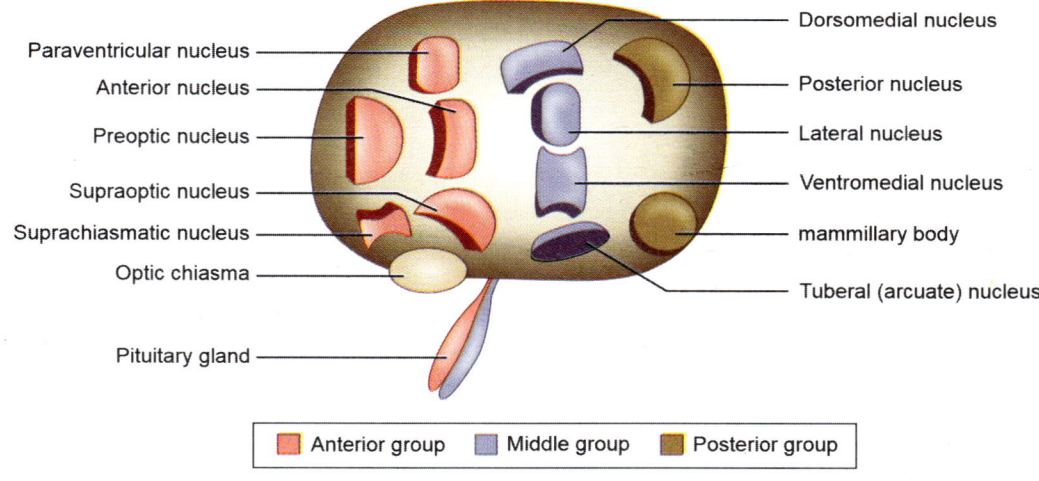

Paraventricular nucleus —
Anterior nucleus —
Preoptic nucleus —
Supraoptic nucleus —
Suprachiasmatic nucleus —
Optic chiasma —
Pituitary gland —

— Dorsomedial nucleus
— Posterior nucleus
— Lateral nucleus
— Ventromedial nucleus
— mammillary body
— Tuberal (arcuate) nucleus

| Anterior group | Middle group | Posterior group |

Fig. 10.36

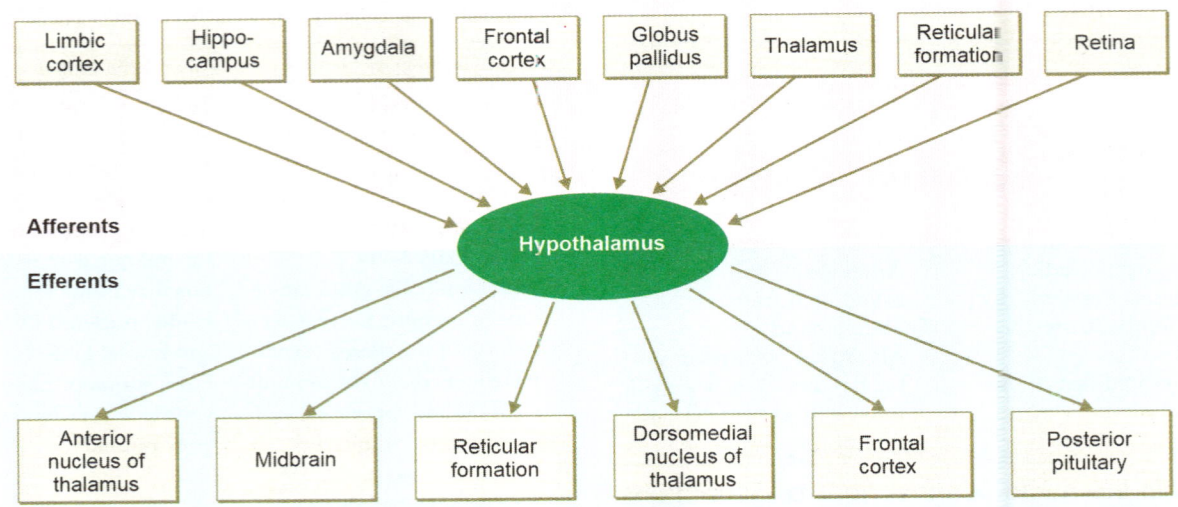

Fig. 10.37

Functions of Hypothalamus

1. Secretion of posterior pituitary hormones
- Supraoptic and paraventricular nuclei secrete the ADH and oxytocin.
- They are transported to the posterior pituitary

2. Control of anterior pituitary hormones
- Through regulating hormones, the hypothalamus controls the release of anterior pituitary hormones

Growth hormone	Growth hormone-releasing hormone (GHRH)
	Growth hormone-inhibiting hormone (GHIH)
	Growth hormone-releasing peptide (GHRP)
Thyroid stimulating hormone	Thyrotropin-releasing hormone (TRH)
Adrenocorticotropin stimulating hormone	Corticotropin-releasing hormone (CRH)
Prolactin	Prolactin inhibiting hormone (PIH)
FSH and LH	Gonadotropin-releasing hormone (GnRH)

3. Control of adrenal cortex and medulla
- Through the effect of CRH, ACTH influences the adrenal cortex to secrete glucocorticoids and mineralocorticoids.
- Also, it controls release of catecholamines through impulses sent through sympathetic nerves.

4. Regulation of autonomic nervous system
- The posterior and lateral nuclei of the hypothalamus are associated with sympathetic control.
- Anterior group of nuclei control the parasympathetic system.

5. Regulation of heart rate and blood pressure
- Through the vasomotor centre, stimulation of the heart rate and blood pressure.
- Stimulation of preoptic area causes a fall in blood pressure.

6. Regulation of body temperature:
It controls the body temperature through heat loss centre (preoptic nuclei) and heat gain centre (posterior hypothalamus)

7. Regulation of hunger
- Food intake is regulated by feeding center and satiety center.
- Feeding centre is formed by the lateral hypothalamus. Stimulation of this area causes excessive food intake and hunger.
- Satiety centre is formed by the ventromedial nucleus. It controls of food intake.
- They are influenced by a number of mechanisms.

8. Regulation of water intake
- The lateral nucleus of the hypothalamus has osmoreceptors. When there is increase in osmolarity of the blood (decrease in ECF volume), thirst center is activated and there is increase in water intake.

- Also, there is stimulation of release of AD which causes water retention in the collecting duct and thus increases ECF volume.

9. **Regulation of sleep and wakefulness**
- Along with melatonin, mammillary body in the posterior hypothalamus forms physiological clock.
- Stimulation of mammillary body causes wakefulness.

10. **Role in behavior**
- Hypothalamus has a role in affective sensations of sensory stimuli—they are designated as pleasant or painful
- Reward center is situated in medial forebrain bundle and ventromedial nucleus of hypothalamus. Electrical stimulation of these areas in animals pleases or satisfies the animals.
- Punishment center is situated in posterior and lateral nuclei of hypothalamus. Electrical stimulation of these nuclei in animals leads to pain, fear, defense.

4. Name the nuclei of the basal ganglia. Describe the connections and functions of basal ganglia. Add a note on Parkinson's disease.
(1 + 2 + 5 + 2 marks)

Nuclei of Basal Ganglia (Fig. 10.38)

Corpus striatum	Substantia nigra	Subthalamic nucleus
Caudate nucleus		
Lenticular nucleus		
• Outer putamen		
• Inner globus pallidus		

Connections of Basal Ganglia

Afferents
- The input into the basal ganglia is mainly through striatum. It receives afferents from the cerebral cortex, thalamus, and locus coeruleus.
- The corticostriate projections originate from all portions of the cerebral cortex like premotor, supplementary motor area and primary somatosensory area.
- Thalamostriate fibers originate from the centromedian nucleus of thalamus.
- Fibers from the pars compacta of the substantia nigra project into the striatum.

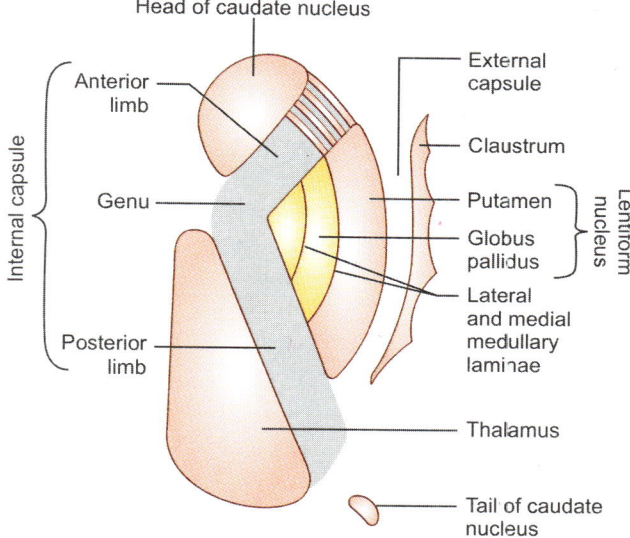

Fig. 10.38

- Projections form the raphe nuclei of reticular system project onto the striatum (serotonergic)
- Locus coeruleus striate fibers (noradrenergic) project onto the striatum.

Projections from Striatum
- The striatum projects into substantia nigra and globus pallidum.
- The projection onto the substantia nigra and globus pallidum is mainly GABAergic and thus inhibitory.

Efferent or Output from Globus Pallidum
Globus pallidum forms the main output site for basal ganglia (Fig. 10.39).

Functions of Basal Ganglia
1. **Control of voluntary muscular activity**
   i. Cognitive control of motor activity
      - When a thought develops in the cortical association area, it is executed by basal ganglia
      - Caudate loop is primarily involved in this activity
   ii. Timing and scaling of movements
      - Basal ganglia act as a centre for coordination of extra-pyramidal activities.
   iii. Subconscious execution of movement
      - Skilled and learnt activities are performed subconsciously
      - It is executed through putamen circuit

Efferent to Thalamus	Efferent to Subthalamic Nucleus	Efferent to Substantia Nigra
• Also called thalamic fasciculus or ansa fasciculus (ventroanterior, ventrolateral and centromedian nuclei) • From thalamus, they project onto prefrontal and premotor cortex.	• From subthalamic nuceli, these fibers project onto substantia nigra	• They project into substantia nigra • Directly, or via subthalamic nucleus or pedunculopotine nucleus/ • From substantia nigra • To reticular formation and spinal cord • Superior colliculus via tectospinal pathway • Habenula

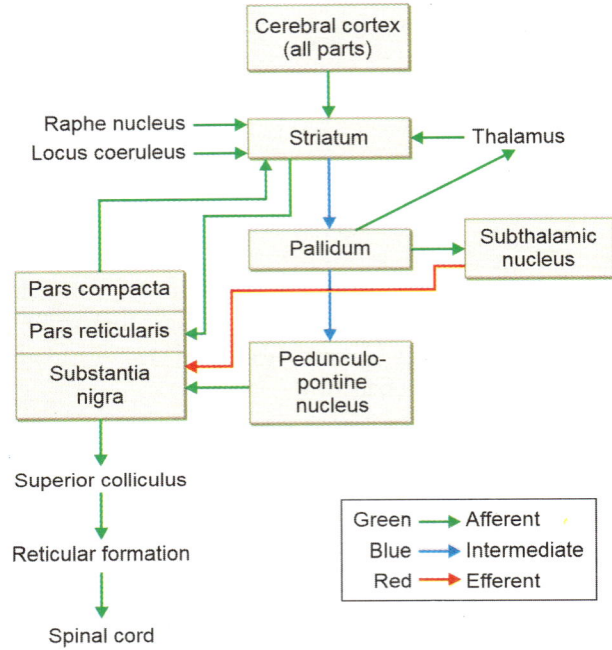

Fig. 10.39

2. **Control of reflex muscular activity:** They have inhibitory effect on spinal reflexes and thus help in maintaining posture.

3. **Control of muscle tone:** Substantia nigra controls the tone of muscle through its effects on muscle spindle and gamma motor neuron.

4. **Role in arousal mechanism:** Due to their connections with the RAS, the basal ganglia have effect on arousal and sleep cycle.

Parkinson's Disease

• It is also called paralysis agitans and is a degenerative condition of the basal ganglia.

• When the aetiology is ageing or idiopathic, it is called Parkinson's disease. If associated with other intracranial causes or secondary to drugs, it is known as Parkinson's syndrome or parkinsonism nigra.

• Its pathophysiology revolves around the basal ganglia.

• A variety of causes leads to degeneration of the basal ganglia. Oxidative stress due to ageing, genetic factors lead to formation of abnormal proteins (Lewy bodies, alpha synuclein) which cause damage to the cells of the substantia nigra and thus there is decrease in production of dopamine from these cells.

• There is loss of inhibition due to deficient dopamine.

• Thus, there is increase in inhibitory output to the external globus pallidus → decreased inhibitory output from the subthalamic nucleus → increased excitatory output to the internal segment of globus pallidus → increased inhibitory output to thalamus → reduction in excitatory drive to the cerebral cortex.

Clinical Features

• There is slowness in initiation of a movement—bradykinesia

• Reduced unconscious facial expression

• Reduced involuntary movements like arm swing

• There is drooling of saliva

• The muscles are hypertonic and there is rigidity. It is called lead-pipe rigidity.

• There is tremor of hands—called resting tremor—called pill rolling tumor

5. Classify the lobes of cerebellum. List the afferent and efferent pathways of cerebellum and their functions.

Lobes of Cerebellum

Anterior lobe	Posterior lobe	Flocculonodular node
Includes lingula, central lobe and culmen	Includes lobulus simplex, declive, tuber, pyramid, uvula and paraflocculi	Nodulus and lateral extension of nodule on either side called flocculus

Connections of Cerebellum

Cerebellum area	Afferent	Efferent
Vestibulocerebellum or archicerebellum	Vestibular nucleus → inferior cerebellar peduncle → through vestibulocerebellar tract	Cerebellovestibular tract (flocculonodular node → inferior cerebellar peduncle → vestibular nuclei → vestibulospinal tract → alpha motor nuclei)
		Fastigiobulbar tract (fastigial nucleus → inferior cerebellar peduncle → vestibular nucleus and reticular formation → vestibulospinal tract → gamma motor neurons)
Spinocerebellum	Dorsal spinocerebellar tract (from Clarke's nucleus)	Fastigiobulbar tract (from fastigial nucelus → reticular formation)
	Ventral spinocerebellar tract (marginal cells)	
	Cuneocerebellar tract (ACC cuneate nucleus)	Cerebelloreticular tract (emboliform and globosus → reticular formation)
	Olivocerebellar tract (inferior olivary nucleus)	
	Pontocerebellar tract (pons)	Cerebello-olivary tract (emboliform and globosus → olivary nucleus → alpha motor nucleus)
	Tectocerebellar tract (superior and inferior colliculi)	
	Trigeminocerebellar tract (mesencephalic nucleus)	
Corticocerebellum	Pontocerebellar (pontine nuclei → crosses midline → corticocerebellum)	Dentothalamic tract (lateral ventral nucleus of thalamus → cerebral cortex)
	Olivocerebellar (inferior olivary nucleus → inferior cerebellar peduncle → corticocerebellum)	Dentorubral tract (red nucleus → lateral ventral nucleus of thalamus → cerebral cortex, RAS and spinal cord)

Functions of Cerebellum

1. **Control of body posture and equilibrium**
   - Vestibulocerebellum is concerned with control of body posture and equilibrium
   - Vestibulocerebellar tracts carry information from vestibular nuclei which bring information from utricle and saccule and semicircular canals.
   - Spinocerebellar and cuneocerebellar tracts bring information about posture and proprioception.
   - The flocullonodular and fastigial nuclei project fibers through inferior peduncle to vestibular nuceli and reticular formation.
   - Also, the vermis sends information to spinal cord.

2. **Control of muscle tone and stretch reflexes**
   - Spinocerebellum is concerned with muscle tone and stretch reflexes.
   - It receives afferents from spinocerebellar, cuneocerebellar and olivocerebellar tracts that have information regarding proprioception and tactile inputs from various parts of the body.
   - The nuceli involved are fastigial, emboliformis and globossus.
   - They project onto the gamma motor neurons through cerebellospinal tracts.
   - They modify the muscle tone by reflex altering the signals to alpha motor neurons.

3. **Control of voluntary movements**
   - Cerebellum controls time, rate, range, force and direction of movements.
   - Corticocerebellum is responsible for control of voluntary movements.
   - Afferent is from cerebro-cerebello-cerebral connection.

4. Comparator function

- Cerebellum is responsible for integration and coordination of various movements of fingers, hands and feet.
- During a planned movement of a joint, the concerned motor cortex sends impulses to the respective muscle through corticospinal tract.
- En route, these fibres relay in the paravermal cerebellum. This part of cerebellum also gets a feedback from the distal parts of the body through proprioceptive receptors from the joints, muscles and tendons.
- The paravermal cerebellum compares the intended movement and the actual movement and sends corrective impulses to the cortex through thalamus and the red nucleus.
- This task gets completed with 20 ms.

5. Damping action

- Even after comparator function is done by the cerebellum, the actions tend to be pendular and may overshoot.
- The corticocerebellum then sends impulses to the motor cortex, so that if any exaggeration of muscular activity is reduced.
- The movements are made smooth.

6. Timing and programming of movements

- This is done by the lateral part of the cerebellum.
- The cerebellum communicates with the premotor and sensory portions of the cerebellum and there is a two-way communication created. A plan is created and is stored in the cerebellum as memory this is the basis for skill development.
- The timing is also decided by the cerebellum, as a result, one function follows the other without overlap.
- Cerebellum also plays an important role in predicting the next outcome through visual and auditory feedback.

7. Control of ballistic movements

- These are rapid alternative movements of the body
- These are also controlled by the cerebellum. This is done by the cerebellum by coordination of actions of the agonist muscles and antagonist muscles.

8. Servomechanism:
When any skilled work is performed, it is performed without any interruption.

SHORT ESSAYS

1. Explain the functions of different lobes cerebral cortex.

The cerebral hemisphere is divided into four lobes:

1. **Frontal lobe:** It is the part of the cerebrum in front of the central sulcus and above the posterior ramus of the lateral sulcus.

Functions

Primary motor area (area 4)
- Functions are initiation of voluntary movements of opposite side of body
- Initiation of speech

Premotor area (6, 8, 44, 45)
- Area 6 is involved in integration of voluntary activities
- Area 44 and 45 are called Broca's motor area—associated with formation of speech. Production of voice and articulation of speech is brought about by dominant hemisphere

Supplementary motor area
- Provides attitudinal movements, fixation movement of different segments of the body and positional movements of head and eyes.

Frontal eye field
- It controls eye movements
- Stimulation causes conjugate movement of eyes to the other side, opening and closure of eyelids, mydriasis and lacrimation

2. Parietal lobe

Functions

Primary sensory area
- Includes Brodmann's area 3,1,2
- Discrimination of sensations takes place in this lobe

Secondary sensory area
- There is a duplicate representation of sensations
- They respond to touch, auditory, visual and nociceptive stimuli.

Sensory association area
- Area 5 and 7
- They are responsible for sensing position of joints, discriminating stimuli

3. Temporal lobe

Functions

Primary auditory area
- Broadman's area 41 and 42
- Perception of sound, information regarding pitch, loudness and source of sound

Auditory association area
- Area 22, 20, 21
- Interpretation and integration of auditory impulses

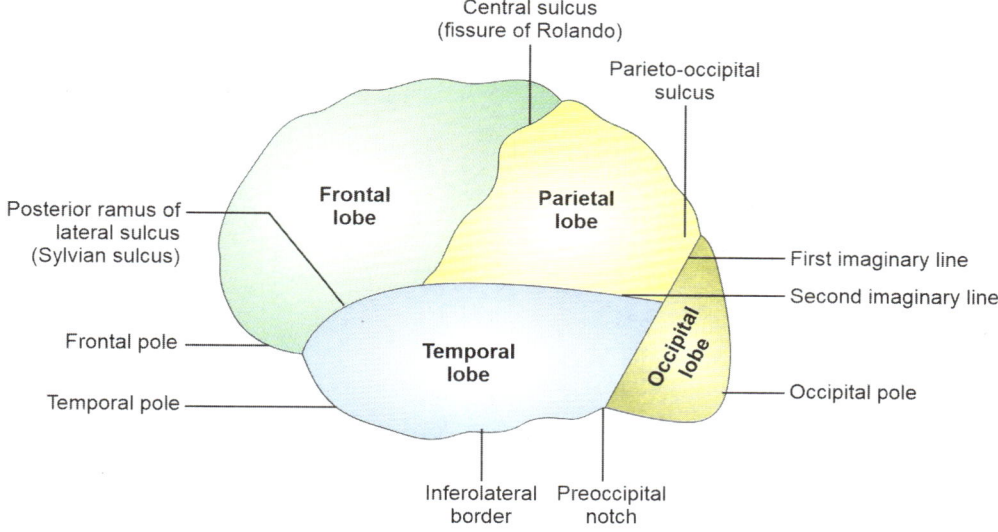

Fig. 10.40

4. Occipital lobe

Functions

Primary visual cortex
- Area 17
- Perception of visual impulses

Visual association area
- Area 18 and 19
- Interpretation of visual impulses
- Recognition and identification

Occipital eyefield area
- Area 19
- Movement of eyeballs

2. A region of the hypothalamus was lesioned in a rat. Over next few weeks the rat grew morbidly obese. Which part of the hypothalamus was lesioned? Explain the various theories behind feeding control.

Part of the Hypothalamus was Lesioned

- The satiety centre has been destroyed in this rat.
- It is formed by the ventromedial nucleus of the hypothalamus.
- Destruction of satiety centre leads to hyperphagia and weight gain.

Theories Regarding Food Intake

1. Glucostatic theory (Fig. 10.41)
- The cells of satiety centres have glucose receptors and thus referred to as glucostats.

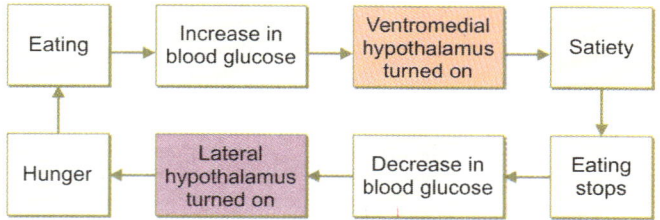

Fig. 10.41

- When there is enough glucose in the body, the satiety centre is activated.
- This increases inhibition of the feeding centre leading to decreased need to eat.
- The reverse happens when glucose levels are low.

2. Lipostatic theory
- The neurons in the feeding centre respond to the levels of fatty acids and amino acids in the blood.
- When there is increase in the volume of adipose tissues, they secrete a hormone called leptin. It enters the blood–brain barrier and inhibits the feeding centre.
- It acts by decreasing the release of neuropeptide YY in the small intestine and it acts by increasing the secretion of pro-ipiomelanocortin.

3. Peptide mechanism (Fig. 10.42)
- Ghrelin is an orexigenic hormone secreted by the cells of the stomach.

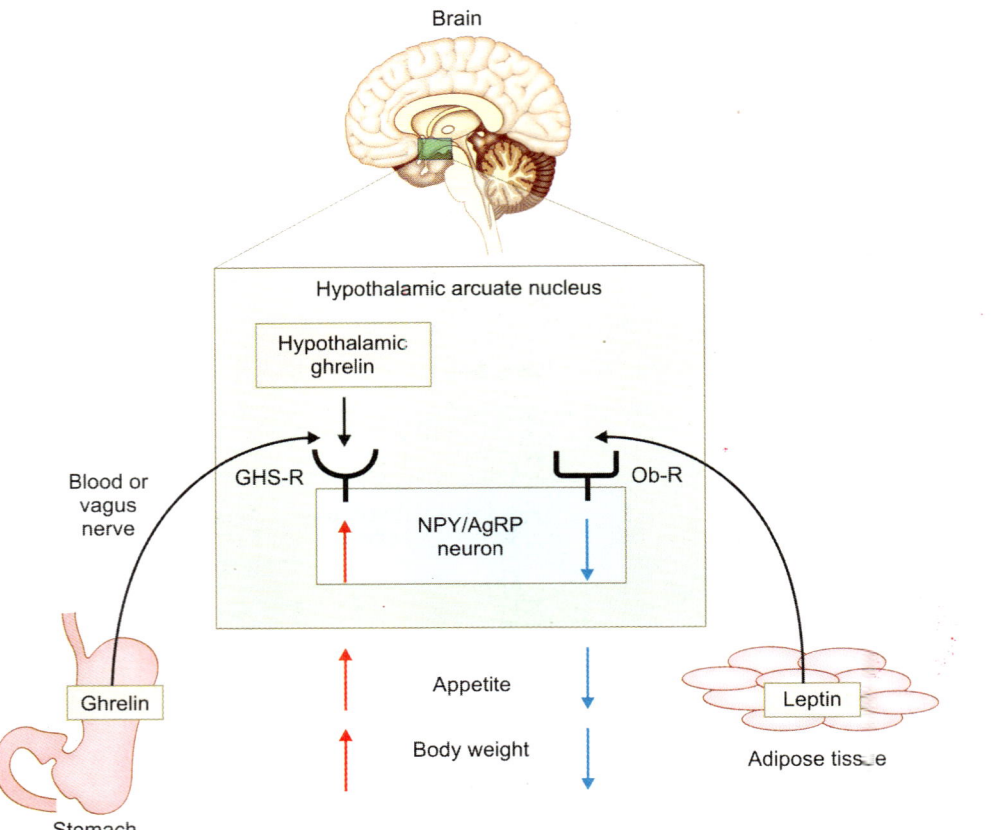

Fig. 10.42

- It acts on the feeding centre and increase appetite.
- Ghrelin acts on the Agouti-related peptide receptor and neuropeptide Y receptor on the arcuate nucleus.
- This causes stimulation of melanocyte stimulating hormone and cocaine–amphetamine related transcripts to be produced proopiomelanocortin neurons.
- MSH activate melanocortin receptors 3 and 4 and cause increased appetite and thus increase weight gain.
4. **Hormonal control:** Some gastrointestinal hormones are involved in inhibiting food intake: Cholecystokinin, oxytocin, glucagon, pancreatic polypeptide.
5. **Thermostatic mechanism**
   - An increase in body temperature causes decrease in food intake
   - Preoptic nucleus may act through feeding centres.

3. List the features of cerebellar lesions and the clinical tests performed for cerebellar dysfunction.

Signs of Cerebellar Lesions

I. *Disturbance in tone and posture*

Atonia or hypotonia: There is reduction in tone of skeletal muscles
Attitude changes: It is seen in unilateral lesions
• Face is turned towards healthy side
• Lowering of shoulder on affected side
• Trunk is bent with concavity on the affected side
• Outward rotation and abduction of leg
Deviation movement
• When eyes are closed and arms extended, they deviate towards the healthy side
Deep tendon reflexes
• Weak pendular reflexes

II. *Disturbance in movements*
- Gait is wide based
- Swaying from side to side

- Unable to maintain the upright posture and falls on closing the eyes (Romberg's sign)
- *Ataxia:* Lack of coordination of movements
- *Decomposition of movements:* Movements seem to occur in stages
- *Asynergia:* Lack of coordination between protagonist, synergist and antagonist muscles
- *Dysmetria:* The brain is unable to guage the distance and thus movements are incorrect in range and direction
- *Intentional tremors:* Tremors become evident during purposeful movements. They are absent at rest
- *Nystagmus:* To and from rhythmic involuntary movements of eyes and occurs even at rest.
- *Dysarthria:* Difficulty in articulation of speech due to incoordination of muscles involved in speech
- *Astasia:* Unsteady voluntary movements.
- *Charcot's triad:* Scanning speech + intentional tremors + nystagmus.

Tests for Cerebellar Functions

1. **Finger-nose test:** The patient is instructed to stretch out his hand, touch the finger shown by examiner and bring it near to touch the nose.
2. **Disdiadochokinesia**
   - Inability to perform alternating movements in a rapid manner.
   - *Example:* Supination and pronation
3. **Rebound phenomenon**
   - When an individual attempts to do something against resistance, and the resistance is suddenly removed, the limb moves in the direction intended.
   - Cerebellum is unable to control its movement.
4. **Gait test**
   - The patient is asked to walk along a straight line with feet in line with each other.
   - He is unable to do so
5. **Past pointing:** The movement usually goes beyond the intended point.

SHORT ANSWERS

1. What is motor and sensory homunculus? Explain.

- Homunculus is a distorted mythological human character.

- The representation of motor function and sensory function in the brain is in the form of homunculus.

Motor Homunculus

- Motor functions which need a lot of neural effort requires larger representation in the motor cortex, example fingers, muscles of chewing, lips have a larger spatial representation.
- They are represented in the area 4.
- Lower parts of the body are represented in the medial surface and upper parts are represented in the lateral side.

Sensory Homunculus

- It is represented in the post-central gyrus
- Different sensory areas of the body are represented in an inverted manner.
- However, face is not represented in inverted fashion.

2. Describe the cause and features associated with thalamic syndrome.

It is an emotional disturbance to sensory experience.

Cause

Ischemic damage to the posteroventral and posterolateral nuclei due to thrombosis of thalamo-geniculate branch of posterior cerebral artery.

Clinical Features

Sensory	Motor
Astereognosis	Due to involvement of
• Loss of tactile localization	posterolateral nucleus
Thalamic phantom limb	Ataxia
• Inability to locate own limb with eyes closed due to loss of proprioception	• Decreased muscle tone
	• Muscular weakness
	Involuntary movements
Thalamic overreaction	• Athetosis
• Decreased threshold for pain, temperature and touch	• Intentional tremors
	Thalamic hand
• Exaggerated sensations	• Abnormal posture of hand—moderate flexion of wrist and hyper-extended fingers

3. Explain Papez circuit. List the functions of limbic system.

Papez Circuit

- A set of interconnections between various parts of the limbic system is called Papez circuit.

- It plays an important role in encoding memory, genesis of EEG and genesis of emotions.

Connections (Fig. 10.43)

- The hippocampus is connected to mammillary bodies of hypothalamus via fornix.
- Mammillary bodies are connected to anterior thalamic nucleus via mammillothalamic tract.
- Anterior thalamic nucleus is connected with cingulate gyrus through medial thalamocortical fibers.
- Cingulate gyrus is in turn connected to hippocampus.

Functions of Limbic System

1. Autonomic regulation through amygdala
2. Regulation of feeding behavior
3. Regulation of sexual function and behaviour
4. Maternal behaviour is expressed through cingulate nucleus
5. Emotional regulation
6. Motivational regulation

4. Describe Klüver-Bucy syndrome, sham rage.

Klüver-Bucy Syndrome

- It is also called temporal lobe syndrome
- It is seen in experimental animals after bilateral ablation of temporal lobes along with amygdala and uncus
- In humans, it is seen due to lesions of this nature.

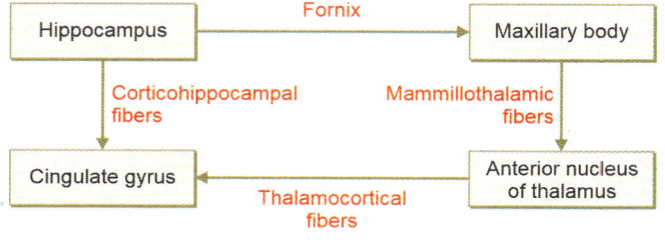

Fig. 10.43

Clinical Features

- Aphasia
- Auditory hallucinations tinnitus—buzzing or ringing
- Disturbances in smell and taste
- Visual hallucination and hemianopia
- Dreamy state—people usually feel unaware of their surrounding

Sham Rage

- It is false rage and occurs pathologically in some conditions.
- Normally, a person is able to find an equilibrium between anger and calm state.
- Until the irritation is major, the person can control his anger or rage
- Sham rage is characterized by increased anger or rage when faced by minor irritations.
- This happens when hypothalamus is released from cortical inhibition.

5. Classify the lobes of cerebellum according to their physiological functions.

Functional Classification

Vestibulocerebellum	Concerned with body posture and equilibrium
Spinocerebellum	Concerned with muscle tone and postural reflexes
Corticocerebellum	Performance of skilled voluntary movements

6. List the structures in the limbic system.

Structures in limbic cortex	Subcortical structures included in limbic system
• Orbitofrontal cortex	• Hypothalamus
• Subcallosal gyrus	• Anterior nuclei of thalamus
• Cingulate gyrus	• Portion of basal ganglia
• Parahippocampal gyrus	• Septum
• Uncus	• Paraolfactory area
	• Amygdala

10.8 DESCRIBE AND DISCUSS BEHAVIOURAL AND EEG CHARACTERISTICS DURING SLEEP AND MECHANISM RESPONSIBLE FOR ITS PRODUCTION

SHORT ESSAYS

1. Describe the physiological basis of EEG. List the different 'waveforms' of EEG and state their characteristics. Add a note on insomnia.

Physiological Basis of EEG

- Electroencephalogram is a collection of spontaneous waveforms of the activity of brain recorded from the scalp.
- These spontaneous discharges are due to continuous activity across thousands of synapses and neuron continuously taking place in various lobes of the brain.
- These graded synaptic potentials are summated and presented in the form of an EEG.
- The electrode placed on the scalp records these potentials through the scalp and skull overlying the neurons.

Waveforms (Table 10.1 and Fig. 10.44)

The normal EEG consists of waveforms of varying frequency and amplitude and represent various stages of alertness of mind.

Insomnia

- It is a disorder of sleep where an individual is unable to have a sufficient amount of sleep even in presence of opportunities for sleep.
- It is quite a common disorder experienced by many people.
- It is caused by stress, anxiety, alcoholism and psychiatric illnesses.
- It can be treated with sleep inducing agents like benzodiazepines. Barbiturates were used previously.

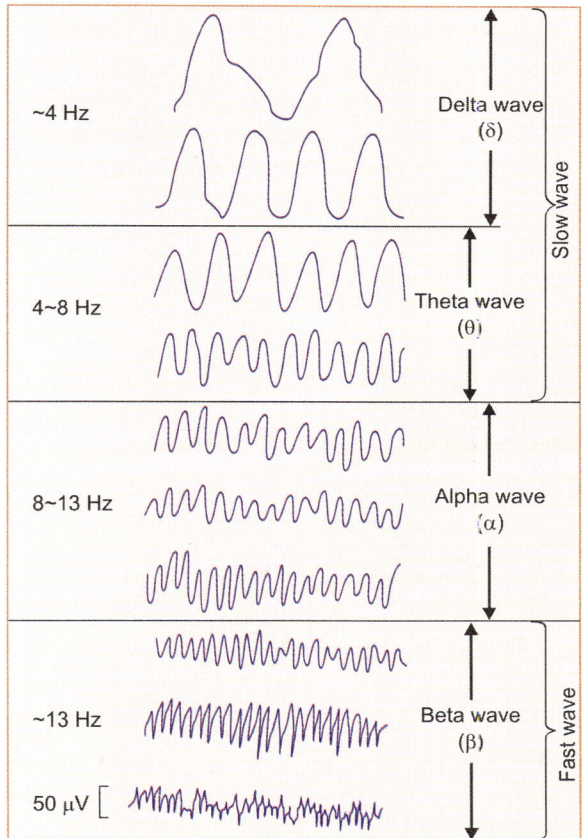

Fig. 10.44

Frequency (hertz)	Name of wave	Amplitude (microvolts)	Remarks
Table 10.1			
14–30	Beta (β)	5–10	• They are most prominent in the parietal and frontal regions • They are seen in tense or during arousal
8–13	Alpha (α)	50	• Most prominent when the individual is awake, but at rest with eyes closed • They are most marked in parieto-occipital area • Disappear during sleep
4–7	Theta (θ)	10	• They are seen during disappointment and frustration • They are seen in infants during crying
1–4	Delta (δ)	20–200	• They are seen in stage III and stage IV of NREM sleep • Infancy • Serious brain damage

2. Explain the stages of NREM sleep.

Non-random Eye Movement Sleep (NREM Sleep)

It is also known as slow wave sleep as the EEG waves in this part of sleep are very slow.

Stages

Stage I	The person is still sensitive to stimuli
	Low amplitude mixed amplitude waves
Stage II	Also called light sleep
	It is characterized by appearances of sleep spindles (10–14 Hz of 50 microvolt amplitude). K complexes are produced by auditory stimuli in this phase in the form of K complex: One or two high voltage waves with followed by a brief 14 Hz activity.
Stage III	Stage of moderate deep sleep
	Characterized by delta waves—high amplitude, low frequency waves
Stage IV	Stage of deep sleep
	Dome-like large delta waves, slower frequency

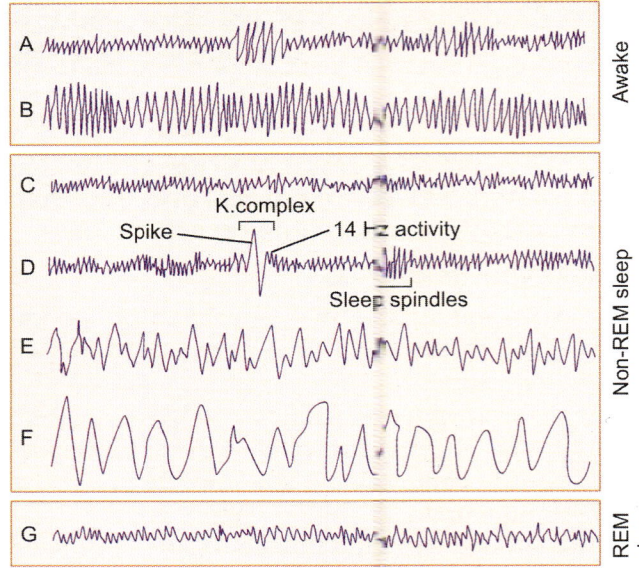

Fig. 10.45

SHORT ANSWER

1. Compare and contrast REM and NREM sleep.

Features	REM sleep	NREM sleep
Rapid eye movements	Present	Absent
Dreams	Present	Absent
Neurotransmitter	Noradrenaline	Serotonin
Arousability	Difficult	Easy
Muscle twitching	Present	Absent
Heart rate and BP	Fluctuating	Stable
Respiration and temperature	Fluctuating	Stable
EEG	Beta rhythm	Has 5 stages of different EEG patterns

10.9 DESCRIBE AND DISCUSS THE PHYSIOLOGICAL BASIS OF MEMORY, LEARNING AND SPEECH

SHORT ESSAYS

1. Describe the key features of classical and operant conditioning.

These are two methods of learning by association.

Classical Conditioning (Fig. 10.46)

- It involves learning by making an association between two stimuli.
- It is also known as Pavlovian conditioning or type 1 conditioned reflex.
- At the first instance, there is no association between the two stimuli.
- With repeated pairing the stimulus with another stimulus, the individual associates the two together.

Example

- For example, salivating by a dog on seeing food is an unconditioned stimulus (US). Ringing a bell is a neutral stimulus (NS).
- When a bell is rung on showing food multiple times, there is development of a temporal association between the US and the NS.
- After the association is learnt, there is salivation by the dog even with just ringing the bell.
- When the association does not continue, there is extinction of the learning.
- Therefore, there must be reinforcement between US and NS.

Operant Conditioning (Fig. 10.47)

- It is also called type II conditioning
- It involves associating a particular behaviour displayed by an organism with a reinforcement event.
- This helps the organism learn and differentiate its actions and behaviour based on the type of reinforcement.
- Thus, it can be associated with a reward or an aversion.
- Therefore, the organism learns which of its actions are responsible for the occurrence of reinforcement event.

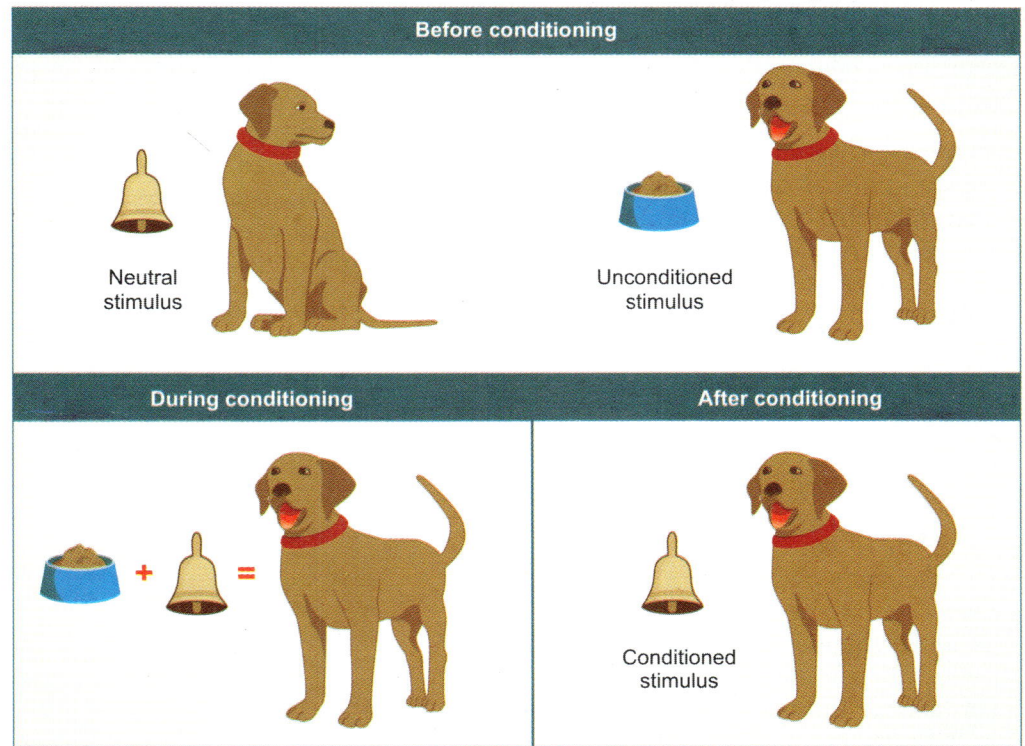

Fig. 10.46

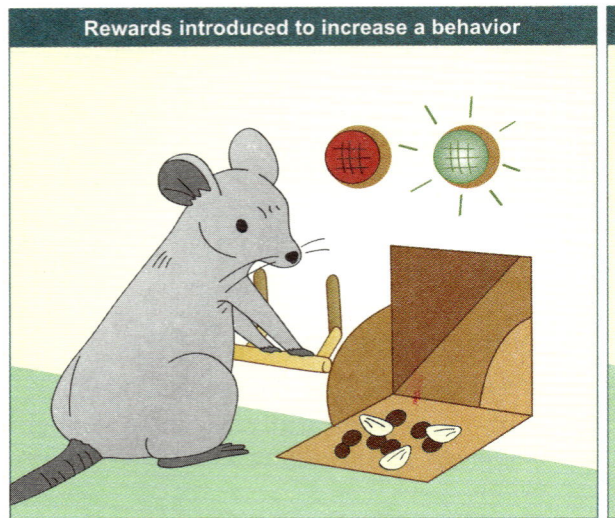

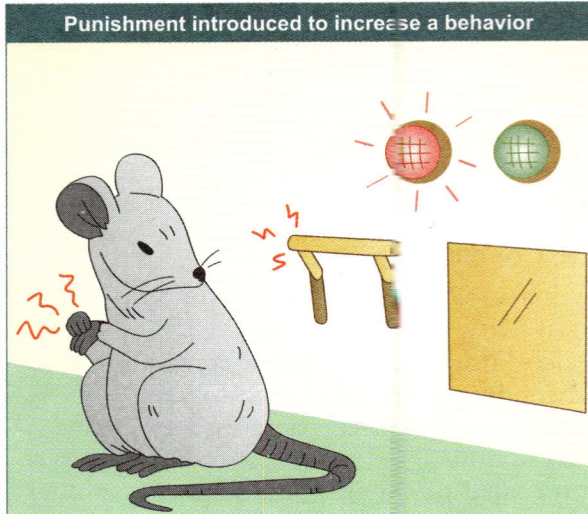

Fig. 10.47

Example
- A rat is placed in a cage with a bar-assisted lever within the wall of the cage.
- By its innate curiosity, the rat presses the lever.
- If the pressing of the lever is associated with entry of food into the cage, the rat is positively reinforced. This encourages the rat to pull the lever again.
- If the pressing of the lever is associated with a mild electric shock, the rat is negatively reinforced and avoids touching the lever again.

2. **A 60-year-old male patient was brought in by his son with complaints of disappearing from the house frequently and also unable to trace his path back to his house since about 2 weeks. On examination, it was observed that the old man had initial stages of dementia and was diagnosed with Alzheimer's disease. What is the pathophysiology of this condition?**

Pathophysiology of Alzheimer's Disease

- It is the most common cause of dementia in the elderly
- Neurodegeneration is central to the pathophysiology of Alzheimer's disease.
- The aetiology is thought to be due to:
  - Formation of senile plaques due to amyloid beta deposition: It may be familial or idiopathic. The amyloid is an extracellular protein which gets deposited in the form of fibrils and plaques.
  - Oxidative stress hypothesis: The reactive oxygen species formed during metabolic activities increase with age. When they are not cleared, they cause lipid peroxidation and death of cells
  - Metal dyes homeostasis: Metals like aluminium, iron, and copper cause damage to the neurons.
  - Cholinergic hypothesis: An age-related choline mediated neurotransmission is thought to cause Alzheimer's disease and this idea is even used to treat Alzheimer's disease.
  - There is global neuronal loss most predominantly in neocortex, entorhinal cortex, hippocampus, amygdala, nucleus basalis, anterior thalamus, locus coeruleus.
  - As a result, there is loss of memory, cognition, loss of spatial orientation and loss of all higher functions.

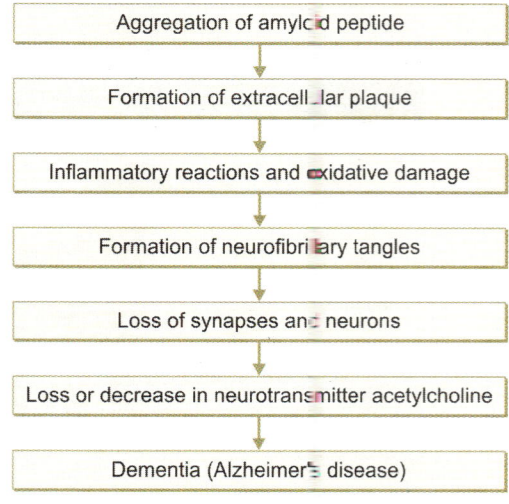

Fig. 10.48

3. What is amnesia? Add a note on Alzheimer's disease.

Amnesia

- Amnesia is partial or complete, reversible, or irreversible loss of memory.
- It can be anterograde or retrograde.
- It can be due to many causes like head injury and concussion, alcohol-induced Wernicke's encephalopathy, Alzheimer's disease and senile dementia.

Alzheimer's Disease

- It is the most common cause of dementia in the elderly
- Neurodegeneration is central to the pathophysiology of Alzheimer's disease.
- The aetiology is thought to be due to:
  - Formation of senile plaques due to amyloid beta deposition: It may be familial or idiopathic. The amyloid is an extracellular protein which gets deposited in the form of fibrils and plaques.
  - Oxidative stress hypothesis: The reactive oxygen species formed during metabolic activities increase with age. When they are not cleared, they cause lipid peroxidation and death of cells.
  - Metal dyes homeostasis: Metals like aluminium, iron and copper cause damage to the neurons.
  - Cholinergic hypothesis: An age-related choline mediated neurotransmission is thought to cause Alzheimer's disease and this idea is even used to treat Alzheimer's disease.

- There is global neuronal loss most predominantly in neocortex, entorhinal cortex, hippocampus, amygdala, nucleus basalis, anterior thalamus, locus coeruleus.
- As a result, there is loss of memory, cognition, loss of spatial orientation and loss of all higher functions.

4. What are the structures involved in speech? Describe sensory and motor aphasia in detail.

Speech (Fig. 10.49)

- The central speech apparatus includes the cortical and subcortical centres.
- For reception and understanding of spoken speech, the following structures are involved
- Intact auditory pathway
- Primary auditory area: Brodmann's areas 41 and 42: located on the superior temporal gyrus.
- For recognition and understanding of spoken words: Auditory association areas 20 and 21—located in the middle and inferior temporal gyrus
- Interpretation of words: Wernicke's area, posterior to areas 41 and 42
- For reception and understanding of written speech
- Intact visual pathway
- Primary visual cortex (area 17) in the occipital cortex around the calcarine fissure
- Interpretation is by visual association area (areas 18 and 19)
- Generation of thoughts/ideas in response to visual stimuli: Dejerine area 39 also called visual speech centre. Along with Wernicke's area, it forms the sensory speech centre.

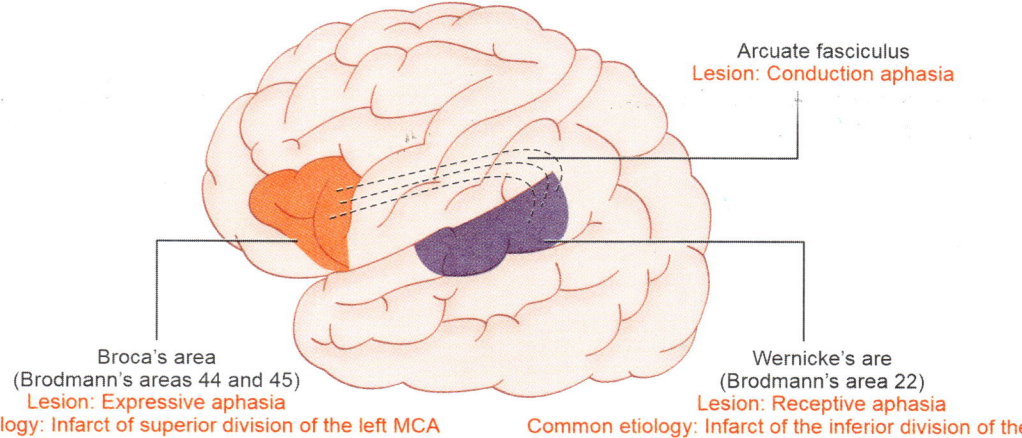

Arcuate fasciculus
Lesion: Conduction aphasia

Broca's area
(Brodmann's areas 44 and 45)
Lesion: Expressive aphasia
Common etiology: Infarct of superior division of the left MCA

Wernicke's are
(Brodmann's area 22)
Lesion: Receptive aphasia
Common etiology: Infarct of the inferior division of the left MCA

Fig. 10.49

- Expression in the form of speech
- Motor speech area or area 44 or Broca's area of the dominant side (left in right-handed people).
- It is situated in the prefrontal cortex in the inferior frontal gyrus.
- It is associated with stimulation of peripheral structures involved in voice production.
- The peripheral speech apparatus includes the larynx, pharynx, nasal cavity, tongue, jaws and lips.

APHASIA

- It is impaired speech due to a neurological cause in absence of mental confusion.
- It is often confused with dysarthria which means difficulty in articulation of words.
- In aphasia, if the patient is asked a question, he is not able to answer it by voice or in written. But in dysarthria, the patient can answer the question in writing as the problem is peripheral in the articulation apparatus—larynx, pharynx, tongue and lips.

Causes

1. Stroke involving any part of the brain associated with speech
2. Head injury
3. Malignancies
4. Infections like encephalitis and meningoencephalitis
5. Degenerative conditions

Sensory Aphasia

- It is also called receptive aphasia or Wernicke's aphasia
- It develops due to a lesion in the Wernicke's area.

Clinical Features

- The affected individual can hear when spoken to but is unable to comprehend speech.
- The individual talks fluently and so sensory aphasia is also called fluent aphasia. However, it may not make much sense
- It may be associated with neologism (formation of new words), anomia (inability to name an object) or paraphasia (use of unintended words)
- He cannot comprehend written language. It is also called word blindness.

- Another variant of sensory aphasia is conduction aphasia, in which the arcuate fasciculus is impaired.
- As a result, the person can comprehend but cannot produce words about what he has been spoken to. But the words flow fluently.

Motor Aphasia

- It is also known as Broca's aphasia
- Results from damage to the Broca's area in the frontal lobe.

Clinical Features

- The person can comprehend when spoken to.
- He cannot form words and speak. He can also not write the answers to questions asked to him.
- With difficulty, the individual may produce a few words.

SHORT ANSWERS

1. Explain Broca's and Wernicke's areas.

Broca's Area

- It is areas 44 and 45
- It is a special region of the premotor cortex and is present in the inferior frontal gyrus.
- It is known as the motor speech area.
- It is associated with stimulation of peripheral structures involved in voice production by activation of vocal cords through respective nerve and movements of jaw and lips to cause speech production.
- Lesion to this area causes Broca's aphasia.

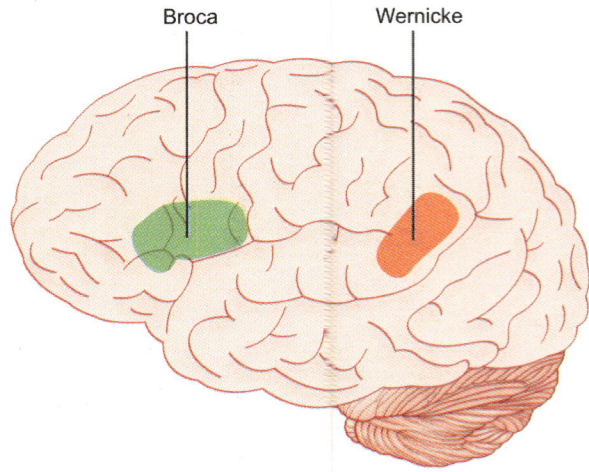

Fig. 10.50

Wernicke's Area

- It is also called auditory association area or area 22.
- It is the sensory speech centre located behind the areas 41 and 42 in the dominant side of the brain.
- It is associated with interpretation and meaning of what is heard.
- It receives signals from the auditory cortex.
- There is also comprehension and formation of ideas in this area.

2. List the types of aphasias and give the salient features of each.

Broca's aphasia	• Results from damage to the Broca's area in the frontal lobe
	• The person can comprehend when spoken to.
	• He cannot form words and speak. He can also not write the answers to questions asked to him.
	• With difficulty, the individual may produce a few words.
Wernicke's aphasia	• It develops due to a lesion in the Wernicke's area.
	• The affected individual can hear when spoken to but is unable to comprehend speech.
	• The individual talks fluently and so sensory aphasia is also called fluent aphasia.
	• However, it may not make much sense
Global aphasia	• There is extensive damage to both the Broca's area and Wernicke's area
	• These individuals cannot comprehend written speech or spoken speech
Conductive aphasia	• Damage to the arcuate fasciculus which connects Wernicke's and Broca's areas
	• As a result, the words can be understood when heard or read.
	• The patient is also able to form sentences
	• But he is unable to answer to the question being asked as there is no communication between Wernicke's and Broca's areas

3. What are the different types of memory?

A. Based on the way in which Information is Stored

1. **Implicit memory**
   - Non declarative memory
   - It is the memory of performing a task or a skill
   - They are acquired by practice and repetition
2. **Explicit memory**
   - Recognition memory
   - Refers to memory about facts like names of people, places
   - It is classified as semantic memory and episodic memory.
3. **Semantic memory:** It is memory of names of objects and spoken words.
4. **Episodic memory:** It is memory of events that an individual's experiences.

B. Based on the Time of Storage of Memory

1. Short-term memory lasts seconds to hours
2. Intermediate term memory: Days to weeks, and is generally lost
3. Long-term memory: Once stored, it can be recalled for lifetime.

4. Classify memory and list the stages and types of memory storage.

Classification

A. Based on the way in which Information is Stored

1. **Implicit memory**
   - Nondeclarative memory
   - It is the memory of performing a task or a skill
   - They are acquired by practice and repetition
2. **Explicit memory**
   - Recognition memory
   - Refers to memory about facts like names of people, places
   - It is classified as semantic memory and episodic memory
3. **Semantic memory:** It is memory of names of objects and spoken words.
4. **Episodic memory:** It is memory of events that an individual's experiences.

B. Based on the Time of Storage of Memory

1. Short-term memory lasts seconds to hours
2. Intermediate term memory: Days to weeks, and is generally lost
3. Long-term memory: Once stored, it can be recalled for lifetime.

Types of Memory Storage

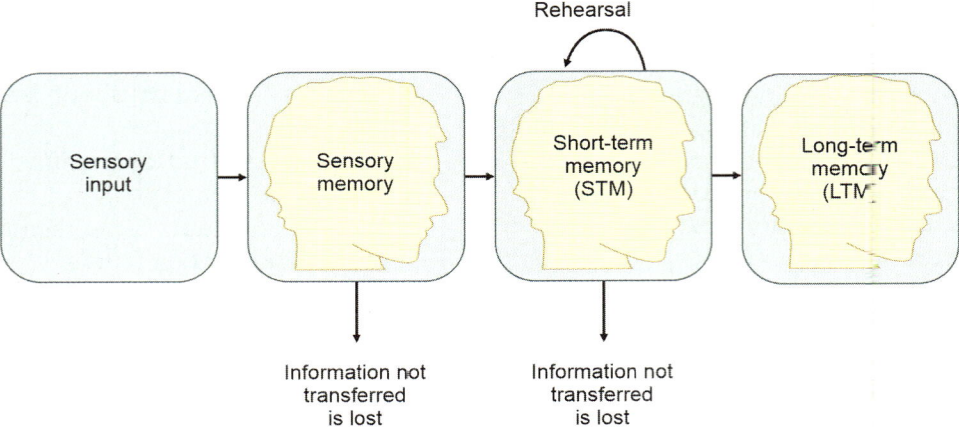

Fig. 10.51

10.10 DESCRIBE AND DISCUSS CHEMICAL TRANSMISSION IN THE NERVOUS SYSTEM
(OUTLINE THE PSYCHIATRY ELEMENT)

SHORT ESSAY

1. Define neurotransmitters. Explain the functions of:
   A. Acetylcholine
   B. Dopamine
   C. Noradrenaline

Neurotransmitter

- Neurotransmitters are substances which cause transmission of a synapse through a synapse.
- They are chemicals by nature.

Acetylcholine

- It is the main neurotransmitter involved in the cholinergic nervous system
- These are:
  - Neuromuscular junction
  - Preganglionic and postganglionic parasympathetic fibers
  - All preganglionic sympathetic fibers
  - Postganglionic sympathetic fibres supplying the sweat glands and skeletal blood vessels.
  - Neurons in forebrain, cortex, and thalamus
  - Neurons of basal ganglia

Functions

1. It is an excitatory neurotransmitter in the brain, cerebral cortex
2. It has a significant role in memory and forms the basis for cholinergic drugs for treatment of Alzheimer's disease.
3. They are involved in cognition, motivation, and perception.
4. ACh is involved in attention and arousal through the RAS.
5. It is an excitatory neurotransmitter involved in basal ganglia.
6. It is also involved in REM sleep through the ponto-geniculo-occipital spike system.

Dopamine

Sites of Release

- Neurons producing dopamine are seen in striatum (nigrostrial pathway)
- Nucleus accumbens
- Limbic system
- Olfactory tubercle

Functions

1. Mainly involved in control of movements in the basal ganglia. It controls the motor functions through the action of corpus striatum.
2. It is involved in mediation of the CTZ causing vomiting.
3. It inhibits production of prolactin and GnRH
4. It also has inhibitory actions in retina
5. It is involved in production of a psychosis called schizophrenia.

Noradrenaline

Sites of Release

- Adrenal medulla
- Post ganglionic sympathetic fibres
- Neurons of cerebral cortex and thalamus
- Noradrenergic neurons in pons and medulla forms the locus coeruleus system and lateral tegmental system.

Functions

1. It is excitatory in most places
2. Norepinephrine acts on alpha receptors and brings about generalised vasoconstriction
3. It also causes increased heart rate and contractility
4. In CNS, it is mainly excitatory.
5. It is involved in dreams, arousal and elevation of mood
6. In hypothalamus, they are involved in regulation of secretion of ADH and oxytocin
7. They also control the secretion of anterior pituitary hormones through the hypothalamo-hypophyseal system
8. It has inhibitory functions in cerebral cortex, cerebellar cortex and thalamus.

10.11 DEMONSTRATE THE CORRECT CLINICAL EXAMINATION OF THE NERVOUS SYSTEM: HIGHER FUNCTIONS, SENSORY SYSTEM, MOTOR SYSTEM, REFLEXES, CRANIAL NERVES IN A NORMAL VOLUNTEER OR SIMULATED ENVIRONMENT

SHORT ANSWER

1. Mention different sensory modalities, the ascending tracts and their functions.

Name of the tract	Origin	Function
Anterior spinothalamic tract	Chief sensory nucleus	Crude touch
Lateral spinothalamic tract	Substantia gelatinosa	Pain and temperature
Ventral spinocerebellar tract	Marginal nucleus	Subconscious kinesthetic sensations
Dorsal spinocerebellar tract	Clarke nucleus	Subconscious kinesthetic sensations
Spinotectal tract	Chief sensory nucleus	Spinovisual reflex
Spinoreticular tract	Intermediolateral cells	Arousal and consciousness
Spino-olivary tract and spino-vestibular tract	No significant origin	Proprioception
Fasciculus dorsolateralis	Posterior nerve root ganglion	Pain and temperature
Fasciculus gracilis	Posterior nerve root ganglion	Stereognosis
Fasciculus cuneatus		Tactile sensation
		Vibration
		Tactile localization and discrimination
		Conscious kinesthetic sensation

10.12 IDENTIFY NORMAL EEG FORMS

SHORT ESSAY

1 Explain the waves of the EEG. What are alpha block and sleep spindles?

- Electroencephalogram is a collection of spontaneous waveforms of the activity of brain recorded form the scalp.
- The normal EEG consists of waveforms of varying frequency and amplitude and represent various stages of alertness of mind.

Waves of EEG (Fig. 10.52, Table 10.2)

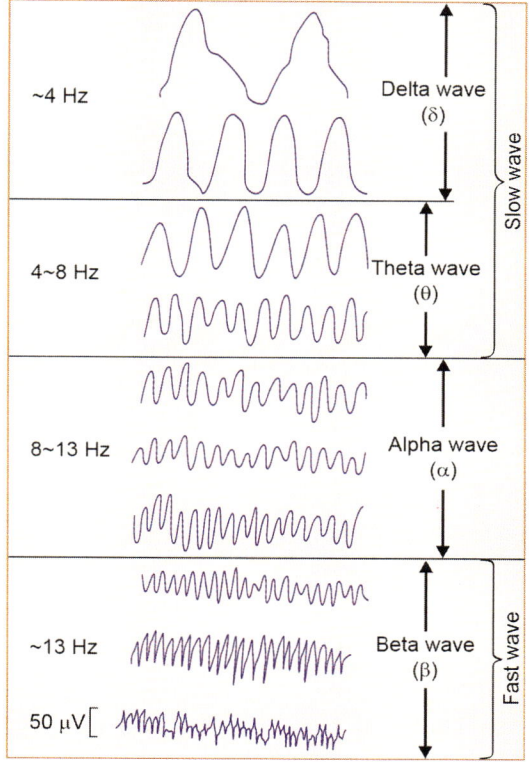

Fig. 10.52

Table 10.2			
Frequency (hertz)	Name of wave	Amplitude (microvolts)	Remarks
1ᴢ–30	Beta (β)	5–10	• They are most prominent in the parietal and frontal regions • They are seen in tense or during arousal
8–13	Alpha (α)	50	• Most prominent when the individual is awake, but at rest with eyes closed • They are most marked in parieto-occipital area • Disappear during sleep
4–7	Theta (θ)	10	• They are seen during disappointment and frustration • They are seen in infants during crying
1–4	Delta (δ)	20–200	• They are seen in stage III and stage IV of NREM sleep • Infancy • Serious brain damage

Alpha Block (Fig. 10.53)

- It is a phenomenon in which wave attenuates and are replaced by the fast, irregular waves of low amplitude.
- It occurs when an individual opens his eyes or when he suddenly engages in conscious mental activity

- It is also termed aroused or alerting response

Sleep Spindles (Fig. 10.54)

- They occur in stage II of NREM sleep
- These are bursts of α-like 10–14 Hz, 50 μV waves, which periodically interrupt the α rhythm.

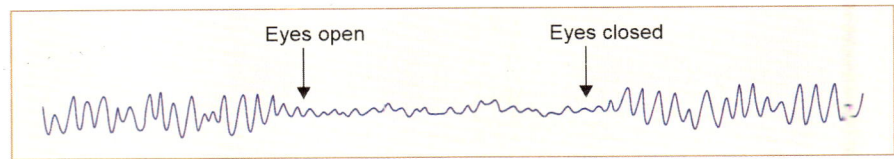

Fig. 10.53

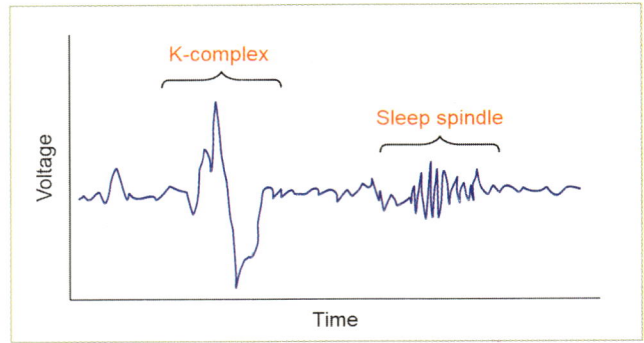

Fig. 10.54

10.13 DESCRIBE AND DISCUSS PERCEPTION OF SMELL AND TASTE SENSATION

LONG ESSAY

1. What are the different types of taste receptors? Explain signal transduction at various receptors, mention the different nerves that carry taste sensation; Trace the taste pathway with the help of a neat diagram.

Taste Receptors (Fig. 10.55)

- Each taste bud has a cluster of taste receptor cells—modified epithelium.
- It contains four types of cells—type I, II, III and IV.
- Type III cells are concerned with taste detection
- Types I and IV are called sustentacular cells.
- The function of type II cells is not known.

Signal Transduction at Various Receptors (Fig. 10.56)

- Type III cells of the taste buds form the receptors. The taste buds have a taste pore through which the juices mixed with food enter.
- These taste receptors like any other cell in the body are negatively charged.
- When exposed to a particular taste, they get polarized due to entry of sodium ions or hydrogen ions and then a potential is generated.
- Binding of a sugar molecule to a receptor cell initiates a signal transduction pathway. This is done by activation of cyclic AMP which further activates protein kinase A.
- As a result, there is closure of K^+ channels in the membrane which causes depolarization.

- Voltage-gated calcium Ca^{2+} channels open, and Ca^{2+} diffuses into the receptor cell.
- Synaptic vesicles release neurotransmitters, sending signals to the sensory neuron which fire the primary afferent nerve.

Nerves that Carry Taste Sensation

1. **Vagus nerve (X):** From taste buds on surface of epiglottis.
2. **Glossopharyngeal nerve (IX):** From posterior one-third of tongue.
3. **Facial nerve (V):** From anterior two-thirds of tongue.

Taste Pathway (Fig. 10.57)

Receptors

- Type III cells of the taste buds form the receptors. The taste buds have a taste pore through which the juices mixed with food enter.
- These taste receptors like any other cell in the body are negatively charged.
- When exposed to a particular taste, they get polarised due to entry of sodium ions or hydrogen ions and then a potential is generated.

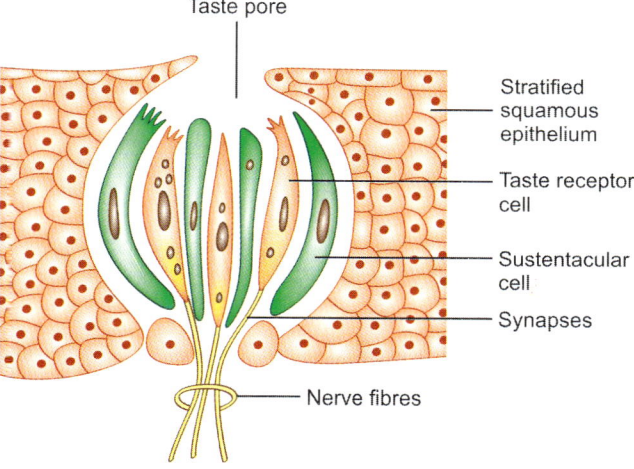

Fig. 10.55

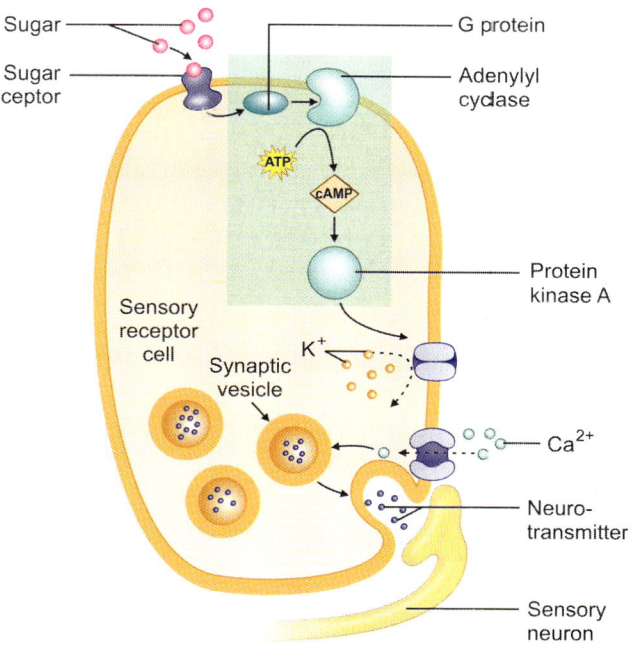

Fig. 10.56

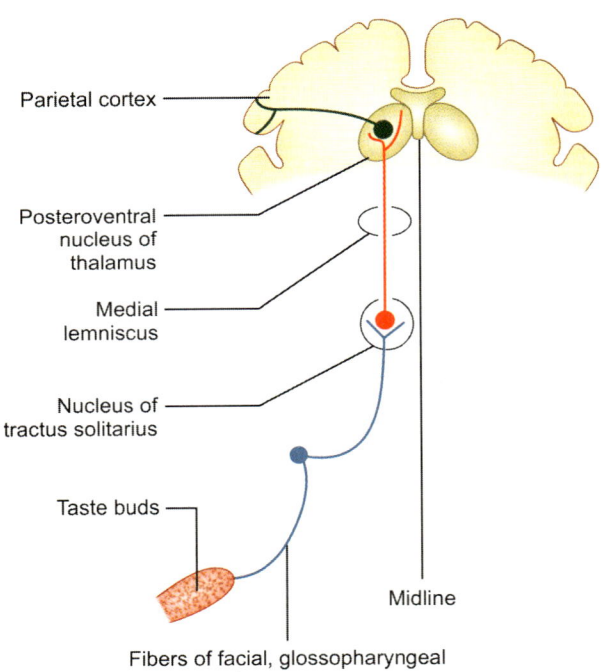

Fig. 10.57

First Order Neurons

- Three different cranial nerves are involved in sending sensory impulses of taste.
- They are chorda tympani of the facial nerve, glossopharyngeal nerve and the vagus nerve.
- The nerve from these regions terminate in the nucleus of tractus solitarius.

Second Order Neurons

- They are in the nucleus of tractus solitarius.
- Fibres from here travel through the medial lemniscus and terminate in the posteroventral nucleus of the thalamus.

Third Order Neurons

- They are in the posteroventral nucleus of the thalamus.
- Axons from here project into the cortex of parietal lobe. The area responsible for taste is opercular insular cortex (lower part of the post-central gyrus).

SHORT ESSAYS

1. 60-year-old female patient had undergone a urological operation under general anaesthesia, 3 months back. After recovery, she observed having altered smell sensation. What is anosmia? What are the different receptors for olfaction?   **(2 + 3 marks)**

Anosmia

- It is the inability to detect any sort of smell.
- It can be temporary or permanent.
- Temporary anosmia is seen in allergic rhinitis and blocked nose.
- Permanent anosmia is seen when there is damage to the olfactory tract and their receptors.

Different Receptors for Olfaction

- Olfactory receptors are modified mucous membrane cells.
- They are present in the upper one-third of the nasal cavity.
  1. Odorant receptors
  2. Vomeronasal receptors
  3. Trace amine associated receptors
  4. Formyl peptide receptors
  5. Membrane guanyl cyclase CD

2. Explain the structure of olfactory receptors and trace the olfactory pathway.   (2 + 3 marks)

Structure of Olfactory Receptors

- Olfactory receptor is a bipolar neuron with an expanded dendritic end forms the olfactory rod.
- From the olfactory rod, about 10–12 nonmyelinated cilia arise.

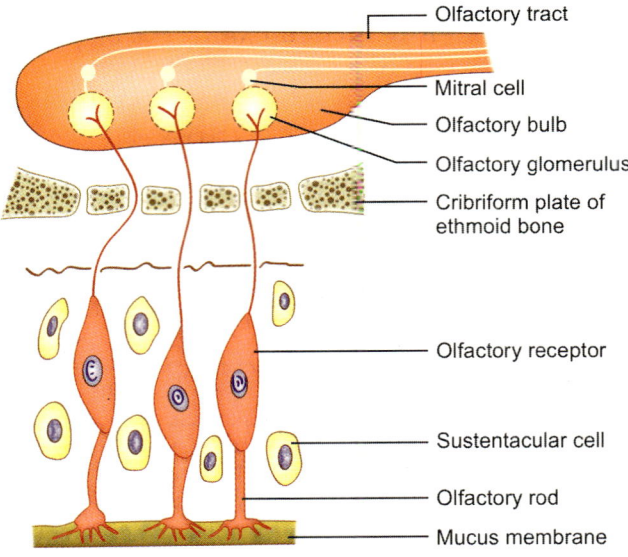

Fig. 10.58

- They enter the olfactory mucosa. They are responsible for detection of olfactory stimuli.
- The proteins present in the mucosa which is renewed continuously is responsible for detection of odoriferous stimuli.

Olfactory Pathway

- It is formed by the axons of the bipolar neurons of the olfactory receptors.

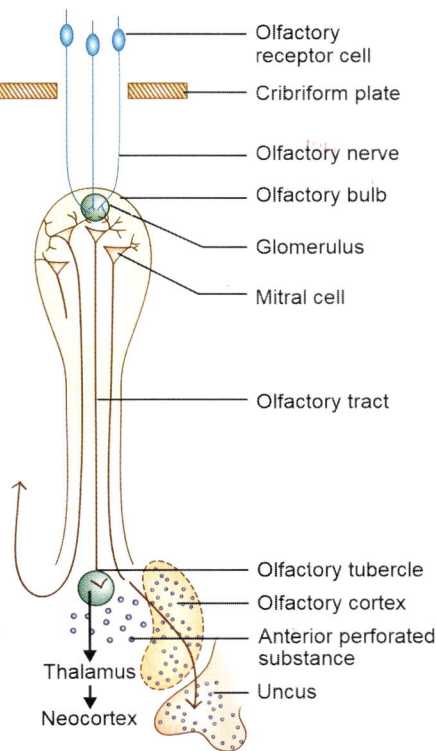

Olfactory receptor cell
Cribriform plate
Olfactory nerve
Olfactory bulb
Glomerulus
Mitral cell
Olfactory tract
Olfactory tubercle
Olfactory cortex
Anterior perforated substance
Thalamus
Uncus
Neocortex

Fig. 10.59

- They pierce the cribriform plate of the ethmoid bone reach the olfactory bulb.
- Here, they synapse with the axons of the mitral cells. These synapses form globular structures called olfactory glomeruli.
- The axons of the mitral cells form the olfactory tract and run backwards to reach the olfactory cortex which is formed by anterior olfactory nucleus, pre-pyriform cortex, olfactory tubercle and amygdala.

3. What is the role of vomeronasal organs?

Vomeronasal Organs

- It is found in lower animals and is also called accessory olfactory organs.
- It is called Jacobson organ as it was discovered by a Danish scientist, Jacobson.

Location

- It is present in a cartilaginous cavity and opens into the base of the nasal septum.
- The olfactory receptors in this organ are susceptible to non-volatile scents like pheromones and scents.
- These are helpful in animals for hunting and help in detection of trace amounts of chemicals.
- Also, they are helpful for mating as they help in detecting pheromones.

Importance in Humans

- They are probably vestigial in humans, but a small area of the olfactory mucosa which functions like vomeronasal organs.
- It is present in the anterior part of nasal septum.
- It is probably involved in sixth sense. They are also helpful in sexual function.

10.14 DESCRIBE AND DISCUSS PATHOPHYSIOLOGY OF ALTERED SMELL AND TASTE SENSATION

SHORT ANSWERS

1. List the disorders of taste and smell.

Disorders of Taste

Ageusia	Loss of taste sensation
	Depending on the nerve involved, the region of tongue becomes insensitive to taste
Hypogeusia	Decrease in taste sensation
Taste blindness	Inability to recognize a taste
	Genetically acquired
Dysgeusia	Temporal lobe syndrome
	Paroxysmal hallucinations of unpleasant taste and smell

Disorders of Smell

Anosmia	Total loss of sense of smell
Hyposmia	Reduced ability to detect smell
Hyperosmia	Increased or exaggerated sensation of smell
Parosmia	Distortion or perversion of smell
	Phantosmia (olfactory hallucination)
	Disagreeable sense of smell even in the absence of olfactory stimulus

2. Describe the clinical tests for taste and smell.

Clinical Tests for Taste

- Here the patient is blindfolded and given various nonodorous solutions for taste.
- The solutions commonly used are 10% sucrose solution (sweet), 15% salt solution (salty), 1% weak acetic acid (sour) and 0.1% quinine sulfate (bitter).
- The subject is asked to rinse his mouth and dry the tongue with a gauze.
- A cotton swab is dipped in sucrose solution and placed on the tip of the tongue. The patient is required to identify the taste. The same procedure is repeated for sides of the tongue, anterior 2/3rds of the tongue, posterior 1/3rd on either side of midline.
- Similarly, the test is repeated for all solutions and record the sensation in various grades.

Clinical Test for Smell

- The subject is asked to close his eyes.
- One nostril is occluded.
- He is given to smell a few strong scents like turpentine oil, oil of wintergreen and alcohol.
- The time till when he cannot perceive the smell is recorded as time for adaptation.
- It is repeated on the other side.

10.15 DESCRIBE AND DISCUSS FUNCTIONAL ANATOMY OF EAR AND AUDITORY PATHWAYS AND PHYSIOLOGY OF HEARING

LONG ESSAY

1. Describe the theories of hearing and trace the auditory pathway.   (4 + 6 marks)

Theories of Hearing

1. **Telephone theory of rutherford**
   - According to this, the cochlea plays the role of a telephone transmitter.
   - The sound waves are converted into electrical impulses and transmitted.
   - Similarly, sound waves are converted into electrical impulses by cochlea and sent to the auditory cortex.

2. **Resonance theory**
   - The basilar membrane of the cochlea has many basilar fibers.
   - These fibers are compared to resonators of piano.
   - When a string of piano is struck, a particular frequency is produced.
   - Similarly, when the sound with a particular frequency is applied, the basilar fibers in a particular portion of basilar membrane are stimulated.

3. **Place theory**
   - According to this theory, nerve fibers at different portions of the basilar membrane on the organ of Corti, respond to various frequencies of sounds.
   - Thus, when the sound with a particular frequency reaches the organ of Corti, the basilar fibers in a particular portion of basilar membrane are stimulated creating a particular sense of hearing.

4. **Travelling wave theory of hearing (Fig. 10.60)**
   - According to the travelling wave theory of von Bekesy, high frequency sounds produce vibrations near the oval window and the waves with low frequency produce vibrations near the apex of the helicotrema.
   - The stapes attached to the oval window.
   - Sound energy is transmitted along the bony ossicles to the footplate of stapes and causes vibration of the oval window.
   - This is transmitted into the perilymph of scala vestibuli.

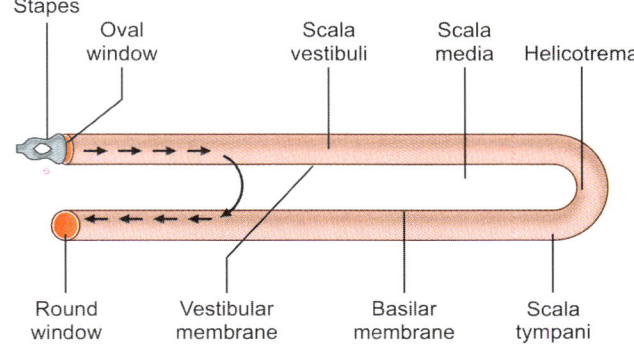

Fig. 10.60

- This causes vibration of the fluid in the scala media and in turn bulging of the basilar membrane
- Resonance point: it is a point on the basilar membrane where the travelling vibration becomes strong enough to cause to and fro motion of the basilar membrane and then the wave does not travel further.
- The bulging of basilar membrane causes vibrations to be transmitted to the perilymph in the scala tympani. This causes vibration of the round window.
- This is called the travelling wave theory.
- The distance between the oval window and the resonance point is determined by the frequency of the sound. It is inversely proportional to the frequency of the sound.
- In practicality, most of the waves travel well before the helicotrema. Only very low frequency waves may occasionally reach the helicotrema.

Auditory Pathway (Fig. 10.61)

Receptors
- Hair cells of the organ of Corti are the receptors.
- Afferent fibres from the hair cells form the cochlear nerve.

First Order Neurons
- Bipolar cells of the spiral ganglion situated in the modiolus of cochlea form the first order neuron.
- Their dendrite forms the afferents from the organ of Corti.

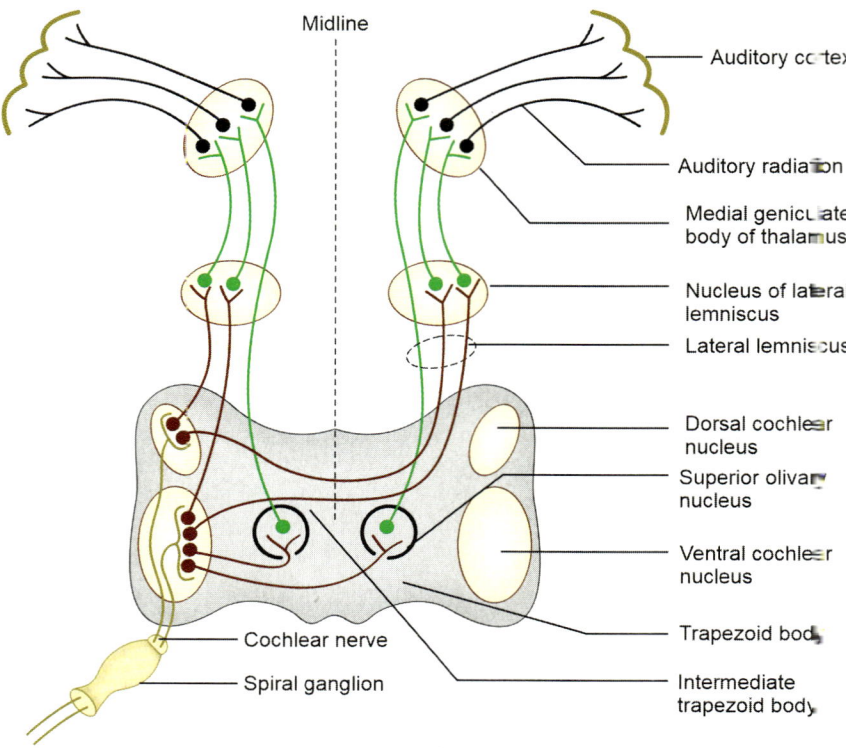

Fig. 10.61

- The longer processes—axons leave the cochlea and enter the medulla oblongata.

Second Order Neurons

- Neurons form the dorsal and ventral cochlear nuclei in the medulla oblongata are the second order neurons.
- One group of neurons relay in the ipsilateral olivary nucleus and the other in contralateral olivary nucleus through respective trapezoid bodies.
- Third group of neurons travel along the ipsilateral lateral lemniscus and terminate in the nucleus of lateral lemniscus.
- Fourth group of neurons cross midline via the intermediate trapezoid fibres and join the contralateral lateral lemniscus.

Third Order Neurons

- Fibres from the nucleus of lateral lemniscus and superior olivary nuclei terminate in the medial geniculate body, also known as the subcortical auditory centres.
- Auditory radiations begin from here and pass through the internal capsule and reach the auditory cortex.
- Some fibres stray from the medial geniculate body to reach the tectum of midbrain—this pathway is important in movement of head towards auditory stimuli.

Cortical Centres

It is formed by the temporal lobe of the cortex.

Primary auditory area	Areas 41 and 42	Perception of auditory impulses	Situated in the anterior transverse gyrus and lateral surface of superior temporal gyrus
	Wernicke's area	Analysis and interpretation of sounds	Upper part of superior temporal gyrus
Secondary auditory area	Area 22 or Auditopsychic area	Analysis and interpretation of sound	Superior temporal gyrus

SHORT ESSAYS

1. Explain the parts and functions of the middle ear.   (2.5 + 2.5 marks)

Structure

- The middle ear is a small, narrow irregular chamber also known as tympanum
- It houses the ossicles, auditory muscles and eustachian tube and is the region between tympanic membrane and oval window.

Tympanic Membrane

- It is a thin translucent membrane which separates external ear from middle ear
- The periphery is fixed to the tympanic sulcus, a fibrocartilaginous ring.
- It consists of an outer cutaneous layer, intermediate fibrous layer and inner mucus layer.
- The tympanic membrane is kept taut by the tensor tympani muscle.

Auditory Ossicles

- The middle ear house three bony ossicles called malleus, incus and stapes.
- Malleus
  - It is called hammer and has a handle, head and neck.
  - The handle of the malleus is in contact with the inner surface of the tympanic membrane.
  - The head of the malleus articulates with the incus which in turn is in contact with the head of the stapes.
- Incus
  - It is also known as anvil and has a long and a short process.
  - The tip of the long process articulates with stapes.

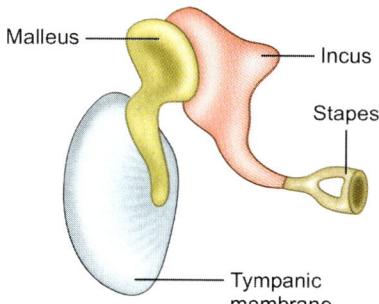

Malleus

Incus

Stapes

Tympanic membrane

Fig. 10.62

- Stapes
  - It is also called stirrup.
  - It has a head which articulates with incus and a foot.
  - The footplate of the stapes is in contact with the membranous labyrinth of the cochlea though the oval window.

Muscles of Middle Ear

Tensor tympani	• Originates from the cartilaginous part of eustachian tube and inserts on the manubrium of the malleus and in turn attaches to the tympanic membrane	• Supplied by mandibular division of trigeminal nerve • Responsible for tympanic reflex
Stapedius	• Smallest skeletal muscle in the body • Originates from the interior pyramid of tympanic cavity and attaches on the posterior surface of the neck of stapes	• It is supplied by facial nerve • It prevents excess movement of stapes and prevents hyperacusis

Eustachian Tube

- It is a flattened canal extending from the anterior wall of middle ear to nasopharynx
- It plays an important role in equalizing pressure on either side.

Functions

1. **Conduction of sound from outer ear to inner ear:** Middle ear converts sound energy into mechanical energy and the mechanical energy to hydraulic energy

2. **Impedance matching**
   - The middle ear house three bony ossicles called malleus, incus and stapes. The tympanic membrane is kept taut by the tensor tympani muscle.
   - The handle of the malleus is in contact with the inner surface of the tympanic membrane. The head of the malleus articulates with the incus which in turn is in contact with the head of the stapes.
   - The footplate of the stapes is in contact with the membranous labyrinth of the cochlea though the oval window.

- Due to this arrangement, the force of movement of the stapes is increased. Thus, there is 1.3 times increase in the force of the stapes.
- Also, the surface area of the tympanic membrane is 17 times more than the foot plate of stapes.
- As a result, there 1.3 × 17 = 22 times increase in energy of the sound waves which covers for the loss of impedance when sound waves enter the fluid medium from air.

3. **Tympanic reflex**
   - It is a protective reflex to loud noise.
   - When there is exposure to loud noise, there is involuntary contraction of the tensor tympani and the stapedius muscle.
   - As a result, the manubrium of the malleus moves inward, and stapes is pulled outward. As a result, there is stiffening of the ossicular system.
   - This causes lesser sound to be transmitted to the inner ear.

4. **Physical protection of the inner ear**

5. **Balance of air pressure between pharynx and the middle ear is done by the eustachian tube**

2. Explain the two mechanisms involved in impedance matching.

Impedance Matching

- When sound waves strike the tympanic membrane, they are converted into mechanical energy and are conducted through the ossicles.
- When sound waves travel from air to a fluid, there is increased resistance offered. This is called impedance.
- The impedance of the cochlear fluid is very high and thus, it causes 0.1% of the sound energy to be transmitted.
- This is called impedance mismatch.

Mechanisms of Impedance Matching

It is an important function of the middle ear.

1. **Lever action of ossicles**
   - The handle of malleus is 1.3 times longer than the long process of incus.
   - This provides a mechanical leverage action and due to this arrangement, the force of movement of the stapes is increased. Thus, there is 1.3 times increase in the force of movement.

2. **Hydraulic action of the tympanic membrane**
   - The vibratory surface area of the tympanic membrane is 45 mm^2. The footplate of the stapes is 3.2 mm^2.
   - This is 17 times more than the footplate of stapes.
   - Thus, this size difference makes the impact of sound concentrate on a smaller area and thus there is 14-fold amplification of sound.
   - As a result, there 1.3 × 17 = 22 times increase in energy of the sound waves which covers for the loss of impedance when sound waves enter the fluid medium from air.
   - If the ossicles and tympanic membrane are removed from the middle ear, very loud sounds are heard as whisper.

3. **A 35-year-old male came with complaint of gait disturbances that increased when he moved in lift or car. He was tested and was found to have defective equilibrium due to lesion in the inner ear. What is the basis of maintenance of equilibrium? Explain the role of semi-circular canals in the same in detail.**

(2 + 3 marks)

Physiological Basis of Equilibrium

- Equilibrium is a state when the line of gravity is in line with that of gravity.
- Equilibrium in the body is maintained by a complex coordination between vestibular apparatus, cerebellum and reticular formation.
- Vestibular apparatus plays an important role in maintaining posture and equilibrium through statokinetic reflexes.
- Statokinetic reflexes are that help in maintaining posture during movement.
- Eyes provide visual inputs for maintaining equilibrium.
- Proprioceptors provide feedback regarding position of joints and muscles with respect to one another.
- These signals are coordinated by the brain and the motor actions are controlled through cerebellum. These signals help control the posture.
- They also relay in the medial longitudinal fasciculus to dictate the movement of eyes.

Role of Semicircular Canals (Fig. 10.63)

- These house the semicircular ducts which are three on each side. They are anterior, lateral, and posterior.
- They represent three axes of movement of the head.
- When the head is bent 30° forwards, the lateral semicircular duct is almost horizontal to the surface of the earth. The anterior duct is 45° forward and posterior duct is 45° backward from the vertical plane.
- Each duct has a dilated end called the ampulla which houses the crista ampullaris. It is the sensory organ of the semicircular ducts.
- Each crista has a gelatinous layer on the surface called the cupula. Thousands of hair cells project into the cupula from the crest. There are many cilia, of which one is longest. It is called kinocilium.

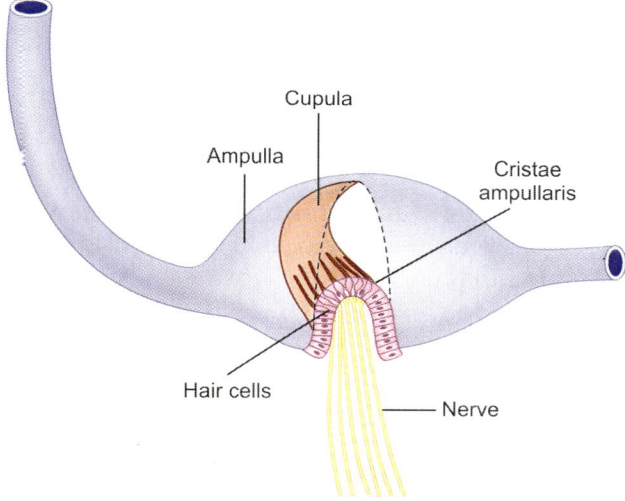

Fig. 10.63

- When the endolymph moves towards the kinocilium, there is depolarization and when it moves away, there is hyperpolarization.
- Semicircular canals are mainly associated with angular motion.
- Based on the movements of the head, there occurs respective depolarization and hyperpolarization in the respective semicircular ducts.

| Lateral semicircular duct | Motion of head along the vertical axis *Example:* "No" movement |
| Vertical semicircular ducts | Motion of head along transverse axis *Example:* "Yes" movement of the head |

Tilting of Head

Example: Ear touches the shoulder.

- Example of working of semicircular ducts:
- When the head moves to right: Hair cells in the right lateral canal are stimulated
- Changes in right canal: Endolymph moves towards ampulla → causing cupula to move towards ampulla → cilia move towards kinocilium → depolarization
- Changes in left canal: Endolymph moves away from ampulla → causing cupula to move away from ampulla → cilia move away from kinocilium → hyperpolarization.

4. Describe travelling wave theory of hearing with neat labelled diagram.

Travelling Wave Theory of Hearing (Fig. 10.64)

- According to the travelling wave theory of von Bekesy, high frequency sounds produce vibrations

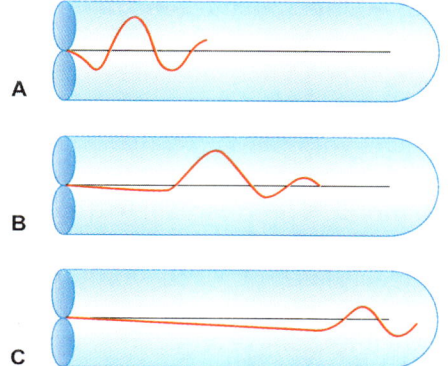

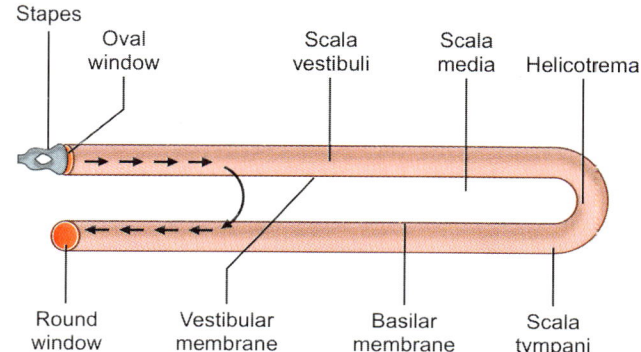

Fig. 10.64

near the oval window and the waves with low frequency produce vibrations near the apex of the helicotrema.

- The stapes attached to the oval window.
- Sound energy is transmitted along the bony ossicles to the footplate of stapes and causes vibration of the oval window.
- This is transmitted into the perilymph of scala vestibuli.
- This causes vibration of the fluid in the scala media and in turn bulging of the basilar membrane.
- Resonance point: It is a point on the basilar membrane where the travelling vibration becomes strong enough to cause to and fro motion of the basilar membrane and then the wave does not travel further.
- The bulging of basilar membrane causes vibrations to be transmitted to the perilymph in the scala tympani. This causes vibration of the round window.
- This is called the travelling wave theory.
- The distance between the oval window and the resonance point is determined by the frequency of the sound. It is inversely proportional to the frequency of the sound.
- In practicality, most of the waves travel well before the helicotrema. Only very low frequency waves may occasionally reach the helicotrema.

SHORT ANSWERS

1. Explain the structure of organ of Corti.

- Organ of Corti is the sensory receptor for hearing and is placed on the basilar membrane of the cochlea.
- It consists of the following parts:
  1. **Border cells:** These are slender columnar cells arranged near the inner hair cells.
  2. **Inner hair cells**
     - These are flask-shaped cells.
     - They appear as a single layer and occupy the upper part of the epithelial layer.
     - The base of these inner hair cells is rounded, and they rest on the inner phalangeal cells.
     - The surface bears a number of short cilia called stercocilia and they are in contact with the tectorial membrane.
     - One of them is longest and is called kinocilium.

- The base of the inner hair cells has nerve endings of cochlear nerve.

3. **Inner phalangeal cells**
   - These are supporting cells for inner hair cells.
   - They rest on the basilar membrane.

4. **Inner and outer pillar cells**
   - They are also called rod cells of Corti
   - The base of the inner pillar cells is in contact with the tympanic lip.
   - They are inclined towards each other and their heads articulate.
   - They form a pillar and an arch—called the tunnel of Corti.

5. **Outer hair cells**
   - They are columnar cells occupying the superficial part of the epithelium of the organ of Corti.
   - Their bases are supported by the outer phalangeal cells.
   - Their structure is similar to that of inner hair cells.

6. **Outer phalangeal cells**
   - They are supporting cells of the outer hair cells.
   - It sends stiff phalangeal processes upward between the hair cells, to form the part of lamina reticularis.

7. **Cells of claudius:** They are cuboidal in nature and line the lower surface of the external spiral sulcus.

8. **Cells of Hensen**
   - They form the outer border of the organ of Corti
   - They are tall columnar cells.
   - They are arranged in several rows.

9. **Tectorial membrane and reticular membrane**
   - Tectorial membrane extends from the vestibular lip to the level of cells of Hensen.
   - It forms the roof of the organ of Corti and is in contact with the stercocilia.
   - When the basilar membrane vibrates, the hair cells move with respect to the tectorial membrane leading to generation of potential.
   - Cuticular plates of all the supporting cells collectively form a reticular membrane, which is known as lamina reticularis. It covers the organ of Corti.

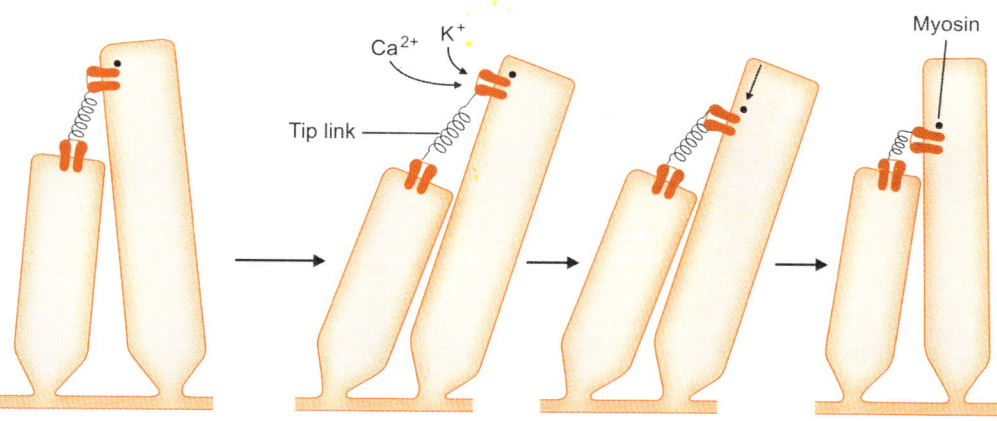

Fig. 10.65

2. Describe the endocochlear potential.

- When the ear is stimulated by sound, two types of potentials are generated—cochlear microphonic potential and action potential of the auditory nerve.
- The spiral organ of Corti is situated on the basilar membrane.
- When the basilar membrane vibrates up and down, there is a resultant movement in the organ of Corti.
- When the basilar membrane moves upward, the tectorial membrane and the stercocilia move away from the limbus and when the basilar membrane moves down, the stercocilia and the tectorial membrane move towards the limbus.
- The gating of potassium channels is controlled by the movement of stercocilia towards or away from the limbus (Fig. 10.65).

Bending of stercocilia away from limbus (upward vibration of the basilar membrane)	Opening of potassium channels ↓ Entry of potassium into the cell ↓ Resultant depolarization
Bending of the stercocilia towards the limbus (downward vibration of the basilar membrane)	Closure of potassium channels ↓ Resultant hyperpolarization

- The sum of receptor potentials of all the activated hair cells thus produced is called cochlear microphonic potential.
- It is recorded by placing microelectrodes in the scala tympani and scala media.

Properties of Cochlear Microphonic Potential

- They have no latency or refractory period. As a result, the hair cells can stimulate by a new vibration when it is still depolarised.
- They do not obey all-or-none phenomenon
- They are resistant to ischemia
- They are resistant to anaesthesia.

3. What is tympanic reflex?

Tympanic Reflex

- It is a protective reflex to loud noise.
- When there is exposure to loud noise, there is involuntary contraction of the tensor tympani and the stapedius muscle.
- As a result, the manubrium of the malleus moves inward, and stapes is pulled outward. As a result, there is stiffening of the ossicular system.
- This causes lesser sound to be transmitted to the inner ear.

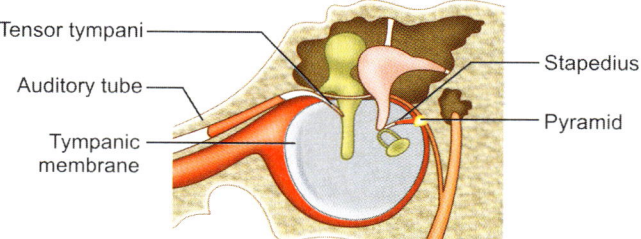

Fig. 10.66

10.16 DESCRIBE AND DISCUSS PATHOPHYSIOLOGY OF DEAFNESS. DESCRIBE HEARING TESTS

SHORT ESSAYS

1. What are the various hearing tests? Describe Weber's test in detail.　　　(2 + 3 marks)

Tests for Hearing

1. **Clinical bedside tests**
   - It includes whisper test and watch test
   - Same word is whispered in both the ears, one at a tie and the patients is asked whether he could appreciate it with same intensity. Similarly, the ticking of a watch can be used.
   - It is a subjective test
2. **Tuning fork tests:** 256 or 512 Hz tuning forks are used to test air conduction and bone conduction of sound.
3. **Sound evoked potentials:** It is performed by stimulating the ear with some sound and recording potentials in the temporal lobe.
4. **Audiometry**

Weber's Test (Fig. 10.67)

- This is a test to compare bone conduction in both ears of the patient.
- The desired (lower frequency first) tuning fork is chosen and thrust at the palm to set it in motion.
- It is placed the forehead of the patient without coming in contact with the forks.
- The patient is asked whether he can hear both the sounds equally.

Interpretation of Results

- If he hears equally, then the bone conduction is equal on both sides.
- In presence of increased hearing on one side, that side has conduction deafness. As a result of conduction deafness, the environmental noise is lesser and thus hears better through conduction of bone.
- In presence of nerve deafness, the subject hears better on the healthy side.

2. Describe the tuning fork tests to assess deafness

- There are three important tuning fork tests.
- They use either 256 Hz or 512 Hz tuning forks.
- Air conduction is normal conduction of sound through the tympanic membrane, ossicles and stimulation of organ of Corti.
- Bone conduction is conduction of sound through the skull to the bony cochlea and organ of Corti.
- Normally, air conduction is better than bone conduction.
  1. **Rinne's test**
     - In this test, a tuning fork is set in motion by striking against the examiner's palm and placed on the patient's mastoid process.
     - The patient hears the sound through bone conduction.
     - After the sound stops, the tuning fork is taken closely to the external auditory meatus.

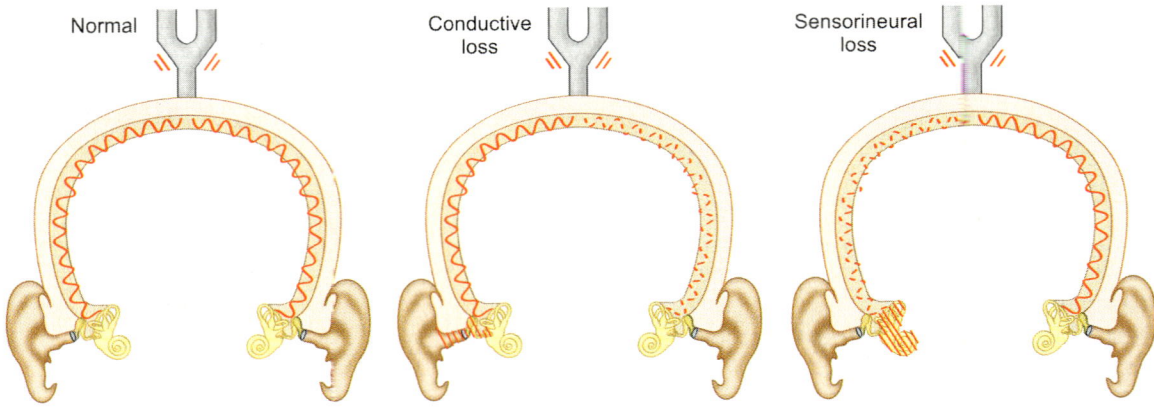

Normal　　　Conductive loss　　　Sensorineural loss

Fig. 10.67

– There is re-appearance of sound as air conduction is better than bone conduction.
– The time duration for which the sound heard is recorded.
– The same is repeated in the other ear.

Results

o *Normal:* Air conduction is more than bone conduction
o *Conductive hearing loss:* Air conduction is lesser than bone conduction.
o *Nerve deafness:* Both air conduction and bone conduction are decreased.

2. **Weber's test**

– This is a test to compare bone conduction in both ears of the patient.
– The desired (lower frequency first) tuning fork is chosen and thrust at the palm to set it in motion.
– It is placed the forehead of the patient without coming in contact with the forks.
– The patient is asked whether he can hear both the sounds equally.

Results

o If he hears equally, then the bone conduction is equal on both sides.
o In presence of increased hearing on one side, that side has conduction deafness. As a result of conduction deafness, the environmental noise is lesser and thus hears better through conduction of bone.
o In presence of nerve deafness, the subject hears better on the healthy side.

3. **Schwabach's test**

– In this test, subject's bone conduction is compared with that of the examiner-assuming the examiner has healthy hearing.
– Set the tuning fork into vibration as before and place its base on the subject's mastoid process.

– Ask the patient to indicate, by raising his hand, when the sound stops.
– After the subject stops hearing the sound, the tuning fork is placed on the examiner's mastoid process.

Results

o If he hears it longer than the patient, the patient as deafness.
o If the examiner hears the tuning fork better, the patient has nerve deafness.
o If the patient hears the tuning fork longer, he has conductive deafness as there is better bone conduction.

SHORT ANSWERS

1. Describe the types of deafness and some common causes.

Types of Deafness

Deafness is mainly of two types.

Common Causes

1. **Conductive deafness:** Deafness is caused by pathology in the external ear or middle ear.

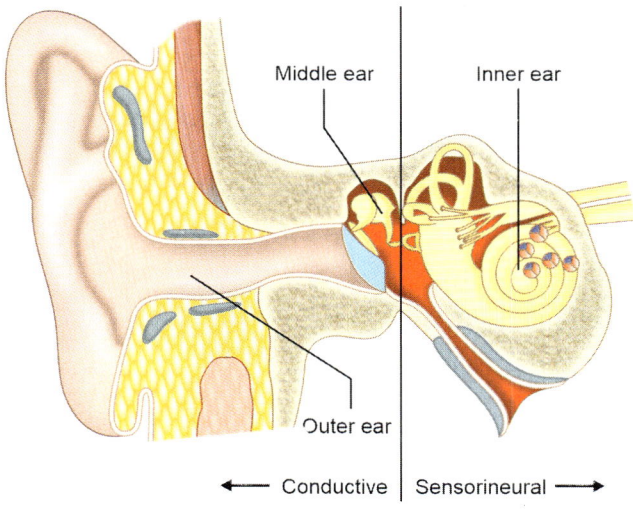

Fig. 10.68

Test	Normal	Conductive hearing loss	Sensorineural hearing loss
Rinne test	AC > BC		
Rinne +ve	BC > AC		
Rinne –ve	AC > BC in partial deafness		
Weber's test	Not lateralized	Lateralized towards affected ear	Lateralized towards healthy ear
Schwabach test	Equal	Better conduction in patient	Better conduction in examiner

Causes

- External ear causes
  - Increased cerumen or wax in the external ear
  - Otitis externa
  - Foreign body in external auditory meatus
  - Perforation of tympanic membrane
- Middle ear causes
  - Otitis media
  - Foreign body in middle ear
  - Middle ear malformation

2. **Sensorineural deafness**

- Deafness due to inner ear causes and central causes
- Presbycusis (age-related)
- Noise-induced hearing loss
- Temporal bone fracture
- Meniere's disease
- Labyrinthitis
- Acoustic neuroma
- Malignancies involving the eighth nerve.

2. Explain audiometry and its indications.

- It is defined as measurement of auditory acuity or sharpness of hearing.
- Audiometry is a technique used to determine the type of hearing loss and its severity
- It consists of an electronic oscillator (which generates a wide range of pure tones or frequency),

an intensity dial (to adjust the threshold intensity) and headphone to deliver the frequencies to each ear separately.

- Pure tone audiometry is a method by which thresholds are tested for air conduction and bone conduction for a varying range of frequencies.
- It is so calibrated that the hearing for air conduction and bone conduction is at 0 dB and there is no gap or difference between the two.
- The amount of intensity raised above the threshold for that particular frequency to be heard correlates with the degree of hearing loss.
- Threshold for bone conduction is a measure of cochlear function. Difference between air and bone conduction threshold gives a measure of conductive deafness.

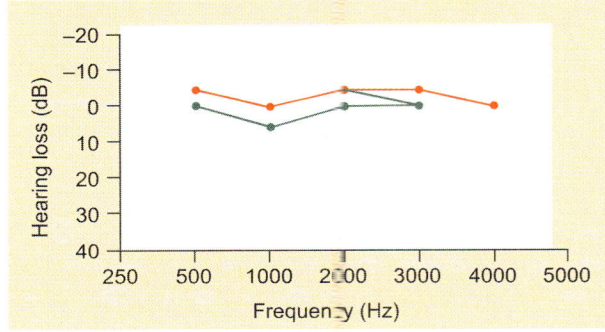

Fig. 10.59

10.17 DESCRIBE AND DISCUSS FUNCTIONAL ANATOMY OF EYE, PHYSIOLOGY OF IMAGE FORMATION, PHYSIOLOGY OF VISION INCLUDING COLOUR VISION, REFRACTIVE ERRORS, COLOUR BLINDNESS, PHYSIOLOGY OF PUPIL AND LIGHT REFLEX

SHORT ESSAYS

1. Describe accommodation reflex

- Accommodation is a process by which divergent rays coming from a near object are converged at a point on the retina with the help of ciliary body, zonules, lens and the pupillary aperture.
- This reflex is necessary to focus proximal objects.
- It is a part of near reflex, which involves convergence of both eyes, miosis and accommodation (Figs 10.70 and 10.71).

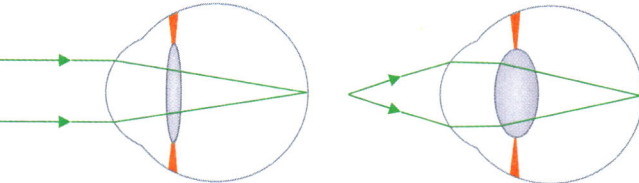

Fig. 10.70

> When rays coming from a proximal object enter the retina. impulses travel along the optic nerve, optic chiasma, optic tract, lateral geniculate body, and visual cortex.
>
> ↓
>
> From the visual cortex, impulses travel to the frontal eye field via the superior longitudinal fasciculus
>
> ↓
>
> The impulses now are conducted to the Edinger-Westphal nucleus and III nerve nucleus through the corticonuclear fibers.
>
> ↓
>
> The parasympathetic fibers from here carry these impulses to the ciliary muscles, and then to the ciliary muscles.
>
> ↓
>
> Von Helmholtz theory: At rest, the lens surface is kept flat by taut zonules, maintaining a large ciliary ring.

2. Describe how aqueous humor is formed and drained. List and describe the different types of glaucoma. (1 + 1 + 3 marks)

Synthesis of Aqueous Humor

- Aqueous is optically clear fluid that occupies the anterior segment, including anterior (0.25 ml) and the posterior (0.06 ml) chamber.
- It is secreted by the ciliary body, enters the posterior chamber, passes through the pupil to reach anterior chamber, and drained out through the angle of anterior chamber.

Production (Fig. 10.72)

- It is secreted from the pars plicata of the ciliary body.
- Each villus has a vascular core with fibrous core.
- Aqueous is formed by diffusion, ultrafiltration, and active secretion. The rate of formation is 2.3 µl/min.

Drainage of Aqueous Humor

- The aqueous flow out into the venous system of the eye through the angle of the anterior chamber.
- The angle is formed at intersection of the cornea and the root of iris. The aqueous is drained by the following two ways:
  1. **Conventional pathway:** Trabecular meshwork → Schlemm's canal → collector channels → aqueous veins → episcleral veins (90% drainage) (Fig. 10.73).
  2. **Uveoscleral pathway:** Anterior chamber → suprachoroidal space → veins of choroid and sclera (10% drainage).

| Contraction of ciliary body | Laxity of the zonules | Increase in anterior curvature of lens | Increase in converging power of lens |

Fig. 10.71

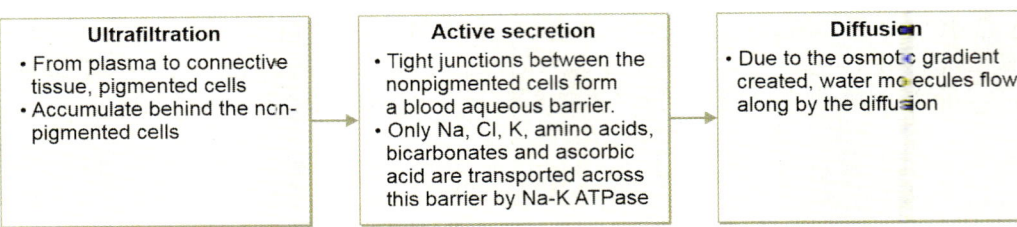

Ultrafiltration	Active secretion	Diffusion
• From plasma to connective tissue, pigmented cells • Accumulate behind the non-pigmented cells	• Tight junctions between the nonpigmented cells form a blood aqueous barrier. • Only Na, Cl, K, amino acids, bicarbonates and ascorbic acid are transported across this barrier by Na-K ATPase	• Due to the osmotic gradient created, water molecules flow along by the diffusion

Fig. 10.72

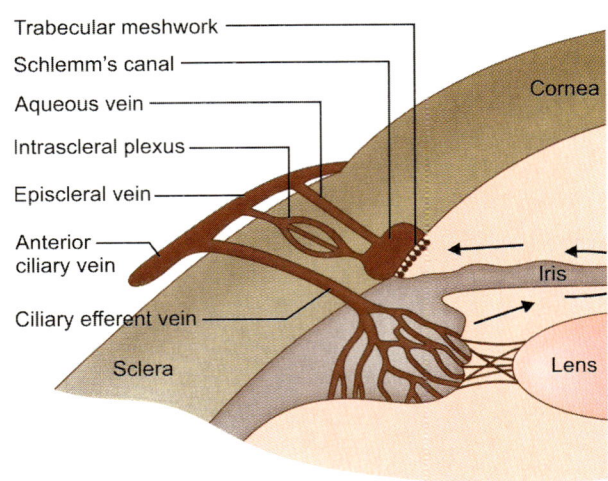

Fig. 10.73

Glaucoma (Table 10.3)

- It is a group of disorders causing optic neuropathy resulting from raised intraocular pressure.
- It is an important cause of irreversible blindness.
- It is classified as in Table 10.3.

3. Describe phototransduction of vision.

Phototransduction

- The rods and cones are the two photoreceptors that serve as sensory nerve endings for visual sensation.

- When light falls on the retina leads to a cascade of photochemical changes which in turn trigger biochemical reactions that result in generation of electrical changes.

Structure of Rods and Cones

- The rods have a cylindrical outer segment and are longer, whereas the cones have a conical outer segment.
- The outer segment contains regularly stacked discs containing rhodopsin and retinal. In cones, such discs are present as in pouching of the cell membrane and it contains photopsin and retinal.
- The inner segment contains the cell body, mitochondria and Golgi body.
- The synaptic ending comes into contact with the bipolar cells. There 120 million rods and 6.5 million cones in one eye.

Photochemical Changes (Figs 10.74 and 10.75)

- Rhodopsin exists as a combination of a colorless protein called opsin coupled with a carotenoid called retinene (vitamin A aldehyde or 11-*cis*-retinal).
- When light falls on the rods, there is conversion of 11-*cis*-retinal component of rhodopsin into all-trans-retinal through various stages.

Table 10.3		
Congenital glaucoma	*Angle closure glaucoma*	*Open angle glaucoma*
• It is an inherited condition due to developmental anomaly of the angle of the anterior chamber • As a result, there is decreased outflow • The eye is enlarged in a child and is referred to as buphthalmos or bull's eye. • The cornea is hazy due to entry of aqueous into the cornea due to breaks in Descemet's membrane	• It can be primary or secondary • It occurs in adults • It is due to decreased depth of the angle of anterior chamber • As a result, there is decreased aqueous drainage and a sharp rise in intraocular pressure. • It is very painful • This causes damage to the ganglion cells and finally atrophy of the optic nerve.	• The depth of the angle is fair enough but there is damage at the trabecular meshwork due to many reasons. • As a result, there is a slow development of increased intraocular pressure • It is asymptomatic condition and there is gradual loss of vision

- The all-*trans*-retinal so formed gets separated from the opsin. (photodecomposition) and this process is called rhodopsin bleaching.
- It is followed by rhodopsin regeneration. It is formed by 11-*cis*-retinal is regenerated from the all-*trans*-retinal separated from the opsin (as described above) and vitamin A (retinal) supplied from the blood. The 11-*cis*-retinal then reunites with opsin in the rod outer segment to form the rhodopsin.
- Bleaching of the rhodopsin occurs under the influence of light, whereas the regeneration process is independent of light.
- Inner segment has an active Na^+ pump which keeps pumping out Na, whereas the outer segment is leaky to Na^+ ions.
- A resting potential of –40 mV is maintained in the rods.
- When there is a configurational change in opsin, the Na+ channels in the outer segments close as a result of inhibition of cGMP.
- There is a hyperpolarization created, which leads to reduced release of synaptic transmitter and then carried further by the bipolar cells.

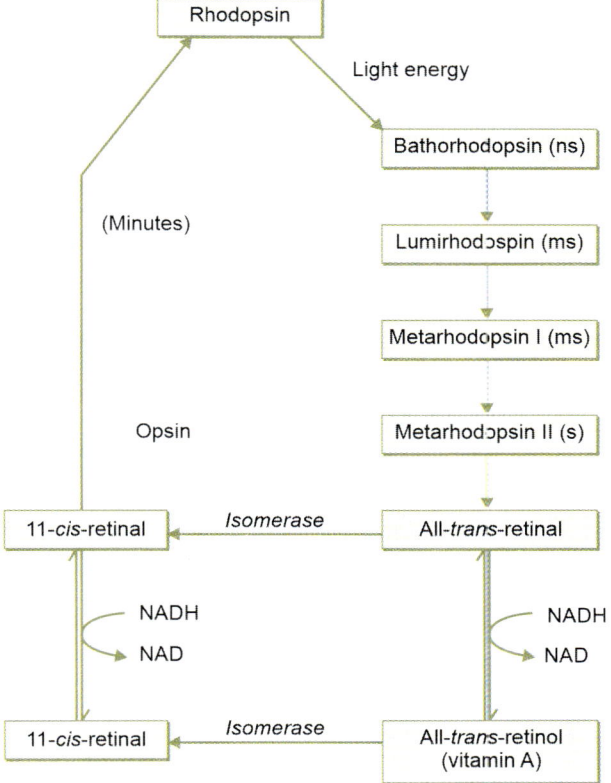

Fig. 10.74

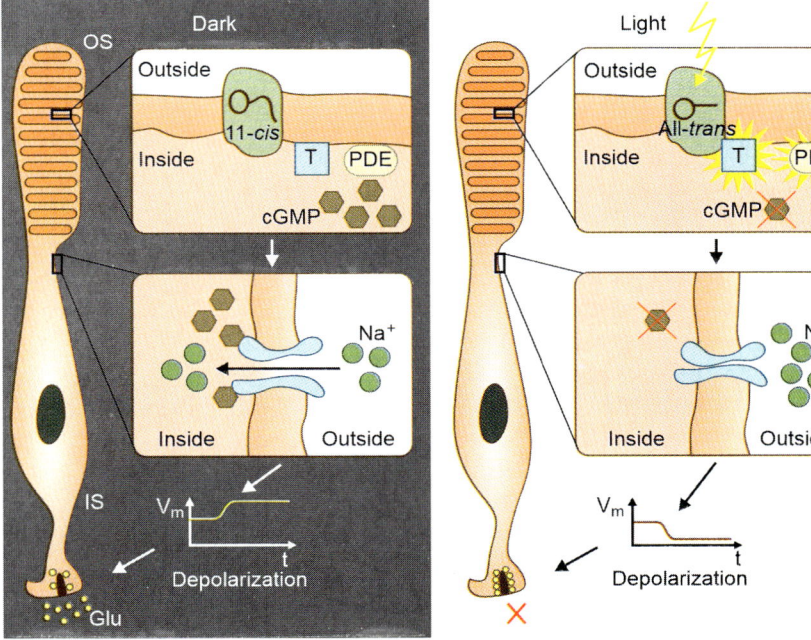

Fig. 10.75

4. A 25-year-old male entered a movie theatre in the afternoon. For about a minute he found it difficult to see the chair numbers and people around. What could be the cause of this loss of vision? What happens after some time that he regains his vision?

The condition is dark adaptation.

Dark Adaptation

- When an individual enters a dark room from a bright room, he/she takes some time to see. This is called dark adaptation time. Its duration is about 20 minutes.
- Dark adaptation is the ability of the eye to habituate itself to sudden dim illumination after being exposed to a significant period of bright light.

Mechanisms that Operate in Dark Adaptation

1. **Dilatation of pupil**
   - It is an immediate response due to abolition of light reflex.
   - This allows more and more light to enter the eye.
2. **Increased sensitivity of rods to dim light**
   - This is the time required for regeneration of rhodopsin
   - During this period, the sensitivity increases 10,000 folds and there is Purkinje shift to sensitivity to blue from sensitivity to red.

After Vision Regain

After the time for dark adaptation has elapsed, the individual is comfortable and can view things around him.

5. An 18-year-old female wanted to be a pilot. During the pre-training medical test, she was unable to identify all the numbers shown in Ishihara's colour chart and her application was thus rejected. She was never tested before using these charts. What is the disorder she has? What is the cause of this disorder? What is Young-Helmholtz theory? (1 + 2 + 2 marks)

The disorder is:
- This patient has congenital colour blindness.
- Since Ishihara chart is used to identify red–green color blindness, this patient has red–green blindness.

Cause for Congenital Colour Blindness

- It is inherited as an X-linked recessive inherited disorder. The genes for the red and green sensitive cones are in q arm of X chromosome and hence transmitted through the mother.
- The female, however, behaves as a carrier. She may manifest the disease if both alleles are affected.
- Due to the defective gene, cones specific for the same color are not produced and thus they are not perceived by the individual leading to color blindness.

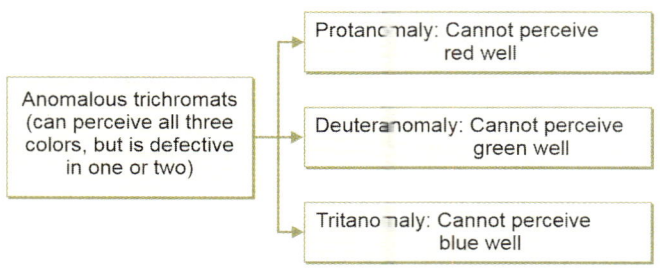

Fig. 10.76

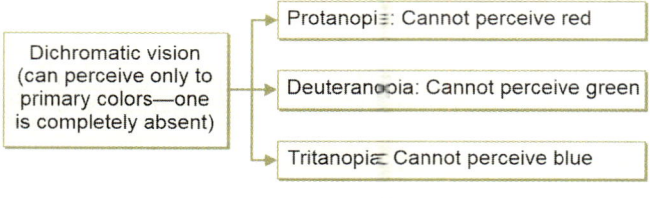

Fig. 10.77

Young-Helmholtz Theory or Trichromatic Theory

- It was put forth by Young and then modified by Helmholtz. They suggested that there are three kinds of cones, each sensitive to a different wavelength.
- The primary colors—red, green, and blue are identified by each type of cone. The sensation of a given color is determined by the relative frequency of each of the cone systems.
  - *Red sensitive cone pigment* (erythrolabe): Absorbs wavelengths of 565 mm.
  - *Green sensitive cone pigment* (chlorolabe): Absorbs wavelengths of 535 nm.
  - *Blue sensitive cone pigment* (cyanolabe): Absorbs wavelengths of 440 nm.

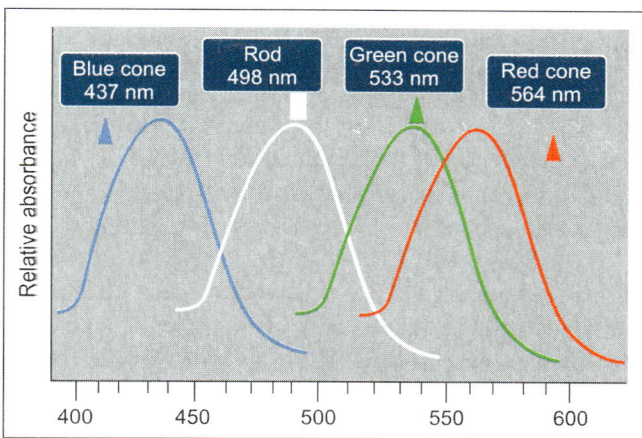

Fig. 10.78

6. Describe central mechanism of vision.

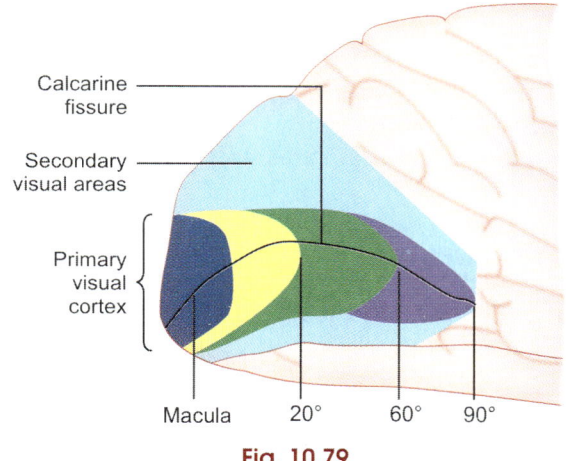

Fig. 10.79

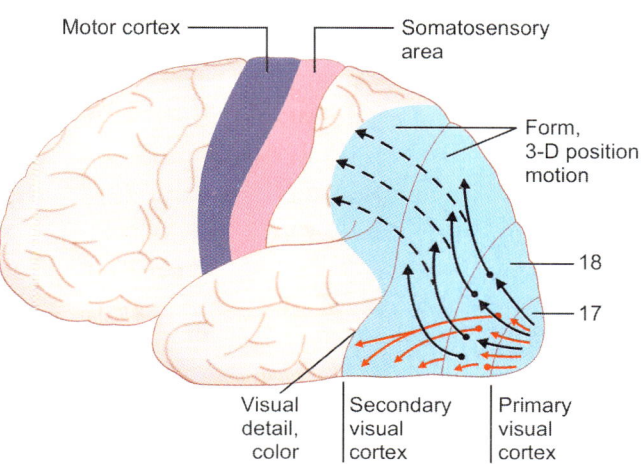

Fig. 10.80

Central Mechanism of Vision

- The lateral geniculate body receives fibres through optic tract and send out impulses through optic radiation. It helps in accurate relay of visual impulses from each eye and gating of impulses to the cortex based on a feedback from reticular areas and mesencephalon.
- The final processing occurs in the visual cortex. This is called visual processing.
- It is an integration of various forms of impulses received by the cortex in the form of light sense, form sense, sense of contrast and colour sense.

Organization of Visual Cortex (Figs 10.79 and 10.80)

1. **Primary visual cortex**
- Also called striate cortex or visual area 1.
- It lies along the calcarine fissure, extending forward from the tip of the occipital lobe on the medial aspect.
- It forms the termination of visual impulses from all points on the retina. signals from macula occupies central and a proportionally large area. It is responsible for visual acuity. It also has highest number of neurons representing the macula.
- Signals from the rest of the periphery terminate in concentric circle around the macular area.
- The representation of retina is reversed, that is, superior part is represented in the lower part of the cortex and vice versa.

2. **Secondary visual cortex**
- It is also called visual association area, peristriate area or visual area 2. It lies anterior, superior, lateral and inferior to the primary visual area.
- They are spread over the lateral aspect of the occipital lobe and the parietal lobe.

Organization of Fibres in the Cortex

- The optic radiation fibres end in the layer IV of the occipital cortex from the corresponding retinae.
- The images formed by the impulses are analysed by two types of cells: Magnocellular and parvocellular pathways. The magnocellular pathway is responsible for detection of form and movement of objects and is conducted through the "Y" ganglia of the retina, where the parvocellular pathway is responsible for colour and fine accuracy of the objects and is conducted through the "X" ganglia of the retina.

- The nerve fibres in the cortex are organized into many vertical columns and each column is taken as a unit.
- Amongst the visual columns are interspersed, colour blobs—they are associated with deciphering of colour sense.
- Finally, there is interspersing of fibers between the columns of the occipital cortex of one eye with the other which helps in forming the concept of 'cyclopean eye' and the concept of binocular singular vision.

Hyper Columns in the Striate Cortex

- The striate cortex is organised into multiple vertical columns, called hyper columns, each housing a number of neurons.
- Each unit is responsible for processing information from one part of retina.
- Each hyper column consists of three types of vertical columns—orientation columns, ocular dominance columns and colour blobs.
- The orientation columns are highly orderly organization of neurons which help in processing information from every part of the visual field and helps in orientation.
- The ocular dominance columns help in attaining binocularity and the color blobs are helpful in deciphering colour.

7. Explain theories of color vision. List the types of color blindness and the methods used to test them.   (2.5 + 1.5 + 1 marks)

Theories of Colour Vision

1. **Trichromatic theory of Young and Helmholtz**
   - They suggested that there are three kinds of cones, each sensitive to a different wavelength.
   - The primary colors—red, green and blue are identified by each type of cone.
   - Stimulation of that particular cone gives perception of that particular color sense.
   - Red sensitive cone pigment (erythrolabe): Absorbs wavelengths of 565 mm.
   - Green sensitive cone pigment (chlorolabe): Absorbs wavelengths of 535 nm.
   - Blue sensitive cone pigment (cyanolabe): Absorbs wavelengths of 440 nm.

2. **Opponent theory of Hering**
   - The opponent color theory says that some colors 'mutually exclusive'.
   - Cones are linked together as pairs. Stimulation of one lead to inhibition of the other.
   - They cannot form a color together.
   - When a cone is stimulated with green color, it inhibits red and when stimulated with wavelength of blue, yellow cones are inhibited.
   - They are red–green and blue–yellow.
   - This theory is applicable at the ganglion cell level.
   - This theory helps us understand congenital dyschromatopsia which usually affect the red–green system or blue–yellow system.

3. **Polychromatic theory**
   - Modern day theory proposed by Granit
   - Dominators are nerve fibers and cones have a wide spectrum of sensitivity (respond to all wavelengths) and thus help in perception of black and white.
   - Modulator nerve fibres are necessary for hue detection.
   - There are 7 receptors—one for each color of the VIBGYOR.

Types of Colour Blindness

1. **Congenital color blindness:** It is seen more in males.

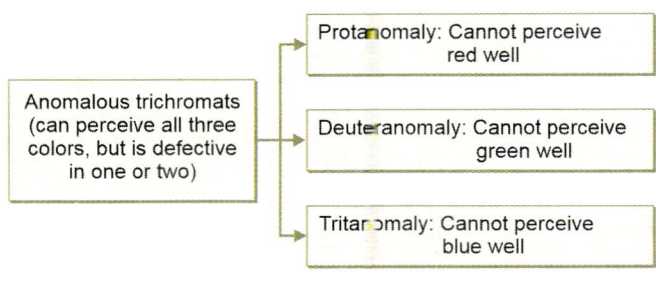

Fig. 10.81

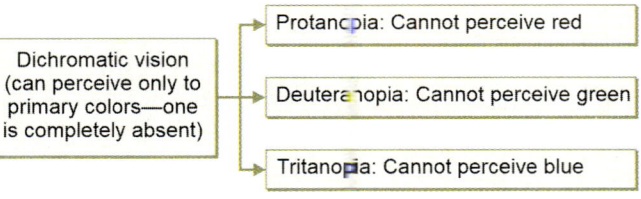

Fig. 10.82

- Achromatopsia: Only one primary color can be perceived. It can be cone monochromatism, characterized by perception of only one color. Rod monochromatism is characterized by total color blindness, day blindness (vision <6/60) and nystagmus.

2. **Acquired color blindness**
   - *Blue–yellow impairment:* Macular pathology like CSR, macular oedema and shallow retinal detachment.
   - *Red–green deficiency:* Optic neuritis, Leber's optic atrophy and compression of the optic nerve.
   - *Blue colour defect (blue blindness):* Dense cataract absorbing blue light.

Tests for Colour Blindness

1. Ishihara's pseudoisochromatic charts
2. Naegel's anomaloscope
3. Edridge green lantern test
4. Farnsworth-Munsell 100 hue test
5. Holmgren's wool test

SHORT ANSWERS

1. What are Purkinje-Sanson images?

- Purkinje-Sanson images are the reflections of an object formed from the structures of the eye.
- Normally four such images are formed:
  1. Anterior surface of cornea
  2. Posterior surface of cornea
  3. Anterior surface of lens
  4. Posterior surface of lens

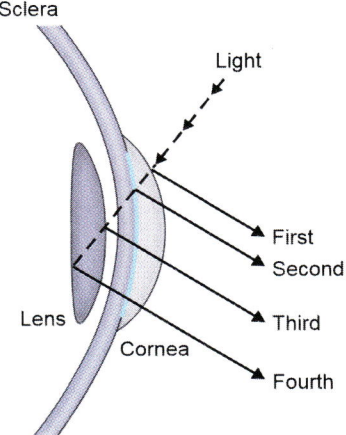

Fig. 10.83

Practical Utility

They are used in eye-tracking procedures.

2. Explain Listing's reduced eye.

- Listing introduced the concept of reduced eye to calculate the total power of the human eye.
- Listing and Gauss's schematic eye had 6 cardinal points.
- Accordingly, the human eye has two principal foci, one nodal point and one principal point.

Total dioptric power of the eye	+60 D
Anterior focal point	15.7 mm in front of the anterior surface of cornea
Posterior focal point	24.4 mm behind the anterior surface of cornea
Principal point	1.5 mm behind the anterior surface of cornea
Nodal point	7.2 mm behind the anterior surface of cornea (posterior capsule of the lens)
Anterior focal length	15.7 mm + 1.5 mm = 17.2 mm
Posterior focal point	24.4 mm – 1.5 mm = 22.9 mm

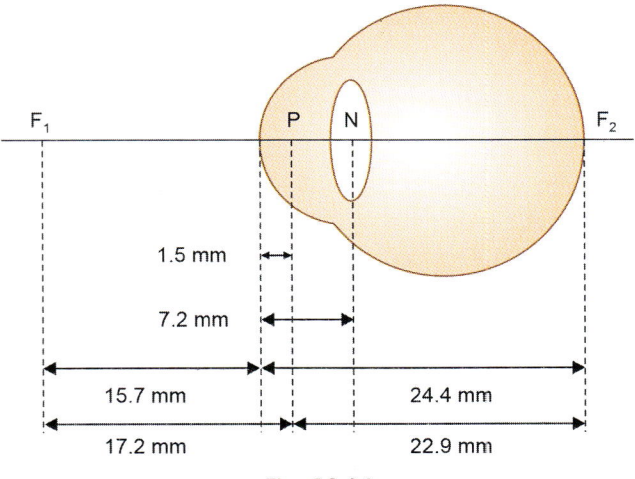

Fig. 10.84

3. List the errors of refraction and how it can be corrected.

Refractive Errors and Correction

These are conditions of the eye where an object cannot be brought to focus at a point on the macula with accommodation being at rest.

Refractive error	Correction
Myopia	
• It is a condition where rays coming from an object of interest from infinity are focussed at a point in front of the retina, with accommodation being at rest	Concave lenses as spectacle and contact lenses
• The converging power of the eye is high	
Hypermetropia	
• It is a condition where rays coming from an object of interest from infinity are focussed at a point behind the retina, with accommodation being at rest	Convex lenses in the form of spectacles or contact lenses
Astigmatism	
• It is a condition where rays coming from an object of interest from infinity are focussed along a line either in front of or behind the retina or both, with accommodation being at rest	Cylindrical lenses in the form of spectacles or contact lenses

4. What is Argyll-Robertson pupil?

• It is characterized dissociation of light and near reflex; light reflex is absent and near reflex is present.
• it was previously known as prostitute's pupil as it was caused by neurosyphilis.

Causes

• It is due to lesion in the region of tectum and was frequently seen as an association of neurosyphilis.

• It can also be seen in demyelinating disorders.
• Encephalitis
• Diabetes
• Wernicke's encephalopathy

Clinical Features

• Both pupils are affected asymmetrically.
• As a result, there is anisocoria or unequal pupils which do not constrict to light.

5. What is the reflex pathway for conjunctival reflex?

Conjunctival Reflex

• It is bilateral blinking response caused by stimulating the conjunctiva with a thin wisp of cotton.
• It is a protective response.

Pathway (Fig. 10.85)

• When the conjunctiva is stimulated with a wisp of cotton, sensory impulses are conducted through the ophthalmic division of the trigeminal nerve
• It relays in the pons
• The efferent travel from the facial nucleus to the orbicularis oculi muscles
• There is bilateral blinking of the eyelids.

6. What are ocular dominance columns?

Ocular Dominance Columns

• The striate cortex is organised into multiple vertical columns, called hypercolumns, each housing a number of neurons.

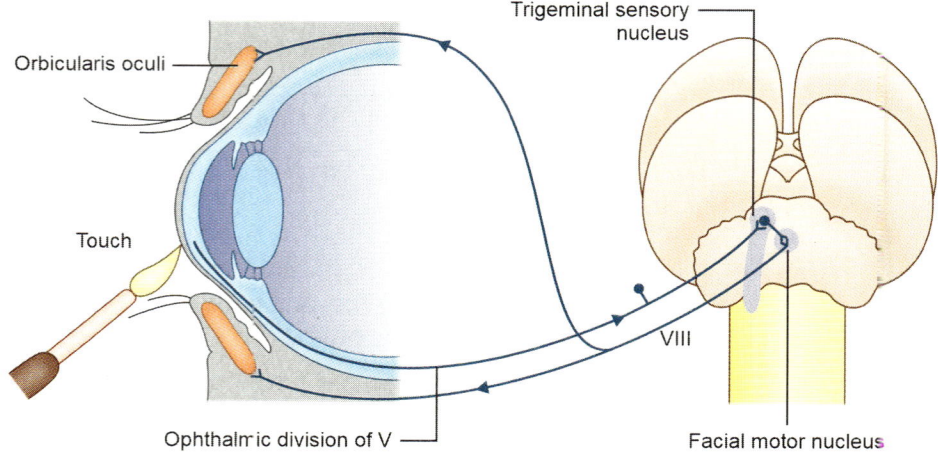

Fig. 10.85

- Each unit is responsible for processing information from one part of retina.
- Each hypercolumn consists of three types of vertical columns—orientation columns, ocular dominance columns and colour blobs.
- Ocular dominance columns are an independent system of columns in the visual cortex.
- They are associated with processing of binocular information.
- Though there is binocularity, there is to an extent, monocular dominance. Thus, the dominant eye may have more ocular dominance columns in the striate cortex. Around 75% of the population have right eye dominance. The knowledge of this lays an important role in providing patient satisfaction in some types of ocular surgeries.
- These columns may play a role in stereoscopy or three-dimensional vision.

7. Why do we observe macular sparing despite of lesion in geniculocalcarine radiation?

Macular Sparing (Fig. 10.86)

- The geniculocalcarine radiation is also known as optic radiation.
- In the posterior visual pathways, whenever there is occlusion to the blood flow, occipital infarct results in a congruent homonymous hemianopia with macular sparing.

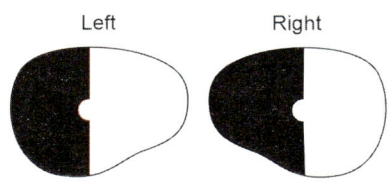

Fig. 10.86

- The reasons for this are:
1. Macula has a very large area of representation in the occipital cortex.
2. Macula has bilateral representation into the visual cortex, i.e. fibres of right macula relay in left and right occipital area and those from left macula also relay in left and right occipital cortex.
3. The collateral blood flow in the later is very strong. The anterior part is through the anterior choroidal artery and posterior is through the posterior choroidal artery. So, in cases of an ischemic event, blood flow is always restored unless the ischemia is global.

8. What is indirect light reflex? How is it elicited?

Indirect or Consensual Light Reflex (Fig. 10.87)

Simultaneous constriction of pupil of the contralateral eye when light is shone on the retina of the ipsilateral eye.

Method of Eliciting an Indirect Light Reflex

- A card is held between the two eyes so that when light is shone on one eye it does not fall on the other.
- A source of light is brought from the temporal side of, say right eye, and the pupil of the left eye is looked at.
- There is simultaneous constriction of pupil.

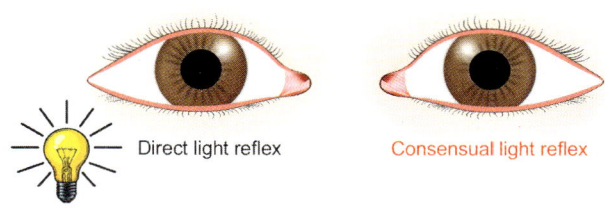

Direct light reflex   Consensual light reflex

Fig. 10.87

10.18 DESCRIBE AND DISCUSS THE PHYSIOLOGICAL BASIS OF LESION IN VISUAL PATHWAY

LONG ESSAY

1. **Draw a neat-labelled diagram of visual pathway. Describe disorders of visual fields in relation to the visual pathway.** (5 + 5 marks)

Anatomy of the Visual Pathway

- Retina → Optic nerve → Optic chiasm → Optic tract → Lateral geniculate body → Optic radiation → Visual cortex.

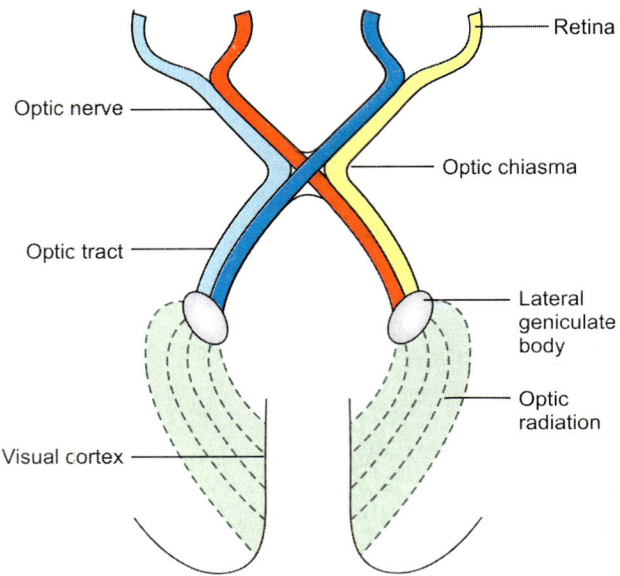

Fig. 10.88

Lesions of the Visual Pathway and Resultant Defects

Lesion at	Causes	Signs	
Optic nerve	Inflammatory Trauma Infectious Compressive Infiltrative	Visual acuity drops Dyschromatopsia Afferent pupillary defect Field loss: Central scotoma: Macular affection Centrocecal: Macula + optic nerve Altitudinal or complete	*Left central scotoma* *Left altitudinal*

Lesion at	Causes	Signs	
Lesions just anterior to optic chiasm	In a post-fixed chiasma, pituitary lesions can compress anterior fibres	Junctional scotoma characterized by ipsilateral complete loss of visual field with contralateral incomplete temporal hemianopia	*Junctional scotoma due to involvement of left optic nerve*
Sagittal lesions at the chiasm	Suprasellar aneurysms, pituitary tumors, craniopharyngioma, suprasellar meningioma, third ventricular dilatation, secondary to hydrocephalus	Bitemporal hemianopia, bitemporal hemianopic loss of pupillary reflexes	*Bitemporal hemianopia*
Lateral lesions at chiasm	Meningiomas, aneurysm of posterior communicating arteries	Binasal hemianopia, binasal hemianopic loss of pupillary reflexes	*Binasal hemianopia*
Optic tract	Syphilitic meningitis, aneurysm of posterior cerebral arteries	Incongruous ipsilateral homonymous hemianopia with contralateral hemianopic pupillary reaction Optic atrophy	*Left-sided lesion*
Lateral geniculate body		Incongruous ipsilateral homonymous hemianopia Pupil spared, partial optic atrophy	*Right-sided lesion, left homonymous hemianopia*
Optic radiation	Tumors, vascular lesions, tumours	Complete homonymous hemianopia Superior quadrantanopia—temporal lobe lesions Inferior quadrantanopia in parietal lobe lesions No loss of pupil reflex No optic atrophy	*Right temporal lobe lesion, left upper quadrantanopia* *Right parietal lesion, left lower quadrantanopia*

Lesion at	Causes	Signs	
Visual cortex	Cortex: Ischemic, trauma, tumors Tip of cortex: Ischemic	Congruous homonymous hemianopia with pupil sparing. Macular homonymous hemianopia May be associated with 'Anton's syndrome'	 *Right cortex lesion, left-sided homonymous hemianopia with macular sparing* *Right tip of occipital cortex lesion*

10.19 DESCRIBE AND DISCUSS AUDITORY AND VISUAL EVOKE POTENTIALS

SHORT ANSWER

1. Discuss the physiological basis and indications of auditory and visually evoked potentials.

Auditory Evoked Potentials

Also called brainstem auditory evoked response (BAER).

Physiological Basis (Fig. 10.89)

- It measures the function of the auditory nerves and pathway
- It is an objective test where the patient is sedated or anaesthetised and sound I is produced in the ear,
- Standard broadband monaural click is used to stimulate the ears and potential is recorded at the brainstem (upper pons) which is the site of reception of impulses.
- It consists of 5 waves:
  1. **Wave 1:** Action potential of VIII nerve
  2. **Wave 2:** Cochlear nucleus
  3. **Wave 3:** Ipsilateral superior olivary nucleus
  4. **Wave 4:** Lateral lemniscus
  5. **Wave 5:** Inferior colliculus

Indications

1. Rule out hearing pathologies in an infant or mentally challenged or comatose patient.
2. Screening for multiple sclerosis and acoustic neuroma.

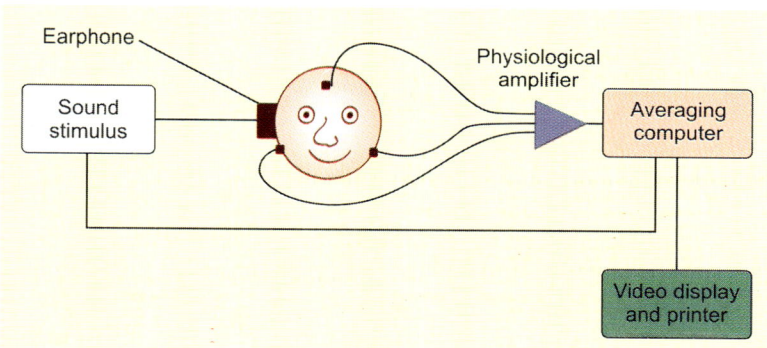

Fig. 10.89

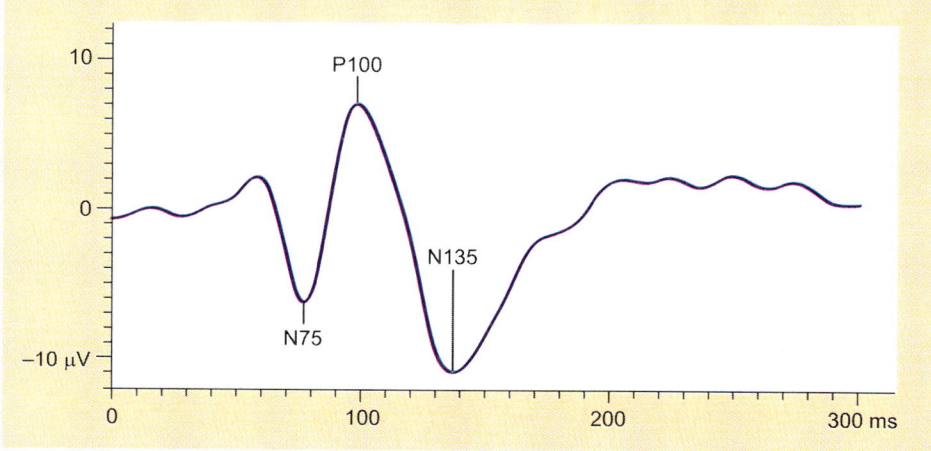

Fig. 10.90

Visually Evoked Potentials

Physiological Basis (Fig. 10.90)

- It is the potential recorded at the occipital cortex when there is an image projected on the retina.
- This principle is used to understand the integrity of the visual pathway when the subjective tests may not be useful.
- The subject is shown a flash of light or a pattern. Based on these, it is said to be flash VEP or pattern VEP.
- The normal visual evoked potential is marked by a period of latency which is the delay which occurs for the light impulse to travel to the cortex.
- Then there is a negative wave at 75 ms and a positive wave at 100 ms.
- The positive wave at 100 ms is called P100. The amplitude is of clinical importance.

Indications

1. To test visual acuity in preverbal infants
2. To rule out malingering
3. To diagnose optic nerve disorders, to follow up (in demyelinating disorders, latency is increased)
4. For medicolegal cases (as it is an objective test).

10.20 DEMONSTRATE (I) TESTING OF VISUAL ACUITY, COLOUR AND FIELD OF VISION, (II) HEARING, (III) TESTING FOR SMELL AND (IV) TASTE SENSATION IN VOLUNTEER/SIMULATED ENVIRONMENT

SHORT ANSWER

1. Give the clinical implications of testing of visual acuity and field of vision.

Visual Acuity Test

- It is a test for assessing the form sense of the visual system—right from retina to the visual cortex.
- It is mainly to test the retinal function.
- It is the ability to differentiate two points separated from a minimum distance as separate.
- It is tested with the help of a Snellen's chart for distance and Jaeger's chart of near vision.
- Distance vision is tested at 6 metres and one eye at a time. Near vision is tested at 25 cm, one eye at a time.
- Normal visual acuity for distance is 6/6 or 20/20 and normal near vision is N6.
- Visual acuity is decreased in various refractive errors, corneal opacities, cataracts, and retinal and optic nerve pathologies.

Field of Vision

- It is defined as an island of vision surrounded by a sea of blindness.
- It is that part or space of the surrounding of an individual that can be seen by the individual.
- Normally, temporally the field is 100°, inferiorly 75°, nasally 60° and superiorly it is 60°.
- It is tested by confrontation method bedside.

- Perimetry is assessment of visual field and can be done by computerised methods.
- Scotoma is a non-seeing area within the visual field.
- Positive scotoma: Perception of a non-seeing dark area. Seen in macular disorders
- Negative scotoma: Non-perception of an area. It is usually not sensed by the patient. It is seen in neurological or visual pathway lesions.
- Causes of decreased field of vision
- Glaucoma: Arcuate scotoma, ring scotoma
- Retinitis pigmentosa—tunnel vision
- Neurological lesions—hemianopias

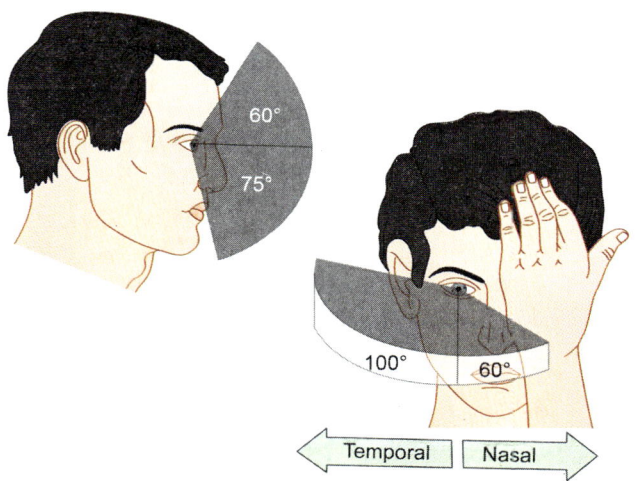

Fig. 10.91

Chapter

11

Integrated Physiology

11.1 DESCRIBE AND DISCUSS MECHANISM OF TEMPERATURE REGULATION

SHORT ESSAY

1. Define the normal range of body temperature. Discuss the modes of temperature regulating mechanism from the body. (2 + 3 marks)

Normal Range of Body Temperature

- It is defined for oral temperature
- Normal body temperature is 98.6° F or 37°C
- It ranges between 35.8 and 37.3°C or 96.4 and 99.1°F

When checked in axilla	0.5–1°F lower than oral
When checked in rectum	0.5–1°F higher than oral
Skin temperature or superficial temperature	85–93°F

Modes of Temperature Regulation (Fig. 11.1)

- It is regulated by various mechanisms of heat loss and heat preservation.
- It is brought about through several mechanisms which are controlled by the hypothalamus.
- The thermoregulatory system consists of thermoreceptors, a thermoregulatory centre and effector mechanisms.

Thermoreceptors

- These are receptors which detect temperature changes.

- They are of mainly two types:
  1. **Peripheral**
     - Cutaneous thermoreceptors detect changes in ambient outside temperature
     - Visceral thermoreceptors detect changes in core temperature.
  2. **Central**
     - These are present in the heat loss centre of the preoptic nucleus of the hypothalamus.

Temperature Regulation

1. **When body temperature increases**
   - When the temperature increases, the thermoreceptors are activated. They in turn activate the preoptic nucleus (heat loss center).
   - This causes heat loss and decreases in production of heat by various mechanisms.
   - By inhibition of the sympathetic system, there is cutaneous vasodilatation. This causes sweating and thus loss of heat through skin.
   - Also, there is inhibition of heat production by inhibition of shivering.
   - Panting is another way of losing heat in many animals.

2. **When body temperature drops**
   - Sympathetic system is activated.
   - There is reduced blood flow to skin.
   - Also, there is cutaneous vasoconstriction under the effect of sympathetic activation.

- Shivering is another effective mechanism by which heat is generated by stimulation of the primary motor cortex. Due to severe muscle contraction, enormous heat is generated.
- Also due to secretion of catecholamines, there is increase in metabolic processes.
- There is increase in production of thyroxine by the action of TRH and TSH. This causes increase in metabolic processes and generation of heat.
- Also, some behavioural changes are initiated like seeking out sources of heat, hyperphagia (excess eating to generate more heat) and hyperactivity (like rubbing of hands and feet).

SHORT ANSWERS

1. Explain the role of the skin in regulation of body temperature.

The skin has a large body surface area and thus can play an important role in thermoregulatory mechanisms.

When Body Temperature Increases

- Heat is lost from skin by radiation (transfer of heat from the body to another object through surrounding air), conduction (loss of heat through contact with another object) and convention (through surrounding gases). Heat loss from skin due to radiation is the most important mechanism and is up to 80% of total heat loss.
- Heat is also lost by evaporation or insensible loss of water.
- The heat loss from skin depends mainly on the temperature gradient between body and surrounding, amount of insulator subcutaneous fat and clothing.
- Under the influence of the hypothalamus, increased blood flows to the skin.
- There is cutaneous vasodilatation and dissipation of heat.
- Also, sweat glands are activated. With production of sweat and evaporation, a lot of heat is lost.

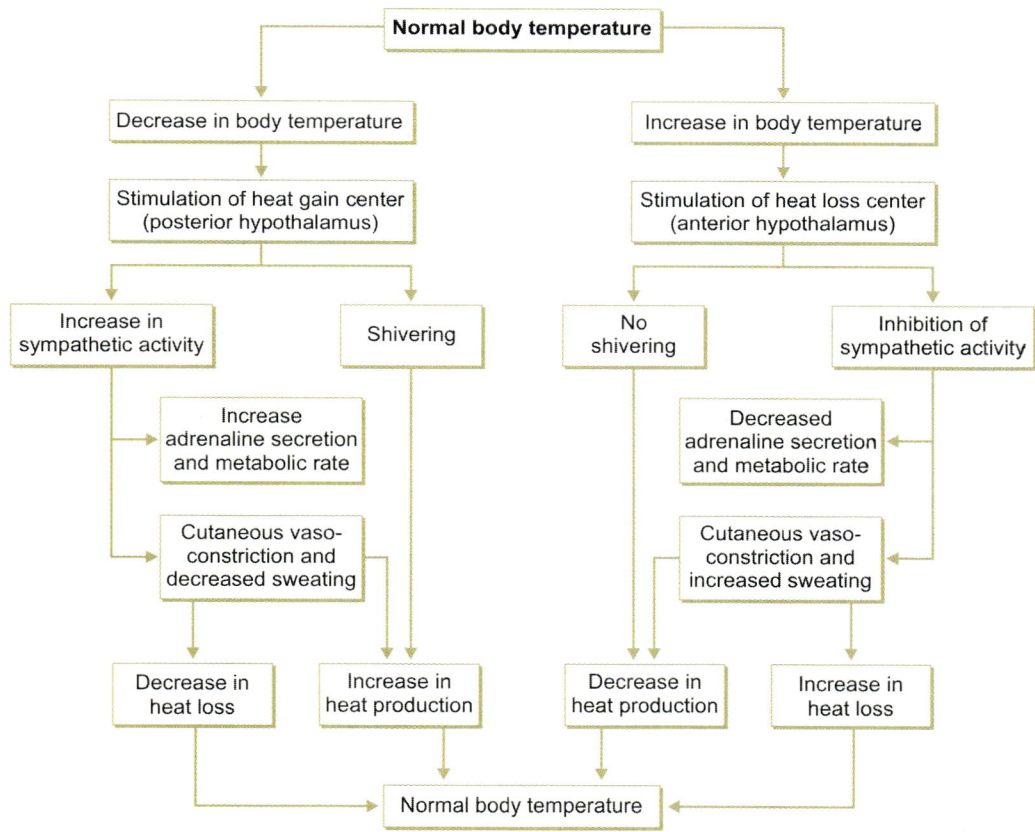

Fig. 11.1

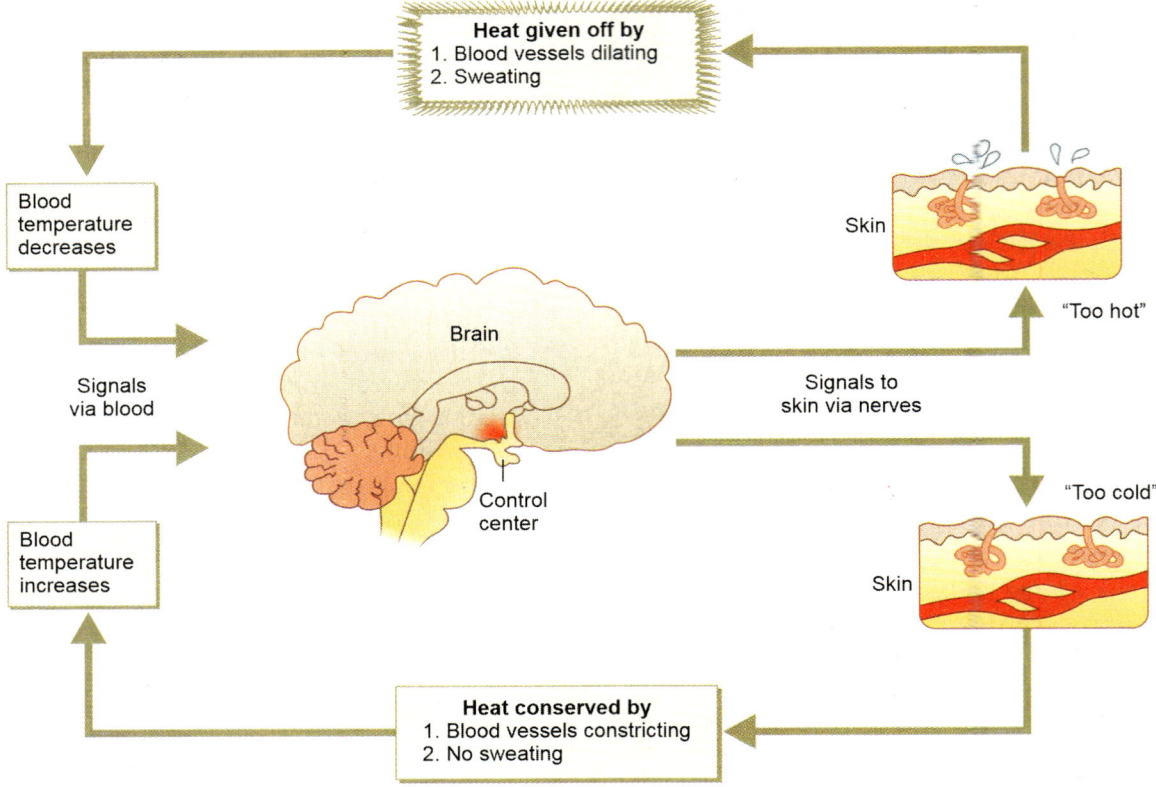

Fig. 11.2

When Body Temperature Decreases (Fig. 11.2)

- When the body temperature decreases, there is activation of the sympathetic system.
- This causes cutaneous vasoconstriction.
- The amount of blood flowing to the body surface is decreased.
- As a result, temperature is controlled.

2. Describe the function of hypothalamus as the thermostat of the body.

- Among many functions of hypothalamus, is temperature regulation.
- It functions as a thermostat.
- A temperature of 98.6°F is defined as "physiological normal" by the hypothalamus.
- Any temperature perceived by thermoreceptors above or below this set point is recognized as abnormal and mechanisms for heat regulation are set in.
- The hypothalamus receives afferents from the peripheral thermoreceptors and central thermoreceptors.

- Peripheral receptors include cutaneous thermoreceptors that detect changes in ambient outside temperature and visceral thermoreceptors detect changes in core temperature.
- Central receptors are present in the heat loss centre of the preoptic nucleus of the hypothalamus.
- The neurons in the anterior hypothalamus are mainly of two types: Heat loss centre and heat gain and conservation center.

Heat Loss Center

- Composed of neurons in the preoptic nucleus
- Stimulation of this area causes cutaneous vasodilatation, sweating, panting and inhibition of shivering.

Heat Production Center

- Stimulation of this area causes conservation of heat by cutaneous vasoconstriction
- Initiates shivering
- Stimulates release of thyroxine

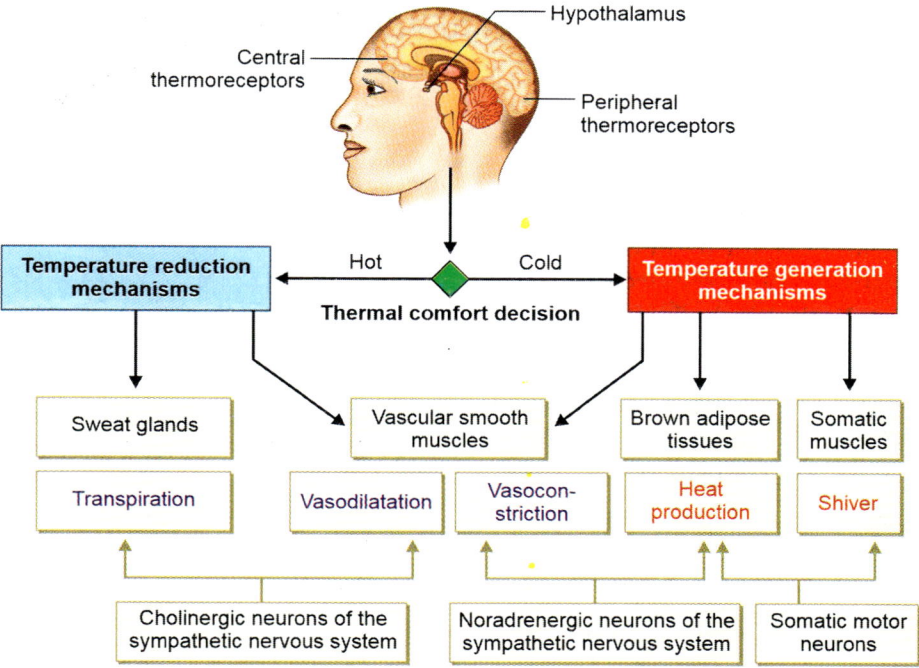

Fig. 11.3

11.2 DESCRIBE AND DISCUSS ADAPTATION TO ALTERED TEMPERATURE (HEAT AND COLD)

SHORT ESSAY

1. Describe the adaptive mechanisms in the body to higher and lower temperatures.

- When the body is exposed to either cold or warm temperature for a short term there are compensatory mechanisms which restore homeostasis in the form of cutaneous vasoconstriction, shivering and chemical heat generation and cutaneous vasodilatation, sweating respectively.
- When the exposure is prolonged, certain physiological changes take place.
- This process is called acclimatization.

Prolonged Exposure to Cold

- It is seen in people residing in the arctic and Southern parts of South America which are exposed to sub-zero temperatures throughout the year.
- They have warmer extremities and a higher core temperature.
- This is attributed to a higher basal metabolic rate almost 200% more than those living at higher temperatures.
- According to Bregmann's rules, there is difference in the body structure based on the climate. The individuals residing in colder climates have a bulkier body and those in warmer climate have a lean and small bodies. Also, it is noted that the people residing in colder climates have shorter extremities (Allen's rule) and thus there is lesser dissipation of heat.
- There is also change in blood flow patterns to various organs and fat insulation around organs to protect from cold.
- Also, some behavioral changes like consumption of high calorie food, drinking alcohol, setting a fire near vicinity, sleeping with bodies closely opposed with each other help in protecting from cold.

Prolonged Exposure to Heat

- These mechanisms are seen in humans residing in the central parts of Africa.
- These individuals have a slower metabolic rate.
- The quantity of salt in the sweat is far less compared to water thus causing salt retention and water loss.
- The extremities and face appear flushed due to prolonged vasodilatation.
- They have smaller body structure with longer limbs to increase loss of heat through periphery.

11.3 DESCRIBE AND DISCUSS MECHANISM OF FEVER, COLD INJURIES AND HEAT STROKE

SHORT ESSAYS

1. A 22-year-old construction worker was diagnosed of malaria. He had fever with chills. He was advised antipyretics. (2 + 1 + 2 marks)

   A. What is fever? What are the types of abnormal body temperature?
   B. What is hypothalamic set point?
   C. What are the actions of pyrogens and antipyretics?

A.

- Fever is raised body temperature. Any temperature above 100.4°F is considered as fever.
- Abnormal body temperature

Parameter	In centigrade	In fahrenheit
Fever		
Low grade	38 to 39°C	100.4 to 102.2°F
Moderate grade	39 to 40°C	102.2 to 104°F
High grade	40 to 42°C	104 to 107.6°F
Hyperpyrexia	> 41.6°C	>107°F
Hypothermia		
Mild	35 to 33°C	95 to 91.4°F
Moderate	33 to 31°C	91.4 to 87.8°F
Severe	<31°C	<87.8°F

B. Hypothalamic Thermostat or Set Point

- It is the servomechanism by which a temperature of 98.6°F is defined as "physiological normal" by the hypothalamus.
- Any temperature perceived by thermoreceptors above or below this set point is recognized as abnormal and mechanisms for heat regulation are set in.

C. Pyrogens and Antipyretics

- Pyrexia is fever. Chemicals or agents which cause increase in body temperature are called pyrogens. Antipyretics are the drugs used to bring down body temperature.
- Usually endotoxins liberated from organisms and other antigens. These are recognized by the mononuclear cells and are phagocytosed.
- They release interleukin 1 which is a pyrogen which acts on the anterior hypothalamus and raises the hypothalamic set point.

- Following increase in the set point, the body tries to raise body temperature by producing heat and preventing heat loss.
- As a result, there is increase in body temperature.
- Antipyretics act by bringing down this thermostat back to normal by decreasing production of prostaglandins.

SHORT ANSWERS

1. Explain the mechanism of fever. What is hypothalamic thermostat?

Mechanism of Fever

- Pyrexia is fever. Chemicals or agents which cause increase in body temperature are called pyrogens.
- Usually endotoxins liberated from organisms and other antigens. These are recognized by the mononuclear cells and are phagocytosed.
- They release interleukin 1 which is a pyrogen which acts on the anterior hypothalamus and raises the hypothalamic set point.
- Following increase in the set point, the body tries to raise body temperature by producing heat and preventing heat loss.
- As a result, there is increase in body temperature.

Hypothalamic Thermostat

- The hypothalamus acts by servomechanism by which a temperature of 98.6°F is defined as "physiological normal" by the hypothalamus.
- Any temperature perceived by thermoreceptors above or below this set point is recognized as abnormal and mechanisms for heat regulation are set in.

2. Explain the pathophysiology of heat stroke.

- Heat stroke occurs as there is immense amount of surrounding heat and physical exhaustion.
- When there is increase in surrounding heat, there is increase in body temperature.
- Compensatory mechanisms are set in, in the form of cutaneous vasodilatation and visceral vasoconstriction.
- If the temperature is regulated by excess sweating and loss of heat, the individual's temperature comes back to normal.

Heat Stroke (Fig. 11.4)

- Normal mechanisms are impaired and core temperature rises to the level of causing tissue damage.
- It is usually seen in the elderly, chronically ill patients and those who cannot care for themselves.
- Heat stroke is a medical emergency.
- There is a shift from compensable phase to a non-compensable phase characterized by continuous rise of core body temperature.
- As a result, cytotoxic injury and systemic inflammatory response is set up which causes a perpetual vicious cycle leading to heat stroke and death.

3. Describe the pathophysiology and management of frost bite.

Pathophysiology of Frost Bite

- It occurs in a localized external surface which is exposed to intense cold temperature.
- Risk factors include severe winters, inadequate shelter, prolonged exposure to cold and wet condition, and malnutrition.
- It occurs usually in fingers and toes.

Direct Injury

Due to cold temperature.

Indirect Injury

- Due to exposure to cold, there is vasoconstriction.
- This causes decreased blood flow to the tissues
- Ischemia thus caused brings about a cascade of inflammatory reactions.
- There is generation of free radicals which causes tissue damage.
- As blood flow is poor, these are not carried away and there is increase in their effect.
- As the blood flow is sluggish, there is a tendency to thrombus formation which is increased by cold, formation of ice crystals, endothelial injury and finally results in frost bite.

Management

- Warm affected extremity.
- Cover exposed areas
- Warm water baths and infusion with warm saline is advised when there is hypothermia
- Pain control by using analgesics
- Thrombolytic therapy is indicated for patients with full thickness injuries and nor restoration after application of warmth.

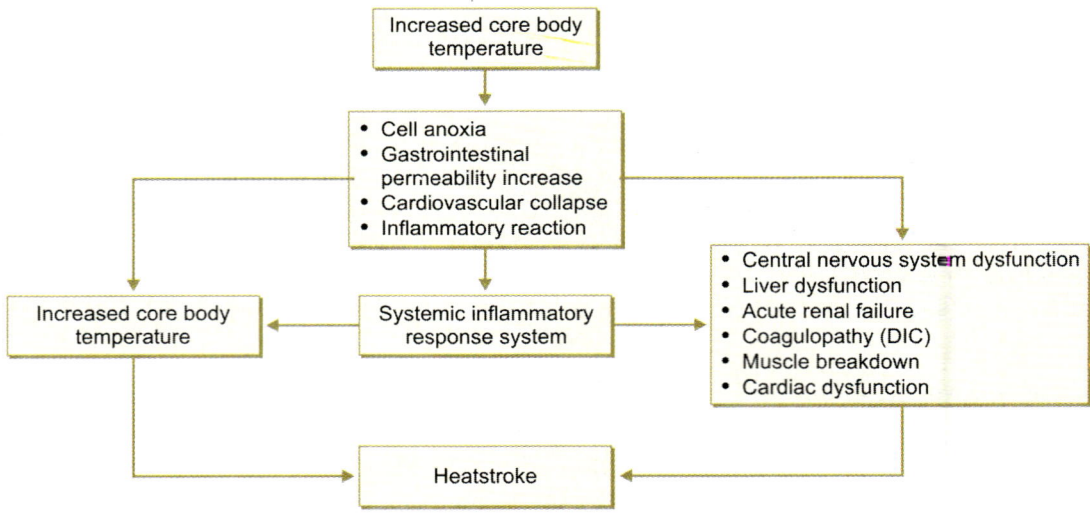

Fig. 11.4

11.4 DESCRIBE AND DISCUSS CARDIORESPIRATORY AND METABOLIC ADJUSTMENTS DURING EXERCISE; PHYSICAL TRAINING EFFECTS

SHORT ANSWERS

1. Explain the reason for reduced oxygen debt in trained athletes.

- Normally, the body contains 2 litres of oxygen available for aerobic respiration even in absence of breathing.
- During intense exercise, there is an increased urgent need for oxygen than what is available as this stored oxygen is readily used up.
- So, at the end of exercise, there is hyperventilation occurring for about 30–45 minutes to restore the used oxygen. This is called oxygen debt.
- In well trained athletes, a few metabolic changes occur in the muscles. Also, the cardiorespiratory changes bring about an increased efficiency.
- Metabolic changes result as there is increased energy stores as the number of mitochondria and mitochondrial enzymes.
- The muscle's ability to extract oxygen as a source of energy also increases.
- So, there is a shift in aerobic respiration during strenuous exercise.
- As a result, more oxygen is available, and the body is more efficient in oxygen extraction.

2. What is oxygen debt? Explain its importance.

Oxygen Debt

- Normally, the body contains 2 litres of oxygen available for aerobic respiration even in absence of breathing.
- During intense exercise, there is an increased urgent need for oxygen than what is available as this stored oxygen is readily used up.
- As a result, glucose is utilized by anaerobic metabolism by glycolysis. This causes lactate production.
- After the period of exercise, extra oxygen is consumed for a period of 30–45 minutes in the form of hyperventilation.
- This causes an increased intake of oxygen. This is called oxygen debt.
- This volume is approximately 11.5 litres

Importance

- This extra oxygen is used to clear up the accumulated lactate, replenish ATP stores and phosphocreatine stores.
- Re-establishes normal concentration of oxygen in hemoglobin and myoglobin.
- Increases oxygen level in the airways to previous normal level.
- This extra amount of oxygen consumed in order to "repay" the deficit oxygen is called oxygen debt. It is proportional to the oxygen deficit produced during the exercise.

3. Explain the cardiorespiratory and metabolic adjustments with physical training.

Cardiorespiratory Adjustments with Physical Training

- Increase in vagal tone with exercise causes a low resting heart rate.
- Regular exercise causes a cardiac hypertrophy which leads to a high stroke volume under resting conditions. It can increase to up to 105 ml from a normal of 75 ml.
- As a result of the above two combinations, a trained athlete can achieve a higher cardiac output easily.
- With training, the maximal oxygen consumption or V_{max} increases by around 5–20%.
- There is also increase in maximal minute ventilation. As a result, the individual has a higher capacity to perform more aerobic exercises.

Metabolic Adjustments with Physical Training

- These result as increased energy stores as the number of mitochondria and mitochondrial enzymes.
- The muscle's ability to extract oxygen as a source of energy also increases.
- So, there is a shift in aerobic respiration during strenuous exercise.
- There is decreased accumulation of lactic acid and products of anaerobic respiration. Thus, the fall in pH is not as much as before.
- Also, there is mobilization of fatty acids instead of glycogen due to increase in aerobic mechanisms.
- Thus, more glycogen is available and endurance increases.

11.5 DESCRIBE AND DISCUSS PHYSIOLOGICAL CONSEQUENCES OF SEDENTARY LIFESTYLE

SHORT ESSAYS

1. Describe the physiological consequences of sedentary lifestyle.

- The amount of exercise done by an individual is measured as MET—minimum energy expenditure test.
- It is the amount of oxygen consumed by an adult per minute.
- One MET is equivalent to 250 ml/min in a male or 200 ml/min in a female adult.
- Sedentary lifestyle is defined when most of the time is spent with MET less than 1.5.
- These activities include watching television or other gadgets, sitting, and driving and other such activities.

Consequences

- The present occupational demands and working style and ease of transport and other changes in lifestyle make an individual prone to sedentary lifestyle.
- It has effects on metabolism, cardiovascular health and others.

1. **Effects on cardiometabolism and cardio-vascular system**
   - There is increase in serum triglyceride level, decreased HDL and increase in insulin resistance
   - They are at increased risk of developing metabolic syndrome
   - So, there are also at an increased risk of developing cardiovascular diseases
   - There is a tendency to pro-thrombotic behaviour of blood.

2. **Effects on bone health**
   - There is reduction in bone mineral density
   - This is due to changes in bone mineral homeostasis

3. **Obesity:** The hours of the day spent in sedentary lifestyle is directly proportional to obesity and increased truncal circumference.

4. **Effect on cancer:** Increased risk of developing ovarian and endometrial cancers in sedentary lifestyle has been reported.

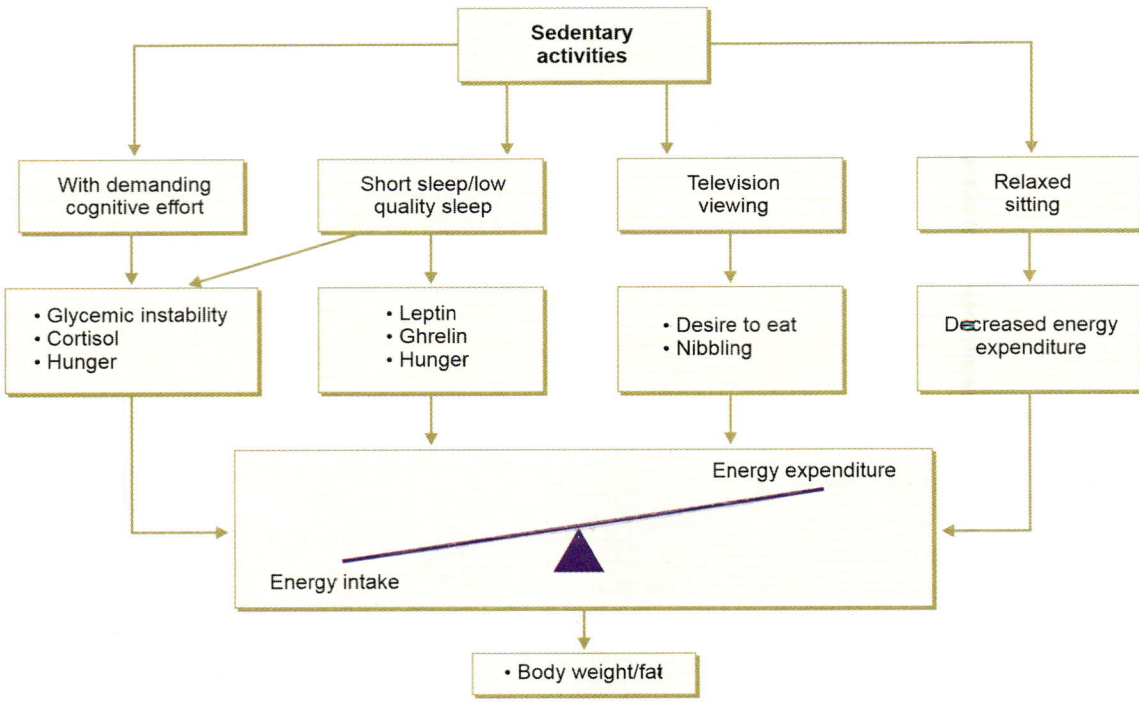

Fig. 11.5

5. **Effects on psychosocial health**
  - Increased physical activity has been reported to cause more satisfaction regarding body image and self-perceptions.
  - Decreased physical activity also can have negative effects on psychosocial component.

2. A young woman with a weight of 90 kg and a known hypertensive comes to the clinic with complaints of breathlessness, easy fatigability, and giddiness. Her work involves sitting for long hours at the computer.
  A. What counselling would you give the patient apart from her diet. (2 marks)
  B. List the risk factors involved in the development of cardiovascular diseases. (3 marks)

A. Counselling

- This patient is living a sedentary lifestyle.
- As her occupation revolves around sitting for most part of the day.
- Inculcation of a routine for exercises, more of aerobic to increase the efficiency of the cardio-respiratory system is advised.
- She should also be advised to perform meditation and yoga for decreasing mental stress.
- Diet should contain less of carbohydrates and lipids and more proteins and fibers.
- Fibers help in decreasing weight and improving healthy cholesterol in blood.
- Drinking adequate amount of water is also necessary to remove toxins and to suppress irregular eating.

B. Risk Factors for Cardiovascular Diseases

Genetic	Concurrent health problems	Environmental
Familial hypercholesterolemia	Hypertension	Sedentary lifestyle
Insulin resistance	Diabetes mellitus	Oily food
Hyperhomocysteinemia	Hypercholesterolemia	consumption
	Insulin resistance	Cigarette
	Protein C deficiency	smoking

SHORT ANSWERS

1. What are current recommendations for Physical activity?

- Physical activity is measured by oxygen consumption per minute.
- It is metabolic energy expenditure (MET). One MET is around 200–250 ml/min.
- Exercises are classified based on the METs consumed (Table 11.1).
- According to American health association, adults should move around more than sit throughout the day.
- At least 150–200 minutes of moderate exercise or 75–150 minutes of vigorous aerobic exercise per week is necessary.
- Additional health benefits are obtained by more exercises being performed.

2. List the methods to assess physical activity of an individual

- Physical activity has four components

Mode	Cycling, walking, sprinting, gardening—aerobic
	Resistance and strength training, push ups—anaerobic
Frequency	Number of sessions per week
Duration	Minutes or hours of exercise
Intensity	Based on oxygen consumed, heart rate, respiratory rate

- Measurement of physical activity
  1. **Subjective**
     - It is the form of questionnaires regarding physical activity
     - Maintenance of physical activity logs
  2. **Objective**
     i. *Indirect calorimetry:* In a room, when a person breathes during exercise, the air of the room is analyzed for concentration of oxygen and carbon dioxide.
     ii. *Doubly labelled water:* In this technique, radiolabelled water is consumed by an

Table 11.1					
Code	Level	Heart rate (beats per min)	Q_1 consumption (L/min)	Relative load index (RLI) (% of max O_3 consumption)	METs
1	Light (mild)	<100	Q.4–0.8	<25	<3
II	Moderate	100–125	Q8–1.6	25–50	3.1–4.5
III	Heavy	125–150	1.6–2.4	51–75	4.6–7
IV	Severe	>150	>2.4	>7.5	>7

individual and the amount of exercise is determined by water loss measured by the machine

iii. **MET**
  – Physical activity is measured by oxygen consumption per minute.
  – It is metabolic energy expenditure. One MET is around 200–250 ml/min.

iv. *Calculation of energy spent*
  – One litre of oxygen consumption is equal to 5 kilocalories of energy spent.
  – Energy expenditure is expressed as kilocalories spent per kg per minute.

3. Describe the pathways through which sedentary lifestyle increases cardiometabolic risk.

- Sedentary lifestyle is becoming the new cause of most of the non-communicable diseases nowadays.

- These individuals have a 30% increase in chances of developing cardiovascular diseases.
- It is a major contributor for cardiovascular diseases.
- Causes obesity and hyperphagia, there is an increased will to eat.
- Due to decreased activity, the cardiorespiratory systems get adjusted to low activity.
- There is decreased leptin generation and therefore decreased satiety.
- All these factors lead to decreased energy expenditure and more energy intake.
- As a result, the carbohydrates are converted into lipids.
- This causes increased chances of venous thrombosis in deep veins and in coronary arteries.

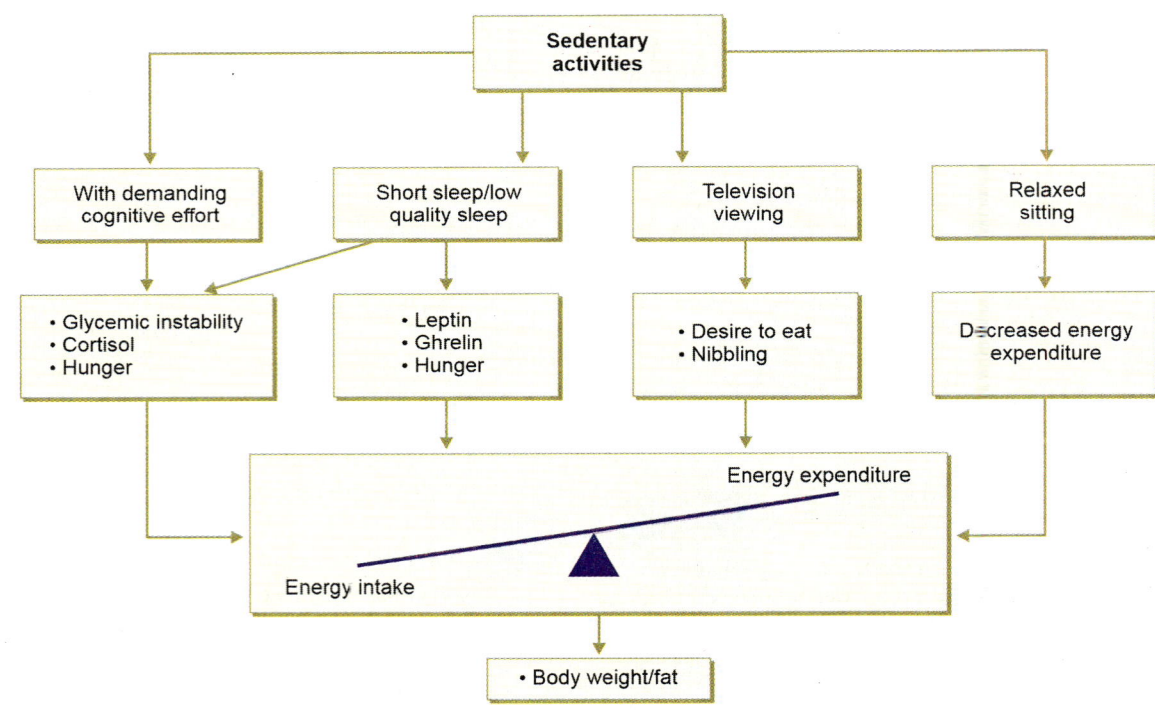

Fig. 11.5a

11.6 DESCRIBE PHYSIOLOGY OF INFANCY

SHORT ANSWER

1. Define the following terms:

   A. Perinatal   B. Neonatal   C. Infancy period

A. Perinatal

It is the time duration around the birth of a child, a few weeks prior to and after birth of a child.

B. Neonatal

Refers to the period of duration from birth of a child to one month.

C. Infancy

Refers to the period of duration from birth of a child to one year of its growth.

11.7 DESCRIBE AND DISCUSS PHYSIOLOGY OF AGING; FREE RADICALS AND ANTIOXIDANTS

SHORT ANSWERS

1. Explain the theories of ageing.

Ageing is a natural process by which there is deterioration of biological efficiency of an individual due to passage of time.

Theories of Ageing

1. **Genetic theories of ageing**
   - According to this, ageing is a controlled process by the genes of the individual
   - It is preprogramed process.
      i. **Programmed senescence theory:** According to this theory, preprogramed expression and non-expression of some genes is associated with ageing and its features.
      ii. **Mutation theory**
         - Mutations occurring in the genome of an animal impair long-term survival.
         - They go one accumulating and bring about their effects.
         - Example, there may be mutation in a gene that causes malignancy of lung in an individual. As the malignancy causes more and more destruction, the lifespan of the individual is decreased.

2. **Random damage theories:** It states that a balance between ongoing damage and repair is impaired which brings about decreased efficiency of ageing.

   i. **Generation of free radicals**
      - Free radicals are generated from oxidative mechanisms though out the life of an individual
      - The capacity of clearing these free radicals by antioxidant mechanisms decreases with age. As a result, there is decrease in biological function.
   ii. **Cell replication theory**
      - There are a few types of cells that always replicate, some replicate under pressure and some do not replicate
      - This theory states that when there is not enough replication to replace damaged cells, ageing results.

2. Describe the role of free radicals and the antioxidants in aging.

- Free radicals are generated during oxidative reactions of the cells (Fig. 11.6).
- They are superoxide, hydroxyl ions.
- Normally they are removed by a scavenging system like enzyme of lysosomes like superoxide dismutase, glutathione and some chemicals which have antioxidant properties like vitamin E, vitamin C.
- When these antioxidant mechanisms are overwhelmed, there occurs an oxidative injury.
- This causes oxidative degeneration of lipids, proteins and nucleic acids.
- This brings down the functioning of an individual and manifests as ageing.

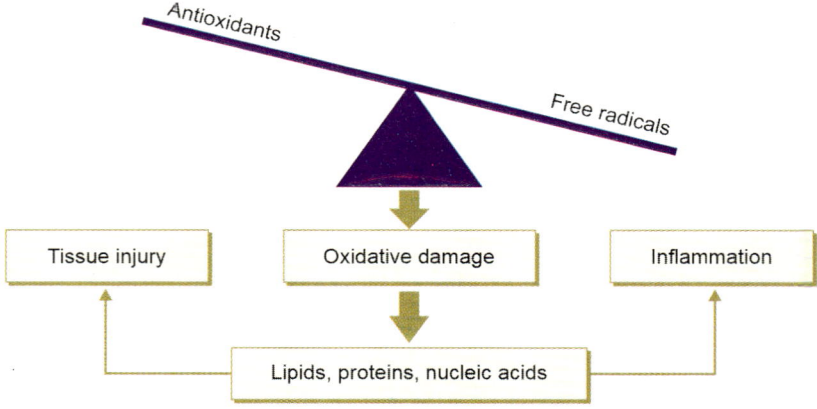

Fig. 11.6

3. List the diseases related with ageing.

They are classified according to the system, they affect

Cardiovascular system	Increased propensity to thrombi formation leads to ischemic heart disease
	Primary hypertension due to stiffening of blood vessels
	Decreased sensitivity to chemoreceptors and baroreceptors
Central nervous system	Age-related atrophy of grey matter: Alzheimer's disease, senile dementia
Special senses	Senile cataract, presbyopia, age-related macular degeneration
	Presbycusis
Respiratory system	Age-related decrease in compliance of lungs and predisposition to collapse
Gastrointestinal system	Decreased motility and absorption
	Decreased tone of abdominal wall predisposes to direct hernia
Renal and urinary	Decreased tubular function
	Increased prostatic size and benign prostatic hyperplasia
Endocrinal system	Impaired glucose tolerance
	Menopause and climacteric
	Decrease in ADH, aldosterone and renin
Blood and immune system	Anemia, senile purpura due to capillary fragility raised ESR

11.8 DISCUSS AND COMPARE CARDIORESPIRATORY CHANGES IN EXERCISE (ISOMETRIC AND ISOTONIC) WITH THAT IN THE RESTING STATE AND UNDER DIFFERENT ENVIRONMENTAL CONDITIONS (HEAT AND COLD)

LONG ESSAY

1. Describe the mechanisms that bring about increased ventilation, before, at the onset, during and after exercise.

Increased ventilation is required for exercise to provide sufficient oxygen for the skeletal muscles which are actively contracting.

Before the Onset of Exercise

- There is anticipatory increase in the rate of respiration initiated by the cerebral cortex by the thought of exercise.
- This is neural mechanism for increase in ventilation prior to the onset of exercise.

At the Onset of and during Exercise (Fig. 11.7)

- At the onset of exercise, there is vasodilatation in the skeletal muscles. Also, there is change in the position of muscles and joints which stimulate the proprioceptors.
- Afferent impulses form these are sent to the respiratory centers which increase the respiratory rate.
- When the exercise continues, there is an increased oxygen demand. Also, there is accumulation of carbon dioxide due to cellular respiration.
- The increased carbon dioxide and decreased oxygen triggers the chemoreceptors in the carotid body which stimulates the respiratory centers.
- This causes tachypnoea.

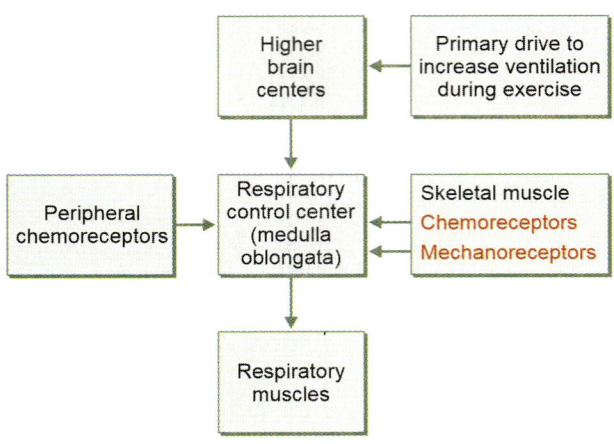

Fig. 11.7

After Exercise (Fig. 11.8)

- After the exercise stops, there is hyperventilation which continues for around 30–45 minutes.
- This is because energy was produced during exercise was mostly anaerobic.
- As a result, there is accumulation of products of anaerobic respiration like lactic acid.
- Thus, a debt of oxygen needs to be repaid. This brings about an increase in respiratory rate and thus increase in pulmonary ventilation.

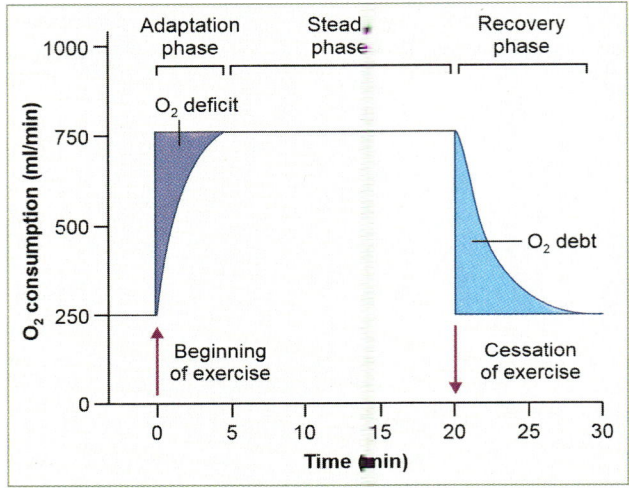

Fig. 11.8

SHORT ESSAY

1. Explain all mechanisms that cause tachycardia during exercise (Fig. 11.9).

1. **Nervous mechanism**
   - The thought of exercise causes tachycardia.
   - This is due to cerebral cortex send impulses to the medullary centers and there is inhibition of the vagal tone.
   - This causes sympathetic activation leading to positive chronotropic effects of catecholamines. This causes stimulation of SA node and thus tachycardia.
2. **Impulses from proprioceptors**
   - Proprioceptors in the joints and muscles send impulses to the brain and medullary centers.
   - These cause vagal inhibition and increase in heart rate.

3. Increased carbon dioxide in blood

- During exercise, a lot of oxygen is exchanged to carbon dioxide by actively contracting muscles for production of ATP.
- This carbon dioxide in blood stimulates the medullary centers.
- These cause vagal inhibition and increase in heart rate.

4. Rise in body temperature because of exercise

- Increase in body temperature stimulates the hypothalamus.
- This has direct effect on the SA node and increases heart rate.

5. Increase in venous return

- Contraction of peripheral muscles causes squeezing of veins and increased venous return to the heart.
- This also causes increased heart rate by Bainbridge reflex.

6. Secretion of catecholamines

- During any stressful condition, there is increased activity of the sympathetic system which stimulates the adrenals.
- The adrenal medulla secretes high amounts of catecholamines, and they have positive chronotropic effect.
- This causes tachycardia.

SHORT ANSWER

1. Attribute for the advice of carbohydrate-rich diet in athletes before a competition.

- The endurance of muscles during an athletic competition depends on the nutritive support to the muscle—mainly formed by muscle glycogen.
- Endurance is the time an individual can sustain a race until complete exhaustion.
- Diet containing high carbohydrates lets an individual store far more glycogen in the muscles than a person on mixed diet or fat diet.
- With different types of diets, the endurance is

High carbohydrate diet	240 minutes
Mixed diet	120 minutes
High fat diet	85 minutes

- The amount of glycogen stored also depends on the type of diet. It is 40 g/kg of muscle of glycogen stored for a high carbohydrate diet, whereas 20 g/kg and 6 g/kg for mixed and fatty diet.
- At the time of an exercise, high amounts of ready-to-consume glycogen is required to overcome the increased need for energy.
- Thus, it is advised to have a carbohydrate-rich diet prior to a competition.

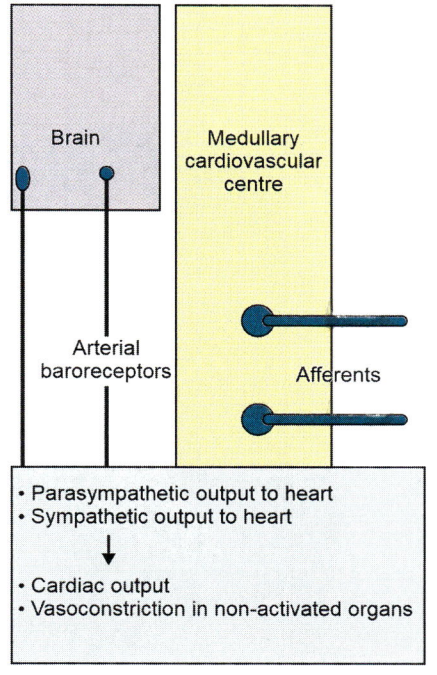

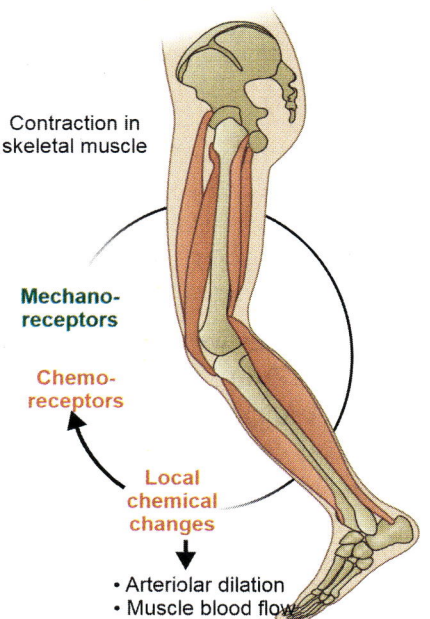

Fig. 11.9

11.9 INTERPRET GROWTH CHARTS

SHORT ANSWERS

1. Explain the growth chart.

- Growth charts are available for length or height-for-age, weight-for-age, weigh-for-height and BMI-for-age (Fig. 11.10).
- There is a separate chart for each sex.
- The X axis is for the age of the child, whereas the Y axis is for weight, height or BMI.
- There are five reference lines for 97th centile, 85th centile, 50th centile, 15th centile and third centile.

Example

- The values of the child are plotted at the particular age. They are assessed in what centile of the growth chart does the value fall.
- When all these points are joined, there should be an upward trend. There should not be flatness or downwards trend.

2. Define stunting, wasting and failure to thrive.

Stunting

- It is impaired growth and development in a child as a result of impaired nutrition, repeated infection and inadequate psychosocial situation.
- It is defined when height for age in a child is less than the expected by two standard deviations or more.

Wasting

- It is severe malnutrition leading loss of fat and muscles due to protein degradation.
- It is defined as weight-for-height.

Failure to Thrive

- When the rate of weight gain is lesser than expected, it is defined as failure to thrive.
- These children have lesser weight and height compared to age-compared children.

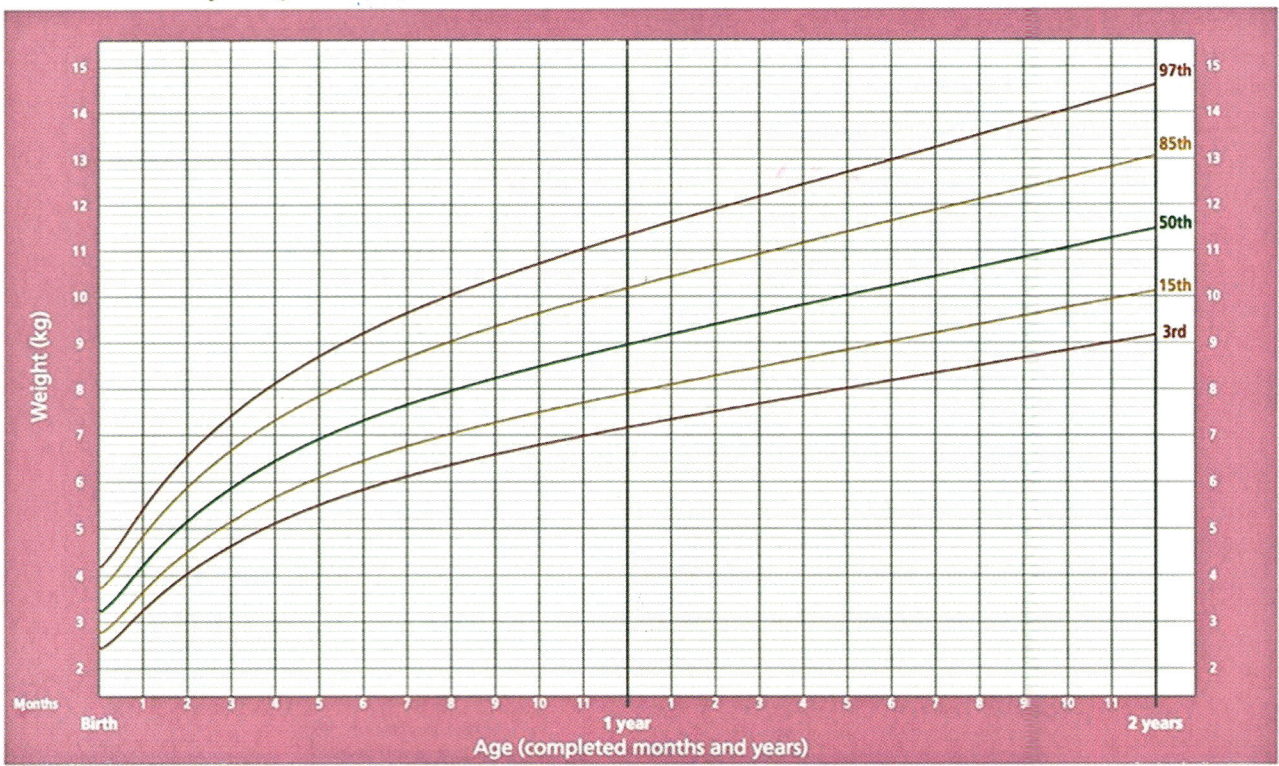

Fig. 11.10

11.10 INTERPRET ANTHROPOMETRIC ASSESSMENT OF INFANTS

SHORT ANSWER

1. List the clinical implications of anthropometric assessments in infants.

- Anthropometry is measurement of body parts and their dimensions.

- They are important for recording progress among infants and are done regularly along with immunization schedules.
- They are some expressed in percentile (the rank position of an individual on a given reference distribution)

Parameter	Implications
Age-dependent anthropometric measurements	
Weight	• Weight is a measure of adequacy of nutrition in a child
	• Acute changes in nutrition or illness reflects on weight of the infant
	• It should be above 50th centile and the chart should be upward progressive
Length or height	• Height is also a measure of adequacy of nutrition over a long period
	• Chronic changes in nutrition and illness is reflected by decrease in height gain
	• Height should also be above 50th centile and progressive
Head circumference	• It is a measure of development and growth of brain and therefore skull
	• It may be less in mentally challenged children
Age-independent anthropometric measurements	
Skin fold thickness	• It is usually measured in the triceps
	• It is also a measure of nutrition
	• It should be more than 10 mm
Weight-for-height	• Weight should be proportional to the height of the child
	• It reflects nutritional status
Midarm circumference	• It is usually measured in the age group of 1–5 years
	• Acute starvation causes decrease in midarm circumference
	• Normal range is from 8.7 to 9.7 cm

11.11 DISCUSS THE CONCEPT, CRITERIA FOR DIAGNOSIS OF BRAIN DEATH AND ITS IMPLICATIONS

SHORT ANSWER

1. Explain the legal issues and organ donation in a brain-dead person.

- Brain death is defined as a condition, where there is irreversible damage to the brain characterized by loss of its functions. The perfusion to the brain is absent.
- However, major organs like heart and lung are functioning with the help of a mechanical ventilation.
- Organs that can be transplanted are heart, lung, liver, pancreas.

Criteria for Brain Death

- Deep unresponsive coma (isoelectric EEG)
- Absent pupillary reflexes, oculovestibular reflexes and corneal reflexes (brainstem reflex)
- Apnea—inability to initiate respiration in presence of raised pCO_2.

Legal Issues and Organ Donation

- Transplant of Human Organ Act was passed by the Government of India in 1994.
- According to this
  1. **Living relative donor**
     - When the donor is living and is kin (parents, sibling, grandparents, issues or spouse)
     - Donation is allowed after providing proof of blood relation
  2. **In brain dead persons**
     - Doctors appointed by the appropriate authority of government of India are eligible to provide brain death certification
     - Two certifications are required at two different occasions, at least 6 hours apart.
     - One of the doctors should be a neurologist
  3. **Regulation of donation is done by an authorizing committee and appropriate authority:** Each state or Union Territory has a committee which overlooks these donation activities.

11.12 DISCUSS THE PHYSIOLOGICAL EFFECTS OF MEDITATION

SHORT ANSWER

1. Describe the physiological changes in autonomic functions due to meditation.

- Meditation is a state of wakeful hypometabolism.
- It is done in a quiet environment, in a comfortable position, with eyes closed and a passive state of mind characterized by non-targeted and non-analytic thinking known as Dhyana.

Changes during Meditation

- There is a decreased heart rate and blood pressure. Better effects have been found with OM chanting.

- There is an increased peripheral or cutaneous vascular resistance which is a marker of psychological alertness in presence of relaxation. (Telles S, Nagarathna R, Nagendra HR. Autonomic changes during "OM" meditation. Indian J Physiol Pharmacol 1995;39(4):418-420.)
- Decrease in oxygen consumption
- Increase in basal metabolic rate is observed within 6 weeks of yoga and meditation
- There is also a decrease in the finger plethysmogram amplitude
- Increased percentage time spent in alpha rhythm of EEG pattern
- Decrease in muscle tone
- Decrease in blood lactate level

11.13 OBTAIN HISTORY AND PERFORM GENERAL EXAMINATION IN THE VOLUNTEER/SIMULATED ENVIRONMENT

SHORT ESSAY

1. Explain clinical implications of general physical examination in the volunteer.

General physical examination includes the following:

1. **Built and nourishment:** It is the general physique of a patient, his height, weight and other features of nutrition allows us to classify quickly if the patient is well or malnourished.

2. **Mental status**
   - It is defined by consciousness, orientation with time, place and person.
   - Decrease in consciousness may be classified as drowsy, stupor and coma. It is a function of cerebral cortex and the reticular system. Any abnormality in consciousness is an indication of underlying damage to cerebral cortex.
   - Disorientation is also seen in acute confusion states like delirium which can be due to organic or metabolic causes.

3. **Pallor**
   - It is tested clinically by looking the lower palpebral conjunctiva or tongue.
   - Appearance of decreased color or paleness in indicative of anemia, systemic illness

4. **Icterus:** It is yellowish appearance of the bulbar conjunctiva and is seen due to increase in blood bilirubin levels due to a number of causes.

5. **Cyanosis**
   - It is bluish appearance of nail bed and peripheries seen when there is excess amounts of carbon dioxide.
   - It is seen in cyanotic congenital heart diseases.

6. **Clubbing:** It is seen as increased thickness of the peripheries of fingers seen in some pulmonary conditions like tuberculosis.

7. **Edema**
   - Accumulation of extracellular fluid in tissues leading to appearance of increased size.
   - It is seen in peripheries usually feet which progress proximally.

8. **Lymphadenopathy**
   - It is swelling of lymph nodes either due to inflammation or cancer of the area they are draining.
   - There are groups of lymph nodes like cervical, axillary, etc.

9. **Pulse**
   - It is the beating of the heart that is felt along the arterial tree in the peripheries.
   - It is an indirect measure of functioning of the heart and allows the examiner to understand the rate, rhythm of heartbeat, volume of cardiac output, and degree of vessel wall thickening.

10. **Blood pressure**
    - It is measured by using a sphygmomanometer.
    - Systolic blood pressure and diastolic blood pressure are measured.
    - Increased systolic blood pressure >120 mmHg is hypertension.
    - Decreased blood pressure is hypotension and causes weakness and giddiness.

11.14 DEMONSTRATE BASIC LIFE SUPPORT IN A SIMULATED ENVIRONMENT

SHORT ESSAY

1. Explain and demonstrate the method of performing basic life support during emergency.

Basic life support is a level of medical care that has to be provided in cases of life-threatening conditions until medical facility arrives.

Indications

1. Cardiac and respiratory arrest
2. Choking
3. Drowning

Method

- Recognize imminent dangers and take the patient away from danger (electric wires/out of water).
- Patient when found unconscious and unresponsive, shake and shout at the patient.
- If unresponsive, call for help (dial for help-104 in India) and people around for help.

ABC of Basic Life Support

1. **Examine airway**
   - Open airway and make sure there are no obstructive elements (foreign bodies) in the airway
   - Clear airway and listen to the sounds of breathing
   - Blocked airway is usually associated with high pitched sounds.

2. **Breathe**
   - Offer two breaths by mouth to mouth resuscitation only airway is clear.
   - Assess for 10 seconds for spontaneous respiration.

3. **Circulation**
   - Assess circulation by peripheral pulses and capillary pressure (palm or feet)
   - If circulation is normal, continue breathe support and check circulation everyone minute
   - If circulation is abnormal, chest compressions are given with two hands. In infants, two fingers are used
   - They are given in the ratio of 15 compressions for every two breaths.

4. **Defibrillation:** At the arrival of ambulance care, defibrillation is done.

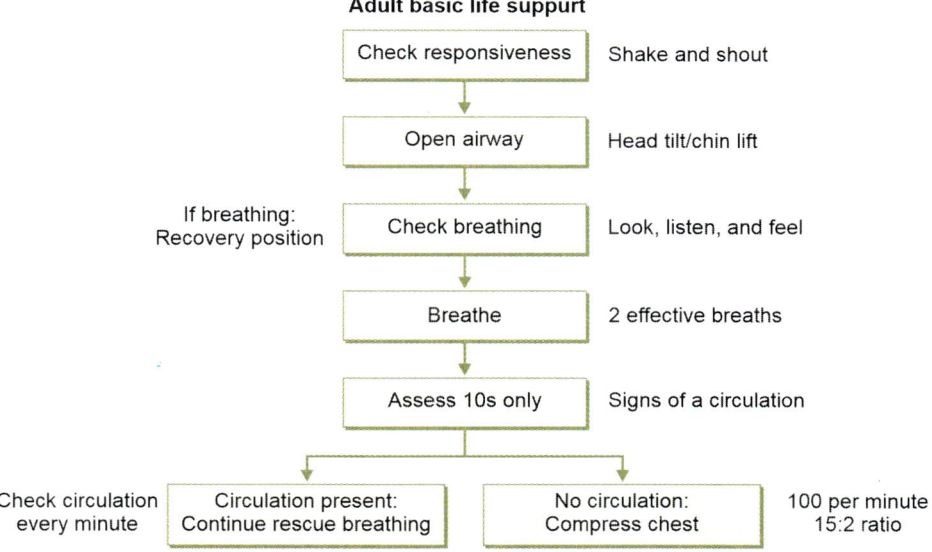

Adult basic life suppurt

Check responsiveness	Shake and shout
Open airway	Head tilt/chin lift
Check breathing	Look, listen, and feel
Breathe	2 effective breaths
Assess 10s only	Signs of a circulation

If breathing: Recovery position

Check circulation every minute — Circulation present: Continue rescue breathing

No circulation: Compress chest — 100 per minute 15:2 ratio

Send or go for help as soon as possible according to guidelines

Fig. 11.11

Multiple Choice Questions

PY 1.1

1. Eukaryotic plasma membrane is made up of all, *except*:
   A. Carbohydrates
   B. Triglycerides
   C. Lecithin
   D. Cholesterol

2. Function of phospholipid in cell membrane is:
   A. Transduction of signals
   B. Transmembrane preparation of protein
   C. DNA replication
   D. Enzyme activation at membrane surface

3. Addition of PUFA in plasma membrane causes:
   A. Membrane becomes rigid
   B. Increase in fluidity of membrane
   C. Decrease in fluidity of membrane
   D. No change in fluidity of membrane

4. All take place in mitochondria, *except*:
   A. Fatty acid oxidation
   B. EMP pathway
   C. Electron transport chain
   D. Citric acid cycle

5. True regarding Golgi apparatus is A/E:
   A. *Cis* is receiving end
   B. *Trans* is secretory end
   C. Non-polarized structure
   D. Situated near nucleus

PY 1.2

6. About the homeostatic mechanism of the body following are true, *except*:
   A. Values revolve around the mean
   B. Value of controlled variable is compared to the reference value
   C. Value of controlled variable oscillates near a set point
   D. System is stabilized by the positive feedback mechanism

7. Positive feedback is seen in A/E:
   A. LH surge
   B. Entry of Ca into sarcoplasmic reticulum
   C. Stimulation of gastric secretion of histamine and gastrin
   D. Thrombolytic activity in coagulation cascade

8. Which of the following is not mediated through negative feedback mechanism?
   A. BP
   B. GH formation
   C. Thrombus formation
   D. ACTH release

PY 1.3

9. The type of membrane junction which plays an important role in electrical conductivity of heart cells and smooth muscle is:
   A. Tight junction
   B. Gap junction
   C. Desmosomes
   D. Pacemaker cells

10. The type of protein that is absent in Charcot-Marie-Tooth disease is:
   A. Connexin in gap junction
   B. Connexin in tight junction
   C. Claudins in gap junction
   D. Claudins in tight junction

11. The types of proteins in tight junctions are all, *except*:
   A. Occludin
   B. Junctional adhesion molecules (JAMs)
   C. Claudins
   D. Connexin

1. B   2. B   3. B   4. B   5. C   6. D   7. C   8. C   9. B   10. A   11. D

PY 1.4

12. **Which of the following is associated with defective apoptosis and increased cell survival?**
    A. Neurodegenerative diseases
    B. Autoimmune disorders
    C. Myocardial infarction
    D. Stroke

PY 1.5

13. **Regarding transport of Ca^{++} across a membrane following are true:**
    A. Ca^{++} calmodulin binding
    B. It is a passive mechanism
    C. Required hydrolysis of ATP
    D. It is a symport
    E. It is an active process

14. **Which of the following characteristics is shared by simple and facilitated diffusion of glucose?**
    A. Occurs down an electrochemical gradient
    B. Is saturable
    C. Requires metabolic energy
    D. Is inhibited by the presence of galactose
    E. Requires a Na^+ gradient

15. **Clathrin is used in:**
    A. Receptor-mediated endocytosis
    B. Exocytosis
    C. Cell-to-cell adhesion
    D. Plasma membrane

16. **In primary active transport:**
    A. The addition of Na^+ on the higher Na^+ concentration will cause movement of molecules into the cell
    B. The covalent bonding will cause conformational modulation of carrier protein.
    C. The use of ATPase enzymes causes high solubility of substrate in lipid bilayer and hence its transport in the cell.
    D. The concentration gradient of Na^+ plays most important role.

17. **The osmolarity of fluid A is twice that of B (A is hypertonic with respect to B) they are separated by a semipermeable membrane the water will move:**
    A. From A towards B
    B. From B towards A
    C. No movement occurs
    D. Can move in either direction

18. **A new drug is developed that blocks the transporter for H^+ secretion in gastric parietal cells. Which of the following transport processes is being inhibited?**
    A. Simple diffusion
    B. Facilitated diffusion
    C. Primary active transport
    D. Cotransport
    E. Countertransport

PY 1.6

19. **The following are true about body water:**
    A. Water constitutes 60% of the body weight
    B. Plasma volume constitutes 10% of the total body water
    C. ECF volume can be determined by dilution methods
    D. 10% is intracellular water

20. **About sodium, true is:**
    A. Normal serum level is 135–145 mEq/L
    B. Daily intake is 150 mmol of NaCl
    C. Major protein is extracellular
    D. Major reserve is skeletal muscle

21. **The interstitial fluid and plasma have essentially the same composition, *except*:**
    A. The plasma contains much higher concentration of fats
    B. The plasma contains much lower concentration of carbohydrates
    C. The plasma contains much higher concentration of proteins
    D. The plasma contains much lower concentration of proteins

12. B   13. C   14. A   15. A   16. B   17. B   18. C   19. A   20. A   21. C

22. **Which of the following methods is not used for measurement of body fluid volumes?**
    A. Antipyrine for total body water
    B. Insulin for extracellular fluid
    C. Evans blue for plasma volume
    D. ^{125}I-albumin for blood volume

PY 1.7

23. **Haemoglobin is the major buffer in blood, bicarbonate ions diffuse out of erythrocyte into plasma in exchange of:**
    A. Potassium
    B. Phosphate
    C. Carbonic acid
    D. Chloride ion

PY 1.8

24. **True about Na$^+$-K$^+$ pump is that:**
    A. Involves ATPase activity
    B. It can move Na$^+$ in and out of cell
    C. Electrically neutral
    D. Pumps out one Na$^+$ for one K$^+$
    E. Pumps 3Na and 2K inside the cell

25. **Upstroke of action potential would lead to:**
    A. Net current in an outward direction
    B. Cell interior becomes more negative
    C. Cell interior becomes less negative
    D. None of the above

PY 1.9

26. **All are locally mediated intercellular communications, *except:***
    A. Gap junctions
    B. Synapse
    C. Autocrine secretions
    D. Endocrine secretions

PY 2.1

27. **The half-life of plasma albumin is approximately:**
    A. 7 days
    B. 20 days

C. 60 days
D. 90 days

28. **Serum is blood plasma without:**
    A. Blood cells
    B. Fibrinogen
    C. Lymphocytes
    D. Plasma colloids

PY 2.2

29. **Which of the following agents is not likely to be found in plasma?**
    A. Thrombin
    B. Fibrinogen
    C. Prothrombin
    D. Calcium ion

30. **The first plasma protein to be generated after severe protein deficiency is:**
    A. Albumin
    B. Globulin
    C. Fibrinogen
    D. Thrombin

PY 2.3

31. **In human the Hb is:**
    A. HbH
    B. HbA
    C. HbM
    D. HbS

32. **Which of the following is correct about delta polypeptide chain of hemoglobin?**
    A. It is present in HbF
    B. It consists of 148 amino acid
    C. Amino acid sequence is same as in β chain
    D. None of the above

33. **Which of the following types of hemoglobin produces crystals called 'tectoids' in hypoxic condition?**
    A. HbA
    B. HbA$_2$
    C. HbS
    D. HbF

22. A   23. D   24. A   25. A   26. D   27. B   28. B   29. D   30. C   31. B   32. A   33. C

PY 2.4

34. Which of the following cell type is not a precursor of erythrocytes?
A. Proerythroblast
B. Normoblast
C. Reticulocyte
D. Myeloblast

PY 2.5

35. The most common oral change due to nutritional anemia is:
A. Enlarged tongue
B. Atrophic glossitis
C. Generalized osteolysis
D. Focal marrow expansion

36. Patient with anemia tends to have all, *except*:
A. Compensatory increase in cardiac output
B. Increased incidence of heart murmurs
C. Pallor of mucous membrane
D. A low pO_2 in arterial blood

PY 2.6

37. Lymphocytes are located in each of the following tissues or organs *except* one. The one exception is:
A. Brain
B. Spleen
C. Lymph nodes
D. Thymus gland

38. The function common to neutrophils, monocytes and macrophages in:
A. Immune response
B. Phagocytosis
C. Release of histamine
D. Destruction of old erythrocytes

39. Immunologically active cells are:
A. Plasma cells
B. Mast cells
C. Eosinophils
D. RBCs

40. In acute infection, which of the following is found:
A. Leucopenia
B. Leucocytosis
C. Neutrophilia
D. Neutropenia

41. MHC class II antigens are located in:
A. Platelets
B. RBC
C. Basophils
D. B cell

PY 2.7

42. Thromboxane is produced mainly by:
A. Liver
B. Platelets
C. Damaged tissue
D. Vascular endothelium

43. Survival time of platelet is approximately:
A. 10 hours
B. 10 days
C. 10 weeks
D. 100 days

44. Which of the following is done for a patient on coumarin (warfarin) therapy?
A. Partial thromboplastin time (PTT)
B. Prothrombin time (PT)
C. Bleeding time (BT)
D. Capillary fragility test (CFT)

PY 2.8

45. Which of them is not affected by vit K deficiency?
A. Factor IX
B. Factor VII
C. Factor II
D. Factor VIII

46. Deficiency of vit K leads to decreased activity of:
A. Platelets
B. Coagulation factors V and VIII
C. Coagulation factors VII, IX and X
D. Fibrinolytic system

---

34. D　35. B　36. D　37. A　38. B　39. A　40. C　41. C　42. B　43. B　44. B　45. D　46. C

47. Thrombosthenin is a:
   A. Coagulation factor
   B. Contractile protein
   C. Thrombosis promoting protein
   D. Regulating platelet protein

43. A 28-year-old woman with history of recurrent abortions, pain in calves for 4 years has deficiency of:
   A. Factor XIII
   B. Protein C
   C. Plasmin
   D. Thrombin

PY 2.9

49. In the blood bank, platelets are stored at:
   A. 18°C for 1 year
   B. 20 to 24°C for 35 days
   C. 20 to 24°C for 3 to 5 days
   D. 2 to 4°C for 35 days

PY 2.10

50. Following are the steps of phagocytosis, *except*:
   A. Chemotaxis
   B. Opsonization
   C. Antigen presentation
   D. Diapedesis

PY 2.11

51. Bleeding time is prolonged in:
   A. von Willebrand's disease
   B. Christmas disease
   C. Hemophilia
   D. Polycythemia

52. Clotting time is prolonged in all, *except*:
   A. von Willebrand's disease
   B. Christmas disease
   C. Hemophilia
   D. Polycythemia

PY 2.12

53. Hematocrit relate to which of the following:
   A. Total blood volume
   B. Total RBC volume
   C. Total WBC volume
   D. Plasma filtrate

54. Which of the following does not change in the old age?
   A. GFR
   B. Glucose tolerance
   C. Haematocrit
   D. Blood pressure

PY 2.13

55. A 40-year-old female on treatment for anemia, the investigation done is:
   A. Reticulocyte count
   B. Platelet count
   C. DLC
   D. TLC

56. PT is useful for:
   A. Detection of clot retraction
   B. Platelet count
   C. In hemophilia
   D. For evaluation in a patient taking anti-coagulant drugs

PY 3.1

57. Axon hillock is a part of neuron which:
   A. Has dense Nissl granules
   B. Has no Nissl granules
   C. Is at commencement of dendrites
   D. Is round in shape

58. Which cell is responsible for myelin sheath production?
   A. Schwann cell
   B. Oligodendrocytes
   C. Neurilemma
   D. Microglia

47. B   48. C   49. C   50. C   51. A   52. A   53. B   54. C   55. A   56. D   57. B   58. A

59. Which of these is responsible for blood–brain barrier?
A. Oligodendrocytes
B. Microglia
C. Astrocytes
D. Schwann cell

60. Identify the neuroglia (in yellow color):

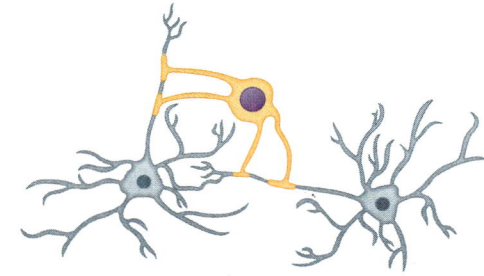

A. Astrocyte
B. Oligodendrocyte
C. Microglia
D. Schwann cell

61. Identify the structure number 6.

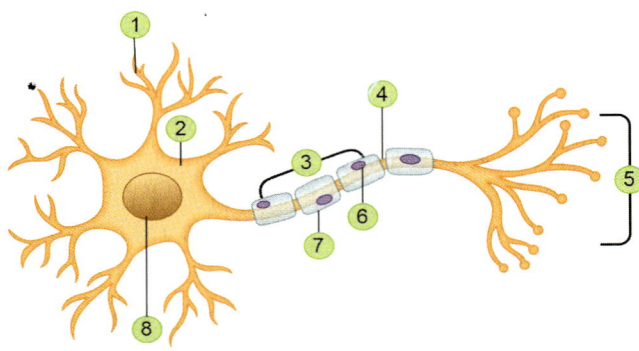

A. Node of Ranvier
B. Soma
C. Schwann cell
D. Telodendron

PY 3.2

62. The type of nerve fiber most susceptible to local anesthetics is:
A. B group
B. Aα group
C. Aβ group
D. C group

63. In which type of nerve fibres is conduction blocked maximally by pressure?
A. Aa
B. Ab
C. Ag
D. C

64. Identify the type of conduction.

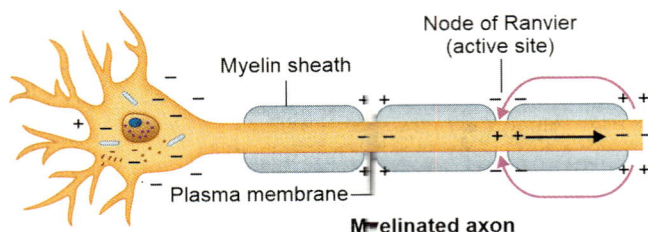

A. Saltatory conduction
B. Electrotonic conduction
C. Myotonic conduction
D. Local endplate potential

65. Match the following:

List I	List II
A. A alpha fibers	I. 15–30 m/s
B. A beta fibers	II. 30–70 m/s
C. A gamma fibers	III. 12–15 m/s
D. A delta fibers	IV. 70–120 m/s

A. A: I, B: II, C: IV, D: III
B. A: IV, B: II, C: I, D: III
C. A: II, B: III, C: I, D: IV
D. A: IV, B: III, C: I, D: I

66. A 28-year-old primigravida at term is posted for caesarean section. She was injected an anaesthetic in the spine. Which sensations of the lower limbs are last to be lost?
A. Pain
B. Fine touch
C. Pressure
D. All sensations are lost at the same pace

67. The correct order of susceptibility of the different types of nerve fibres to local anesthetics is:
A. B>C>A
B. A>B>C
C. C>A>B
D. C>B>A

59. C   60. B   61. C   62. D   63. B   64. A   65. B   66. C   67. D

PY 3.3

68. Axonotmesis includes discontinuity in:
A. Perineurium
B. Epineurium
C. Endoneurium
D. Axon
E. Myelin sheath

69. Neuronal degeneration is seen in all of the following, *except:*
A. Crush nerve injury
B. Fetal development
C. Senescence
D. Neuropraxia

70. A 40-week gestation 4.2 kg baby was delivered by forceps assistance. The duration of delivery was very long. After delivery, the attitude of the child's right hand was in the following manner.

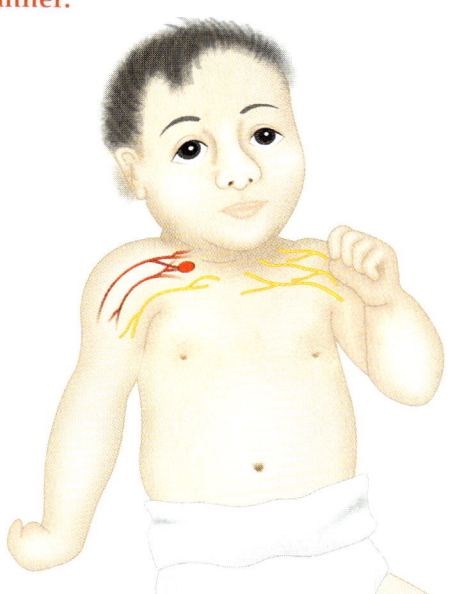

The parents are apprehensive. What is the treatment needed?
A. Perform nerve suturing
B. Give neurotrophic agents
C. Wait and watch
D. Provide a cast

71. Match the following:

List I	List II
A. First degree injury	I. Only perineurium intact
B. Second degree injury	II. Perineurium and epineurium intact
C. Third degree injury	III. Only myelin is lost
D. Fourth degree injury	IV. Nerve damage with intact endoneural tube

A. A: III, B: IV, C: II, D: I
B. A: II, B: I, C: IV, D: III
C. A: I, B: II, C: IV, D: III
D. A: IV, B: II, C: III, D: I

72. All the following are important for regeneration of a cut nerve, *except:*
A. Distance between the cut ends
B. Presence of myelin sheath
C. Presence of neurilemma
D. Presence of an integral nucleus

PY 3.4

73. A patient complains of muscle weakness. On administration of neostigmine it disappears. The mechanism of action of the drug is:
A. It blocks action of acetylcholine
B. It interferes with the action of amine oxidase
C. It interferes with the action of carbonic anhydrase
D. It interferes with the action of acetylcholine esterase

74. The endplate potential at the neuromuscular junction:
A. Obeys all-or-none law
B. Can be easily recorded
C. Is a localized potential
D. Is a hyperpolarizing potential

75. Myaesthenia gravis presents with ptosis and double vision in a majority of patients. The reason for this is:
A. Eye muscle weakness is easily visible
B. They have less ACh receptors
C. Eye muscles have more antibodies
D. Eye muscles are fast twitch fibers

68. D   69. D   70. C   71. A   72. B   73. D   74. D   75. D

76. Deep in the Jungles of Amazon rain forest, a tribe uses arrows dipped in a liquid to hunt animals. This compound is called curare. Mechanism of action of curare is:

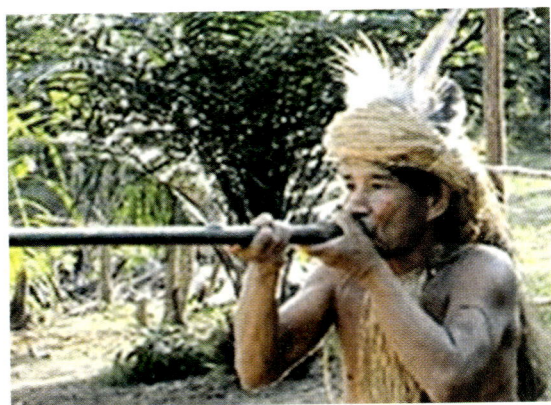

   A. Prevents action potential from reaching the synaptic junction

   B. Prevents release of ACh from vesicles

   C. Binds with acetylcholine receptor on the post-synaptic membrane and prevents action of ACh

   D. Binds with calcium channels and prevents entry of calcium influx into the cells

77. A 68-year-old man, smoker from 50 years, complains of weakness in the proximal parts of the limbs, along with xerostomia and absent deep tendon reflexes. Chest CT scan showed a carcinoma. All the following features differentiate myaesthenia gravis from Lambert-Eaton syndrome, *except:*

   A. Involvement of skeletal muscles

   B. Loss of deep tendon reflexes

   C. Autonomic involvement

   D. All of the above

PY 3.5

78. Which of the following is a presynaptic blocking agent of neuromuscular junction?

   A. D-tubocurarine

   B. Succinylcholine

   C. Botulinum toxin

   D. Physostigmine

79. Malignant hyperthermia is a complication of use of succinylcholine. It occurs in some individuals who have mutation of gene responsible for:

   A. ACh receptor

   B. Ryanodine receptor

   C. SERCA calcium pumps

   D. Na channel

80. .... is an example for rapidly acting neurotransmitter.

   A. Somatostatin

   B. Calcitonin

   C. Substance P

   D. Glycine

81. A 44-year-old actress wants to conceal her crow's feet. Her cosmetologist suggests her to use a neuromuscular blocking agent. Which of the following is used?

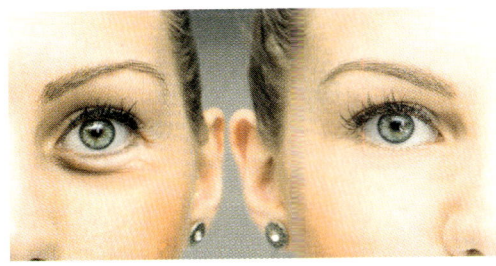

   A. Bungarotoxin

   B. Curare

   C. Botulinum toxin

   D. Succinylcholine

82. All the following are therapeutic indications of botulinum toxin, *except:*

   A. Squint

   B. Essential blepharospasm

   C. Remove wrinkles

   D. GI hypermotility

PY 3.6

83. Which tumor is usually associated with myaesthenia gravis?

   A. Small cell carcinoma of lung

   B. Thymoma

   C. Hepatoma

   D. All of the above

76. C   77. A   78. C   79. B   80. D   81. C   82. D   83. B

84. In myasthenia gravis:
A. There is lack of ACh
B. Lack of ACh receptors
C. There is isometric contraction
D. Muscles are rigid and tough

85. The nicotinic receptors are found in:
A. Neuromuscular junctions of skeletal muscles
B. Smooth muscles
C. Glands
D. Preganglionic cell bodies of autonomic system.

86. Which of the following is definitive treatment for myasthenia gravis?
A. Neostigmine
B. Edrophonium
C. Systemic steroids
D. Thymectomy

87. An EMG on a single muscle fiber showed the following result:

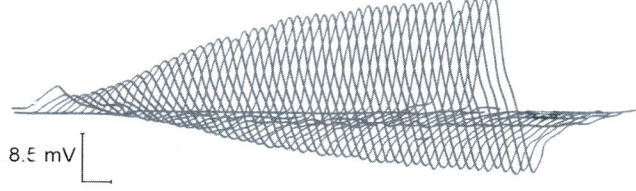

8.5 mV

A. Myaesthenia gravis
B. Lambert-Eaton syndrome
C. Myotonus dystrophica
D. Cannot comment without clinical picture

PY 3.7

88. Twitch of a single motor unit is called:
A. Myoclonic jerk
B. Fasciculation
C. Tremor
D. Chorea

89. In muscle contraction all are true, *except*:
A. A band remains unchanged
B. H zone disappears
C. I band becomes wider
D. Two Z lines come closer

90. The real reason for Frank-Starling's law is:
A. Increase in length causes more calcium influx
B. Increase in length causes more potential to flow in
C. Increase in length causes exposure of more myosin heads
D. Increase in length causes more ATP to be produced

91. Identify the structure marked by red arrow:

The structure marked by red arrow

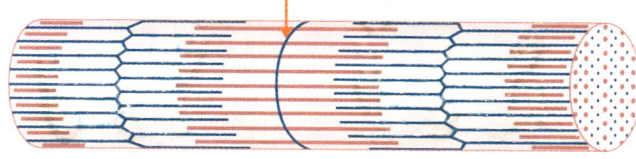

A. H zone
B. A zone
C. M line
D. Z line

92. The part of the muscle between two Z lines is called.
A. Myofibril
B. Endomysium
C. Perimysium
D. Sarcomere

PY 3.8

93. The skeletal muscle action potential:
A. Is not essential for contraction to occur
B. Has a prolonged plateau phase
C. Spreads inwards to all parts of the muscle via the t-tubule system
D. Begins with an inward movement of K^+ ions

94. The strength of contraction of a skeletal muscle does not depend on:
A. Total number of motor units stimulated
B. Duration of action potential in the motor nerve
C. Frequency of action potential in each motor nerve
D. Amount of summation in each motor unit

84. A   85. A   86. D   87. B   88. B   89. C   90. C   91. C   92. D   93. C   94. B

95. The force of muscle contraction can be increased by all of the following, *except*:
   A. Increasing the frequency of activation of motor units
   B. Increasing the number of motor units activated
   C. Increasing the amplitude of action potentials in the motor neurons
   D. Recruiting larger motor units

96. A 33-year-old man was found dead in his apartment. His body was charred and the limbs were in flexed position. What is this condition called?
   A. Rigor mortis
   B. Burn mortis
   C. Heat rigor
   D. None of the above

97. What is the ionic basis for phase 4?

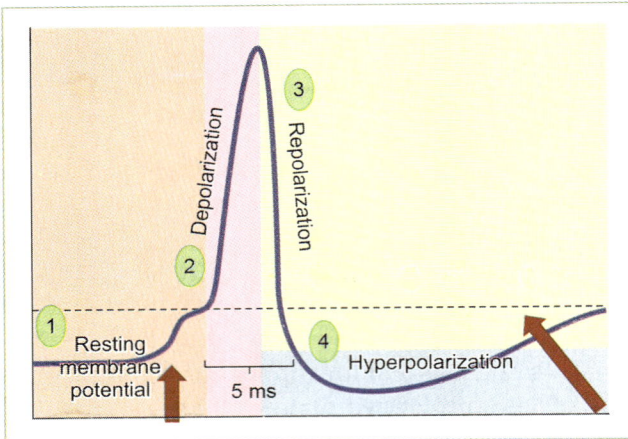

   A. Opening of fast sodium channels
   B. Closure of sodium channels
   C. Opening of calcium channels
   D. Closure of potassium channels

98. Rigor mortis results after death due to:
   A. Failure of acetylcholine to diffuse
   B. Failure of ATP supply
   C. Failure of break down of calcium bridges
   D. None of the above

99. True regarding excitation contraction coupling in smooth muscles is:
   A. Presence of troponin is essential
   B. Sustained contraction occurs with high calcium concentration
   C. Phosphorylation of actin is required for contraction
   D. Presence of cellular calcium is essential to cause muscle contraction

100. Following are differences between skeletal and smooth muscle contraction, *except*:
   A. The store of calcium is intracellular in skeletal muscle and extracellular in smooth muscle
   B. Troponin is the regulatory protein in skeletal muscle and calmodulin in smooth muscle
   C. There is association between actin and myosin in skeletal muscle, whereas actin and desmin in smooth muscle
   D. Contraction in a skeletal muscle is rapid, whereas it is slow and sustained in smooth muscle

101. Which property of a smooth muscle helps the stomach to accommodate varying amounts of food?
   A. Tonic contraction
   B. Plasticity
   C. Elasticity
   D. Auto-rhythmicity

95. C   96. C   97. D   98. B   99. D   100. C   101. B

102. A 22-year-old woman was suffering from achalasia cardia. She was advised injection of botulinum toxin into the lower esophageal sphincter. What is the basis for this?

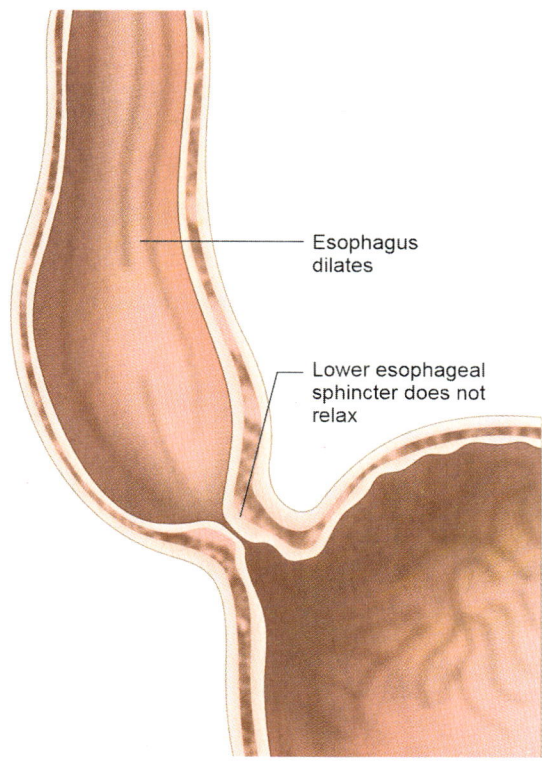

Esophagus dilates

Lower esophageal sphincter does not relax

A. Botulinum toxin improves tone of smooth muscle
B. Botulinum toxin causes necrosis of mucosa
C. Botulinum toxin relaxes smooth muscles
D. Botulinum toxin causes lysis of muscles

PY 3.10

103. A 28-year-old woman wants to loose belly fat after her delivery. She was advised 30 seconds plank exercise. What is the type of exercise?

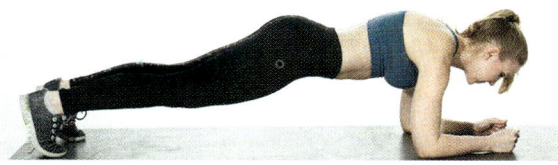

A. Isotonic exercise
B. Isometric exercise
C. Aerobic exercise
D. None of the baove

104. In an isotonic contraction of the muscles:
A. The muscles move a load through a distance
B. The muscle is not able to move the load
C. The latent period of contraction is shorter than isometric contraction
D. The length of muscle is increased

105. A 21-year-old has recently started exercising. He experiences burning sensation in the abdominal muscles while doing pull-ups. The reason is:
A. Accumulation of carbon dioxide
B. Stimulation of phrenic nerve
C. Stimulation of sympathetic nerves
D. Accumulation of lactic acid

106. Which of the following is not an isotonic exercise?
A. Jumping jacks
B. Plank
C. Weight lifting
D. Push ups

107. Match the following:

List I	List II
A. Resting heat	I. Heat produced by metabolic processes to restore metabolic state
B. Heat of activation	II. Heat produced by contraction of muscle
C. Heat of shortening	III. Heat produced by entry of calcium ions
D. Heat of recovery	IV. Heat produced due to ongoing basal metabolic process

A. A: I, B: III, C: II, D: IV
B. A: III, B: II, C: I, D: IV
C. A: IV, B: III, C: II, D: I
D. A: I, B: IV, C: III, D: II

PY 3.11

108. The first site to undergo fatigue in a nerve muscle preparation is:
A. Nerve
B. Neuromuscular junction
C. Muscle
D. All at the same time

102. C   103. B   104. A   105. D   106. A   107. C   108. B

109. In resting state of muscle, which molecule helps as a reservoir of ATP?
A. Creatine
B. Creatinine
C. Myoglobin
D. All of them

110. During intense exercise, a person uses reserved oxygen which is around 2 L. The following act as a reservoir of energy, *except:*
A. Oxyhemoglobin
B. Myoglobin
C. Lactic acid
D. Glycogen

111. An athlete is caught using recombinant human erythropoietin for enhancing endurance. False about EPO is:
A. It increases hematocrit
B. It increases propensity to bleed
C. It enhances endurance
D. It can be detected in urine.

112. Which of the following is not a doping agent?
A. Erythropoietin
B. IGF-1
C. Testosterone
D. Estrogen

PY 3.12

113. Heavy exercise consumes how many METs?
A. <3
B. 3.1–4.5
C. 4.6–7
D. >7

114. The average value of VO_2 max in a nontrained adult is:
A. 50 ml/kg/min
B. 75 ml/kg/min
C. 100 ml/kg/min
D. 125 ml/kg/min

115. Following adjustments occur with training, *except:*
A. Decrease in oxygen demand
B. Increase in cardiac contractility
C. Increase in VO_2 max
D. Decrease in mitochondrial enzymes

116. Following is true about blood circulation during exercise:
A. Increase in blood flow to kidney
B. Increase in blood flow to brain
C. Decrease in blood flow to viscera
D. Decrease in blood flow to heart

PY 3.13

117. Which of the following is not a sarcolemmal protein?
A. Sarcoglycan
B. Dystrophin
C. Dystroglycan
D. Perlecan

118. A 3-year-old boy is brought with delayed motor milestones. On attempting to stand, the following picture is seen.

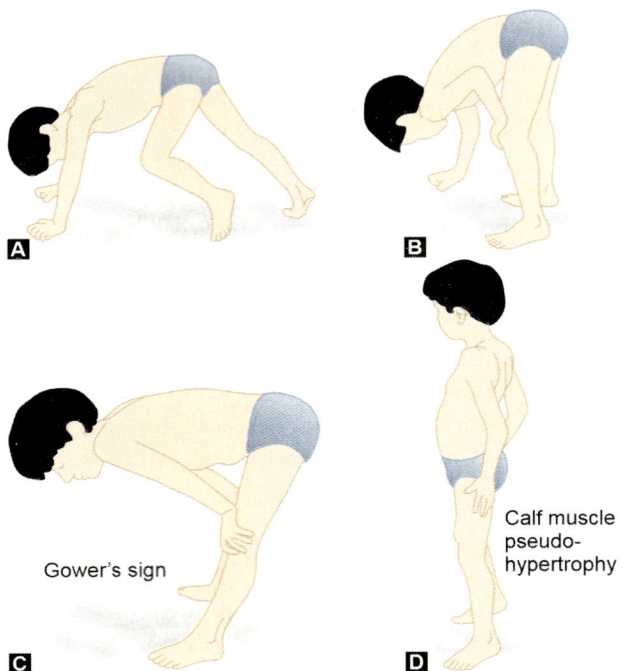

Gower's sign

Calf muscle pseudo-hypertrophy

What is the genetic inheritance of this condition?
A. X-linked recessive
B. Autosomal dominant
C. Autosomal recessive
D. Polygenic inheritance

109. A   110. C   111. B   112. D   113. C   114. B   115. D   116. C   117. D   118. B

119. **Which of these features differentiates myasthenia gravis from oculopharyngeal dystrophy?**
    A. Adult onset
    B. Proximal muscle weakness
    C. Ptosis and diplopia due to ophthalmoplegia
    D. Presence of creatine kinase in blood

120. **A 19-year-old has been on and off on oral steroids for autoimmune renal disorder. She develops fatigue and weakness while getting up from squatting position. The reason for this is:**
    A. Steroid-induced osteoporosis
    B. Steroid-induced nerve degeneration
    C. Steroid-induced hyperglycemia
    D. Steroid-induced myopathy

121. **The protein deficient in Duchenne muscular dystrophy is:**
    A. Dystrophin
    B. Troponin
    C. Tropomyosin
    D. Actin

PY 3.14

122. **Fatigue is:**
    A. Decrease in amplitude of the contraction due to increased instensity of stimuli
    B. Decrease in amplitude of the contraction due to repeated stimuli
    C. Decrease in the number of contractions due to increased voltage
    D. All of the above

123. **The normal range of an EMG is:**
    A. 1–5 mV
    B. 0.5–1 mV
    C. 0.1–0.5 mV
    D. 0–0.1 mV

124. **A surface electrode patch is used to perform EMG. All the following are true, *except:***

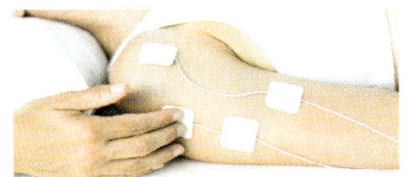

A. It potentiates spread of infection
B. It helps in studying a group of fibers
C. It is pain-free
D. It is inexpensive

125. **Which of these can be diagnosed on EMG?**
    A. Alzheimer's disease
    B. Parkinsonism
    C. Huntington's chorea
    D. Myaesthenia gravis

126. **Following is a feature of myaesthenia gravis on EMG:**
    A. Incremental response
    B. Decremental response
    C. Tetanus
    D. All the above occur at various time intervals

PY 3.15

127. **Following changes occur during exercise, *except:***
    A. Increase in heart rate
    B. Decrease in blood pressure
    C. Increase in cardiac output
    D. Increase in stroke volume

128. **A 66-year-old smoker experiences shooting pain in abdomen during exercise. He was diagnosed of mesenteric ischemia. The reason why it manifested during exercise is:**
    A. Exercise leads to dislodging of a clot from heart valves into mesenteric circulation
    B. During exercise there is vasospasm which causes ischemia
    C. During exercise there is decrease in blood flow to the visera which increases ischemia
    D. All of the above

129. **After performing a sprint, a woman was hyperventilating for 30–40 minutes after exercise. The reason for this is:**
    A. Oxygen dissociation
    B. Oxygen debt
    C. Oxygen deficit
    D. Oxygen doubling

119. D   120. D   121. A   122. B   123. C   124. A   125. D   126. B   127. B   128. C   129. B

130. Treadmill stress test is used as a screening for:

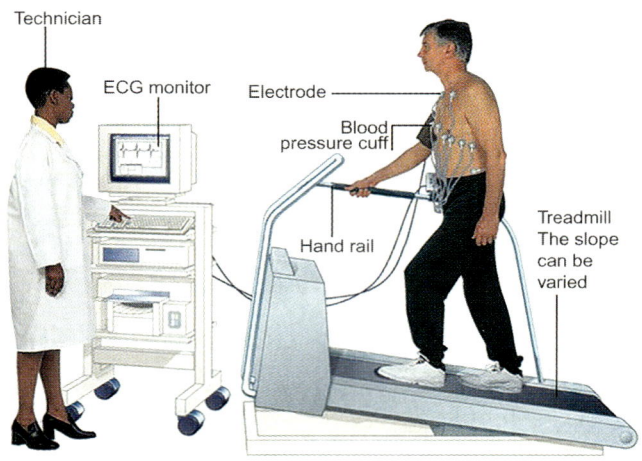

A. Coronary artery disease
B. Cardiac valvular disease
C. Myocarditis
D. Pericarditis

131. All contribute to tachypnoea during exercise, *except:*

A. Increase in blood carbon dioxide
B. Increased need for oxygen
C. Increased pulmonary resistance
D. Increased oxygen gradient

PY 3.16

132. Identify the test.

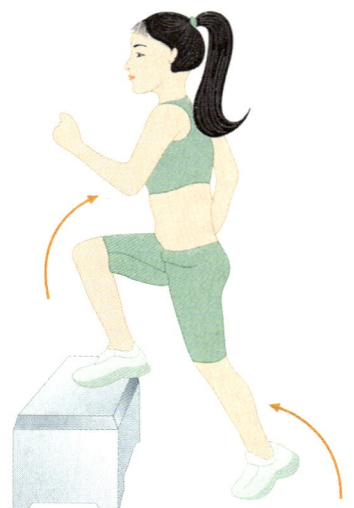

A. Brickben step test
B. Harvard step test
C. Mississippi stress test
D. None of the above

133. All are true about Harvard stress test, *except:*

A. It is a pulmonary stress test
B. The height of the step is 50 cm
C. It is a measure of endurance
D. A rate of 30 steps per minute must be maintained.

134. A person performs Harvard step test at the rate of 30 steps per minute for 5 minutes and gets exhausted. The total number of heartbeats counted at designated is 200. What is the fitness index?

A. 60
B. 70
C. 75
D. 80

135. Which of these is not a cardiac stress test?

A. Plethysmography
B. Treadmill test
C. Harvard stress test
D. Myocardial perfusion imaging

PY 3.17

136. Identify number 1.

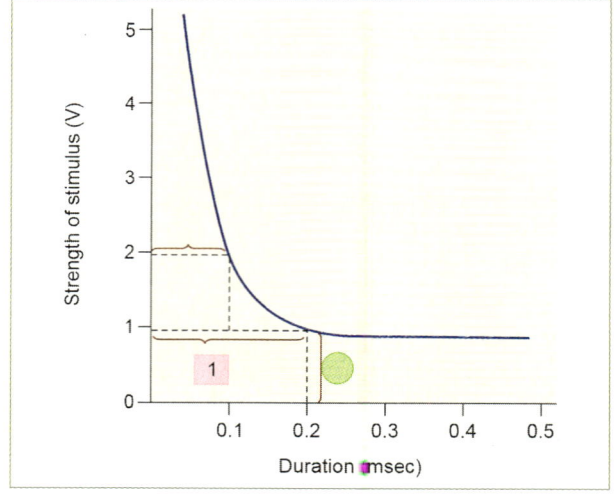

A. Chronaxie
B. Rheobase
C. Utilization time
D. Minimum time

130. A   131. C   132. B   133. A   134. C   135. A   136. C

137. **Rheobase is defined as:**
    A. Minimum strength of stimulus that can excite the tissue
    B. Minimum time for which minimum strength stimulus should act
    C. Index of excitability
    D. Minimum time required for 2 times the minimum strength to excite a tissue

138. **Rheobase is measured in:**
    A. Amps
    B. Watts
    C. Volt
    D. J/second

139. **If a stimulus of strength lower than rheobase is applied to a tissue:**
    A. There is fasciculation
    B. There is no excitement
    C. The excitement is same for all strengths of stimuli
    D. The time required for stimulus is longer, but the same amplitude can be produced

140. **Cronaxie is measured in:**
    A. Volts
    B. Amps
    C. Seconds
    D. Joules/second

PY 3.18

141. **Most commonly used nerve muscle preparation in a frog is:**
    A. Radial nerve—triceps
    B. Sciatic nerve—gastrocnemius
    C. Musculocutaneous nerve—biceps
    D. Femoral nerve—quadriceps

142. **Identify the equipment:**

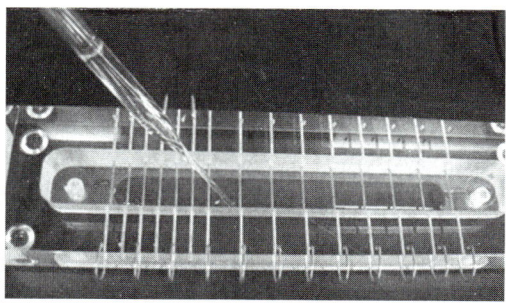

    A. Nerve bath
    B. Cathode ray oscilloscope
    C. Hemoglobinometer
    D. Induction coil

143. **The reason for preferring sciatic nerve—gastrocnemius to sartorius is:**
    A. Easy to dissect
    B. Sartorius fatigues easily
    C. Gastrocnemius has a larger cross-sectional area
    D. Gastrocnemius contracts even after dissection

144. **The nerve muscle preparation is suspended in:**
    A. Balanced salt solution
    B. 5% dextrose
    C. Isotonic saline
    D. Ringer's solution

145. **Pithing is:**
    A. Fixing the animal to a log
    B. Destroying the brain without hurting it
    C. Giving a blow on the head to make it unconscious
    D. Cutting the skin of the frog

146. **Identify the graph:**

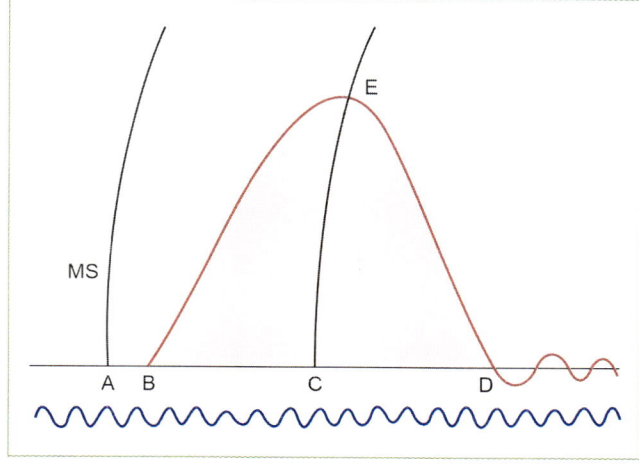

    A. Single muscle twitch
    B. Action potential of a smooth muscle
    C. Action potential of a skeletal muscle
    D. Action potential of a nerve

137. A   138. C   139. B   140. C   141. B   142. A   143. C   144. C   145. B   146. A

PY 4.1

147. Brunner's gland is characteristic of which of the following parts of gastrointestinal tract?
A. Large intestine
B. Stomach
C. Small intestine
D. Appendix

148. Crypts of Lieberkühn are which types of the following glands?
A. Tubuloalveolar gland
B. Simple tubular gland
C. Compound tubuloalveolar gland
D. Simple alveolar gland

149. Which of the following about gastrointestinal smooth muscles is not true?
A. They are connected by gap junctions
B. Act as syncytium
C. Are sensitive hormones
D. Do not change in length by stretching

150. All of the following are differences between spike potentials of nerves and gastrointestinal smooth muscles, *except*:
A. The spike rarely crosses the isoelectric base in nerves but in GI smooth muscles, it overshoots the isoelectric base
B. The duration of action potential in smooth muscle is longer
C. The resting membrane potential in a smooth muscle is undulating between –40 and –50 mV
D. The spike is caused by influx of calcium in smooth muscles and sodium in nerves

151. Which of the following structures does not have a muscularis mucosa?
A. Mouth
B. Esophagus
C. Ileum
D. Duodenum

PY 4.2

152. Maximum potassium ions secretion is seen in:
A. Saliva
B. Gastric secretions
C. Jejuna secretions
D. Colonic secretions

153. The amount of saliva secreted per day is:
A. 0.5–0.75 L
B. 1–2 L
C. 1–2.5 L
D. 2.5–3.5 L

154. All of the following enzymes are present in saliva, *except*:
A. Amylase
B. Lipase
C. Dextrinase
D. Maltase

155. A 11-week pregnant lady has been craving for chocolate cake. When she is about to place the cake in her mouth, she feels a strange feeling below her chin. This is due to:
A. Contraction of tongue
B. Contraction of the sublingual acini
C. Contraction of the muscles of mastication
D. Psychological feeling due to excess craving

156. A 19-year-old girl was chased by a stranger with a knife in his hand. She was petrified and when she reached a night guard, she could not narrate her story and her mouth fell dry. The reason for this is:
A. She lost a lot of fluid due to sweat and was thirsty
B. She ran with her mouth open and the saliva dried away
C. Sympathetic stimulation causes decrease in saliva secretion
D. She swallowed a lot of saliva and her mouth became dry

157. A 35-year-old man is stressed about his work and is always on the run. He starts experiencing heart burn before every meal. He was diagnosed of gastritis. The cause for increased secretion of gastric juices is:
A. Stress
B. Idiopathic
C. Probable tumor secreting gastrin
D. Irregular feeding habits

147. C   148. B   149. D   150. A   151. A   152. A   153. A   154. C   155. B   156. C   157. A

158. Which of the following is essential for B$_{12}$ absorption?
A. Pepsin
B. Gastrin
C. Intrinsic factor
D. Extrinsic factor

159. Which phase of GI secretion does this image explain?

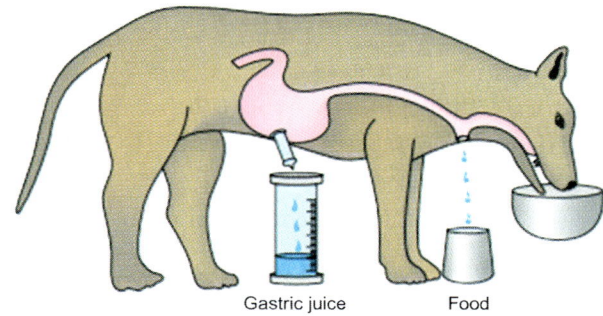

Gastric juice   Food

A. Cephalic phase of salivation
B. Oral phase of salivation
C. Cephalic phase of gastric acid secretion
D. Gastric phase of gastric acid secretion

160. Secretin is secreted by:
A. Duodenum
B. Pancreas
C. Liver
D. Stomach

PY 4.3

161. There are mainly two types of GI contractions—slow waves and action potentials. In which part of the GIT is the frequency of these slow waves the highest?
A. Stomach
B. Duodenum
C. Ileum
D. All are at same frequency

162. During swallowing, pressure recorded due to muscles contraction are lowest at:
A. Gastro-oesophageal sphincter
B. Oesophagus
C. Pharynx
D. Pharyngo-oesophageal sphincter

163. The aim of which of the following deglutination stages is to avoid the entry of bolus into the respiratory tract?
A. Buccal stage
B. Esophageal stage
C. Pharyngeal stage
D. Both of the above

164. In earlier days, ether was placed on the abdomen when there was absolute constipation. What is the rationale?
A. Cold temperature stimulates abdominal movements
B. The smell of ether causes abdominal movements
C. Ether gets absorbed through skin and increases GI movements
D. All of the above

165. Which of the following is false?
A. Meissner's plexus is responsible for gastrointestinal motility
B. Auerbach's plexus is present in the muscular layer
C. Sympathetic nerves inhibit the nervous system and thus decrease movements
D. Parasympathetic system is responsible for watery secretion

166. A 66-year-old man with constipation was advised to consume hemicellulose along with water. The reason is:
A. Hemicellulose is osmotic, and attracts water
B. Hemicellulose is indigestible, so increases bulk of the feces
C. Hemicellulose stimulates the muscles of the GIT chemically
D. All of the above

PY 4.4

167. Trypsin is an activator of all of the following enzymes, *except*:
A. Chymotrypsinogen
B. Pepsinogen
C. Proelastase
D. Procarboxypeptidase A and B

158. C   159. C   160. A   161. B   162. A   163. C   164. A   165. A   166. B   167. B

168. **Which of the following correctly describes bile lipid?**
A. Bile lipid = Bile acid + Phosphoprotein + Cholesterol
B. Bile lipid = Bile acid + Cholesterol
C. Bile Lipid = Bile acid + Fatty acids excluding cholesterol
D. None of the above

169. **Digestion of carbohydrates begins in:**
A. Mouth
B. Stomach
C. Duodenum
D. Ileum

170. **A 6-day-old baby presents with vomiting and loose stools. She was consuming only mother's breast milk. This condition is probably due to:**
A. Hirschsprung disease (congenital megacolon)
B. Congenital lactase deficiency
C. Botulism
D. Imperforate anus

171. **Amino acids are absorbed into the intestinal epithelium as co-transport with:**
A. Calcium ions
B. Phosphorus ions
C. Potassium ions
D. Sodium ions

172. **A 36-year-old obese lady complains of fatty feces which floats in the pot and is difficult to flush. She was diagnosed of steatorrhea. What is expected on an ultrasound of the abdomen?**
A. Dilated bile duct
B. Pancreatic mass
C. Calculi in the common bile duct
D. All of the above

PY 4.5

173. **Secretin does not cause:**
A. Bicarbonated secretions
B. Augments the action of CCK
C. Contraction of pyloric sphincter
D. Gastric secretion increase

174. **All of the following are GIT hormones, *except* one, that is:**
A. Gastrin
B. Secretin
C. Enterokinase
D. Cholecystokinin

175. **A 61-year-old lady complains of epigastric pain and watery diarrhoea. A dueodenal ulcer was found on endoscopy. Her serum gastrin levels were 820 pg/ml (normal is <100 pg/ml). The most probable cause is:**
A. Zollinger-Ellison syndrome
B. *H. pylori*-induced dueodenal ulcer
C. Stress ulcers
D. Aspirin-induced dueodenal ulcer

176. **Match the following:**

List I	List II
A. Gastrin	I. S cells
B. Secretin	II. G cells
C. Cholecystokinin	III. K cells
D. Gastric inhibitory peptide	IV. I cells

A. A: IV, B: II, C: III, D: I
B. A: II, B: I, C: IV, D: III
C. A: III, B: II, C: I, D: IV
D. A: I, B: III, C: II, D: IV

177. **A hormone secreted by hypothalamus which can be therapeutically used in neuroendocrine tumors is:**
A. Leptin
B. Prolactin inhibiting hormone
C. Growth hormone inhibiting hormone
D. Gonadotropin-releasing hormone

PY 4.6

178. **The gut brain axis involves all the following, *except*:**
A. Hypothalamopituitary adrenal axis
B. Central nervous system
C. Hypothalamopituitary gonadal axis
D. Enteric nervous system

168. D   169. A   170. B   171. D   172. D   173. D   174. C   175. A   176. B   177. C   178. C

179. **Improvement of hepatic encephalopathy by administration of oral antibiotics is an evidence of:**
    A. Gut–hepatic axis
    B. Gut–colon axis
    C. Gut–adrenal axis
    D. Gut–brain axis

180. **Norepinephrine released during surgery favors growth of an organism—pseudomonas in the gut and predisposes to sepsis. This is an example for:**
    A. Gut–brain interaction
    B. Gut–hormone interaction
    C. Hormone–microbe interaction
    D. All of the above

181. **False about gut–brain axis is:**
    A. It is bidirectional interaction
    B. Removal of microbiota from the gut causes sudden loss of cognition
    C. Vagus nerve is the most important pathway for communication
    D. Gut microbiota are involved in secretion of hormones in the GIT

182. **Match the following:**

List I	List II
A. Prebiotics	I. Substances which contain both prebiotics and probiotics
B. Probiotics	II. Substrate that is selectively utilized by host microorganism
C. Synbiotics	III. Substances which inhibit growth of bacteria
D. Antibiotics	IV. Live microorganisms when administered in adequate amounts are beneficial to the host organisms

    A. A: II, B: III, C: I, D: IV
    B. A: II, B: IV, C: I, D: III
    C. A: I, B: III, C: II, D: IV
    D. A: III, B: IV, C: II, D: II

PY 4.7

133. **Production of bile takes place in:**
    A. The gall bladder
    B. Kupffer cells
    C. Hepatic duct
    D. Hepatocytes

184. **In jaundice, there is an unconjugated hyperbilirubinemia which is most likely due to:**
    A. Hepatitis
    B. Cirrhosis
    C. Obstruction of canaliculi
    D. Increased breakdown of red cells

185. **A sonographer instructs a patient to be empty stomach while performing an ultrasound of the abdomen to look for gall bladder pathology. What is the reason?**
    A. The patient's distended stomach may block view of the gall bladder
    B. The gall bladder empties itself after food enters due to the action of CCK
    C. The stones are same density as the food so cannot be differentiated
    D. The stones recede back into the gall bladder from the duct and may be difficult to localize

186. **A patient has generalized itching and yellowish discoloration of urine. On examination, he was found to have icterus. What is expected in his blood picture?**
    A. Hemolysis
    B. Increased unconjugated bilirubin
    C. Increased conjugated bilirubin
    D. Anemia

187. **A 54-year-old was diagnosed of gall stones, and so underwent cholecystectomy. What is the effect of this on his digestive system?**
    A. Improvement of lipid profile
    B. Increase in the frequency of stools
    C. Sphincter of Oddi dysfunction
    D. All of the above

PY 4.8

188. **Van den Bergh reaction is directly positive in which of the following types of jaundice?**
    A. Haemolytic jaundice
    B. Obstructive jaundice
    C. Toxic jaundice
    D. Infective jaundice

179. D   180. A   181. B   182. B   183. D   184. D   185. B   186. C   187. D   188. B

189. Which of the following shows the bilirubin concentration above which jaundice is clinically detectable?
    A. 1 mg/100 ml
    B. 1.5 ml /100 ml
    C. 2 gm/100 ml
    D. 2 mg/100 ml

190. A 29-year-old female with high BMI (26 kg/m²) came with severe pain in the abdomen of acute onset.

Serum amylase	330 IU/L (normal <115 IU/L)
Serum lipase	177 IU/L (normal < 82 IU/L)
Blood glucose (random)	122 mg/dl
Serum triglycerides	355 mg/dl (normal <150 mg/dl)
AST	35 IU/L
ALT	24 IU/L

   What is the diagnosis?
    A. Acute hepatitis
    B. Acute pancreatitis
    C. Acute mesenteric ischemia
    D. Acute hepatic failure

191. Which of the following is not a hepatic function test?
    A. Blood urea
    B. Serum bilirubin
    C. Serum albumin
    D. AST

192. A 63-year-old undergoes the following test. What is it used to diagnose (*see* Figure given in 2nd col. at top)
    A. *H. pylori* infection
    B. Duodenal ulcer
    C. Small intestine bacterial overgrowth
    D. Intestinal obstruction

PY 4.9

193. Opening of which of the following sphincters marks the end of deglutition?
    A. Lower pharyngeal sphincter
    B. Upper pharyngeal sphincter
    C. Upper esophageal sphincter
    D. Lower esophageal sphincter

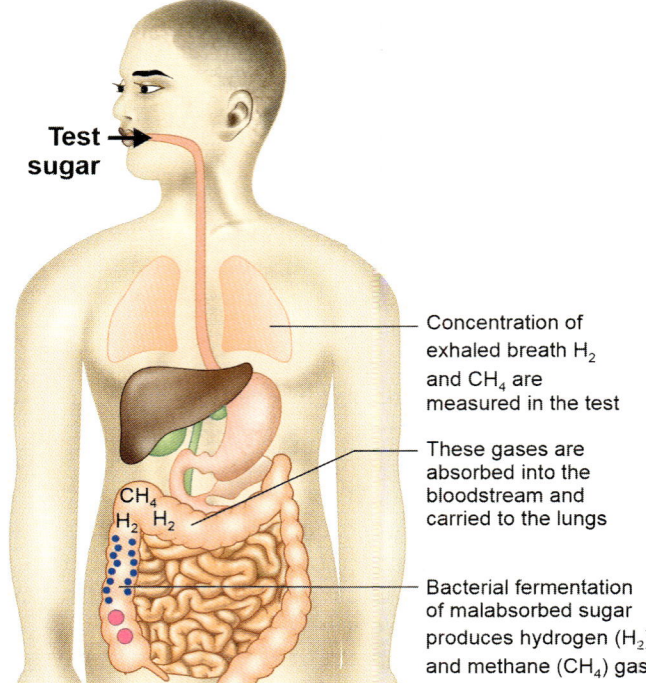

Test → sugar

Concentration of exhaled breath H_2 and CH_4 are measured in the test

These gases are absorbed into the bloodstream and carried to the lungs

Bacterial fermentation of malabsorbed sugar produces hydrogen (H_2) and methane (CH_4) gas

CH_4
H_2 H_2

194. A person with high intraocular pressure is given oral glycerol. What is its effect on gastro-intestinal system?
    A. Causes constipation
    B. Causes watery diarrhea
    C. Does not cause any problem
    D. Gets absorbed through the mucosa

195. Congenital megacolon is also called.......... .
    A. Hirschsprung disease
    B. Imperforate anus
    C. Volvulus
    D. Intussusception

196. A 44-year-old underwent an uneventful surgery under spinal anaesthesia. He was told that he may have difficulty in passing stools for 3–6 hours. What is the cause?
    A. Paralytic ileus
    B. Intestinal perforation
    C. Intestinal obstruction
    D. Damage to spinal cord

189. D   190. B   191. A   192. C   193. D   194. B   195. A   196. A

197. A 38-week pregnant lady complains of difficulty in eating food as she feels burning sensation after every meal. She was advised to have frequent spaced smaller meals. What is the cause for this symptom?

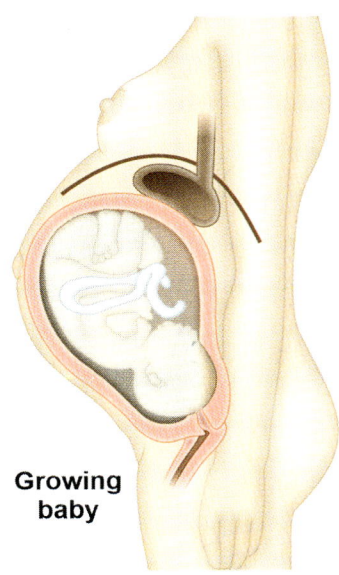

Growing baby

A. Progesterone causes laxity of sphincter in pregnancy
B. The growing baby presses the stomach against the esophagus
C. Both A and B
D. Placenta secretes gastrin which causes increased acidity

PY 4.10

193. Which side of the subject is best suited for a left-handed examiner, to be while examining?
A. Right
B. Left
C. Near the head
D. Near the feet

199. Inspection of abdomen includes all of the following, *except:*
A. Shape of the abdomen
B. Position of umbilicus
C. Position of the apex beat
D. Appearance of any other pulsations

200. Which parameter has to be assessed last in palpation?
A. Size of mass
B. Movement with respiration
C. Palpation of pulsation
D. Tenderness

201. An obese lady presented with pain in abdomen. On examination, the umbilicus was seen pushed upward. Where is the probable location of an abdominal mass?
A. Superior abdomen
B. Inferior abdomen
C. Posterior to umbilicus
D. Flanks

202. A 16-year-old female presents with pain abdomen in the right iliac fossa. On examination there is tenderness. What are the structures that cause presentation in this fossa?
A. Appendix
B. Cecum
C. Fallopian tube and ovary
D. All of the above

PY 5.1

203. Left ventricular mass is more compared to right ventricular mass because:
A. Increased blood flow to the left ventricle through left coronary artery
B. Left ventricle does more work to pump out the blood
C. The valve consists of only two cusps which allow increased accumulation of blood
D. The systemic arteries offer lesser resistance to the blood flow

204. ACh decreases the sinus nodal discharge by:
A. Increasing permeability of the fibre membrane to K^+ ions
B. Decreasing permeability of the fibre membrane to K^+ ions
C. Increasing permeability of the fibre membrane to Na^+ ions
D. Decreasing permeability of the fibre membrane to Na^+ ions
E. Increasing permeability of the fibre membrane to Ca^{++} ions

197. C   198. B   199. C   200. D   201. B   202. D   203. B   204. A

205. **Fourth heart sound is caused by:**
    A. Closure of aortic and pulmonary valves
    B. Vibration of ventricular wall during systole
    C. Last rapid filling phase
    D. Retrograde flow in vena cava

206. **At each intercalated disc in cardiac muscle, the cell membranes have:**
    A. Tight junctions
    B. Gap junctions
    C. Desmosomes
    D. Hemidesmosoms

207. **Accentuation of first heart sound occurs in:**
    A. Hypertension
    B. Acute myocardial infarction
    C. Constrictive pericarditis
    D. Obesity

PY 5.2

208. **The plateau phase of cardiac muscle action potential is due to:**
    A. Slow influx of Na^+ ions
    B. Slow influx of Ca^{++} ions
    C. Slow efflux of Na^+ ions
    D. Slow efflux of Ca^{++} ions

209. **Why cardiac muscle cannot be tetanized?**
    A. Complete summation of contractions occurs
    B. It has a long refractory period
    C. Muscle fibers are arranged in a syncytial fashion
    D. It responds to subthreshold stimulus

210. **Which experimental evidence proves that cardiac muscle acts as pacemaker?**
    A. SA node becomes electrically positive before any other part of the atria
    B. Local cooling of SA node increases the heart rate
    C. Local warming of SA node decreases the heart rate
    D. SA node becomes electrically positive before any other part of the atria

211. **Delay in the conduction of heart impulse occurs maximally at:**
    A. SA node
    B. AV node
    C. Bundle of His
    D. Purkinje fibers

212. **What changes occur in the cardiac muscle action potential when ECF sodium concentration decreases?**
    A. Cardiac muscle action potential increases
    B. Cardiac muscle action potential decreases
    C. No change occurs
    D. Becomes unstable

PY 5.3

213. **During cardiac cycle opening of aortic valve takes place at the:**
    A. Beginning of systole
    B. End of isovolumetric contraction
    C. End of diastole
    D. End of diastasis

214. **Dicrotic notch on the aortic pressure curve is caused by:**
    A. Closure of mitral valve
    B. Closure of tricuspid valve
    C. Closure of pulmonary valve
    D. Bouncing of blood at aortic valve

215. **What changes occur in JVP in patients with complete heart block?**
    A. Giant C wave
    B. Gaint A wave
    C. Absent C wave
    D. Absent A wave

216. **The last rapid filling phase of ventricular diastole coincides with:**
    A. Atrial systole
    B. Atrial diastole
    C. Prodiastole
    D. Isovolumic relaxation phase

205. C   206. B   207. A   208. B   209. B   210. D   211. B   212. C   213. B   214. D   215. B   216. A

217. **How do you differentiate between atrial and ventricular premature beats?**
    A. Presence of A wave in the atrial premature beats
    B. Presence of A wave in the ventricular premature beats
    C. Presence of C wave in the atrial premature beats
    D. Presence of C wave in the ventricular premature beats

PY 5.4

218. **The self-excitatory discharge rate of Purkinje fibres is:**
    A. 15–40/min
    B. 40–60/min
    C. 70–80/min
    D. 90–100/min

219. **The plateau phase of cardiac muscle action potential is due to:**
    A. Influx of Na^+ ions
    B. Influx of Ca^{++} ions
    C. Efflux of K^+ ions
    D. Efflux of Ca^{++} ions

220. **The component of cardiac tissue having highest propagation velocity:**
    A. Purkinje fibers
    B. AV node
    C. Ventricular muscle
    D. Atrial muscle

221. **In normal healthy adults the ratio of left to right ventricular thickness is:**
    A. 1:3
    B. 2:3
    C. 3:1
    D. 3:2

222. **Papillary muscles:**
    A. Originate from chordae tendineae
    B. Help in closure of AV valves
    C. Help in opening of AV valves
    D. Prevent bulging of AV valves into atria during ventricular contraction

PY 5.5

223. **In lead II of the standard bipolar limb lead of ECG:**
    A. The negative terminal is connected to the right arm and positive terminal to the left arm
    B. The negative terminal is connected to the left leg and positive terminal to the right arm
    C. The negative terminal is connected to the right arm and positive terminal to the left leg
    D. The negative terminal is connected to the left arm and positive terminal to the left leg

224. **Long QT syndrome occurs due to genetic abnormality which blocks:**
    A. Sodium channels
    B. Potassium channels
    C. Calcium channels
    D. Chloride channels

225. **If the duration of PR interval is <0.12 sec, expected is:**
    A. Decrease in the heart rate
    B. Increase in the heart rate
    C. Impulse has probably arisen from AV node
    D. Normal

226. **Normal QRS complex duration is:**
    A. 0.02 sec
    B. 0.04–0.06 sec
    C. 0.08-0.12 sec
    D. 0.1–0.15 sec

227. **ST segment:**
    A. Extends from end of S wave to end of T wave
    B. Extends from end of S wave to beginning of T wave
    C. End of the P wave to beginning of QRS complex
    D. End of the P wave to end of QRS complex

217. A   218. A   219. B   220. A   221. C   222. D   223. C   224. B   225. C   226. C   227. B

PY 5.6

228. Presence of an aberrant bundle that bypasses the AV node and enters the intraventricular conducting system distal to node is seen in:
- A. Wenckebach phenomenon
- B. Sick sinus syndrome
- C. Stokes-Adams syndrome
- D. Lown-Ganong-Levine syndrome

229. 50-year-old diabetic and a chronic smoker presented with the history of chest pain and vomiting. On examination, pulse rate was 110 bpm and blood pressure was 180/100 mm Hg. What changes do you expect in ECG to confirm the diagnosis of MI?
- A. ST segment elevation
- B. T wave elevation
- C. Tall R waves
- D. Low voltage QRS complex

230. Identify the condition with the help of ECG feature.

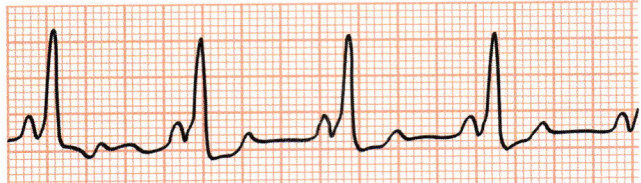

- A. Myocardial ischemia
- B. Wolff-Parkinson white syndrome
- C. Lown-Ganong-Levine syndrome
- D. Left bundle branch block

231. In Mobitz type 1 block:
- A. PR interval is shortened
- B. Ventricular beats occur in every 2 or 3 atrial beats
- C. Also called complete heart block
- D. PR interval progressively prolonged until the next beat is dropped

232. Sinus bradycardia occurs in:
- A. Cardiac failure
- B. Acute carditis
- C. Fever
- D. Obstructive jaundice

233. Prolonged QT interval is seen in:
- A. Hypernatremia
- B. Hyponatremia
- C. Hypercalcemia
- D. Hypocalcemia

PY 5.7

234. Which scientific principle is the basis for thermodilution method used in measuring cardiac output by pulmonary catheter?
- A. Hagen-Poiseuille's principle
- B. Stewart-Hamilton principle
- C. Bernoulli's principle
- D. Universal gas equation

235. Lymph flow from the foot is:
- A. Increased when an individual rises from supine to standing
- B. Increased by massaging the foot
- C. Increased when capillary permeability is decreased
- D. Decreased when the valves of leg veins are incompetent

236. All are true about Poiseuille's law, except:
- A. Flow is directly proportional to pressure gradient
- B. Flow is inversely proportional to the length of the vessel
- C. Flow of fluid varies directly as the fourth power of the diameter
- D. Flow varies inversely with the viscosity of fluid

237. Arm to lung circulation time is:
- A. 15 sec
- B. 6 sec
- C. 24 sec
- D. 80 sec

238. Why capillaries are less prone to rupture though they are thin?
- A. They require lesser tension to balance the distending pressure
- B. They require greater tension to balance the distending pressure
- C. They have a greater radius
- D. They are enormous in number

228. D   229. A   230. B   231. D   232. D   233. D   234. B   235. B   236. C   237 B   238. A

PY 5.8

239. A patient with increased BP and decreased heart rate is likely to have:
A. Increased intracranial tension
B. Brain tumor
C. Head trauma
D. Any of the above

240. Activation of chemosensitive vagal C fibers in the cardiopulmonary region causes:
A. Bezold-Jarisch reflex
B. Cushings reflex
C. Somatosympathetic reflex
D. Hering-Breur reflex

241. Maximal baroreceptor nerve activity occurs at about:
A. 50 mm of Hg
B. 80 mm of Hg
C. 100 mm of Hg
D. 200 mm of Hg

242. The pressure difference between the heart and aorta is least in the:
A. Left ventricle during systole
B. Left ventricle during diastole
C. Right ventricle during systole
D. Right ventricle during diastole
E. Left atrium during systole

243. What happens when both carotid arteries are ligated proximal to the carotid sinus?
A. Blood pressure decreases
B. Heart rate decreases
C. Blood pressure increases
D. No change in the heart rate and blood pressure

PY 5.9

244. Isovolumetric relaxation phase of cardiac cycle ends with:
A. Peak of C wave
B. Opening of AV valve
C. Closure of semilunar valve
D. Beginning of T wave

**245. All are determinants of arterial blood pressure, *except:*
A. Stroke volume
B. Arterial muscular content

C. Arterial blood volume
D. Heart rate

246. Heart rate is accelerated by:
A. Increased activity of atrial stretch receptors
B. Expiration
C. Increased activity of arterial baroreceptors
D. Increased intracranial pressure

247. If cardiac output is 5 L/min and body surface area is 1.5 m², cardiac index is equal to:
A. 3.3 L/min/m²
B. 4.3 L/min/m²
C. 2.5 L/min/m²
D. 5.3 L/min/m²

248. The term vis-a-tergo refers to:
A. Increased venous return to the heart due to decrease in intrathoracic pressure
B. Force from front to attract blood in the veins towards heart
C. Propelling force in the blood which drains the blood forward
D. Rhythmic contraction of leg muscles that squeeze the blood out m²

PY 5.10

249. The volume of blood, spinal fluid and brain in the cranium at any given time must be relatively constant. This is:
A. Monro-Kellie doctrine
B. Bell-Magendie law
C. Law of projection
D. Weber-Fechner's law

250. Oxygen consumption is more for:
A. Basal ganglia
B. Cerebellum
C. Medulla oblongata
D. Pons

251. What keeps the alveoli dry:
A. Low pulmonary capillary hydrostatic pressure
B. Presence of lymphatics
C. Low pulmonary colloidal osmotic pressure
D. Low pulmonary arterial pressure

239. D 240. A 241. D 242. A   243. C 244. B 245. C 246. A   247. A   248. C 249. A   250. A   251. A

252. Why does fluid accumulate in the tissue?
   A. Due to increased precapillary vascular resistance
   B. Due to decreased postcapillary vascular resistance
   C. Due to increased venous pressure
   D. Due to decreased plasma osmotic pressure

253. Phasic coronary blood flow refers to:
   A. Almost zero flow through coronary arteries
   B. Maximum blood flow through coronaries
   C. Increase in blood flow during systole
   D. Variation in blood flow with reference to cardiac cycle

PY 5.11

254. Decreased pumping ability of heart due to massive myocardial infarction leads to:
   A. Hypovolaemic shock
   B. Cardiogenic shock
   C. Vasogenic shock
   D. Obstructive shock

255. Which type of heart failure is most likely associated with pulmonary edema?
   A. Heart failure due to arteriovenous fistula
   B. High output heart failure
   C. Left heart failure
   D. Right heart failure

256. After hemorrhage, restoration of blood volume is due to:
   A. Arteriolar constriction
   B. Shift of intracellular fluid to extracellular space
   C. Increased venous return
   D. Intravenous infusion

257. Warm shock is the term applied to the:
   A. Hypovolumic shock
   B. Cardiogenic shock
   C. Low resistance shock
   D. Surgical shock

258. Frank-Starling mechanism fail to operate in late stages of heart failure due to:
   A. Shock
   B. Cardiomegaly
   C. Cardiac ischemia
   D. Conduction disturbance

PY 6.1

259. Total number of alveoli in both the lungs are:
   A. 100 million
   B. 200 million
   C. 300 million
   D. 600 million

260. Lack of motility of cilia in ciliated epithelium of tracheobronchial tree is observed in:
   A. Bronchial asthma
   B. Chronic bronchitis
   C. Kartagener's syndrome
   D. Cushing's syndrome

261. Diffusion of gases depends upon:
   A. Difference in the partial pressure of gases
   B. Difference in the temperature of gases
   C. Difference in the water vapour content
   D. Difference in the number of molecules

262. How the foreign particles reaching the bronchus are expelled out:
   A. By activation of tissue macrophage system
   B. By bronchodilatation
   C. By ciliary escalator action
   D. By deglutition reflex

263. The conducting zone:
   A. Extends from 17th generation
   B. Consists of respiratory bronchioles
   C. Volume is approximately 4 litres
   D. Consists of terminal bronchioles

PY 6.2

264. How do diaphragmatic movements constitute for 75% of tidal volume in eupnoea?
   A. Contraction causes decent of diaphragm sucking in 200–300 ml of air
   B. Causes decrease in the vertical diameter thereby increasing the capacity of the lungs
   C. Contraction increases the convexity of the dome towards thorax
   D. Decreases the intra-abdominal pressure thereby pulling down the lower ribs

252. D 253. D 254. B 255. C 256. B 257. C 258. C 259. C 260. C 261. A 262. C 263. D 264. A

265. Compliance of the lungs is:
A. 0.22 L/mm Hg
B. 0.13 L/mm Hg
C. 0.22 L/cm H_2O
D. 0.13 L/cm H_2O

266. Pressure at the lower end of oesophagus (intra-oesophageal pressure) is same as:
A. Intrapulmonary pressure
B. Intrapleural pressure
C. Transpulmonary pressure
D. Atmospheric pressure

267. Why is vital capacity higher in standing position compared to lying down position?
A. Due to decreased pulmonary blood flow
B. Due to increased pulmonary blood flow
C. Due to decreased inspiration
D. Due to increased venous return

268. V/Q ratio in the subject with alveolar ventilation of 3.5 L/min and pulmonary blood flow of 5 L/min is:
A. 0.8
B. 0.9
C. 1.0
D. 0.7

269. Work done by the respiratory muscle is to overcome:
A. Elastic resistance
B. Viscous resistance
C. Airway resistance
D. All of the above

270. Preterm female baby weighing 1.2 kg was delivered due to prolonged rupture of membranes. The baby cried immediately after birth but was pale, hypothermic and tachypneic. SPO_2 was 60%. Which of the following is a false statement?
A. Commonly called as respiratory distress syndrome
B. Is caused due to surfactant deficiency
C. More common in newborns born after 37 weeks
D. Corticosteroids when given to mothers before delivery lowers the severity

PY 6.3

271. Loading of blood with oxygen causes un-loading of carbon dioxide. This is called:
A. Bohr's effect
B. Haldane's effect
C. Hamburger phenomenon
D. Hering-Breur reflex

272. All of the following shift the Hb–oxygen dissociation curve (ODC) to the right, except:
A. Increased temperature
B. Increased carbon dioxide.
C. Increased pH
D. Increase in 2,3-BPG

273. Observed haematocrit value is more in:
A. Arterial blood
B. Venous blood
C. Blood of pulmonary vein
D. Anemia

274. Why is the dissociation curve of myoglobin rectangular hyperbola?
A. Rate of association of myoglobin with oxygen is very slow
B. Rate of association of myoglobin with oxygen is very fast
C. Contains two heme group with one polypeptide chain
D. Contains one heme group with two polypeptide chain

275. Higher th P50:
A. Lower affinity of hemoglobin for oxygen
B. Higher affinity of hemoglobin for oxygen
C. No change in the affinity
D. Affinity of hemoglobin to oxygen is zero

276. Oxygen dissociation curve during exercise:
A. Shifts to left
B. Shifts to right
C. Does not affect
D. Is hyperbolic

PY 6.4

277. A person can ascend safely up to:
A. 4000 mt
B. 5000 mt
C. 3000 mt
D. 6000 mt

265. C 266. B 267. A 268. D 269. D 270. C 271. B 272. C 273. B 274. B 275. A 276. B 277. C

278. **Acclimatization is possible due to:**
    A. Increase in pulmonary ventilation
    B. Decrease in pulmonary ventilation
    C. Decrease in hemoglobin concentration
    D. Decreased vascularity of hypoxic tissues

279. **Explain why nitrogen bubbles are formed in the tissue when diver comes to the surface:**
    A. Due to sudden increase in the pressure
    B. Due to sudden decrease in the pressure
    C. Due to gradual increase in the pressure
    D. Due to gradual decrease in the pressure

280. **Caisson's disease is due to:**
    A. Air embolism
    B. Fat embolism
    C. Amniotic fluid embolism
    D. Plasma embolism

281. **Complete obstruction of blood vessel leads to:**
    A. Local asphyxia
    B. Hypocapnea
    C. General asphyxia
    D. Acclimatization

PY 6.5

282. **Cerebral cortex develops irreversible damage if oxygen supply is stopped for:**
    A. 2 min
    B. 3 min
    C. 1 min
    D. 5 min

283. **What do you do to expel the air that enters the stomach during artificial respiration?**
    A. Stop the procedure
    B. Apply pressure on the epigastrium
    C. Apply pressure over the sternum
    D. Apply pressure over sternoclavicular joint

284. **Oxygen therapy is of no use in:**
    A. Anemic hypoxia
    B. Hypoxic hypoxia
    C. Histotoxic hypoxia
    D. Stagnant hypoxia

285. **A 25-year-old Sham is in excellent physical condition, runs 2 km daily and is a national level volley ball player. What changes occur in him when he ascents to high altitude?**
    A. Respiratory rate decreases
    B. Percentage saturation of hemoglobin is increased
    C. P50 decreases
    D. Pulmonary arterial pressure is increased

PY 6.6

286. **Stimulation of vagus nerve produces apnoea by:**
    A. Stimulating the inhibitory center
    B. By inhibiting the expiratory center
    C. By inhibiting apneustic center
    D. By inhibiting inspiratory center

287. **Why cardiac failure patients are comfortable in sitting rather than lying down position?**
    A. Lying down causes increased pulmonary congestion
    B. Lying down causes decreased pulmonary congestion
    C. Lying down causes decreased pulmonary ventilation
    D. Lying down causes decreased venous return

288. **Why does the blood volume decrease in sea water drowning?**
    A. Sea water is hypertonic
    B. Sea water is hypotonic
    C. Glottis contract decreasing entry of water
    D. Glottis contract causing retention of water

289. **Patients with Cheyne-Stokes breathing have:**
    A. Increased PCO_2 at the end of apnoea
    B. Decreased PO_2 at the end of apnoea
    C. Increased sensitivity to CO_2
    D. Increased sensitivity to O_2

290. **Why does exposure to severe cold not cause cyanosis?**
    A. Oxygen hemoglobin dissociation curve shifts to right
    B. Oxygen hemoglobin dissociation curve shifts to left
    C. Oxygen consumption of the tissue increases
    D. Reduced hemoglobin content increases

278. A 279. B 280. A 281. A 282. D 283. B 284. C 285. D 286. D 287. A 288. A 289. C 290. B

PY 6.7

291. The volume of the air that can be expired rapidly by maximal expiratory effort after maximal inspiration is:
A. Slow vital capacity
B. Forced vital capacity
C. Peak expiratory flow rate
D. Functional residual capacity

292. The following cannot be measured by simple spirometer:
A. Vital capacity
B. Tidal volume
C. Residual volume
D. Functional residual capacity

293. 70-year-old male chronic smoker complained of shortness of breath, easy fatigability. Auscultatory findings revealed prolonged expiratory phase and expiratory wheeze. What changes would you expect in the pulmonary function test?
A. Increased residual volume, decreased vital capacity
B. Decreased residual volume, decreased vital capacity
C. Decreased residual volume, increased vital capacity
D. Decreased residual volume, decreased functional residual capacity

PY 7.1, 7.2 and 7.3

294. Which of the following parts is not present in cortical nephrons?
A. Proximal convoluted tubule
B. Thin ascending limb of loop of Henle
C. Thick ascending limb of loop of Henle
D. Distal convoluted tubule

295. Principal cells (P cells) involved in sodium reabsorption present in which of the following segment of nephron?
A. Proximal convoluted tubule
B. Loop of Henle

C. Distal convoluted tubule
D. Collecting ducts

296. Efferent arteriole of cortical nephrons drains into:
A. Peritubular capillaries
B. Vasa recta
C. Both peritubular capillaries and vasa recta
D. None of the above

297. Juxtaglomerular apparatus consists of the following cells, *except*:
A. Lacis cells
B. Macula densa
C. Mesangial cells
D. Juxtaglomerular (JG) cells

298. Which of the following cells of juxtaglomerular apparatus releases renin?
A. Lacis cells
B. Macula densa
C. Mesangial cells
D. Juxtaglomerular (JG) cells

299. Filtered load of NaCl across distal convoluted tubule is detected by which of the following cells?
A. Lacis cells
B. Macula densa
C. Mesangial cells
D. Juxtaglomerular (JG) cells

300. Which of the following causes increase to secretion of renin?
A. Decreased renal perfusion
B. Decreased renal blood pressure
C. Sympathetic stimulation
D. All of the above

301. In physiological conditions which of the following pressure is zero (0) mm Hg?
A. Bowman capsule hydrostatic pressure
B. Bowman capsule oncotic pressure
C. Glomerular hydrostatic pressure
D. Glomerular oncotic pressure

291. B   292. D   293. A   294. B   295. D   296. C   297. A   298. D   299. C   300. D   301. B

302. Match the following:

List I	List II
a. Proximal convoluted tubule	i. Tubuloglomerular feedback
b. Loop of Henle	ii. Glomerulotubular balance
c. Distal convoluted tubule	iii. No brush border
d. Collecting/ducts	iv. Na-K-2Cl symporter

    A. a: ii, b: iv, c: i, d: iii
    B. a: iv, b: iii, c: ii, d: i
    C. a: i, b: iii, c: ii, d: iv
    D. a: iii, b: iv, c:I, d: ii

303. Plasma glucose is 450 mg/dl, GFR is 120 ml/min, Tm for glucose is 375 mg/min. What is the excretion rate of glucose?
    A. Zero (0) mg/min
    B. 100 mg/min
    C. 165 mg/min
    D. 180 mg/minrrds

304. Which of the following does not make part of filtering barrier of a nephron?
    A. Capillary endothelial cell
    B. Podocyte
    C. Basement membrane
    D. Mesangial cell

305. Which of the following substance is not freely filtered across glomerular membrane?
    A. Albumin
    B. Bicarbonate
    C. Creatinine
    D. Glucose

306. Facultative reabsorption of water takes place in the following segments of nephron, *expect*:
    A. Proximal convoluted tubule
    B. Proximal part of distal convoluted tubule
    C. Distal part of distal convoluted tubule
    D. Collecting ducts

307. Match the following:

List I	List II
a. Proximal convoluted tubule	i. Na-K-2Cl symporter
b. Loop of Henle	ii. Aquaporin-2
c. Distal convoluted tubule	iii. SGLT (sodium-dependent glucose transporter)
d. Collecting ducts	iv. Na-H antiporter

    A. a: iii, b: I, c: iv, d: ii
    B. a:i, b:iii, c:ii, d:iv
    C. a:iv, b:ii, c:i, d:iii
    D. a: I, b: iii, c:iv, d: ii

308. Site of action for aldosterone:
    A. Glomerulus
    B. Proximal convoluted tubule
    C. Loop of Henle
    D. Collecting ducts

309. Which of the following is true?
    A. Acidosis increases potassium excretion
    B. Acidosis decreases potassium excretion
    C. Acidosis increases glucose excretion
    D. Acidosis decreases glucose excretion

310. Which of the following segment of nephron does not take part in countercurrent mechanism?
    A. Proximal convoluted tubule
    B. Descending loop of Henle
    C. Thin ascending loop of Henle
    D. Thick ascending loop of Henle

311. Obligatory volume of urine is:
    A. 200 ml/day
    B. 300 ml/day
    C. 400 ml/day
    D. 500 ml/day

312. Kidneys can concentrate the urine up to:
    A. 500 mOsm/L
    B. 700 mOsm/L
    C. 1000 mOsm/L
    D. 1200 mOsm/L

313. Which of the following statement is not correct?
    A. Loop of Henle acts as countercurrent multiplier
    B. Peritubular capillaries act as countercurrent exchanger
    C. 50% of medullary interstitial osmotic gradient is due to urea
    D. Minimum urine osmolality achieved by kidneys is 50 mOsm/L

302. A 303. C 304. D 305. A 306. A 307. A 308. D 309. B 310. A 311 D 312. D 313. B

PY 7.4

314. If substance 'X' is freely filterable and its excretion rate is nil, which of the following statement best characterizes substance 'X':

A. 'X' is not reabsorbed

B. 'X' is partially reabsorbed

C. 'X' is completely reabsorbed

D. 'X' is completely secreted

315. Measure the plasma clearance of given substance 'X'. Plasma concentration of 'X' is 25 mg/dl, concentration of 'X' in the urine is 100 mg/dl and urine flow rate is 2.5 ml/min.

A. 0.025 ml/min

B. 0.25 ml/min

C. 2.5 ml/min

D. 25 ml/min

316. Which of the following substance can be used to measure renal plasma flow?

A. Inulin

B. Para-aminohippuric acid

C. Mannitol

D. D_2O

317. The para-aminohippuric acid (PAH) clearance of a 65-year-old female with chronic kidney disease is 196 ml/min, extraction ratio of PAH is 70%, hematocrit is 30. Her renal blood flow is approximately:

A. 200 ml/min

B. 300 ml/min

C. 400 ml/min

D. 500 ml/min

318. Which of the following clearance method is clinically preferred to measure the glomerular filtration rate (GFR)?

A. Inulin clearance

B. Creatinine clearance

C. Iodine clearance

D. Sucrose clearance

PY 7.5

319. Homeostatic management of body water and its osmolality is attained by adjusting the following:

A. Water-input and salt excretion

B. Water-output and urea reabsorption

C. Water-output and salt excretion

D. All of the above

320. When the osmolality of urine is maximum, the greatest amount water is reabsorbed in:

A. Proximal tubule

B. Inner medullary collecting ducts

C. Outer medullary collecting ducts

D. Distal tubule

321. Intracellular water content is determined by its:

A. Na^+

B. K^+

C. H^+

D. Ca^{2+}

322. Maximum pH of urine achieved by kidneys is:

A. 3.5

B. 4.5

C. 5.5

D. 6

323. Secretion of H^+ in distal tubules and collecting tubules is:

A. Dependent of Na^+ exchange

B. Dependent of K^+ exchange

C. Relatively independent of Na^+ exchange

D. Relatively independent of K^+ exchange

324. Removal of free H^+ from the tubular fluid depends on which of the following reaction/s?

A. Bicarbonate to form CO_2 and H_2O

B. HPO_4^{2-} to form H_2PO_4

C. NH_3 to NH_4^+

D. All of the above

314. C   315. D   316. B   317. C   318. B   319. C   320. A   321. A   322. B   323. C   324. D

325. **The principal mechanism by which H⁺ secreted into proximal tubule is:**
 A. Na^+-H^+ exchanger
 B. K^+-H^+ exchanger
 C. H^+-Ca^{++} exchanger
 D. Direct H^+ secretion

326. **If pH of blood is high, bicarbonate levels are low and PCO_2 is low, what is the compensatory response of kidney?**
 A. Increased renal excretion of H^+
 B. Increased renal excretion of HCO_3^-
 C. Decreased renal excretion of HCO_3^-
 D. None of the above

PY 7.6

327. **The spinal centre that controls micturition is located at:**
 A. Lumbar spinal cord (L_{1-2})
 B. Lumbar spinal cord (L_{3-4})
 C. Sacral spinal cord (S_{1-2})
 D. Sacral spinal cord (S_{2-4})

328. **Main sensory motor supply to the urinary bladder up to the internal urethral sphincter is provided by:**
 A. Sympathetic nerves of L_{1-2}
 B. Parasympathetic nerves of S_{2-4}
 C. Pudendal nerve
 D. None of the above

329. **The urge to void urine in a healthy adult is first felt at a bladder volume of about:**
 A. 150 ml
 B. 200 ml
 C. 250 ml
 D. 300 ml

330. **In a healthy adult, the volume of urine in the bladder that no longer voluntary hold is not possible:**
 A. 100 ml
 B. 150 ml
 C. 200 ml
 D. 400 ml

PY 7.7

331. **Removal of waste substances and water by circulating blood outside the body through an external filter, called a dialyzer is:**
 A. Peritoneal dialysis
 B. Intestinal dialysis
 C. Hemodialysis
 D. None of the above

332. **Which of the following compatibility test is must for kidney transplantation?**
 A. ABO blood grouping
 B. HLA matching
 C. Both of the above
 D. None of the above

PY 7.8

333. **A 49-year-old male patient renal function tests results are 24-hour urine volume is 6.2 L and presence of ketones, glucose and proteins is nil. Which of the following condition/disease is closely associated?**
 A. Diabetes mellitus
 B. Diabetes insipidus
 C. Dehydration
 D. Nephrosis

334. **A 53-year-old female patient renal function tests results are 24-hour urine volume is 1.6 L; presence of proteins is 4⁺ and presence of ketones, glucose is nil. Which of the following condition/disease is closely associated?**
 A. Diabetes mellitus
 B. Diabetes insipidus
 C. Dehydration
 D. Nephrosis

335. **A 24-year-old male patient renal function tests results are 24-hour urine volume is 400 ml and presence of ketones, glucose and proteins is nil. Which of the following condition/disease is closely associated?**
 A. Diabetes mellitus
 B. Diabetes insipidus
 C. Dehydration
 D. Nephrosis

325. A   326. B   327. D   328. B   329. A   330. D   331. C   332. C   333. B   334. D   335. C

PY 7.9

356. Study of relationship between the urinary bladder volume and pressure is:
A. Spirometry
B. Perimetry
C. Angiogram
D. Cystometry

357. The recording of urinary bladder pressure–volume relationship is called.
A. Cystometrogram
B. Spirogram
C. Angiogram
D. None of the above

PY 8.1

338. Positive calcium balance is seen in:
A. Normal healthy individual
B. Growing children
C. Women during pregnancy
D. Women during lactation

339. Cells of mesenchymal origin that proliferate and convert themselves into osteoblasts are called....... .
A. Osteocytes
B. Osteoprogenitor cells
C. Osteoclasts
D. Endosteal cells

340. Match the different forms of calcium with their normal values:

List I	List II
1. Total plasma calcium	A. 4 mg/ dl
2. Ionized calcium	B. 10 mg/dl
3. Bound to albumin	C. 5 mg/ dl

A. 1-B, 2-C, 3-A
B. 1-A, 2-B, 3-C
C. 1-C, 2-B, 3-A
D. 1-A, 2-C, 3-B

341. Plasma calcium regulates the synthesis of vitamin D through:
A. Prolactin
B. Plasma phosphate

C. Parathyroid hormone
D. Calcitonin

342. Identify the following signs:

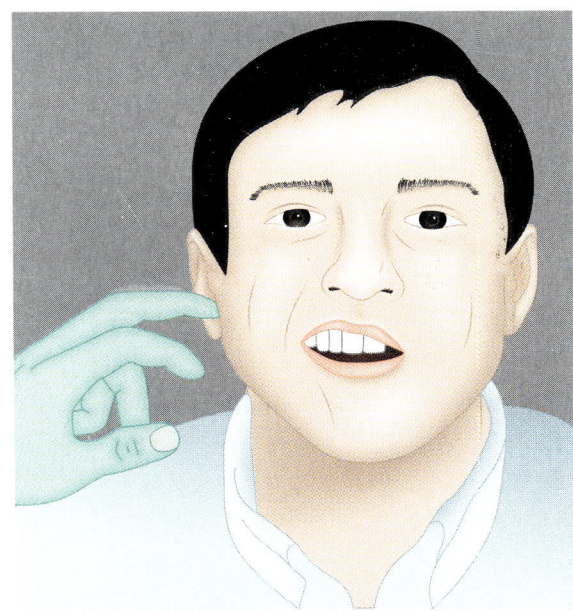

A. Chovstek's sign
B. Trousseau's sign
C. Carpal spasm
D. Carpopedal spasm

PY 8.2

343. What causes release of growth hormone from anterior pituitary?
A. Influx of Ca^{2+} into pituitary cells
B. Efflux of Ca^{2+} into pituitary cells
C. Influx of Na^+ into pituitary cells
D. Efflux of Na^+ into pituitary cells

344. Why you won't grow if you don't sleep well?
A. Secretion of growth hormone peaks 1–2 hr before NREM sleep
B. Nocturnal sleep bursts account for 30% of daily GH secretion
C. Secretion peaks only stage II slow wave sleep
D. Secretion peaks 1–2 hr after deep sleep

336. D   337. A   338. B   339. B   340. A   341. C   342. A   343. A   344. D

345. How growth hormone promotes growth due to its effects on carbohydrate metabolism?
A. By decreasing gluconeogenesis
B. By increasing glycolysis
C. By Increasing insulin secretion
D. By Increasing glucagon secretion

346. Identify the clinical condition.

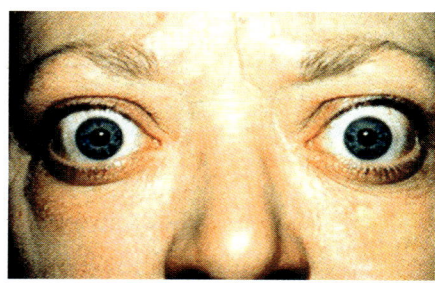

A. Gigantism
B. Acromegaly
C. Cushing's syndrome
D. Graves' disease

347. In syndrome of inappropriate ADH secretion:
A. ADH secretion is increased despite hyperosmolality
B. ADH secretion is increased despite hypo-osmolality
C. ADH secretion is increased despite iso-osmolality
D. ADH secretion is decreased despite hypo-osmolality

348. How does thyroid hormone behave in physiological doses?
A. Act as anabolic hormones
B. Act as catabolic hormones
C. Cause negative nitrogen balance
D. Effect is same both at physiological and higher concentrations

349. Match the ophthalmological signs with their respective names:

List I	List II
1. Lid retraction leading to staring look	A. Stellwag's sign
2. Lid lag	B. Dalrymple's sign
3. Infrequent and incomplete blinking	C. Von Graefe's sign

A. 1-B, 2-C, 3-A
B. 1-C, 2-A, 3-B
C. 1-A, 2-B, 3-C
D. 1-B, 2-A, 3-C

350. Somatomedin deficiency causes:
A. Pituitary dwarf
B. Laron dwarf
C. Hypothyroid dwarf
D. African dwarf

351. Hyperparathyroidism is characterized by all, except:
A. Increase in serum calcium
B. Decrease in serum calcium
C. Decrease in serum phosphate
D. Nephrocalcinosis

352. What is effect of cortisol in diabetic patients?
A. Increases plasma lipid levels
B. Decreases plasma lipid levels
C. Increases insulin secretion
D. Decreases ketone body formation

353. Cortisol exhibits its anti-inflammatory effect by:
A. Increasing the activity of phospholipase A2
B. Stabilizing the lysosomal membrane
C. Increasing collagen formation
D. Stimulating phagocytosis

354. A female patient failed to take hormone therapy post-bilateral adrenalectomy. What would you expect in her?
A. Cushing's syndrome
B. Conn's disease
C. Addison's disease
D. Adrenogenital syndrome

355. Why norepinephrine and not epinephrine is used in patients with shock?
A. It causes decreased heart rate, increased mean blood pressure
B. It causes increased heart rate, increased mean blood pressure
C. It causes increased heart rate, decreased mean blood pressure
D. It causes decreased heart rate, increased cardiac output

345. C   346. D   347. B   348. A   349. A   350. B   351. B   352. A   353. B   354. C   355. A

356. The stimulus for producing insulin is:
A. Decreased blood glucose
B. Decreased amino acids
C. Epinephrine
D. Increased fatty acids

357. In between meals:
A. Free fatty acid level decreases
B. Glucose level increases
C. Glucose becomes the chief fuel for energy
D. Free fatty acid becomes the chief fuel for energy

358. To exert calorigenic effect, glucagon requires:
A. Insulin
B. Glucocorticoids
C. Mineralocorticoids
D. Somatostatin

359. False statement regarding hypothalamus:
A. Functions as master co-ordinator of hormonal action
B. Situated below the thalamus
C. Provides link between endocrine system and nervous system
D. Serves its endocrinal functions through endothelial cells

360. A 43-year-old school teacher complained of weight gain despite eating less. On detailed enquiry said that she fatigues easily, always feels cold, is constipated and has heavy menstrual flow every month. Laboratory investigations revealed decreased serum T3 and T4 and increased TSH. How do you explain the cause for weight gain in this patient?
A. Increased leptin levels
B. Decreased basal metabolic rate
C. Loss of hypothalamic control
D. Sedentary lifestyle

361. Identify the condition from the below diagram:
A. Cushing's syndrome
B. Addison's disease
C. Cretinism
D. Acromegaly

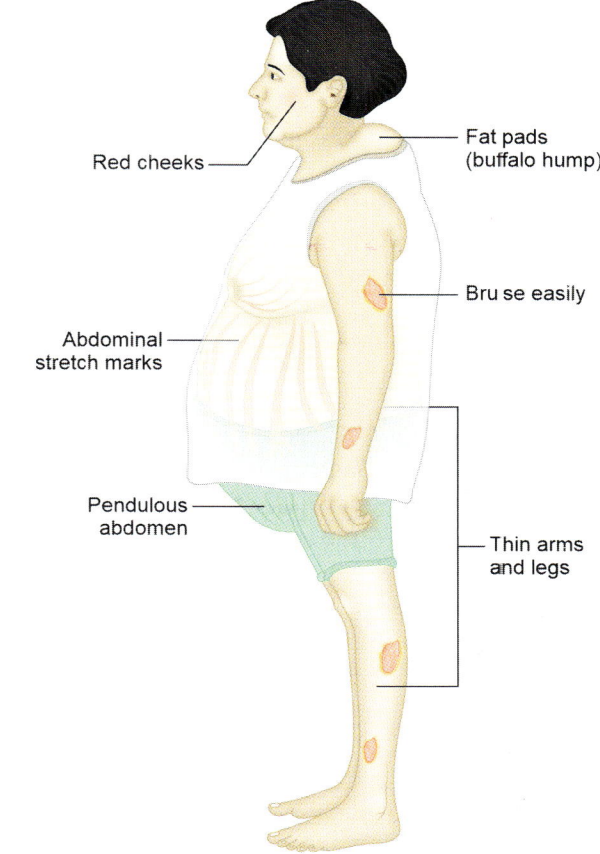

Red cheeks

Fat pads (buffalo hump)

Bru se easily

Abdominal stretch marks

Pendulous abdomen

Thin arms and legs

PY 8.3

362. Removal of thymus three months after birth does not affect cell-mediated immunity. Why?
A. Proliferation of T cells occurs between three months before and three months after birth
B. Proliferation of T cells occurs between three months before birth
C. Proliferation of T cells occurs between three months after birth
D. Thymosin produces antibodies up to three months after birth

363. Melatonin is secreted by:
A. Hypothalamus
B. Pineal gland
C. Anterior pituitary
D. Posterior pituitary

356. D   357. D   358. B   359. D   360. B   361. A   362. A   363. B

364. Pineal gland is called neuroendocrine transducer because:
- A. Secretes hormone in response to nervous activity
- B. Exerts its effect on nerve
- C. Its actions are controlled by nerve activity
- D. It lacks blood–brain barrier

PY 8.4, 8.5

365. What happens to BMR in hyperthyroidism
- A. Increases slightly
- B. Decreases
- C. Does not alter
- D. Increases markedly

366. Which is the best test widely used for diagnosis of various thyroid disorders?
- A. Measurement of free T3, T4 and TSH levels
- B. Thyroid scan
- C. Radioactive iodine uptake
- D. Fine needle aspiration cytology

367. Fine needle aspiration of thyroid helps in the diagnosis of:
- A. Hashimoto's thyroiditis
- B. To detect malignancy in nodular goiter
- C. Differentiate between hypo- and hyeper-thyroidism
- D. Toxic nodular goiter

368. An increase in 24 hr urinary excretion of vanillylmandelic acid is a characteristic feature of:
- A. Pheochromocytoma
- B. Addison's disease
- C. Cushing's syndrome
- D. Hyperaldosteronism

369. A 25-year-old pregnant woman of 26 weeks gestation with family history of diabetes was advised for glucose tolerance test. The results revealed—FBS ≥126 mg/dl, PPBS ≥200 mg/dl. What is your probable diagnosis?
- A. Normal
- B. Impaired glucose tolerance
- C. Pregestational diabetes
- D. Gestational diabetes

370. Metabolic syndrome is also known as:
- A. Raven syndrome
- B. Insulin sensitivity syndrome
- C. Insulin resistance syndrome
- D. Beer belly syndrome

371. According to IDF criteria for diagnosis of metabolic syndrome, the following is included, *except*:
- A. Central obesity
- B. Hyperglycemia
- C. Hypertension
- D. High HDL

372. BMI >40 mg/dl, true statements include all, *except*:
- A. Classified as severe obesity
- B. Increased risk of major depression
- C. Depression more common in women
- D. Depression improves with weight loss and not recur with weight gain

373. How does obesity oppose insulin actions?
- A. Increases muscle glucose uptake
- B. Decreases hepatic gluconeogenesis
- C. Increases hepatic gluconeogenesis
- D. Decreases free fatty acid levels

374. A 50-year-old female presents with easy fatigability. She weighed 98 kg and had waist circumference of 42 inches. Her blood pressure values were high, lab investigations revealed hypertryglyceridemia and high blood sugar levels. What is the most likely diagnosis?
- A. Metabolic syndrome
- B. Hyperthyroidism
- C. Obesity
- D. Hypothyroidism

PY 8.6

375. What kind of chemical signaling is this?

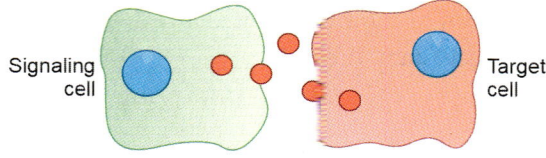

- A. Neurocrine
- B. Endocrine
- C. Paracrine
- D. Autocrine

---

364. A   365. D   366. A   367. B   368. A   369. D   370. A   371. D   372. D   373. C   374. A   375. C

376. Match the following:

List I	List II
1. Amine hormone	A. Testosterone
2. Steroid hormone	B. Oxytocin
3. Peptide hormone	C. Epinephrine

A. 1-A, 2-C, 3-B
B. 1-C, 2-A, 3-B
C. 1-B, 2-C, 3-A
D. 1-A, 2-B, 3-C

377. Example of periodic hormone secretion:
A. Secretion of GnRH
B. Secretion of ACTH
C. Secretion of gonadotrophins
D. Secretion of melatonin

378. Less responsiveness on subsequent exposure is known as:
A. Desensitization
B. Downregulation
C. Upregulation
D. Mutation

PY 9.1

379. Differentiation of external genitalia in males requires:
A. Dihydrotestosterone
B. 5α-reductase
C. Testosterone
D. Aromatase 3

380. Testosterone production by the fetal Leydig cells is stimulated by:
A. FSH
B. LH
C. Chorionic gonadotropin
D. GnRH

381. An individual was brought with ambiguous genitalia. For sex determination, some blood cells were seen under microscope (*see* Figure below).

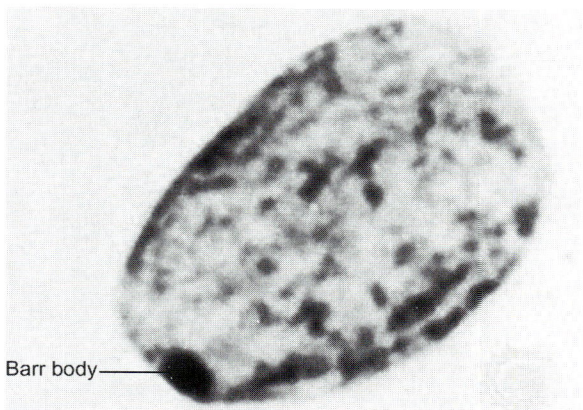

Barr body

What is the sex of the individual?
A. Genotype female
B. Genotype male
C. Cannot comment without karyotyping
D. Hyper female

382. Which of these is aneuploidy?
A. Deletion of long arm of 5th chromosome
B. Trisomy 21
C. Translocation between 11 and 21
D. Replacement of valine by leucine gene

383. A 35-year-old primigravida (pregnant for the first time), at 16 weeks is apprehensive as there is family history of death of her maternal uncle due to cystic firbsois, a genetic disorder characterized by repeated pulmonary infections. Which test is appropriate?
A. Fetal lung biopsy
B. Antenatal ultrasound
C. Chorionic villus biopsy
D. Amniocentesis

376. B   377. C   378. A   379. A   380. C   381. A   382. B   383. D

384. A 17-year-old female presents with primary amenorrhea. On examination, she is short stature, has webbed neck and broad chest. What do you expect in karyotyping?

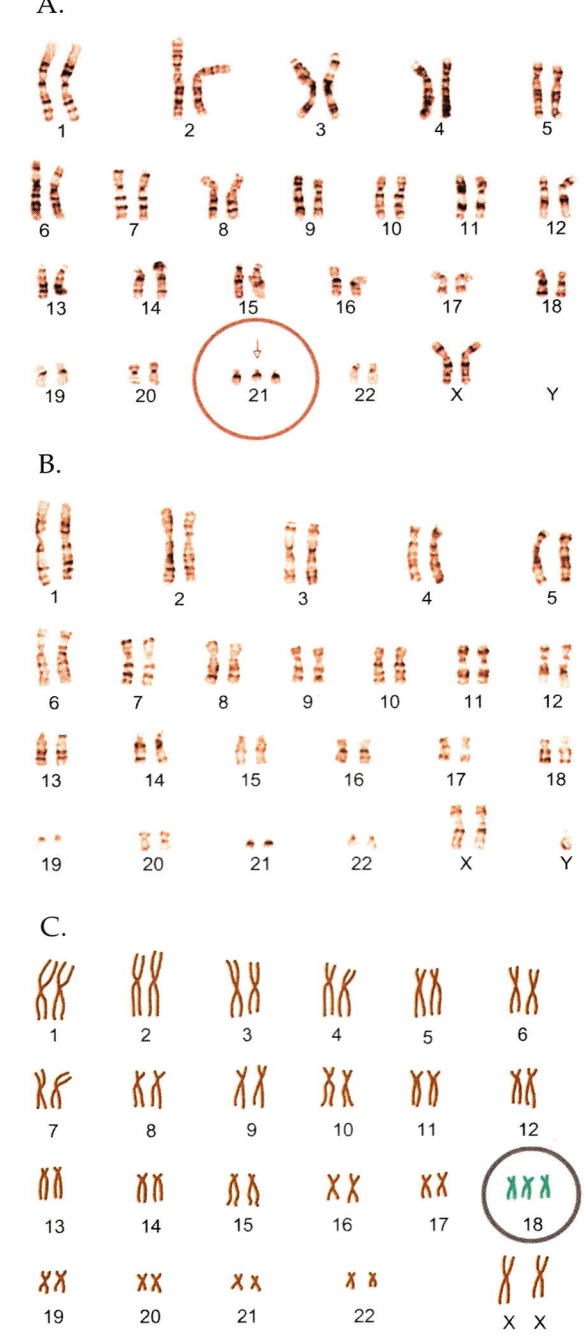

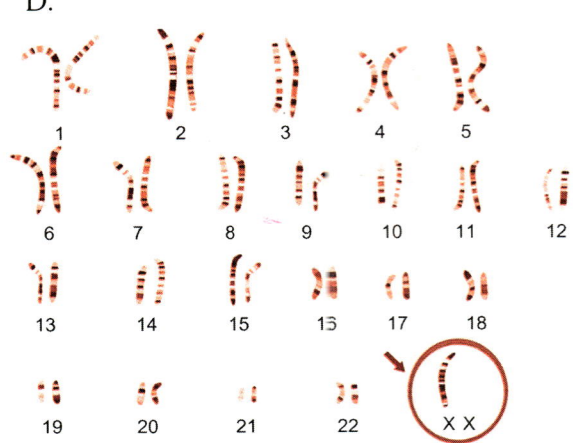

385. A 15-year-old female presents with primary amenorrhea. On examination, her secondary sexual characteristics are well developed. On hysteroscopy, vagina ended blindly and there was no cervix and uterus. Imaging of the abdomen showed tumor of undescended testis. Diagnosis is:

A. Female pseudohermaphroditism
B. True hermaphroditism
C. Testicular feminization syndrome
D. Congenital adrenal hyperplasia.

PY 9.2

386. Arrange the following in the order of occurrence during puberty:

A. Menarche
B. Thelarche
C. Development of secondary sexual characteristics
D. Pubarche
A. A, B, C, D
B. B, C, A, D
C. B, D, A, C
D. D, C, B, A

387. Precocious puberty is defined in a boy when he attains puberty before the age of:

A. 7 years
B. 8 years
C. 9 years
D. 10 years

384. A   385. A   386. C   387. B

388. Which of the following is not a feature of precocious puberty?
  A. Extremely tall compared to others of same age
  B. Bone age higher than actual age
  C. Development of secondary sexual characteristics like breasts before the age of 8 years
  D. Development of facial hair in boys before the age of 8 years.

389. A 16-year-old girl was brought by parents for evaluation of primary amenorrhea. On examination, she had the following features:

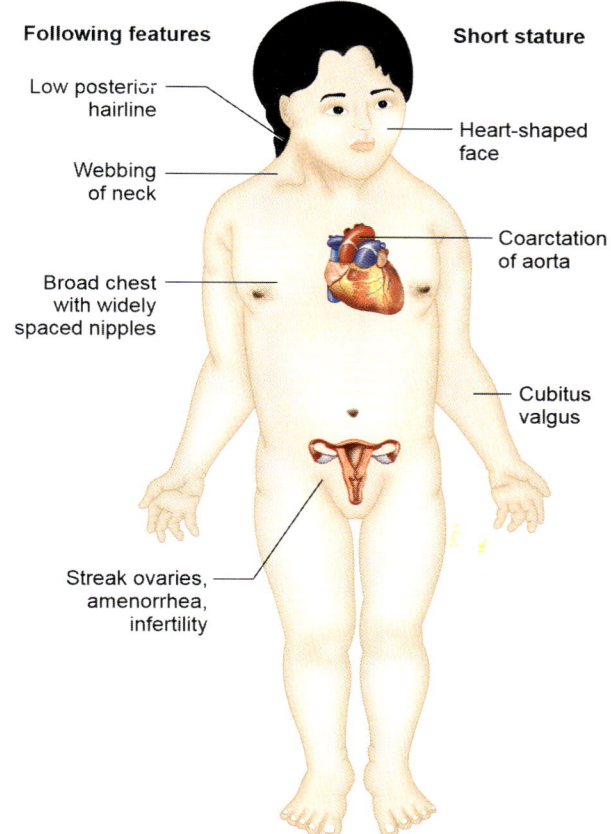

Following features

Short stature

Low posterior hairline

Heart-shaped face

Webbing of neck

Coarctation of aorta

Broad chest with widely spaced nipples

Cubitus valgus

Streak ovaries, amenorrhea, infertility

How do you confirm the diagnosis?
  A. Echocardiogram
  B. Ovarian biopsy
  C. Abdominal ultrasound
  D. Karyotyping

390. Which of the following are known to hasten puberty?
  A. Meningitis
  B. Bulimia nervosa
  C. Malnutrition
  D. Recurrent infections

PY 9.3

391. LH receptors in males are present on:
  A. Leydig cells
  B. Sertoli cells
  C. Primary spermatocyte
  D. Spermatozoa

392. Full development and function of seminiferous tubule requires:
  A. Somatostatin and LH
  B. LH and oxytocin
  C. Androgens and FSH
  D. Oxytocin and FSH

393. Give the correct order of spermatogenesis
  A. Primary spermatocyte → spermatogonia → secondary spermatocyte → spermatids → spermatozoa
  B. Spermatogonia → primary spermatocyte → secondary spermatocyte → spermatids → spermatozoa
  C. Primary spermatocyte → secondary spermatocyte → spermatogonia → spermatids → spermatozoa
  D. Spermatids → primary spermatocyte → spermatogonia → secondary spermatocyte → spermatozoa

394. A 28-year-old gets infected by mumps. Also he notices there is pain and redness in both scrotal region. What is the possible outcome of this infection?
  A. Possible future testicular tumor
  B. No sequel, it heals well
  C. Possible future impotence
  D. Possible future infertility

388. A   389. D   390. A   391. A   392. C   393. B   394. D

395. All of the following are functions of Sertoli cells, *except*:
A. Mechanical support for spermatozoa
B. Secretion of aromatase
C. Secretion of testosterone
D. Secretion of inhibin

396. What are the complications of undescended testis?
A. Development of sterility
B. Development of malignancy
C. Torsion
D. All of the above

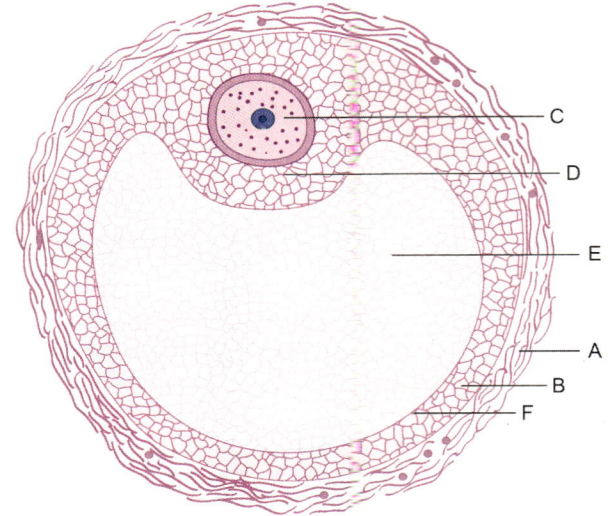

PY 9.4

397. Fern pattern of cervical mucus is due to:
A. The action of estrogen
B. The action of progesterone
C. Action of both estrogen and progesterone
D. Secretory changes in the endometrium

398. Secretory phase of endometrium is due to the action of:
A. Estradiol
B. LH
C. FSH
D. Progesterone

399. A 30-year-old woman with hypothyroidism complains that she gets her period once in more than 37–40 days. What is this condition called?
A. Polymenorrhoea
B. Oligomenorrhoea
C. Menorrhagia
D. Metrorrhagia

400. Identify 'D' in this diagram of graafian folloicle:
A. Theca interna
B. Membrana granulosa
C. Antrum
D. Cumulus oophorus

401. Theca cells secrete all of the following, *except*:
A. Inhibin
B. Leutinizing hormone
C. Estrogen
D. Androgens

402. Which of the following is not a specific test for ovulation?
A. Basal body temperature
B. LH surge
C. Ultrasound showing empty follicle along with fluid is cul de sac
D. None of the above

403. Ovulation occurs how many hours after LH surge?
A. 24 hours
B. 48 hours
C. 9 hours
D. 2 hours

PY 9.5

404. The hormone that is responsible for pigmentation of areola is:
A. Estrogen
B. Progesterone
C. Melatonin
D. LH

395. C   396. D   397. A   398. D   399. B   400. D   401. B   402. A   403. C   404. A

405. The placental hormone which reduces the possibilities of fetal rejection is:
A. hCG
B. Estrogen
C. Progesterone
D. Relaxin

406. Which of the following is true?
A. GnRH is secreted by the hypothalamus in a continuous form
B. Estrogen causes relaxation of smooth muscles of uterus
C. Progesterone causes pigmentation of skin around nipple
D. FSH helps in growth of follicle

407. Match the following:

List I	List II
A Testosterone	I. Induces growth of secondary sexual characteristics in a female
B Estrogens	II. Helps in maintaining pregnancy
C Progesterone	III. Inhibits development of uterus
D MIS	IV. Stimulates descent of testes

A. A: IV, B: I, C: II, D: III
B. A: I, B: III, C: IV, D: II
C. A: I, B: II, C: III, D: IV
D. A: III, B: II, C: I, D: IV

408. An endometrial biopsy was performed in a woman with dysfunctional bleeding. It showed increased number of endometrial glands. Which hormone is responsible for this type of endometrium?

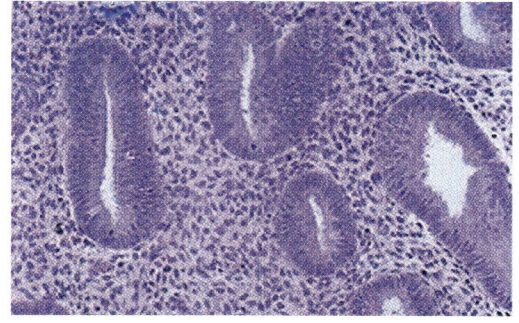

A. Oestrogen
B. Progesterone
C. FSH
D. LH

409. A newly married young healthy couple come for advice on contraception. Best method is:
A. Barrier method
B. Calendar method
C. Oral contraceptives
D. Tubectomy

410. Rhythm method includes abstaining from intercourse during:
A. The day of ovulation
B. 1–8th day of cycle
C. 8–18th day of cycle
D. 18–28th day of cycle

411. An unmarried couple who are living together approach for medical termination of pregnancy at 6 weeks of menorrhea. Best way to manage is:
A. Medical termination of pregnancy
B. Dilatation and curettage
C. Shun them away
D. Tubectomy

412. Identify the contraceptive:

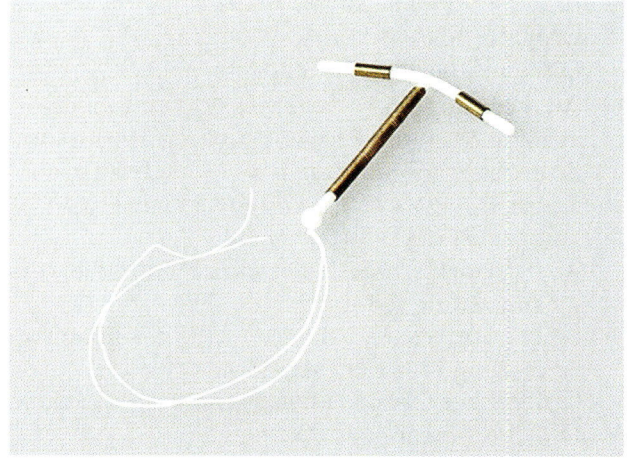

A. Lippe's loop
B. Copper T
C. Nonoxynol
D. Female condom

413. Match the following advantages of contraceptives:

List I	List II
A. Condom	I. Prevents menorrhagia and dysmenorrhoea
B. Oral contraceptive	II. Permanent solution
C. Vasectomy	III. Long duration of action
D. Progesterone injection	IV. Prevents sexually transmitted disease

A. A: I, B: II, C: IV, D: III
B. A: III, B: II, C: I, D: IV
C. A: IV, B: I, C: II, D: III
D. A: II, B: III, C: IV, D: I

PY 9.7

414. Following syndromes may be associated hypogonadism, *except*:
A. Klinefelter's syndrome
B. Turner syndrome
C. Bardet-Biedl syndrome
D. Albinism

415. Following are features of eunuchoidism, *except*:
A. Well developed testes
B. Absence of secondary sexual characters
C. High-pitched voice
D. Feminine shape of body

416. A 26-year-old lady with bilateral endometriotic cysts in ovary underwent surgery for the same. She was given intramuscular goserelin (GnRH agonist). After ten days she experienced hot flushes. What is the reason?
A. It suppresses the heat centre in hypothalamus simulating fever
B. It suppresses estrogen and progesterone leading to GnRH secretion
C. It causes vasodilatation by increasing estrogen
D. All of the above

417. If oophorectomy is done at a pre-menopausal age in a woman, what is she at a risk of developing?
A. Breast cancer
B. Endometrial cancer
C. Osteoporosis
D. All of the above

PY 9.8

418. Peak level of hCG in urine is attained by .... weeks of pregnancy.
A. 2–3 weeks
B. 9–12 weeks
C. 16–20 weeks
D. 20–24 weeks

419. A lady with single gestation has nausea during pregnancy less than a lady with twin gestation. The cause for this is:
A. Due to emotional stress
B. Due to increased weight gain
C. Due to higher levels of beta hCG
D. Due to higher levels of placental lactogen

420. A 37-week gestation pregnant lady complains of feeling of tightness in her abdomen and is anxious that she is in labor. The doctor says it is Braxton Hicks contractions. Which features help in differentiating Braxton Hicks from normal labor?
A. Cervical dilatation
B. Pain
C. Duration of contraction
D. All of the above

421. A 21-year-old newly married lady presents with amenorrhea of 4 weeks duration. But the transvaginal scan confirms that the fetus is 6 weeks old and cardiac activity is detected. But the lady is quite sure she had bleeding 4 weeks back, but lasted only a few hours and was minimal. What is the diagnosis?

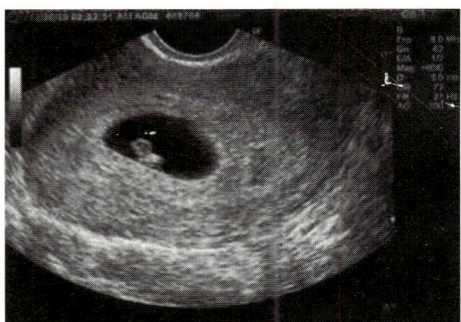

A. Irregular cycle
B. Implantation bleed
C. Twin gestation
D. Wrong dates

422. Following endocrine related changes occur during pregnancy, *except*:
A. Decreased functioning of thyroid gland
B. Increased functioning of the anterior pituitary
C. Increased synthesis of cortisol
D. Increased blood glucose

PY 9.9

423. Azoospermia is:
A. Decreased number of sperms
B. Decreased number of viable sperms
C. Absence of sperms
D. Decreased motility of sperms

424. Testosterone causes
A. Increase in sperm motility
B. Increase in scalp hair
C. Negative nitrogen balance
D. Protein anabolism

425. What is the diagnosis?

Semen examination	
Test	*Result*
Semen analysis	
Physical examination	
Colour	Creamy white
Consistency	Thin
Reaction	Alkaline
Liquefaction	30 min at 370
Microscopic examination	
PUS cells/WBC	08–10/HPF
RBCs	04–06/HPF
Epithelial cells	Rare/HPF
Sperm count	NIL
Active	NIL
Sluggish	NIL
Dead	NIL

A. Oligospermia
B. Azoospermia
C. Teratospermia
D. Teratozoospermia

426. Which factors can cause decreased sperm count?
A. Actively involved in sports
B. Eating healthy food
C. Varicocele
D. Lycopene supplements

427. Which type of sperm motility is not preferred?
A. Linear forward movement
B. Zigzag forward movement
C. Linear sideways movement
D. Circular movement

PY 9.10

428. Immunological test of pregnancy is based on the urinary detection of:
A. hCG
B. Estrogen
C. Progesterone
D. Estrogen and progesterone

429. The purpose of adding latex to sheep RBC agglutination test is:
A. To sensitize the serum
B. To activate the hCG
C. To make agglutination visible
D. All of the above

430. What is the mode of increase in the serum of levels of beta hCG in pregnancy?
A. Algebraic progression
B. Geometric progression
C. Harmonic progression
D. All of the above

431. A 28-year-old lady was practicing contraceptive methods but has missed her period and 4 days have passed. She did a blood beta hCG and it came as 120 mIU/ml. What is the level of hCG in blood in nonpregnant individuals?
A. 0–5 mIU/ml
B. 0–25 mIU/ml
C. 0–100 mIU/ml
D. 0–150 mIU/ml

422. A   423. C   424. D   425. B   426. C   427. D   428. A   429. C   430. B   431. A

432. Identify the test.

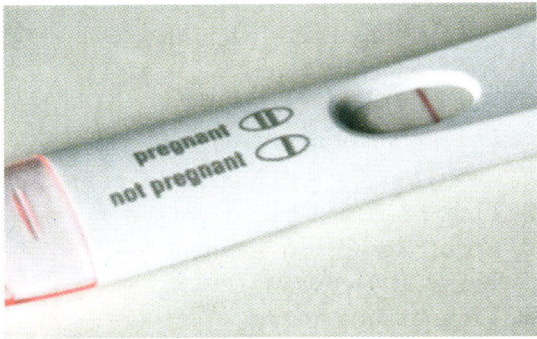

A. Ovulation test
B. Urine pregnancy test
C. Urine test for sugars
D. Urine test for protein

PY 9.11

433. GnRH is secreted from:
A. Hypothalamus
B. Anterior pituitary
C. Posterior pituitary
D. Adrenal cortex

434. A 49-year-old lady, otherwise healthy, starts experiencing irregular periods. The cause for this:
A. Hyperthyroidism
B. Estrogen-progesterone imbalance
C. Stress related
D. All of the above

435. Following are indications for hormone replacement therapy, *except:*
A. Intolerable menopausal symptoms
B. High risk of osteoporosis
C. High risk of coronary artery disease
D. High risk of breast cancer

436. A 56-year-old is prescribed hormone replacement therapy for menopausal symtpoms. She develops breast tenderness. Which drug is causing this?
A. Estrogen
B. Progesterone
C. GnRH analogs
D. GnRH antagonists

437. Menopause in men is called ....
A. Andropause
B. Menopause
C. Climacteric
D. Adrenarche

PY 9.12

438. Which of the following decreases fertility in a woman?
A. Advancing age
B. Obesity
C. Hypothyroidism
D. All of the above

439. To define infertility, the couple should have regular unprotected intercourse for at least:
A. 1 month
B. 6 months
C. 1 year
D. 2 years

440. Which of these procedures can help an infertile couple?
A. Ovulation induction
B. Intrauterine insemination
C. *In vitro* fertilization
D. All of the above

441. A 26-year-old married lady was unable to conceive. On hysterosalpingography, there was bilateral cornual block. What is the best possible treatment for this lady?
A. Adoption
B. Intrauterine insemination
C. *In vitro* fertilization
D. Surrogacy

442. A couple with infertility underwent examination and the husband was found to have oligospermia due to varicocele. What is the next logical decision considering that the wife has normal ovulation and no structural abnormalities?
A. Adoption
B. Surrogacy
C. Surgery for varicocele
D. Artificial insemination from donor

432. B   433. A   434. B   435. D   436. A   437. C   438. D   439. C   440. D   441. C   442. C

PY 10.1

443. Lamina II of dorsal grey column corresponds to:
A. Substantia gelatinosa
B. Posteromarginal nucleus
C. Nucleus proprius
D. Dorsal nucleus

444. Match the following divisions of the brain with their structures:

List I	List II
A. Prosencephalon	1. Cerebral peduncles
B. Mesencephalon	2. Medulla
C. Rhombencephalon	3. Thalamus

A. A-3, B-1, C-2
B. A-1, B-3, C-2
C. A-2, B-1, C-3
D. A-3, B-1, C-2

445. Cells that provide myelin sheath to the axons in the CNS are called ....
A. Schwann cells
B. Microglia
C. Oligodendrocytes
D. Astrocytes

446. Why neurons once destroyed cannot be replaced?
A. It does not contain centrosome
B. Contains only one or two nucleoli
C. Contains Nissl bodies
D. It does not contain nucleoli

447. Give an example for pseudounipolar neuron:
A. Spinal motor neurons
B. Primary sensory neurons
C. Retinal bipolar cells
D. Neurons in the embryonic stage

448. A 40-year-old female presented with gradual cognitive decline, loss of memory since 2 years. Since two months she reported that she needed frequent reminders for household routine works. Which nerve cell component is altered in this patient?
A. Nissl bodies
B. Dendrites

C. Neurofibrillae
D. Pigment granules

PY 10.2

449. Depolarization of presynaptic membrane causes opening of:
A. Voltage-gated Ca^{++} channels
B. Voltage-gated Na^+ channels
C. Voltage-gated K^+ channels
D. Voltage-gated Cl^- channels

450. In occlusion effect the response obtained by simultaneous stimulation of two presynaptic neurons:
A. Is greater than the sum total response obtained when they are stimulated separately
B. Is lesser than the sum total response obtained when they are stimulated separately
C. There is no change whether stimulated separately or stimulated simultaneously
D. There is no response at all when stimulated separately

451. What causes postsynaptic inhibition occur without the development of inhibitory postsynaptic potential?
A. Greater influx of K^+ and Cl^- ions along with Na^+
B. Greater efflux of K^+ along with Na^+
C. Greater efflux of Cl^- along with Na^+
D. Greater efflux of Na^+

452. Why presynaptic receptors are called auto-receptors?
A. They sense and control the rate of secretion of neurotransmitters
B. They synthesize neurotransmitters released at presynaptic terminal
C. They stimulate the destruction of their own
D. They allow calcium ions to enter the pre-synaptic neuron causing hyperpolarization

453. Receptor potential in the pacinian corpuscle occurs due to opening of:
A. Stretch sensitive sodium channels
B. Stretch sensitive potassium channels
C. Voltage-gated sodium channels
D. Voltage-gated potassium channels

443. A 444. D 445. C 446. A 447. B 448. C 449. A 450. B 451. A 452. A 453. A

454. The following is an example of a phasic receptor:
A. Baroreceptor
B. Muscle spindle
C. Nociceptor
D. Pacinian corpuscle

455. How do you explain the condition where in the patient complains of pain in the limb that actually does not exist?
A. Occurs due to recruitment of sensory unit
B. Law of projection
C. Weber-Fechner law
D. Bell-Magendie law

456. In myocardial ischemia, why is the pain referred to the left shoulder and arm?
A. Afferent fibers from heart and the left shoulder converge onto the same second order neuron
B. Due to process of radiation
C. Pain fibers of the heart facilitates the fibers supplying the arm
D. Both heart and left shoulder have same segmental origin

457. Primary endings of the muscle spindle are called ....
A. Annulospiral endings
B. Flower spray endings
C. Plate endings
D. Trial ending

458. All of the following are features of withdrawal reflex, *except:*
A. Response is nonlinear and widespread
B. Has short latency
C. Reflex activity continues even after withdrawal of stimulus
D. Involves many muscle groups

PY 10.3

459. What type of sensation is carried by lateral spinothalamic tract?
A. Vibration
B. Stereognosis
C. Fine touch
D. Temperature

460. Why does the slow pain keep the person awake?
A. Due to its connection with limbic system
B. Projection to the reticular formation
C. Due to hypothalamic connections
D. Due to nonspecific projections to the cortex

461. The sensation to be affected early in the cortical lesions is:
A. Touch
B. Vibration
C. Pain
D. Proprioception

462. Why is touch sensation preserved while temperature sensation is lost in syringomyelia?
A. Dorsal column fibers are present close to the central canal
B. Fibers of dorsal cross to the opposite side and lie away from the central canal
C. Fibers of spinothalamic tract cross to the opposite side and lie close to the central canal
D. Fibers of spinothalamic tract cross to the opposite side and lie away from the central canal

463. Paleospinothalamic tract carries:
A. Fast pain
B. Slow pain
C. Fine touch
D. Proprioception

464. In pain inhibiting mechanism, the collateral fibers of fine touch enhance the activity of:
A. Substantia gelatinosa of Rollando
B. Nucleus proprius
C. Clarkes column
D. Ventral horn cells

465. A 30-year-old female complains of intense pain in the absent limb which was operated two years back. What type of pain do you suspect in this patient?
A. Radiating pain
B. Projected pain
C. Somatic pain
D. Visceral pain

454. D   455. B   456. D   457. A   458. B   459. D   460. B   461. B   462. C   463. B   464. A   465. B

PY 10.4

466. Which one of the following regions of the body has the largest representation in cortical area?
A. Trunk muscle
B. Muscles of forearm
C. Muscles of back
D. Digits and hand

467. Static response is the response to the:
A. Muscle stretch
B. Rate at which the muscle is being stretched
C. Sustained stretch
D. Velocity of lengthening

468. How does inverse stretch reflex prevent muscle rupture when muscle is stretched to greater extent?
A. By allowing the muscle to contract
B. By allowing the muscle to relax
C. By keeping the muscle activity at rest
D. By monitoring the muscle length

469. Prolongation of response due to prolonged and repetitive firing of the target motor neurons is called ....
A. Prepoint
B. Local sign
C. After discharge
D. Facilitation

470. What percentage of corticospinal tract fibers decussate in the midline to reach the opposite side?
A. 60
B. 50
C. 80
D. 90

471. What is the role of cerebellum in maintenance of muscle tone?
A. Discharges inhibitory impulses to spinal motor neurons
B. Receives impulses from cerebral cortex and inhibits bulboreticular inhibitory area
C. Acts as a site of alpha–gamma linkage
D. Maintains tonic discharge from gamma motor neurons

472. Chief center for the righting reflex is:
A. Red nucleus
B. Spinal cord
C. Vestibular nuclei
D. Reticular nuclei

473. All are the characteristic features of classical decerebrate rigidity, *except:*
A. Caused due to transection of brainstem between superior and inferior colliculi
B. Exhibits clasp knife effect
C. Rigidity is due to increased activity of gamma motor neurons
D. Rigidity is due to increased activity of alpha motor neurons

474. Why is cupula unaffected by linear acceleration force?
A. It has same specific gravity as that of endolymph
B. Has increased specific gravity as that of endolymph
C. It has same specific gravity as that of perilymph
D. Has increased specific gravity as that of perilymph

475. Identify the postural reflex.

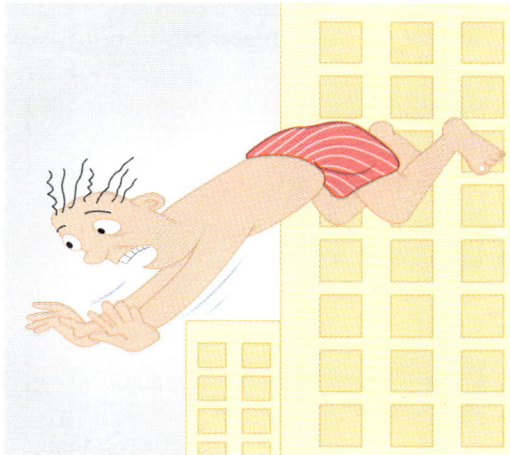

A. Tonic neck reflex
B. Tonic labyrinthine reflex
C. Long loop stretch reflex
D. Crossed extensor reflex

466. D   467. A   468. B   469. C   470. D   471. C   472. A   473. D   474. A   475. A

476. **A 45-year-old woman suddenly fainted and became unconscious, and when consciousness returned, she was unable to move her left arm and leg. On examination, there was spastic paralysis of the left arm and leg with increased muscle tone and exaggerated tendon reflexes. What is the most likely diagnosis?**
   A. Left-sided hemiparesis
   B. Left-sided hemiplegia
   C. Left-sided peripheral neuropathy
   D. Left-sided vascular thrombosis

PY 10.5

477. **Increased activity of reticular facilitatory area results in:**
   A. Direct increase in α motor neuron discharge
   B. Decreased tone of extensor muscles
   C. Reflexely inhibits cerebellum
   D. Increased γ motor neuron discharge

478. **Reticulospinal tract regulates posture through:**
   A. Stimulation of extensor group of muscles
   B. Inhibition of extensor group of muscles
   C. Stimulation of extensor group of muscles
   D. Inhibition of extensor group of muscles

479. **Seventh cranial nerve sends preganglionic fibers to:**
   A. Otic ganglion
   B. Superior salivary nucleus
   C. Pterygopalatine ganglion
   D. Dorsal nucleus

480. **How does sympatholytic drug act?**
   A. By stimulating the synthesis of norepinephrine
   B. Blocking alpha and beta receptors
   C. By increasing the reuptake of norepinephrine
   D. Causing transmission of nerve impulse through sympathetic ganglion

481. **Match the following which shows the distribution of preganglionic neurons and postganglionic fibers:**

Segmental level of preganglionic neurons	Area of distribution of postganglionic fibers
1. T_1, T_2	A. Thoracic viscera
2. T_3, T_4	B. Head and neck
3. T_5 to T_9	C. Lower limb
4. T_{10} to L_2	D. Upper limb

   A. 1-B, 2-A, 3-D, 4-C
   B. 1-A, 2-B, 3-C, 4-D
   C. 1-B, 2-C, 3-1, 4-D
   D. 1-D, 2-B, 3-C, 4-D

PY 10.6

482. **The most common cause of complete transection of spinal cord is:**
   A. Accidental injuries
   B. Subacute combined degeneration of spinal cord
   C. Syringomyelia
   D. Gunshot injury

483. **Recovery of reflex excitability is due to the development of:**
   A. Babinski's reflex
   B. Dennervation hypersensitivity
   C. Improved sympathetic tone
   D. Improved muscle tone

484. **Which sensation is preserved on the side of the lesion in Brown-Sequard syndrome?**
   A. Touch
   B. Vibration
   C. Muscle sense
   D. Temperature

485. **Subnormal temperature after complete transection of spinal cord is due to:**
   A. Inactive sympathetic neurons
   B. Inefficient thermoregulation
   C. Muscle contraction
   D. Muscle paralysis

476. B   477. D   478. A   479. C   480. B   481. A   482. D   483. B   484. D   485. D

486. In paraplegic patients, certain degree of bladder control can be achieved by:
A. Flexor reflex
B. Mass reflex
C. Phillipson's reflex
D. Crossed extensor reflex

437. A 53-year-old female presented with the history of weakness and wasting of right forearm since 1 year. She also complained of paresthesias of all four limbs and impaired pain and temperature sensation in the right upper limb. What could be your possible diagnosis?
A. Syringomyelia
B. Multiple sclerosis
C. Dorsal nerve root lesion
D. Right-sided hemiplegia

PY 10.7

488. Kluver-Bucy syndrome is characterized by all, *except*:
A. Visual agnosia
B. hyperphagia
C. Decreased sexual activity
D. Omniphagia

489. Why the emotional response usually is prolonged even after the end of the stimuli?
A. Emotional response is voluntary
B. Due to prolonged after discharge
C. Due to facilitation
D. Due to synaptic plasticity

490. The only sensory modality which does not reach the thalamus is:
A. Proprioception
B. Taste
C. Olfaction
D. Pain and temperature

491. Illusion felt by the patient that his limb is absent is called ....
A. Astereognosis
B. Thalamic hand
C. Amelognosis
D. Thalamic phantom limb

492. The satiety center is located in the:
A. Dorsomedian nucleus of hypothalamus
B. Ventromedian nucleus of hypothalamus
C. Perifornical region
D. Lateral hypothalamic area

493. What causes rage?
A. Strong stimulation of punishment center
B. Strong stimulation of reward center
C. Strong stimulation of feeding center
D. Strong stimulation of satiety center

494. Flocculonodular lobe of cerebellum is concerned with:
A. Equilibrium
B. Coordination
C. Baroreceptor reflex
D. Chemoreceptor reflex

495. Smoothening and coordination of movement is the function of:
A. Vestibulocerebellum
B. Spinocerebellum
C. Neocerebellum
D. Corticocerebellum

496. A 69-year-old man goes to consult his physician. As he sits in the waiting room, he is observed to have tremors in his hands. His face seemed unexpressive, he had difficulty in standing up and walked slowly into the room, while walking his arms did not swing appreciably, his speech was monotonous. On examination, muscles exhibited rigidity. Which part of nervous system is affected?
A. Cerebellum
B. Basal ganglia
C. Thalamus
D. Hypothalamus

PY 10.8

497. The EEG rhythm with lowest frequency is:
A. Alpha
B. Beta
C. Gamma
D. Delta

486. B   487. A   488. C   489. A   490. C   491. C   492. B   493. A   494. A   495. D   496. B   497. D

498. Sleep spindles in EEG appears during:
A. Stage I NREM sleep
B. Stage II NREM sleep
C. Stage III NREM sleep
D. Stage IV NREM sleep

499. Why is sleep considered as an active state though bodily functions does not occur?
A. Eye balls role up and out during sleep
B. Sweat secretion increases
C. Consumes energy similar to awake state
D. Pulsatile release of growth hormone occurs

500. Neurons necessary for shifting of REM to NREM sleep include:
A. Cholinergic neurons
B. Adrenergic neurons
C. Serotonergic neurons
D. Dopaminergic neurons

501. Identify the type of EEG wave.

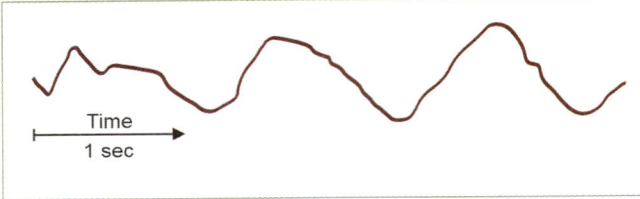

A. Alpha
B. Beta
C. Gamma
D. Delta

502. Uncontrollable urge to sleep during daytime with loss of muscle tone is called ....
A. Insomnia
B. Somnambulism
C. Narcolepsy
D. Cataplexy

PY 10.9

503. Which neurotransmitter deficiency causes Alzheimer's disease?
A. Dopamine
B. GABA
C. Serotonin
D. ACh

504. Motor aphasia is characterized by:
A. Alexia
B. Agraphia
C. Dyslexia
D. Word blindness

505. Match the steps of Pavlov's experiment with response:

List I	List II
1. Introduction of food into dog's mouth	A. Reflex salivation (conditioned)
2. Ringing of the bell alone	B. Reflex salivation (unconditioned)
3. Ringing of bell just before food after repeated episodes of combining food with ringing of bell	C. No salivation

A. 1-A, 2-B, 3-C
B. 1-B, 2-C, 3-A
C. 1-A, 2-C, 3-B
D. 1-C, 2-B, 3-A

506. What happens when conditioned stimulus is not followed with an unconditioned stimulus?
A. Internal inhibition occurs
B. External inhibition occurs
C. Internal reinforcement occurs
D. External reinforcement occurs

507. In retrograde amnesia:
A. Recent and remote memory is lost
B. Recent memory is preserved, remote memory is lost
C. Remote memory is preserved, recent memory is lost
D. Both recent and remote memory is preserved

508. True statement regarding inborn reflexes is:
A. Also called conditioned reflex
B. Present in newborns with brain disorders
C. Does not include superficial and deep reflexes
D. Includes organic reflexes

498. B   499. C   500. A   501. D   502. C   503. D   504. B   505. B   506. A   507. C   508. D

PY 10.10

509. **What is the role of serotonin in the control of movements?**
  A. Has inhibitory effect on motor pathway
  B. Has inhibitory effect on sensory pathway
  C. Has inhibitory effect on cholinergic neurons
  D. Has stimulatory effect on cholinergic neurons

510. **True statement regarding nitric oxide is:**
  A. Released from nerve endings
  B. Also called endothelium derived relaxing factor
  C. Has stimulatory effects in cerebellum
  D. Has inhibitory effects in hippocampus

511. **Which neurotransmitter regulates pain?**
  A. Substance P
  B. Glycine
  C. Serotonin
  D. Endorphin and enkephalin

512. **Neurotransmitter responsible for schizophrenia is:**
  A. ACh
  B. Dopamine
  C. Epinephrine
  D. Norepinephrine

513. **Name the neurotransmitter released from spinal nerve endings whose cell bodies are located in raphe nucleus:**
  A. Glycine
  B. Dopamine
  C. Endorphin
  D. Serotonin

PY 10.11

514. **Which papilla does not contain taste buds?**
  A. Fungiform
  B. Filiform
  C. Vallate
  D. Foliate

515. **Sustentacular cells in the taste buds are:**
  A. Supporting cells
  B. Gustatory receptors
  C. Taste cells
  D. Modified epithelial cells

516. **The piriform cortex is concerned with:**
  A. Coordination of input from contralateral olfactory cortex
  B. Coordination of input from ipsilateral olfactory cortex
  C. Olfactory discrimination and conscious perception
  D. Emotional response to olfactory stimuli

517. **For difference in odor to be detected the concentration of odour producing substance should be changed by about:**
  A. 30%
  B. 50%
  C. 20%
  D. 60%

518. **Explain why the perception of odor declines and ceases over time.**
  A. Threshold of receptors decreases
  B. Intensity of stimuli decreases
  C. Concentration decreases
  D. Receptors adapt rapidly

PY 10.12

519. **Condition where the person shows insensitivity to the taste of certain substance, whereas perception of other tastrants remains unaltered is called ....**
  A. Taste blindness
  B. Dysguesia
  C. Xerostomia
  D. Paraguesia

520. **Patients with adrenal insufficiency exihibit:**
  A. Increased sensitivity for smell
  B. Decreased sensitivity for smell
  C. No change in the sensitivity
  D. Absent sensitivity

509. B   510. B   511. D   512. B   513. D   514. B   515. A   516. C   517. A   518. D   519. A   520. A

PY 10.13

521. How tympanic reflex protects from damage to the inner ear?
A. Reduces the vibrations transmitted to the inner ear through ossicles
B. Increases the vibrations transmitted to the inner ear through ossicles
C. Keeps the articulation sites loose
D. Relaxes the tensor tympani and stapedius muscle

522. Lever-like arrangement of ear ossicles increases the sound pressure by:
A. 20-fold
B. 22-fold
C. 15-fold
D. 18-fold

523. Hair cells of organ of Corti are depolarized due to influx of:
A. K^+
B. Na^+
C. Ca^{2+}
D. Cl^-

524. Intensity of sound for normal conversation is:
A. 30dB
B. 90 dB
C. 120 dB
D. 60 dB

525. Why the maximum rate of discharge through auditory nerve fiber is 1000 impulse/sec?
A. Refractory period is 1 ms
B. Refractory period is 2 ms
C. Refractory period is 3 ms
D. Refractory period is 4 ms

PY 10.14

526. Causes of sensorineural deafness include:
A. Acoustic neuroma
B. Otitis media
C. Otosclerosis
D. Wax in the external ear

527. Broad band noise which contains all frequencies in the audible spectrum is called ....
A. White noise
B. Speech noise
C. Soft noise
D. Narrow noise

528. Match the interpretation of tuning fork tests with the type of deafness:

List I	List II
A. Rinne test: AC>BC	i Normal
B. Rinne test: BC>AC	ii Sensorineural hearing loss
C. Weber test: Not lateralized	iii Conductive hearing loss

A. A-i, B-ii, C-iii
B. A-ii, B-iii, C-i
C. A-iii, B-ii, C-i
D. A-i, B-ii, C-ii

529. Self recording audiometry where various pure tone frequencies move from low to high:
A. Pure tone audiometry
B. Speech audiometry
C. Bekesy audiometry
D. Impedance audiometry

530. Disruption of ear ossicles causes:
A. Deafness
B. Conductive hearing loss
C. Sensorineural hearing loss
D. Presbycusis

PY 10.15

531. Presbyopia is due to:
A. Loss of elasticity of lens
B. Opacity of the cornea
C. Increase in anteroposterior length of the eyeball
D. Decrease in anteroposterior length of the eyeball

521. A   522. A   523. A   524. D   525. A   526. A   527. A   528. B   529. C   530. B   531. A

532. In myopia:
A. Near point of vision moves further away
B. Distant objects can be seen clearly
C. Near objects can be seen clearly
D. Accommodative convergent squint occurs

533. Colour perception is a function of:
A. Rods
B. Cones
C. Visual association area
D. Lateral geniculate body

534. Reading for long period can cause severe headache due to:
A. Muscular fatigue caused by accommodation
B. Muscular fatigue caused by extraocular muscles
C. Tension in the lens
D. Activation of pain fibers

535. In binocular vision of normal subjects, diplopia is not present, because the images are formed:
A. On non-corresponding points of both retinae
B. On corresponding points of both retinae
C. In front of retina
D. Behind the retina

536. All of the following are true for dark adaptation, *except*:
A. Pupils are dilated
B. Maximum adaptation is by rods
C. Faster adaptation is by cones
D. Sensitivity of rods to light is decreased because of increased concentration of rhodopsin

537. Nyctalopia is due to deficiency of:
A. Retinol
B. Cyanocobalamin
C. Ascorbic acid
D. Calciferol

538. Cells which increase the retinal sensitivity by improving contrast are called ....
A. Amacrine cells
B. Horizontal cells
C. Bipolar cells
D. Ganglion cells

539. Accommodation reflex constitutes the following features, *except*:
A. Contraction of ciliary muscle
B. Constriction of pupil
C. Dilatation of pupil
D. Convergence of visual axes

PY 10.16

540. Lesion at optic tract results in:
A. Anopia
B. Bitemporal hemianopia
C. Binasal hemianopia
D. Homonymous hemianopia

541. Bitemporal hemianopia is observed in the lesion of:
A. Optic nerve
B. Optic tract
C. Optic chiasma
D. Occipital lobe

542. Central lesions of chiasma occur in:
A. Optic neuritis
B. Suprasellar aneurysms
C. Optic atrophy
D. Occlusion of posterior cerebral artery

PY 10.17

543. While recording auditory evoked potentials reference electrode is placed:
A. On the right mastoid process
B. On the left mastoid process
C. In front of vertex
D. At the occiput

544. In which conditions wave II is absent:
A. Peripheral nerve
B. Cochlear nucleus
C. Lateral lemniscus
D. Inferior colliculi

545. What should be the stimulus intensity for recording auditory potentials?
A. 40–70 dB
B. 80–100 dB
C. 20–30 dB
D. 100–120 dB

532. C 533. B 534. A 535. B 536. D 537. A 538. B 539. C 540. D 541. C 542. B 543. C 544. B 545. A

546. **If there is a visual field defect what needs to be done for recording visual evoked potentials:**
    A. Use mydriatic before testing
    B. Vary the filter setting
    C. Use additional lateral electrodes
    D. Decrease the electrode impedance

547. **Drugs that decrease P100 latency include:**
    A. Pilocarpine
    B. Phospholine
    C. Carbachol
    D. Atropine

PY 11.1

548. **Average oral body temperature is:**
    A. 36°C
    B. 98.6°F
    C. 96.8°F
    D. 95.6°F

549. **The hypothalamic thermostat is located in the:**
    A. Supraoptic nucleus
    B. Preoptic nucleus
    C. Paraventricular nucleus
    D. Median eminence

550. **A Komodo dragon consumes far less food than required by a tiger of same weight. The reason is:**
    A. Komodo dragon generates energy by glycolysis
    B. Komodo dragon walks slower than a tiger
    C. Komodo dragon lives in a warm climate
    D. Komodo dragon is a poikilothermic, so less energy is needed.

551. **A lean individual feels cold easily than a well-nourished individual. The reason is:**
    A. The lean person has a hypothalamus that does not function well
    B. The lean person has less subcutaneous fat which acts as insulation
    C. The lean person has less muscles which cannot generate heat
    D. The well nourished individual can generate more heat as they have more mitochondria in cells

552. **A portion of hypothalamus of the rat was transected. After that, the rat there is drop in the body temperature of the rat. Which part of the hypothalamus was removed?**
    A. Preoptic nucleus
    B. Supraoptic nucleus
    C. Ventromedial nucleus
    D. Posterior nucleus

PY 11.2

553. **Shivering starts when the core temperature falls to:**
    A. 36.5°C
    B. 35.5°C
    C. 31°C
    D. 32°C

554. **The following statements regarding temperature regulation are correct, *except*:**
    A. Eccrine sweat glands are supplied by sympathetic cholinergic fibres
    B. One feels hotter on a dry day than on a humid day
    C. Insensible water loss amounts to 50 ml/hour normally
    D. Atropine does not inhibit secretion from apocrine glands

555. **A 55-year-old lady is going through menopause. Which of these symptoms is attributed to the hypothalamic GnRH release?**
    A. Hot flushes
    B. Mood swings
    C. Decreased sexual drive
    D. Dysfunctional uterine bleeding.

556. **A Gorkha in Nepal has rosy cheeks. What is the reason for this?**
    A. High altitude causes plethora due to polycythemia
    B. Racial attributes
    C. Due to dryness of skin
    D. Due to cutaneous vasodilatation as a climatic adaptation

---

546. C   547. D   548. B   549. B   550. D   551. B   552. D   553. B   554. B   555. A   556. D

557. Match the following:

List I	List II
A. Shivering	i. Chemical thermeognesis
B. Thyroxine	ii. Decreases heat loss
C. Sweating	iii. Increases heat production
D. Cutaneous vasoconstriction	iv. Increases heat loss

A. A: iii, B: i, C: iv, D: ii
B. A: iii, B: ii, C: iv, D: i
C. A: i, B: ii, C: iii, D: iv
D. A: iv, B: ii, C: i, D: iii

PY 11.3

558. Hypothermia produces all the following, *except*:
A. Increase in blood pressure
B. Decrease in heart rate
C. Loss of consciousness
D. Decreased O_2 needs of tissues

559. Cytokines that act as endogenous pyrogens are produced by:
A. Monocytes and marcrophages
B. Lymphocytes
C. Hepatocytes
D. Endothelium

560. A newborn preterm baby is placed in an incubator. The pediatrician advises not to use wet cloth to clean the baby's skin. The reason for this is:
A. To prevent others from touching the baby
B. To prevent hypothermia
C. To prevent the baby catching on a cold
D. The cloth in the hospital is not clean

561. A 66-year-old destitute was found in a drink state in a mall road in Nainital, on a snowy night. A picture of his toe is shown.

What is the diagnosis?
A. Heat stroke
B. Frostbite
C. Dry gangrene
D. Wet gangrene

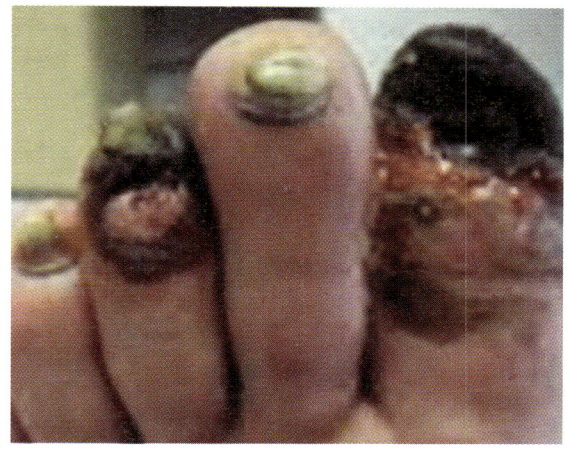

562. Which of the following conditions can cause hyperpyrexia?
A. Thyrotoxicosis
B. Cushing's syndrome
C. Conn's syndrome
D. Addison's disease

563. Mutations in the gene coding for ryanodine receptor in muscles lead to:
A. Frostbite
B. Heatstroke
C. Hypothermia
D. Malignant hyperthermia

PY 11.4

564. The cardiac output during heavy exercise can go up to:
A. 15 L/min
B. 20 L/min
C. 25 L/min
D. 30 L/min

565. Which of the following is not a cause for increased heart rate during exercise?
A. Increase in venous return
B. Increase in circulating catecholamines
C. Decreased cardiac output
D. Bainbridge reflex

557. A   558. A   559. A   560. B   561. B   562. A   563. D   564. C   565. C

566. **A 19-year-old man complains of pain in burning pain in calf within the first 10 minutes of exercise. He has always had a sedentary life. What is the reason for this?**
    A. Stimulation of sympathetic fibers
    B. Accumulation of lactic acid
    C. Accumulation of carbon dioxide
    D. Deficiency of vitamin E

567. **Which of the following hormonal changes does not take place during exercise?**
    A. Increase in anti-diuretic hormone
    B. Increase in cortisol
    C. Increase in endorphins
    D. Increase in insulin secretion

568. **An 18-year-old is undergoing athletic training for a sprint. What kind of diet is he advised immediately prior to his sprint?**
    A. Carbohydrate-rich diet
    B. Fat-rich diet
    C. Protein-rich diet
    D. Balanced diet

PY 11.5

569. **One MET in an adult female is equivalent to:**
    A. 50 ml of oxygen consumed in one minute
    B. 100 ml of oxygen consumed in one minute
    C. 150 ml of oxygen consumed in one minute
    D. 200 ml of oxygen consumed in one minute

570. **Following is not an effect of sedentary lifestyle:**
    A. Increase in high density lipoprotein
    B. Increase in insulin resistance
    C. Increase in truncal circumference
    D. Decrease in bone mineral density

571. **Ritu, a 35-year-old software engineer, who spends more than 10 hours of working in sitting position, complains of increased weight gain and difficulty in walking for long distances. Following changes in her lifestyle should be advocated, *except*:**
    A. Increase in carbohydrate content in diet
    B. Decrease in fatty food intake
    C. Increase in physical activity
    D. Short gaps in between work to walk around

572. **Which hormone is responsible for satiety?**
    A. Gastrin
    B. Ghrelin
    C. Leptin
    D. Renin

573. **Which of the following diseases does sedentary lifestyle promote?**
    A. Diabetes
    B. Hypertension
    C. Coronary artery disease
    D. All of the above

574. **A 33-year-old woman weighs 60 kg and is 5'4" tall. How is her BMI calculated?**
    A. $33 \times 60/(5.4)^2$
    B. $60/(5.4)2$
    C. $33 \times 60/(1.62)^2$
    D. $60/(1.62)^2$

PY 11.6

575. **The function of umbilical vein is:**
    A. Transport of oxygenated from placenta to the fetus
    B. Transport of deoxygenated blood from fetus to placenta
    C. Transport of deoxygenated blood from fetal organs to the fetal heart
    D. Transport of oxygenated blood from fetal heart to fetal organs

576. **Normal fetal circulation is:**
    A. Right atrium → foramen ovale → left atrium → left ventricle → aorta
    B. Right atrium → right ventricle → pulmonary artery → lungs → pulmonary veins → left atrium → left ventricle → aorta
    C. Right atrium → right ventricle → pulmonary atery → ductus arteriosus → aorta
    D. A and C

577. **A 24-month-old child is brought with recurrent lower respiratory tract infections. He was diagnosed of atrial septal defect. The cause for this is:**
    A. Patent foramen ovale
    B. Patent foramen pellucidum
    C. Patent ductus venosus
    D. Patent ductus arteriosus

566. B　567. D　568. A　569. D　570. A　571. A　572. C　573. D　574. D　575. A　576. D　577. A

578. A 28-week gestation pregnant lady is brought to the hospital with severe pregnancy induced hypertension. She was warned that they might perform a C-section to prevent further harm due to hypertension if the BP was not getting controlled. She was advised control of blood pressure and an intramuscular injection of betamethasone (synthetic corticosteroid) was given. What is the reason for steroid injection?
    A. To control blood pressure
    B. To cause fetal lung maturity
    C. To fight against infections
    D. To tide over stress

579. Which of the following is a reason for difficult temperature control in infants?
    A. They have a larger surface area
    B. They have a higher basal metabolic rate
    C. Sweating mechanisms are not fully developed
    D. All of the above

PY 11.7

580. The branch of medicine which deals with elderly indivduals is called ....
    A. Paediatrics
    B. Geriatrics
    C. Orthopaedics
    D. Gynaecology

581. Which of the following features is associated with ageing?
    A. Increased thickness of blood vessels
    B. Increased rigidity of heart valves
    C. Decreased colon motility
    D. All of the above

582. An 89-year-old gentleman (Mr. M) says he has difficulty in remembering his food that he ate at breakfast. Another 89-year-old gentleman (Mr. N) says he has difficulty in remembering what he did in the morning. Based on these, what is your conclusion?
    A. M has age-related memory deficit, N has Alzheimer's disease
    B. M has Alzheimer's disease, N has age-related memory deficit

C. Both have Alzheimer's disease
    D. Both have age-related memory deficit

583. The present day pandemic affects the elderly more adversely. What may be the reasons?
    A. More chances of comorbidities
    B. Decreased immune response
    C. Decrease in elasticity of lungs with age
    D. All the above

584. An 80-year-old male complains of difficulty in reading his newspaper noticed since 20 days. Which of the following not a possibility?
    A. Age-related macular degeneration
    B. Cataract
    C. Arcus senilis
    D. Progression of glaucoma

585. Which of the following is an age-related disorder of the bones and joints?
    A. Rickets
    B. Osteomalacia
    C. Osteoporosis
    D. None of the above

PY 11.8

586. Following are the causes for tachypnoea during exercise, *except:*
    A. To repay oxygen debt
    B. Increase in blood carbon dioxide levels
    C. Decrease in ATP and oxygen
    D. Increased impulses from proprioceptors

587. Which of the following is an isometric exercise?
    A. Walking
    B. Cycling
    C. Push ups
    D. Running

588. Which of the following diets gives a runner highest endurance?
    A. Carbohydrate-rich diet
    B. Fat-rich diet
    C. Protein-rich diet
    D. Fiber-rich diet

578. B   579. D   580. B   581. D   582. A   583. D   584. C   585. C   586. A   587. C   588. A

589. Bainbridge reflex is:
A. Increase in cardiac contractility due to increase in venous return
B. Increase in cardiac conductance due to sympathetic overactivity
C. Increase in ventilation due to increase in carbon dioxide
D. Increase in heart rate due to increase in venous return

590. Roger Federer, takes a break during his play. He is seen eating a Robusta banana in the interval. What is the reason behind this?

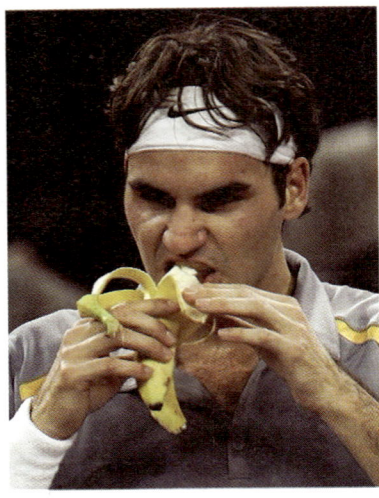

A. He likes banana
B. To compensate for potassium loss
C. To provide quick energy through carbo-hydrates
D. It helps in digestion

PY 11.9

591. Following are uses of growth charts:
A. Helps know whether the anthropometric measurement is adequate for age or not
B. Know the centile value of the child's growth
C. Is a good tool to keep track
D. All of the above

592. A child's weight is between 50th–97th centile. What does it mean?
A. He is 50–97% of expected weight
B. He has to gain 50–97% of more weight to be normal
C. In age matched children, arranged in the order of weight, this child is somewhere between 50th to 97th number
D. All of the above

593. Tippu, an year old boy was brought for his vaccination. While charting his weight, it was found that the curve in the growth chart was deflecting downward. What does it mean?
A. He is not gaining weight at all
B. His weight gain is not adequate for his age
C. He is losing weight
D. All of the above

594. Which parameters can be plotted in a growth chart?
A. Weight for age
B. Height for age
C. Weight for height
D. All of the above

595. Stunting refers to:
A. Impaired growth and development in a child
B. Loss of fat and muscles due to protein degradation
C. Rate of weight gain is lesser than expected
D. All of the above

PY 11.10

596. Length of a baby is measured by:
A. measuring tape
B. Infantometer
C. Stadiometer
D. Ruler

589. D   590. C   591. D   592. C   593. B   594. D   595. A   596. B

597. Identify the anthropometry.

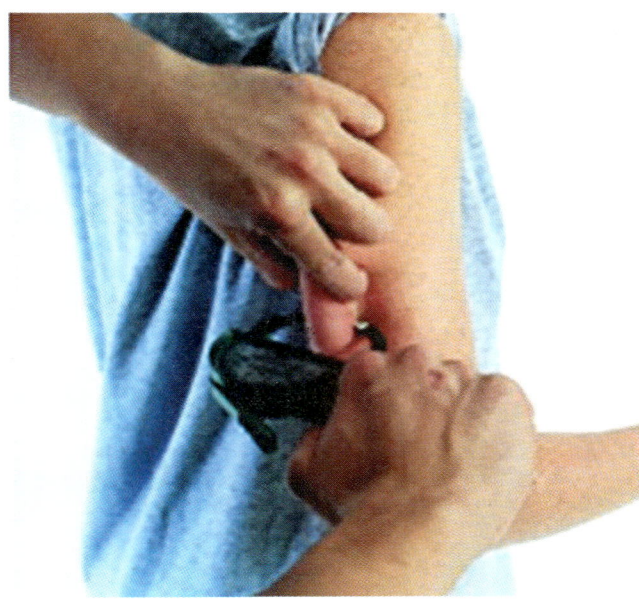

A. Midarm circumference
B. Skin fold thickness
C. Triceps muscle thickness
D. None of the above

598. Normal midarm circumference in a child up to the age of 5 years is:
A. 10–12 cm
B. 15–17 cm
C. 20–22 cm
D. 25–27 cm

599. Brachiocephaly refers to:
A. Short AP diameter of head
B. Long AP diameter of head
C. Small circular head
D. Frontal bossing

600. The anterior fontanelle is the space between:
A. Two frontal plates
B. Two parietal plates
C. Frontal and parietal plates
D. Frontal and temporal plates

PY 11.11

601. Which of these is not a criterion for brain death?
A. Absence of pupillary reflexes
B. Deep coma
C. Inability to initiate respiration
D. Decreased capillary filling time

602. Eye donation should be performed within:
A. 10 minutes of death
B. 3 hours of death
C. 6 hours of death
D. 24 hours of death

603. Organs that can be harvested from a living donor are:
A. Kidney
B. Liver
C. Pancreas
D. All the above

604. The Human Transplantation of Organs Act was passed in:
A. 1994
B. 1995
C. 1996
D. 1997

605. A person dies of road traffic accident and he is declared brain dead by the resident in the ICU. He is on ventilator. True about this scenario is:
A. His organs can be harvested only after declaration by a doctor appointed by appropriate authority
B. His organs can be harvested after declaration by any doctor
C. His organs can be harvested after declaration by 2 doctors appointed by appropriate authority, 6 hours apart, one of them being an anaesthetist
D. His organs can be harvested after declaration by 2 doctors appointed by appropriate authority, 6 hours apart, one of them being a neurologist.

597. B   598. B   599. A   600. C   601. D   602. C   603. D   604. A   605. D

PY 11.12

606. True about meditation:
- A. Began in ancient India
- B. Is a state of hypometabolism
- C. Passive state of mind
- D. All of the above

607. Following are seen during meditation, *except*:
- A. Increase in heart rate
- B. Decrease in blood pressure
- C. Decrease in oxygen consumption
- D. Increase in basal metabolic rate

608. Meditation brings about:
- A. Arousal
- B. Deep sleep
- C. Mass response
- D. Relaxation

609. Which of the following is not an effect of meditation on autonomic system?
- A. Increased sympathetic activity
- B. Decreased parasympathetic activity
- C. No effect on autonomous system
- D. Increased parasympathetic activity

610. Which are the requirements for meditation?
- A. Calm surroundings
- B. Clear mind
- C. Comfortable seating
- D. All of the above

PY 11.13

611. A person says he underwent a limb surgery 8 years back. Which type of history is this?
- A. Present history
- B. Past history
- C. Family history
- D. Personal history

612. On examination, you find pallor in a patient. What is the next logical step?
- A. Prescribe her iron tablets
- B. Complete your examination
- C. Send her for hemoglobin estimation
- D. All of the above

613. Central cyanosis is seen in:
- A. Extreme cold temperatures
- B. Cervical rib
- C. Cyanotic heart diseases
- D. All of the above

614. Which of the following points in general examination can be gathered from examining the eyes?
- A. Pallor
- B. Cyanosis
- C. Clubbing
- D. Lymphadenopathy

615. What is the examiner performing?

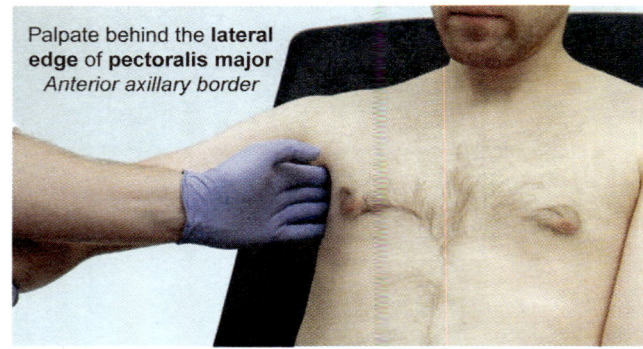

Palpate behind the **lateral edge** of **pectoralis major**
Anterior axillary border

- A. Palpating axillary artery
- B. Palpating the median nerve
- C. Palpating axillary group of lymph nodes
- D. All of the above

PY 11.14

616. Following are indications for basic life support, *except*:
- A. Myocardial infarction
- B. Choking
- C. Drowning
- D. Electrocution

617. Who is entitled to give BLS?
- A. A cardiologist
- B. Any doctor
- C. Any health care worker
- D. Anyone who knows BLS

606. D   607. A   608. D   609. D   610. D   611. B   612. B   613. C   614. A   615. C   616. A   617. D

618. What is the first step in BLS?
A. Clear airway
B. Shout for help
C. Dial 911/104 or national helpline number
D. Remove from danger

619. You are jogging along a beach line and you find a bunch of people surrounding a collapsed person. When you enquire, you know he has been rescued from drowning. There is a strong pulse and feeble movement of chest. What is the logical sequence to be followed?
A. Check for airway occlusion and give mouth to mouth resuscitation
B. Ask an on-looker to dial the ambulance and clear airway and give mouth to mouth for 15 cycles
C. Ask an on-looker to dial the ambulance and turn head to side to remove water, clear airway and give mouth to mouth for 15 cycles and check pulse again
D. First give chest compressions to remove water from airways, ask an on-looker to dial the ambulance and clear airway and give mouth to mouth for 15 cycles

620. How do you give chest compressions to a neonate?
A. Use base of palm
B. Use tips of two fingers
C. Use a twig
D. Use elbow

621. Identify the instrument.

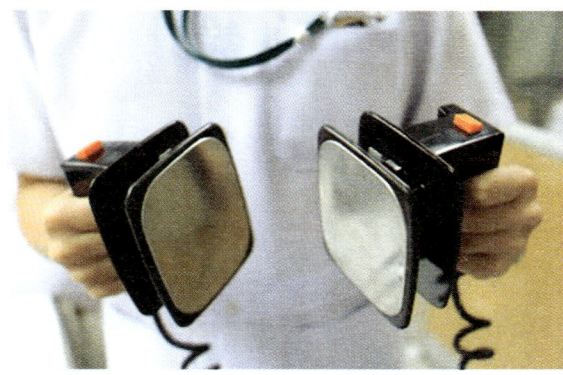

A. Paddles of a defibrillator
B. Magnetic electrodes to initiate heart beat
C. Electrocautery machine
D. None of the above

618. D   619. C   620. B   621. A